Atlas of Gastrointestinal Endoscopy & Endoscopic Biopsies

T. S. Emory
H. A. Carpenter

C. J. Gostout
L. H. Sobin

Atlas of Gastrointestinal Endoscopy & Endoscopic Biopsies

Theresa S. Emory, MD
Armed Forces Institute of Pathology

Herschel A. Carpenter, MD
Mayo Clinic

Christopher J. Gostout, MD
Mayo Clinic

Leslie H. Sobin, MD
Armed Forces Institute of Pathology

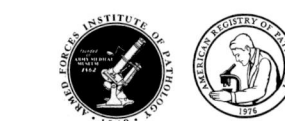

Armed Forces Institute of Pathology
American Registry of Pathology
Washington, DC
2000

Theresa S. Emory, MD
Division of Gastrointestinal Pathology
Department of Hepatic and Gastrointestinal Pathology
Armed Forces Institute of Pathology
Washington, DC 20306
emorypath@aol.com

Herschel A. Carpenter, MD
Consultant, Department of Laboratory Medicine and Pathology
Associate Professor of Pathology
Mayo Medical School
Mayo Foundation
Rochester, MN 55905

Christopher J. Gostout, MD
Director of Endoscopy
Associate Professor of Medicine
Division of Gastroenterology and Hepatology
Mayo Foundation
Rochester, MN 55905
gostout.christopher@mayo.edu

Leslie H. Sobin, MD
Chief, Division of Gastrointestinal Pathology
Department of Hepatic and Gastrointestinal Pathology
Armed Forces Institute of Pathology
Washington, DC 20306
sobin@afip.osd.mil

Available from
American Registry of Pathology
Armed Forces Institute of Pathology
Washington, DC, 20306-6000
www.afip.org

ISBN: 1-881041-64-6
2000

The use of general descriptive names, registered names, trademarks, etc., in this publication does not imply, even in the absence of a specific statement, that such names are exempt from the relevant protective laws and regulations and therefore free for general use.

The views of the authors do not purport to reflect the positions of the Department of the Army or the Department of Defense.

Preface

The aim of this atlas is to facilitate clinicopathologic correlative diagnosis and enhance communication between gastroenterologist and pathologist. Endoscopic examination and biopsy play a major role in the diagnosis of diseases of the gastrointestinal tract and accurate diagnosis depends on clinicopathologic correlation. A close working relationship between gastroenterologist and pathologist is essential, particularly as endoscopic findings are often nonspecific and histologic patterns may reflect several pathogenetic mechanisms rather than a specific disease state.

The book is arranged by anatomic site (esophagus, stomach, small intestine, and large intestine). Each chapter begins with sections on endoscopic examination and histology. Patterns-of-injury discussions describe the typical reaction patterns seen on mucosal biopsy and allow the pathologist to suggest potential causes for the histologic patterns. Each topic begins with a brief text: morphology, endoscopic features, clinical features, and differential diagnosis. The text is meant to provide helpful features for the endoscopist and pathologist to facilitate accurate diagnosis or develop a broad differential diagnosis.

Ideally, the gastroenterologist should send, along with the biopsy specimen, a copy of the endoscopy report, clinical details, the clinical differential diagnosis, and the questions to be answered by the biopsy. Endoscopic photographs are often helpful and sometimes essential. Pathology reports should be concise, clear, and answer the clinical questions. The histologic pattern should be identified and, when possible, accompanied by a list of possible clinicopathologic diagnoses. Standardized formats help to provide a clear and useful report. A standardized reporting format used successfully at the Mayo Clinic is in appendix 2.

We believe that the atlas will be useful in training both gastroenterologists and pathologists, that it will fill a need in clinical practice, and stimulate effective interaction between gastroenterologists and pathologists in the best interest of the patient.

Acknowledgements

Numerous endoscopists and pathologists provided endoscopic and histologic material; this atlas could not have been completed without their contributions. The authors especially wish to acknowledge the endoscopists of the Division of Gastroenterology and Hepatology, Mayo Clinic, for their photographs, Eric Van Os, MD, former Mayo advanced endoscopy fellow, who helped organize the photographs and reports, and Larry Brandt, MD.

The authors thank the pathologists of the GI working group, Mayo Clinic, for contributing cases to the GI endoscopic biopsy teaching files and for their contributions to the Mayo Clinic GI diagnostic abbreviations and templates. Special thanks go to Sandy Dawsey, MD, and Robert Karnei, MD, for contributions of endoscopic biopsy specimens and photographs.

The authors would particularly like to acknowledge Mary Lou Howard, Lois A. Macken, and Linda L. Smith, for organizing endoscopic materials and for their secretarial support. We also wish to thank JoAnn Mills, Bonnie Casey, and Roger E. Emory, MD, for their valuable editorial review, and to gratefully acknowledge Fran Card for book design and layout and Ken Stringfellow for color separation. This atlas could not have been accomplished without their invaluable assistance.

The photographic illustrations were prepared with Olympus endoscopes and microscopes. The financial support of the Olympus Corporation is gratefully acknowledged.

Table of Contents

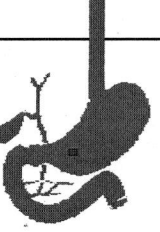

ESOPHAGUS

Endoscopic examination 2
Histology 3
Normal esophagus 5
Rings, webs, hernias 8
Mallory-Weiss tear and diverticula 11
Gastric heterotopia/inlet patch 13
Glycogenic acanthosis 14
Varices 16
Esophagitis 18
Reflux esophagitis 19
Inflammatory polyps associated with reflux 23
Squamous papillomas associated with reflux 23
Eosinophilic esophagitis 26
Candida esophagitis 28
Herpes esophagitis; Herpes simplex virus 30
Cytomegalovirus esophagitis 31
Bizarre stromal cells 33
Chemical injury 34
Pill esophagitis 35
Radiation injury 36
Granulomatous esophagitis 38
Dysmotility disorders 40
Barrett's esophagus 42
Barrett's esophagus with squamous islands 44
Dysplasia in Barrett's esophagus 46
Barrett's esophagus, dysplasia variations 48
Barrett's esophagus, high-grade dysplasia 48
Barrett's esophagus, reactive atypia versus dysplasia 51
Barrett's esophagus, dysplasia, stricture, ulcer, mass 53
Adenocarcinoma 55
Squamous dysplasia 58
Squamous cell carcinoma 61
Malignant melanoma 64
Metastatic tumors 66
Vascular lesions 68
Fibrovascular polyp 70
Granular cell tumor 72
Stromal tumors 74

STOMACH

Endoscopic examination	78
Histology	79
Normal stomach	80
Patterns of injury: gastritis and gastropathy	84
Acute gastritis	87
Active chronic gastritis	88
Focal atrophy/metaplasia and chronic atrophic gastritis	92
Lymphocytic gastritis	95
Eosinophilic gastritis	95
Granulomatous gastritis	98
Acute erosive gastropathy	101
Reactive gastropathy	103
Reactive gastropathy, bile reflux	108
Xanthelasma	111
Gastropathy, radiation/chemotherapy	113
Portal hypertensive gastropathy	115
Watermelon stomach	117
Hypertrophic gastropathy and gastritis	119
Cytomegalovirus gastropathy	122
Miscellaneous infections	122
Benign ulcers	125
Cameron erosion	129
Dieulafoy lesion	131
Varices and vascular malformations	132
Atrophic gastritis with carcinoid tumors	135
Carcinoid tumor	137
Pancreatic heterotopia and metaplasia	139
Fundic gland polyp	141
Hyperplastic polyp	143
Juvenile polyp and Peutz-Jeghers polyp	145
Inflammatory fibroid polyp	147
Dysplasia	149
Adenoma	151
Malignant ulcer	153
Adenocarcinoma	155
Signet-ring cell carcinoma	159
Malignant lymphoma	161
Stromal tumors (smooth muscle/stromal, neurogenic, lipomatous)	165
Metastatic tumors	171

SMALL INTESTINE

Endoscopic examination	174
Histology	175
Normal small intestine	176
Normal ileum	179
Patterns of injury	181
Duodenitis	182
Ulcers and erosions	184
Ileal ulcers/erosions	186
Eosinophilic enteritis	188
Granulomatous enteritis/Crohn's disease	190
Infections with normal mucosal pattern	193
Giardiasis	194
Cryptosporidia	196

Microsporidia 197
Isospora belli 198
Viral infections 199
Infections within histiocytes: *Mycobacterium avium-intracellulare*, Whipple disease 201
Infections within histiocytes: leishmania, histoplasma, typhoid 204
Candida infection 206
Parasites, worms 207
Common variable immunodeficiency/hypogammaglobulinemia 208
Lymphoid hyperplasia 210
Malabsorption 212
Cronkhite-Canada syndrome: protein-losing enteropathy 216
Lymphatic dilatation 218
Congenital lymphatic dilatation 218
Vascular lesions 221
Vasculitis 224
Hemorrhagic enteropathy 226
Ischemia 227
Collagen vascular disease 230
Amyloid 231
Intussusception 232
Ostomy, diverticula 234
Anastomotic ulcers 236
Pouchitis 237
Pigments 239
Submucosal inflammatory mass lesion 241
Heterotopic gastric mucosa 242
Brunner gland lesions 244
Lipoma 246
Hyperplastic polyps 247
Inflammatory fibroid polyp 248
Peutz-Jeghers polyps 250
Pancreatic heterotopia 252
Gangliocytic paraganglioma 254
Schwannoma 256
Neurofibroma 257
Carcinoid tumor 258
Adenoma 260
Ampullary adenomas 263
Adenocarcinoma 265
Malignant lymphoma 267
Smooth muscle/stromal tumors 271
Benign vascular neoplasms 272
Vascular malignancies 272
Lymphangioma 275
Metastatic tumors 276

LARGE INTESTINE

Endoscopic examination 280
Histology 281
Normal large intestine 282
Patterns of injury 289
Insufflation artifact (pseudolipomatosis) 293
Histiocyte infiltrates 294
Near-normal colonic mucosa with pathogenic organisms 296
Specific infectious agents 298
Parasites 301
Acute colitis 303

Pseudomembranous colitis	306
Ischemia	307
Radiation injury	310
Active chronic destructive colitis	312
Dysplasia and adenocarcinoma in ulcerative colitis	318
Dysplasia-associated lesion/mass (DALM)	318
Crohn's colitis	321
Adenocarcinoma arising in Crohn's disease	321
Granulomatous colitis	325
Chronic nondestructive colitis	329
Eosinophilic colitis	331
Graft-versus-host disease	332
Diversion colitis	334
NSAID ileocolitis/ulcers	335
Melanosis coli	337
Diverticular disease	338
Stricture/anastomosis	342
Vascular lesions	344
Hemorrhoids/varices	349
Vasculitis	351
Fibrosing colopathy	353
Amyloidosis	354
Dysmotility syndromes	356
Lymphoid hyperplasia	357
Pneumatosis coli	359
Endometriosis	361
Inverted appendix	362
Rectal prolapse syndrome and inflammatory cloacogenic polyp	363
Barium granuloma and oleogranuloma	367
Hypertrophied anal papilla/skin tag	369
Inflammatory polyps	370
Hyperplastic polyp	373
Combined adenoma/hyperplastic polyp	376
Serrated adenoma	376
Juvenile polyp	379
Peutz-Jeghers polyp	381
Cowden syndrome	383
Ganglioneuroma	384
Cronkhite-Canada polyps	386
Granular cell tumor	387
Lipoma	388
Lipohyperplasia of ileocecal valve	388
Adenomas	391
Adenoma with pseudoinvasion	395
Familial adenomatous polyposis	397
Flat adenoma	399
Adenocarcinoma arising in an adenoma	401
Adenocarcinoma	403
Carcinoma variants	406
Mucinous adenocarcinoma	406
Signet-ring cell and small cell carcinomas	406
Recurrent adenocarcinoma	409
Metastatic tumors	410
Carcinoid tumor	412
Smooth muscle/stromal tumors	414
Kaposi sarcoma	416
Malignant lymphoma	417
Malignant melanoma	419
Squamous lesions	421

Appendices

Appendix 1: Selected reference texts
    Gastroenterology 427
    Pathology 427

Apendix 2: Mayo Clinic GI Working Group Abbreviations 428

Index 437

CHAPTER 1

ESOPHAGUS

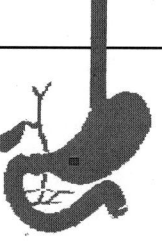

Endoscopic examination 2	Granulomatous esophagitis 38
Histology 3	Dysmotility disorders 40
Normal esophagus 5	Barrett's esophagus 42
Rings, webs, hernias 8	Barrett's esophagus with squamous islands 44
Mallory-Weiss tear and diverticula 11	Dysplasia in Barrett's esophagus 46
Gastric heterotopia/inlet patch 13	Barrett's esophagus, dysplasia variations 48
Glycogenic acanthosis 14	Barrett's esophagus, high-grade dysplasia 48
Varices 16	Barrett's esophagus, reactive atypia versus dysplasia 51
Esophagitis 18	Barrett's esophagus, dysplasia, stricture, ulcer, mass 53
Reflux esophagitis 19	
Inflammatory polyps associated with reflux 23	Adenocarcinoma 55
Squamous papillomas associated with reflux 23	Squamous dysplasia 58
Eosinophilic esophagitis 26	Squamous cell carcinoma 61
Candida esophagitis 28	Malignant melanoma.. 64
Herpes esophagitis; Herpes simplex virus 30	Metastatic tumors 66
Cytomegalovirus esophagitis 31	Vascular lesions 68
Bizarre stromal cells 33	Fibrovascular polyp 70
Chemical injury 34	Granular cell tumor 72
Pill esophagitis 35	Stromal tumors... 74
Radiation injury 36	

ENDOSCOPIC EXAMINATION

The tubular esophagus begins 16 cm from the incisors and ends at the junction with the stomach, which is usually 35 to 40 cm from the incisors, depending on torso length. There are natural compression points where adjacent structures (aorta, left main bronchus) cross over the esophagus. At these locations in the midesophagus, large and/or caustic pills are likely to lodge and cause ulcers. This is also the area where infections and neoplasms invade from contiguous tracheobronchial lymph nodes.

During the initial passage of the endoscope, swallowed secretions and aggregated topical anesthetic solutions often make a meticulous examination of the esophagus difficult. The examination may be easier after the stomach and duodenum have been viewed and accumulated materials have passed through or been suctioned. The location of the squamocolumnar junction (Z line) and any abnormalities should be recorded relative to the distance from the incisors. The location of the squamocolumnar junction relative to the esophagogastric junction is important in Barrett's esophagus and in patients with hiatal hernias. An irregular Z line may be an indication of short-segment Barrett's esophagus and warrant biopsies. Biopsies should be taken immediately distal to the Z line. The cervical esophagus should be examined during passage for webs and during withdrawal of the endoscope until the upper sphincter is passed. Otherwise, proximal neoplasms and gastric inlet patches may be overlooked.

All mucosal abnormalities should be biopsied. This may be done using several methods, depending upon the abnormality. The tangential approach to mucosal biopsies presents a technical challenge to tissue sampling, especially in the more proximal esophagus. Standard-sized pinch avulsion biopsy forceps may be used for the vast majority of abnormalities, whether focal or widespread. The margins of ulcerating lesions should be sampled. Jumbo biopsy forceps offer advantages for surveillance of Barrett's esophagus. The use of the jumbo biopsy forceps is optional but preferred because they yield larger samples, making it more likely the pathologist will detect dysplasia. Whether jumbo or standard biopsy forceps are used, the same number of biopsies are required. Random samples should be taken from 4 quadrants every 2 cm throughout the Barrett's esophagus, beginning at the esophagogastric junction. Additionally, any endoscopic abnormality, particularly raised mucosal nodules, strictures, or ulcers should be biopsied. Directed biopsy of Barrett's esophagus is enhanced by the use of chromoscopy or dye staining. Dye staining may be performed by 2 methods—vital staining, during which dye agent is selectively absorbed by normal tissues, or contrast staining, during which the dye is not absorbed by the mucosa and instead enhances the surface features of the mucosa. The latter technique is best used with high-resolution video endoscopes and magnification video endoscopes. Lugol's iodine, toluidine blue, and methylene blue are the most commonly used dyes in the esophagus. Vital dye staining is very well-suited to surveillance of Barrett's esophagus. Biopsies are directed at areas without staining.

Mucosectomy is a method of tissue sampling that may provide specimens of up to 2 cm in diameter. This technique allows complete removal of focal lesions and is preferred when neoplasia is suspected, including suspected dysplastic lesions. Mucosectomy may be performed several ways. The mucosal area to be removed should first be isolated by creating a submucosal cushion of fluid, typically normal saline, by direct injection. The tissue is then removed by snare excision with the saline-isolated tissue drawn into the open snare using suction, or else by grasping the tissue with a biopsy forceps and pulling it into the snare. This requires the use of a 2-channel therapeutic endoscope. Suction is applied in a standard fashion, or else a cylindrical cap is retrofitted onto the tip of the endoscope to allow the tissue to be drawn into the cap and then excised. A snare is specially predeployed just within the tip of the suction cap to permit excision of the isolated tissue. Alternatively, mucosectomy is performed after the saline-isolated tissue has been banded using a variceal band ligator and amputated by a snare immediately above the level of the band.

Brush cytology may be used for screening, but biopsy is the preferred sampling method. Brushing in situations of suspected infection for culture and direct microscopy is useful.

HISTOLOGY

The esophagus is lined by stratified squamous mucosa. The junction of the squamous mucosa and the gastric mucosa (squamocolumnar junction) is irregular (Z line) and may move upward with healing following injury. Most esophageal carcinomas are squamous cell carcinomas. However, when gastric mucosa extends into the tubular esophagus and undergoes intestinal metaplasia (Barrett's esophagus), the risk for adenocarcinoma increases. The squamocolumnar junction is not the same as the anatomic gastroesophageal junction, but is usually 1 to 2 cm proximal to that point. The gastroesophageal junction is judged endoscopically and in resection specimens by determining the point at which the gastric folds end.

The mucosa consists of stratified squamous epithelium lying on a vascular connective tissue bed that is separated from the submucosal vascular connective tissue by the muscularis mucosae. Uncommonly, the lamina propria and submucosa give rise to lipomas, fibrovascular polyps, or vascular tumors.

The lower border of the squamous epithelium has a gently undulating profile. The basal layer of immature cells is the proliferative zone, and the cells are recognized not only by location but also by their scant cytoplasm. Being almost all nucleus, they look basophilic on low magnification. Normally, there are only 1 to 3 layers of basal cells which acquire characteristic abundant, glycogen-rich cytoplasm with maturation. Mild chronic acid reflux sometimes stimulates epithelial proliferation before causing inflammation. As the squamous epithelium thickens, the gentle undulation of the lower edge becomes a dramatic serration and the lamina propria forms fibrovascular papillae that appear to extend well into the epithelium, but probably mark the original interface. The basal layer also thickens.

The immune system consists of intraepithelial lymphocytes (T-suppressor) and lymphoid follicles near the muscularis mucosae (B- and T-helper). Intraepithelial T-lymphocytes increase in reflux esophagitis.

The smooth muscle of the muscularis mucosae is not uniform but usually 2 layers thick. Individual smooth muscle cells anchor and order the mucosa, but this is seldom apparent from individual histologic sections. When the mucosa is destroyed and replaced by squamous mucosa or by metaplastic gastric epithelium, the muscularis mucosae, especially the inner layer, becomes thickened, disorganized, and fibrotic. This is sometimes detected on ultrasonic examination as uniform thickening of the mucosa.

There are 2 sets of accessory glands distinguished by their location either in lamina propria (cardiac glands) or in submucosa (esophageal glands). Both are mainly mucus-secreting glands that provide lubrication and assist in pH modulation. The submucosal glands are distributed uniformly throughout the esophagus, but the cardiac glands are located irregularly in the proximal and distal esophagus. The ducts of these glands open onto the surface and are lined by a transitional-type epithelium. Duct epithelium may participate in healing erosions or ulcers, e.g., squamous island formation in Barrett's esophagus. Rarely, salivary gland tumors develop from these glands. Pancreatic-type glands, referred to as pancreatic metaplasia, can be found throughout the mucosa of the distal esophagus, stomach, and biliary tract. It is probably a normal feature of the upper gastrointestinal tract.

The muscularis propria consists of 2 layers—an inner circular and outer longitudinal layer. In the upper third of the esophagus, striated muscle replaces the smooth muscle present in the rest of the esophagus. At the gastroesophageal junction, the layers of smooth muscle split, develop a diagonal orientation, and blend with the muscularis propria of the stomach; the sling-type arrangement provides some control over gastric content. The distal several centimeters of muscularis propria is thickened and forms an ill-defined but important area known as the lower esophageal sphincter. Sphincter function is important in preventing reflux. Smooth muscle tumors arise from either muscularis propria or muscularis mucosae. Diseases affecting smooth muscle (scleroderma, hollow visceral myopathy) or striated muscle (dermatomyositis) adversely affect esophageal function and predispose to reflux and aspiration.

There is a rich neural network in the submucosa and muscularis propria similar to other areas of the gastrointestinal tract. Defects or imbalance in neural transmission (e.g., achalasia) also predispose to dysphagia, reflux, and aspiration.

The esophagus is well-vascularized, being fed by a myriad of arteries coming directly from the aorta. Esophageal ischemia is thus extremely rare, unless small vessels are obliterated, as in radiation injury. The venous outflow connects with the portal as well as the systemic circulation via collaterals and is affected by elevated chronic portal venous pressure (varices).

NORMAL ESOPHAGUS

- Endoscopic features .... The major features of the normal esophagus include the upper sphincter area, uniform pale squamous mucosa, lower esophageal sphincter area, squamocolumnar junction, and diaphragmatic hiatus. The upper sphincter region lies posterior to the airway and vocal cords (Fig. 1-3). This region is seen best during withdrawal of the endoscope, appearing as a rosette composed of contracted mucosal folds. The Z line is a discrete circumferential boundary between the squamous mucosa and columnar mucosa of the stomach (Fig. 1-4). There may be some irregularity in the course of the Z line. The lower esophageal sphincter, similar to the upper esophageal sphincter, is an estimated area in the very distal esophagus. Although the orderly progression of esophageal contraction from proximal to distal can be seen, the specific contractile activity of the lower esophageal sphincter cannot be visualized. The diaphragmatic hiatus appears as a contracted lumen and rosette of folds composed of esophageal and gastric mucosa. Swallowed secretions are typically present in the normal esophagus.

    Variant appearances of the normal esophageal lumen and mucosa include the pale nodularity of acanthotic glycogenosis, venous blebs (Fig. 1-6), and focal extrinsic compression by the aortic arch.

- Differential diagnosis ...... Endoscopic: If the Z line is irregular, biopsies are necessary to exclude short-segment Barrett's esophagus (Fig. 1-7).

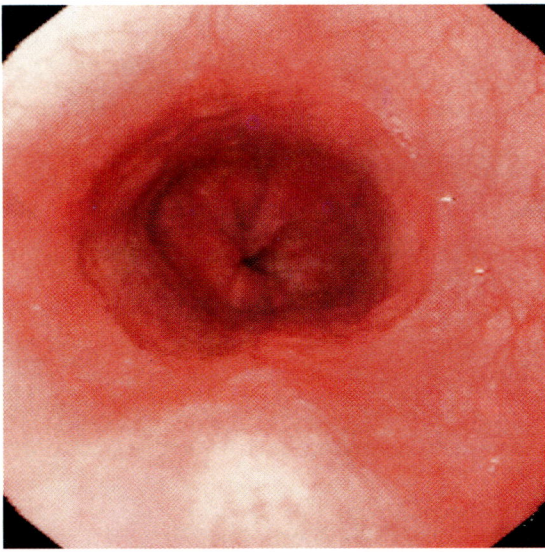

Figure 1-1: **Esophagus. Normal.** Uniform pale mucosa proximal, normal squamocolumnar junction and gastric folds distally.

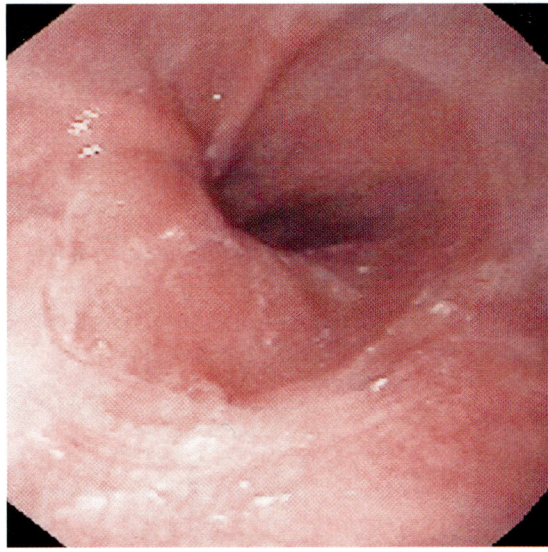

Figure 1-2: **Esophagus. Normal.** A normal squamocolumnar junction. The Z line is discrete and without irregularities in its circumferential path.

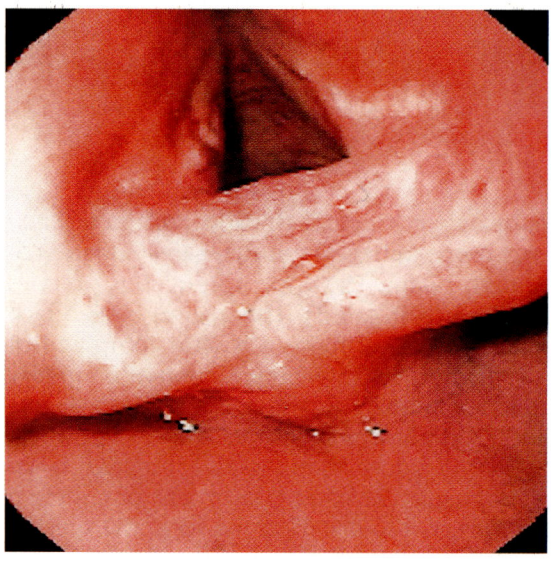

Figure 1-3: **Esophagus. Normal.** Upper esophageal sphincter is located just distal to the larynx.

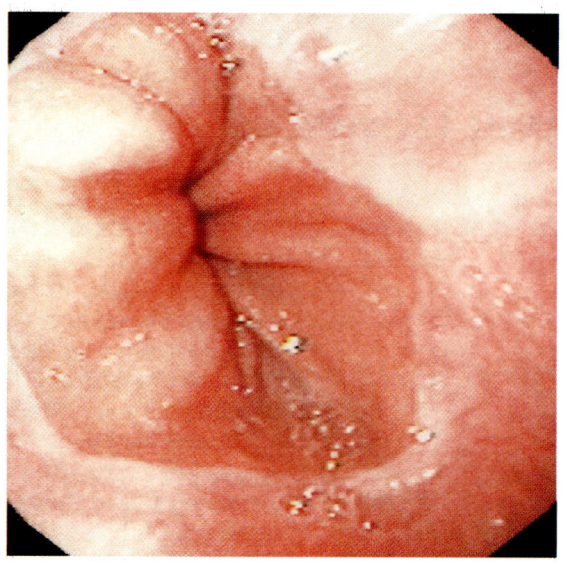

Figure 1-4: **Esophagus. Normal.** Z line circumferential and well-demarcated.

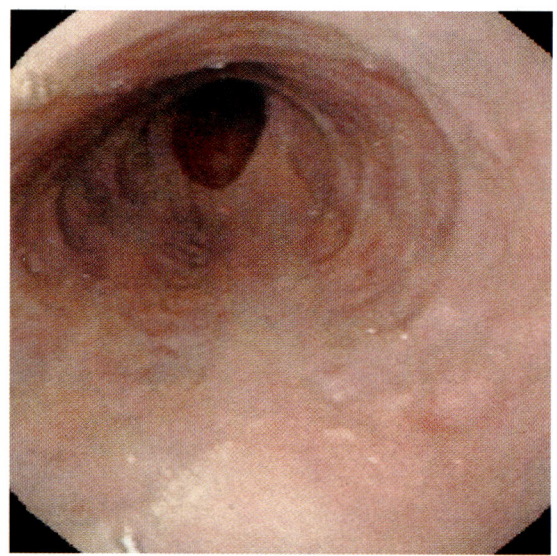

Figure 1-5: **Esophagus. Normal.** Contractile waves course through the esophagus.

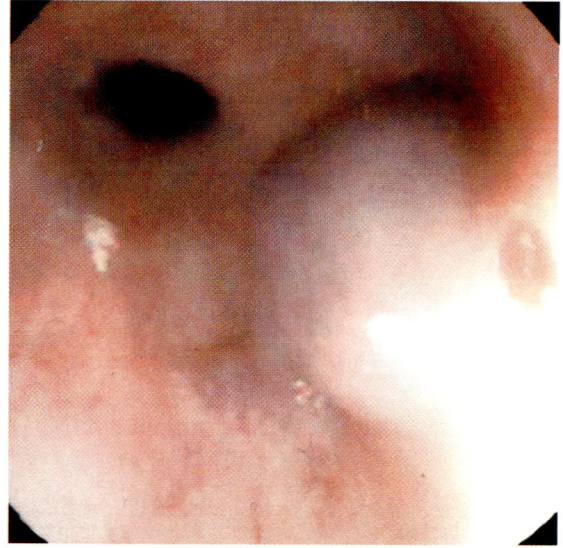

Figure 1-6: **Esophagus. Normal.** Small venous nodule/bleb beneath the squamous mucosa.

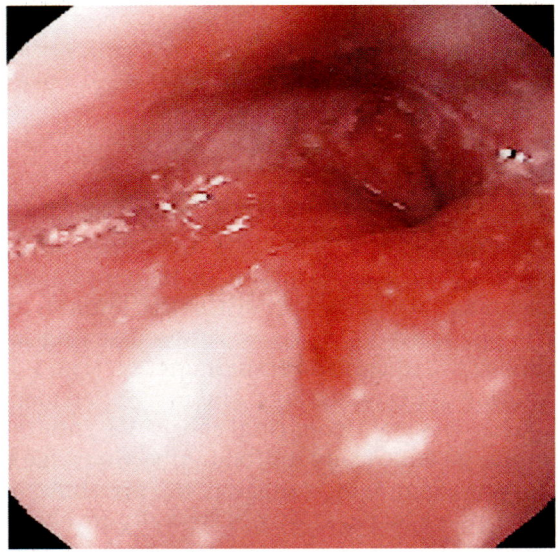

Figure 1-7: **Esophagus. Normal.** Irregular Z line may be normal or represent a focus of short-segment Barrett's esophagus.

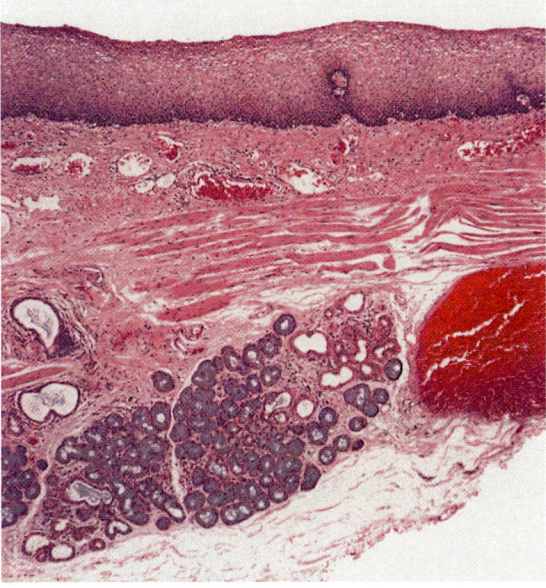

Figure 1-8: **Esophagus. Normal.** Stratified squamous epithelium supported by lamina propria is separated from the submucosa by muscularis mucosae. The lower edge of the epithelium is slightly undulated. A submucosal gland is present. Oblique sections through a duct extending toward the surface. There are numerous vessels in the lamina propria and submucosa.

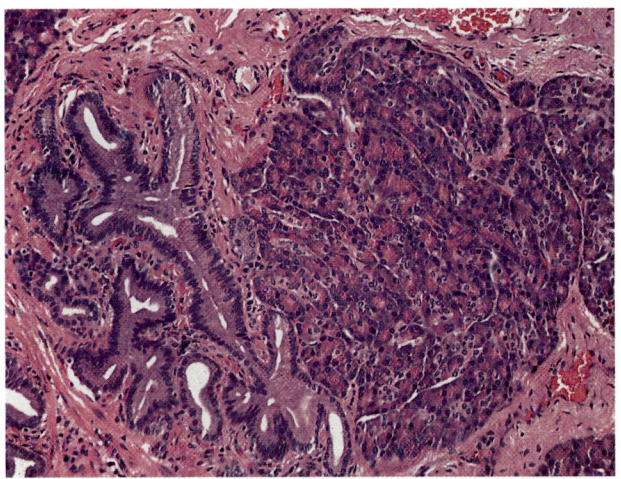

Figure 1-9: **Esophagus. Pancreatic-type Tissue in the Distal Esophagus.** Gland and duct with histologic features of pancreatic acinar tissue.

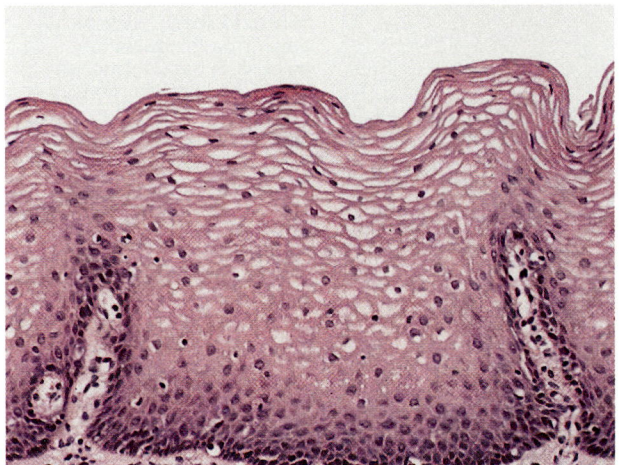

Figure 1-10: **Esophagus. Normal.** Immature basal cells with little cytoplasm form basophilic layer of 1 to 3 cells beneath more mature squamous cells with abundant clear (glycogen-rich) cytoplasm. The invaginations of lamina propria form vascular papillae that extend into the epithelium for a distance equal to half the epithelial thickness.

RINGS, WEBS, HERNIAS

- Morphology .... *Rings* are concentric structures that narrow the esophageal lumen. *Webs* are eccentric, thin, membranous rims. The Schatzki ring is classified as A and B types. The Schatzki B ring is a concentric structure at the esophagogastric junction, at the squamocolumnar junction. This distinctive lesion is a cause of intermittent dysphagia. The Schatzki A ring is a muscular ring located approximately 1 to 2 cm above the squamocolumnar junction (Fig. 1-13). It is evanescent, rarely seen during upper endoscopy, and more often identified during barium swallow. This less common ring can cause intermittent dysphagia. Patients who undergo endoscopy for food impactions due to the A ring typically have a normal exam, which suggests the possibility of the ring. Rings are usually not biopsied. Schatzki B rings typically are covered by squamous mucosa on the proximal and gastric mucosa on the distal side. Schatzki A (muscular) rings are covered by squamous mucosa on both sides. Cervical and midesophageal rings are either congenital or acquired and sometimes associated with proximal esophagitis and anemia. Congenital midesophageal stenosis may manifest as multiple rings (Fig. 1-15). Unlike Schatzki rings, hiatal hernias are covered by gastric cardia and fundic mucosa.

- Endoscopic features .... Esophageal rings are discrete, focal, and circumferential. Webs form only partial eccentric ridges.

- Clinical features .... Intermittent dysphagia may be caused by rings and webs. Large hiatal hernias can contribute to nonspecific meal-related dyspepsia. They may be complicated by bleeding from linear Cameron ulcers located on top of the rugal folds of the distal hernia rosette (See page 129).

- Differential diagnosis ...... Endoscopic: The major differential diagnosis of the B-type Schatzki ring is that of a reflux-induced distal esophageal stricture. While this distinction may be impossible, the presence of a hiatal or diaphragmatic hernia or esophagitis supports a reflux-induced ring or web.

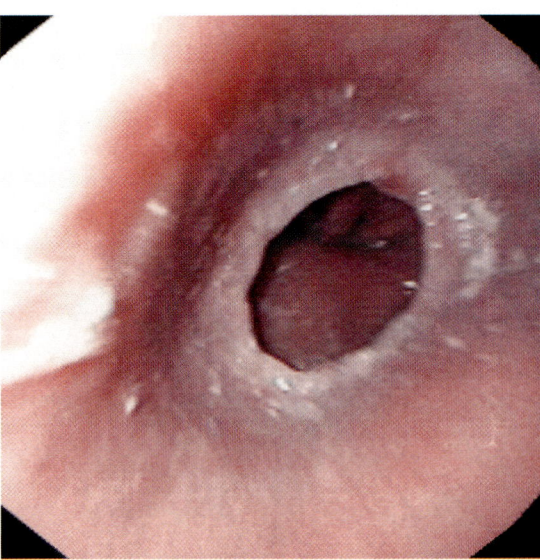

Figure 1-11: **Esophagus. Schatzki Ring.** A typical-appearing, uniform and weblike Schatzki mucosal ring. The lumen is compromised (less than 13 mm). A tiny erosion at the upper portion of the ring suggests superimposed GERD.

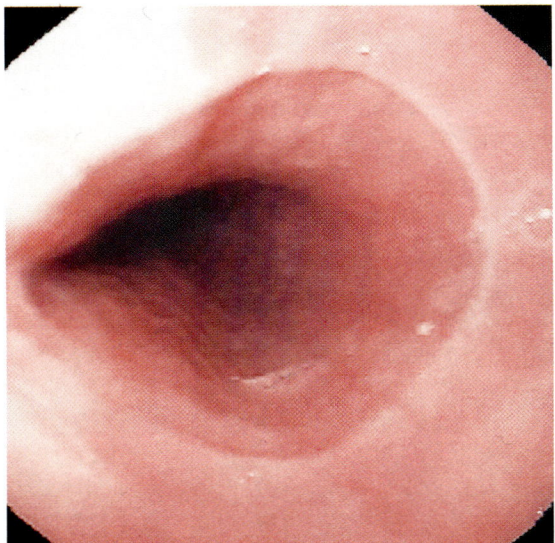

Figure 1-12: **Esophagus. Schatzki Ring.** The Schatzki ring may have a subtle presentation, as in this patient, where it appears as a small circumferential ridge of tissue.

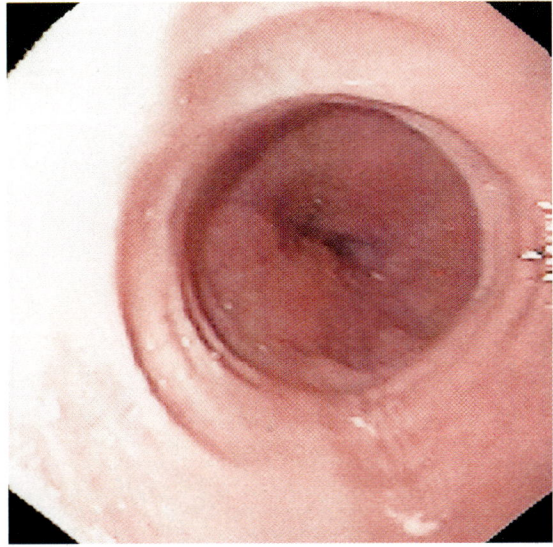

Figure 1-13: **Esophagus. Schatzki Ring.** The A-type (muscular) ring is seen in this view. Although these may give rise to symptoms of intermittent dysphagia, they are typically difficult to identify. In addition to the distal ring, there are several more proximal but incomplete contractile rings seen here. The esophagus in the absence of the contractions appears normal in these patients.

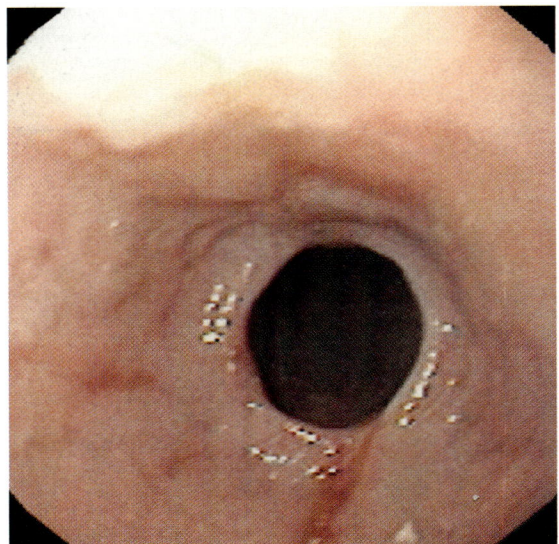

Figure 1-14: **Esophagus. Ring.** Distal esophageal ring associated with reflux-related ulceration. The distinction between a B-type Schatzki ring and a reflux-induced stricture may be difficult to establish.

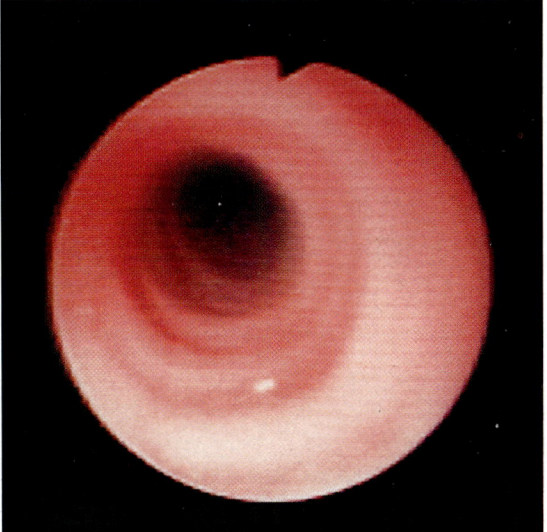

Figure 1-15: **Esophagus. Ring.** Multiple concentric rings in the midesophagus. Congenital stenosis.

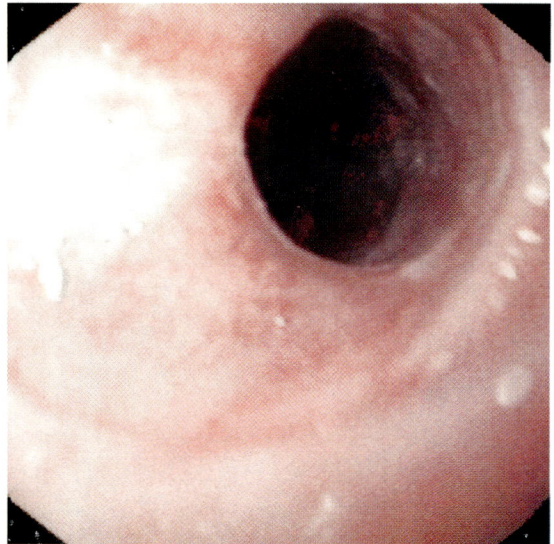

Figure 1-16: **Esophagus. Web.** This cervical esophageal web is not circumferential and arose in a patient with a distant history of radiation therapy.

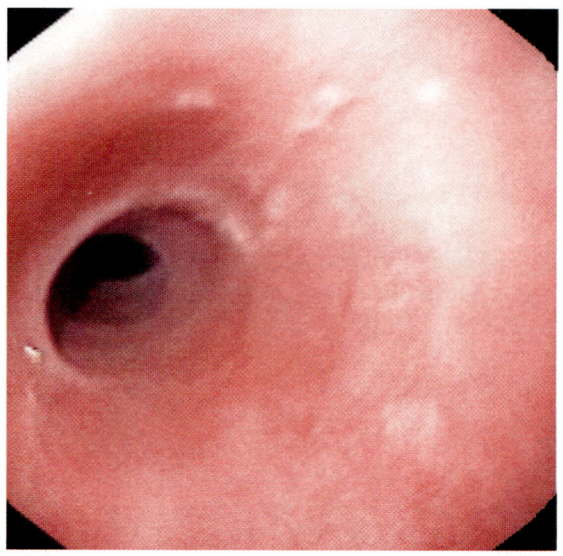

Figure 1-17: **Esophagus. Ring.** Incomplete idiopathic midesophageal ring.

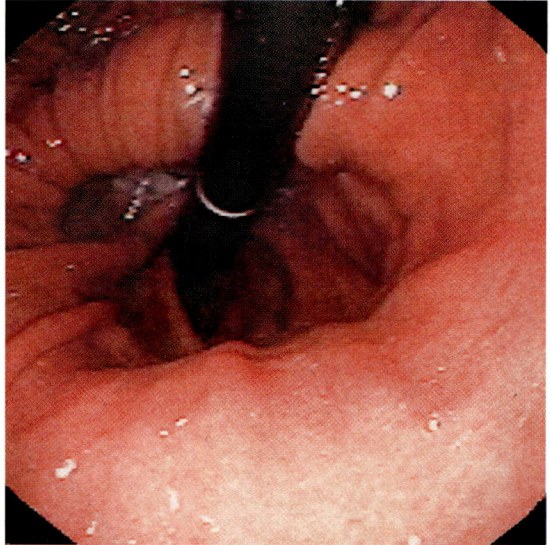

Figure 1-18: **Esophagus. Hiatal Hernia.** A hiatal hernia is well-seen during the retroflexed examination of the stomach. In this view, the hiatal interface is prominent. The patulous distal esophagus with the endoscope emanating from it can also be seen well in the center of the photograph.

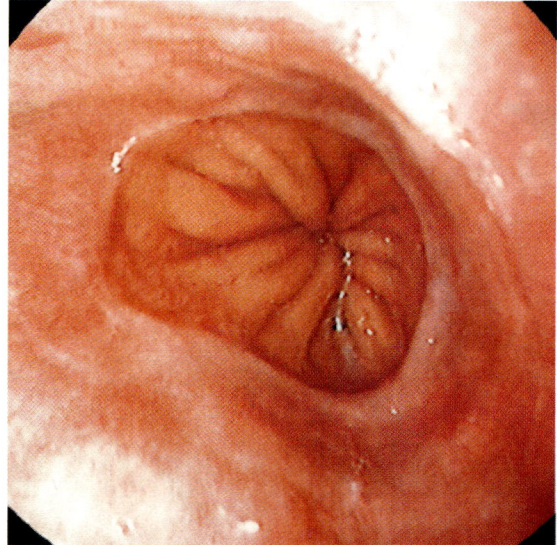

Figure 1-19: **Esophagus. Hiatal Hernia.** The view through an open distal esophagus reveals a small diaphragmatic or hiatal hernia. The diaphragmatic hiatus seen at the distal end of this hernia presents itself in a typical rosette made of longitudinal gastric folds.

MALLORY-WEISS TEAR AND DIVERTICULA

- Endoscopic features .... The Mallory-Weiss tear is an acute lesion that, when viewed soon after the tear occurs, has the appearance of an edematous and irregular split in the mucosa. Bleeding is usually multifocal, but can arise from an exposed intramural artery branching off the left gastric artery. A Mallory-Weiss tear encountered later on remains edematous but presents as a linear ulcer. The Mallory-Weiss tear is either localized to the gastric side of the squamocolumnar junction or extends across the Z line into the esophagus.

   Diverticula occur at any point within the esophagus and are single or multiple. The latter typically are associated with gastroesophageal reflux disease (GERD). Isolated diverticula may be large and wide-mouthed. They usually do not have an inflammatory component, such as ulceration or erosions. Large diverticula may contain food and retained debris.

- Clinical features .... The classic presentation for the Mallory-Weiss tear is a sequence of events beginning with nausea and vomiting, followed soon by hematemesis.

   Esophageal diverticula in the setting of GERD may be asymptomatic. With severe advanced reflux disease they are symptomatic due to an associated stricture. Large wide-mouthed diverticula at other locations are associated with dysphagia.

- Differential diagnosis ...... Endoscopic: The Mallory-Weiss tear can be confused with GERD with distal esophageal ulceration and an ulcerating neoplasm, especially if there is a large submucosal hematoma.

   Esophageal diverticula are straightforward, with the exception of confusing a proximal esophageal diverticulum with a Zenker diverticulum.

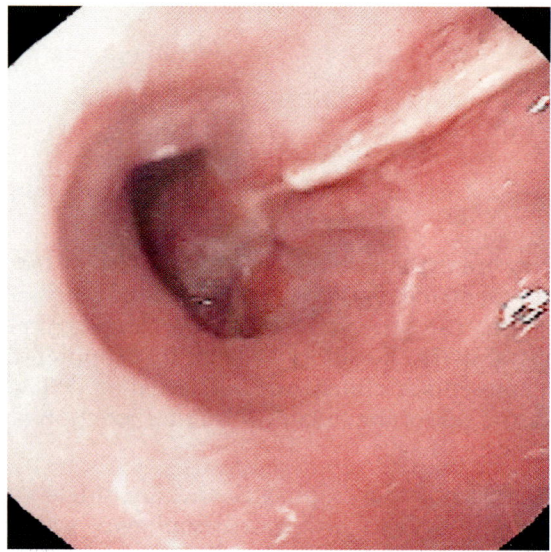

Figure 1-20: **Esophagus. Mallory-Weiss Tear.** A long and characteristic linear tear in the distal esophagus can be followed across the gastroesophageal junction into the cardia. A whitish exudate covers the exposed submucosal tissues. The distribution of this acute lesion (cardia to the distal esophagus) is typical.

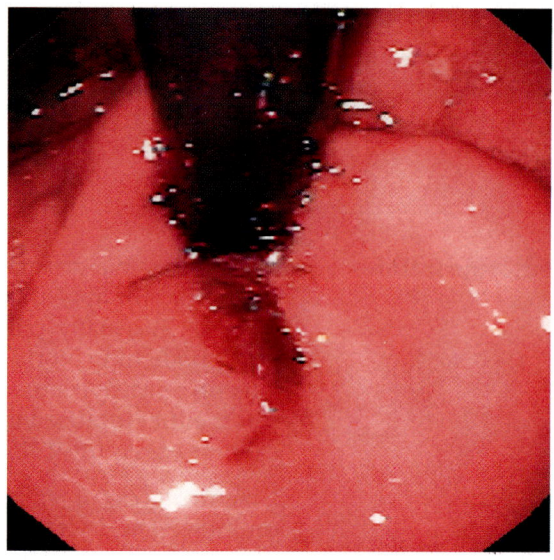

Figure 1-21: **Esophagus. Mallory-Weiss Tear.** The cardia component of an acute tear.

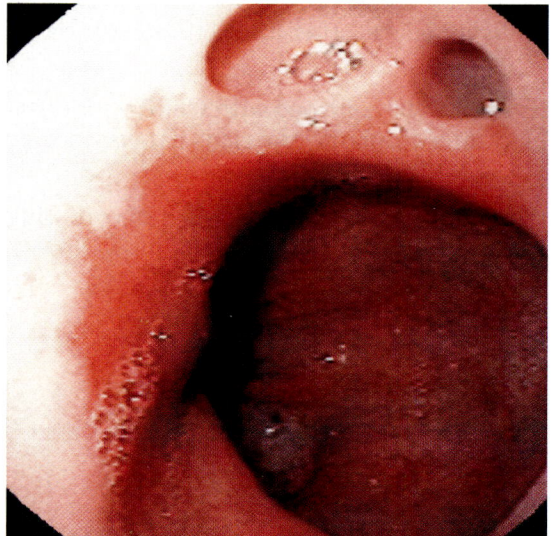

Figure 1-22: **Esophagus. Diverticula.** The distal esophagus just above the esophagogastric junction contains 2 small epiphrenic diverticula. There is also a mild related stricture at this level. These findings can be encountered in long-standing severe GERD.

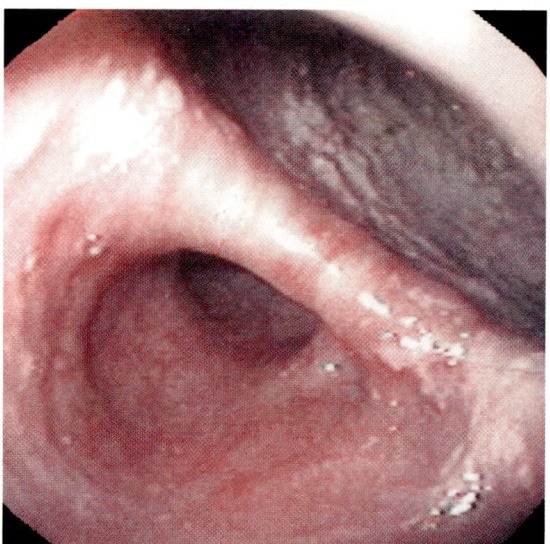

Figure 1-23: **Esophagus. Diverticulum.** A large distal esophageal diverticulum occupies the upper portion of the photo. The diverticulum is large-mouthed, with a scant amount of retained debris. The esophageal lumen is slightly displaced by the distal margin of the diverticulum. This, plus the size of the diverticulum, contributed to the patient's dysphagia.

GASTRIC HETEROTOPIA/INLET PATCH

- Morphology .... Ectopic gastric mucosa is typically located in the proximal esophagus. Most often it is of fundic type, but may consist of cardia-type mucosa or a mixture of gastric mucosal types. It may be inflamed but rarely develops intestinal metaplasia.

- Endoscopic features .... A gastric inlet patch is a discrete localized collection of gastric mucosa in a spherical or ellipsoid configuration. The margins are sharp and at times may have a slightly raised appearance, although the heterotopic gastric tissue is flat. These patches rarely exceed 2 cm in size. The gastric inlet patch is typically an incidental finding. Ulceration and stricture are rare.

- Clinical features .... Usually incidental and asymptomatic but may cause a burning sensation or dysphagia.

- Differential diagnosis ...... Endoscopic: Distinguished from Barrett's esophagus by the cervical esophageal location.

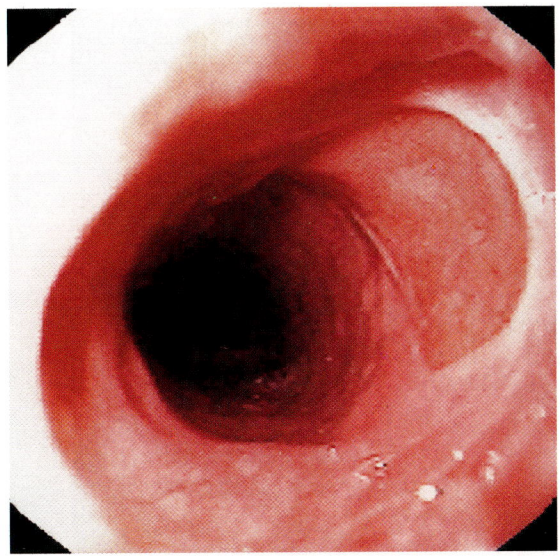

Figure 1-24: **Esophagus. Gastric Inlet Patch.** A patch of heterotopic gastric tissue on the right side of the esophageal lumen. The discrete margins and gastric mucosal (salmon) coloring are classic features.

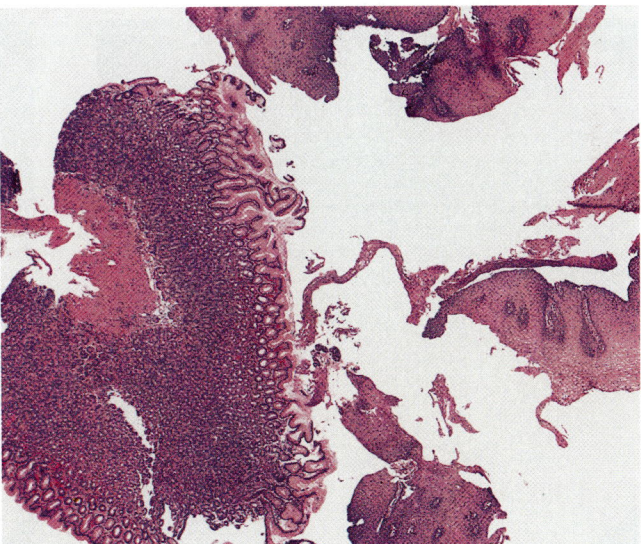

Figure 1-25: **Esophagus. Gastric Heterotopia.** Normal squamous and gastric fundic mucosa.

GLYCOGENIC ACANTHOSIS

- Morphology .... These nodules or plaques result from accumulation of excess glycogen in mature squamous cells of the upper epithelium. The diagnosis is often difficult to establish on biopsy, unless normal mucosa is also present for comparison.
- Endoscopic features .... Glycogenic acanthosis is typically distributed throughout the length of the esophagus, concentrated mostly in the proximal two thirds. The appearance is that of discrete white or pale nodules, plaques (Fig. 1-27), or exudates (Fig. 1-28). The number, size, and distribution of the lesions depicted here are characteristic of glycogenic acanthosis.
- Clinical features .... None. This condition is asymptomatic and an incidental finding.
- Differential diagnosis ...... Endoscopic: *Candida* or ectopic salivary gland tissue.

    Histologic: Normal mucosa, epithelial edema, and human papillomavirus.

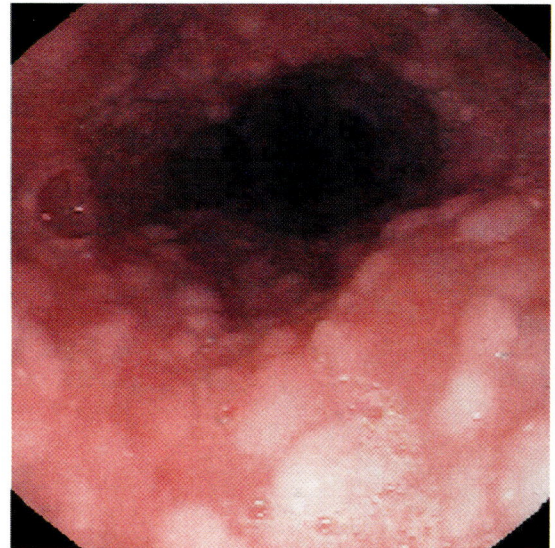

Figure 1-26: **Esophagus. Glycogenic Acanthosis.** Numerous whitish nodules or plaques throughout the length of the esophagus.

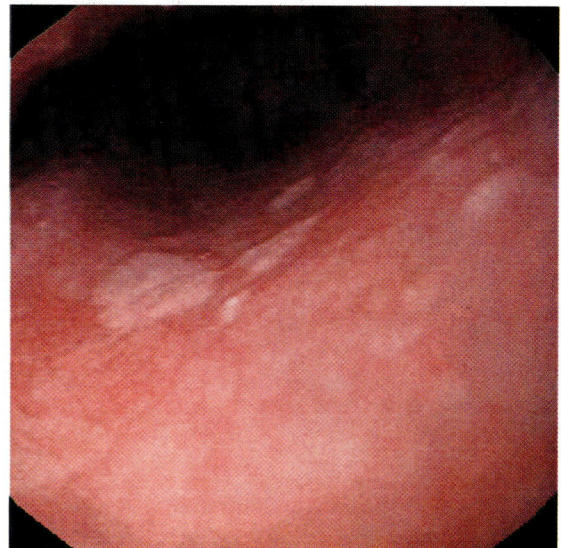

Figure 1-27: **Esophagus. Glycogenic Acanthosis.** Pale, slightly elevated plaques.

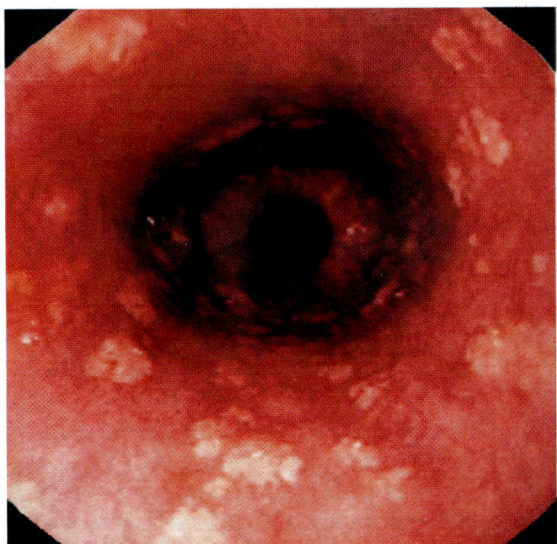

Figure 1-28: **Esophagus. Glycogenic Acanthosis.** White lesions appear exudative.

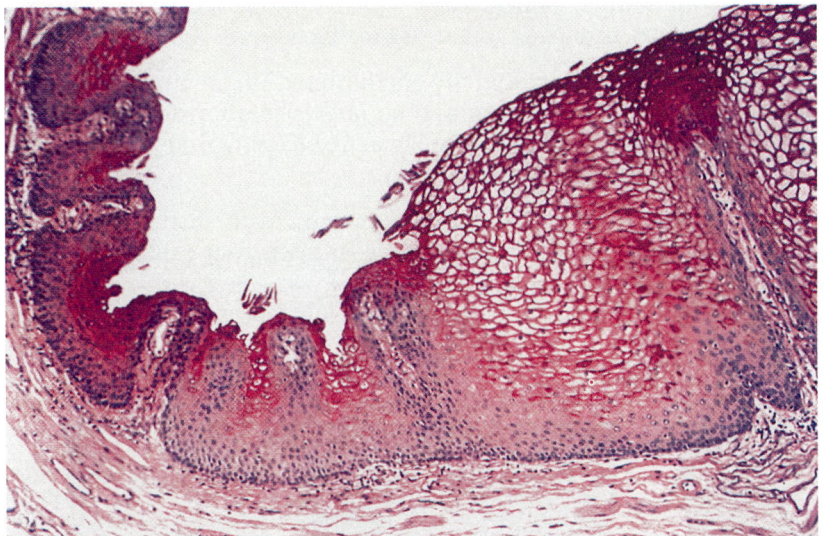

Figure 1-29: **Esophagus. Glycogenic Acanthosis.** This PAS-stained section shows an area of mucosal thickening due to enlarged mature squamous cells with clear or PAS-positive (glycogen-rich) cytoplasm. This contrasts with the adjacent normal epithelium.

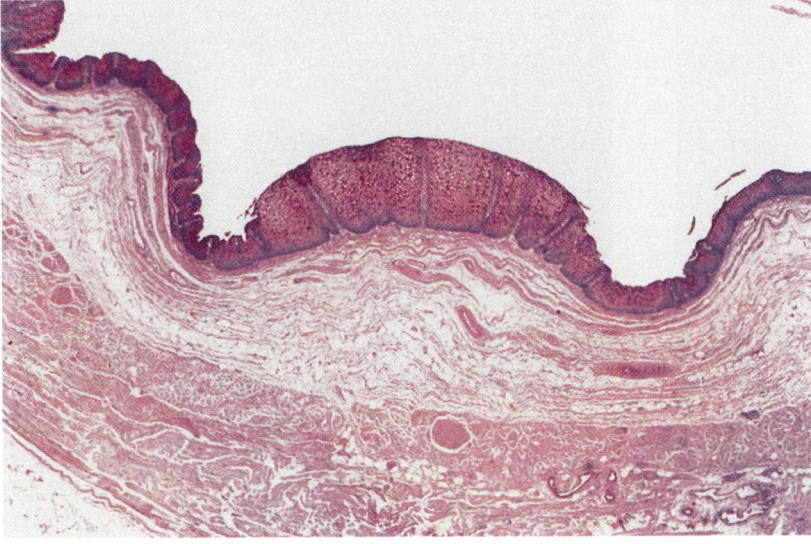

Figure 1-30: **Esophagus. Glycogenic Acanthosis.** Low magnification shows well-demarcated elevated lesion.

VARICES

- Morphology .... Large, tortuous, thick and focally thin-walled submucosal veins bulge into the esophageal lumen. Biopsy is avoided.

- Endoscopic features .... The mucosa overlying a varix may be normal, especially when varices are small or have been injected with sclerosing agents. Red color signs are used to classify varices that may be at high risk for bleeding. Red color signs include the discrete small, round hemocystic spot and linear or serpiginous red wale marking, an indicator of significant risk of bleeding. Esophageal varices otherwise are classified according to their size using a grading system, or else noted as being small or large. An example of a grading system is: size of esophageal varices within 5 cm from the esophagogastric junction (with air inflation)—grade 1, flat; grade 2, one fourth of lumen obliterated; grade 3, one half of lumen obliterated; and grade 4, greater than one half of lumen obliterated. Large size indicates added risk for bleeding.

- Clinical features .... Esophageal varices may be incidentally encountered in patients with portal hypertension from any cause. Despite their large size, they do not give rise to dysphagia. Their main clinical feature is acute bleeding that presents with hematemesis and/or melena/hematochezia.

- Differential diagnosis ...... The appearance and distribution of esophageal varices are distinctive. Some patients may have prominent distal esophageal veins that can be confused with very small esophageal varices.

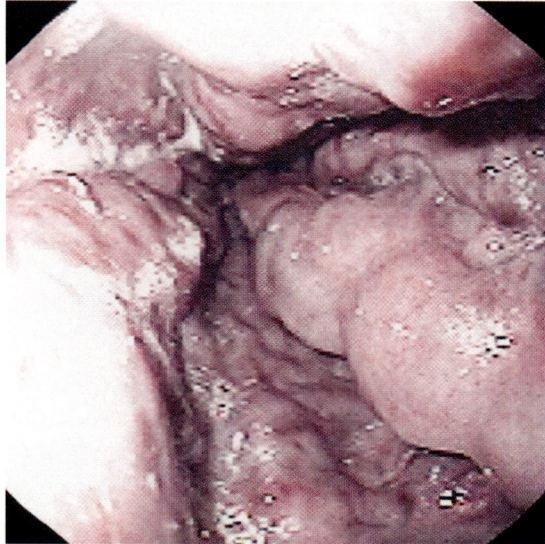

Figure 1-31: **Esophagus. Varices.** Large, irregular esophageal varices. There are multiple trunks, nearly occluding the esophageal lumen, extending down to the gastroesophageal junction.

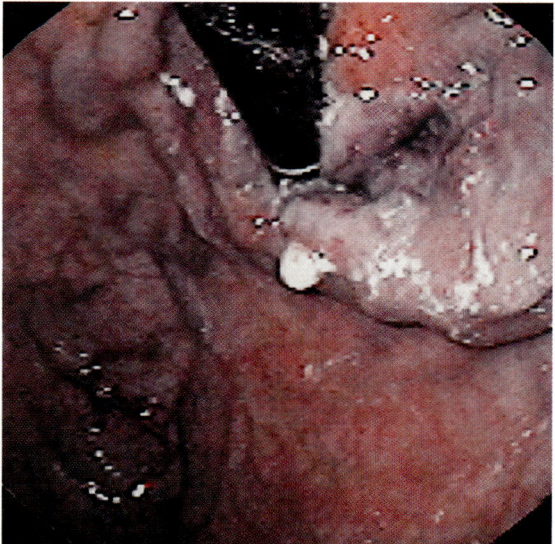

Figure 1-32: **Esophagus. Gastroesophageal Junction Varices.** Retroflexion of the gastroesophageal junction of patient in Fig. 1-31. Varices can be seen extending into the cardia.

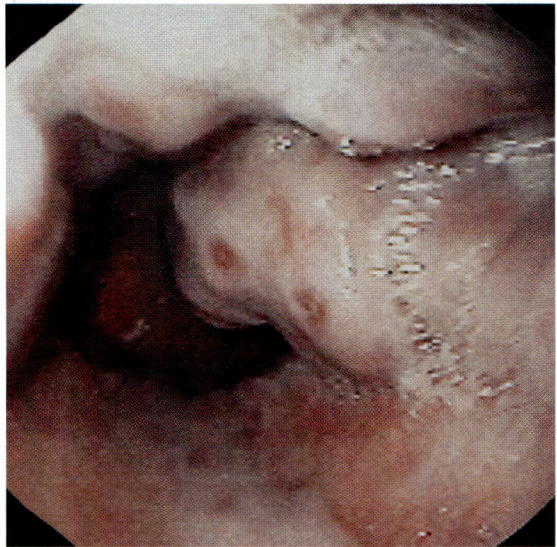

Figure 1-33: **Esophagus. Varices.** A prominent esophageal variceal trunk with a variety of red color signs. There are 2 discrete hemocystic spots visible.

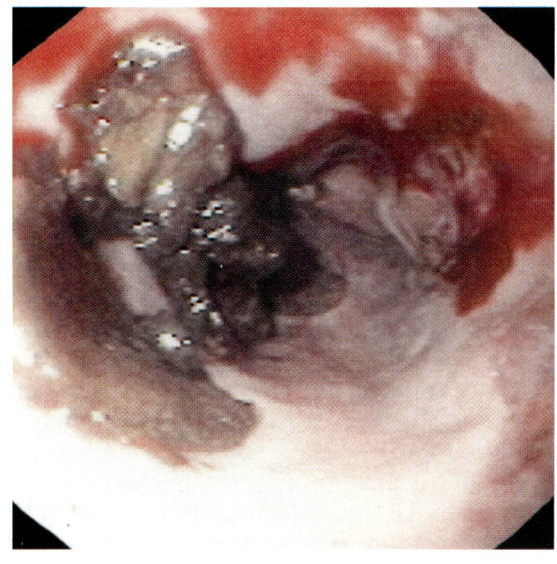

Figure 1-34: **Esophagus. Bleeding Varix.** Fresh and altered blood overlie varix.

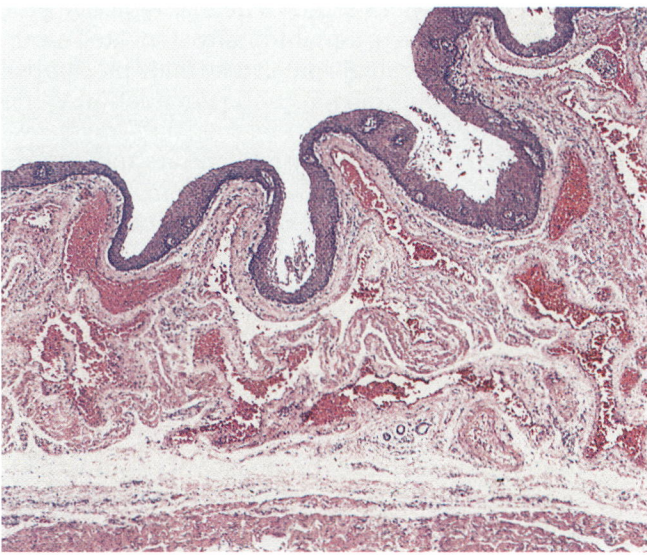

Figure 1-35: **Esophagus. Varices.** The veins and venules in the submucosa and lamina propria are markedly ectatic and thick-walled.

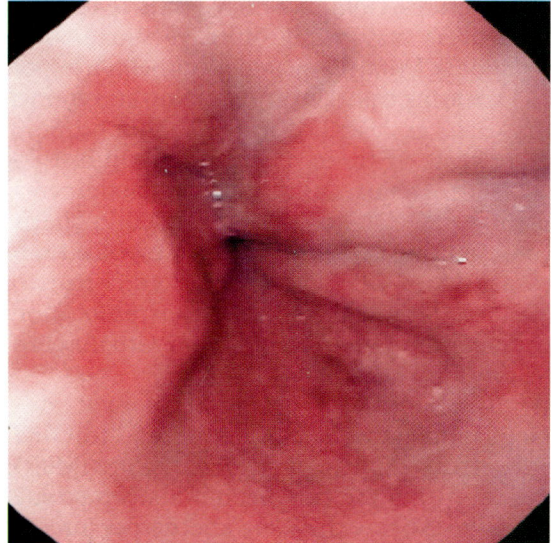

Figure 1-36: **Esophagus. Varices.** Irregular tongues of salmon-colored mucosa (Barrett's esophagus) associated with varices.

ESOPHAGITIS

The most common cause of esophagitis is reflux. The histologic changes are not specific. Correlation with gross endoscopic findings is necessary for diagnosis. On endoscopic examination, erosions and ulcerations are superficial and extend upward as tongues from the region of the squamocolumnar junction. Histologic findings may include epithelial swelling, superficial epithelial necrosis and neutrophilic infiltrates, erosions, and ulcers. This is followed by healing, i.e., granulation tissue formation and re-epithelialization. Re-epithelialization begins with the migration of squamous epithelial cells with huge, round, uniform macronucleoli. This single layer becomes multilayered and forms narrow, elongated, penetrating epithelial trabeculae that broaden as the epithelium matures. Oblique sections from re-epithelializing areas may mimic invasive squamous cell carcinoma. Irritated squamous epithelium responds by increasing basal cell proliferation and epithelial thickness, as described in the section on normal esophagus. At times, this is the only histologic evidence of reflux. Other changes include increases in intraepithelial T cells and eosinophils. The most common cause of eosinophils in esophageal mucosa is reflux. Pill esophagitis lacks differentiating features. It is recognized by an isolated location in the midesophagus in conjunction with the clinical history.

Infections are the next most common cause of esophagitis. Most infections are due to *Candida* species, herpesvirus, or cytomegalovirus. Multiple infections are the rule in immunocompromised patients. Whereas *Candida* and herpes infections occur in nonimmunosuppressed persons, cytomegalovirus infection is usually seen in immunocompromised individuals.

When *Candida* is suspected, biopsy samples should be from areas covered by yellow-white inflammatory exudate. Special stains may be necessary to identify the typical budding yeast and pseudohyphae, which are located in the superficial epithelial layer and exudate. Brushings and washings are diagnostic more often than biopsy samples.

Herpes causes multiple small, shallow, round, and often confluent ulcers. Nuclear inclusions and other characteristic changes such as multinucleation and molding are best seen in ulcer edges and debris.

Cytomegalovirus infects endothelial and other stromal cells rather than esophageal squamous epithelium. Endothelial cell involvement predisposes to thrombosis and ischemia, typically producing large, deep, longitudinally elongated ulcers that are usually single but can be multiple. Biopsy samples should come from the granulation tissue at the base of the ulcer.

Other forms of esophagitis are rare and include eosinophilic esophagitis and granulomatous esophagitis. Eosinophilic esophagitis may be part of an ill-defined clinical syndrome: young men with dysphagia and midesophageal eosinophilic infiltrates. It may also be a manifestation of a systemic hypereosinophilic syndrome, idiopathic eosinophilic gastroenteritis, or an allergic type of hypersensitivity response to food, drugs, or parasites. Granulomatous esophagitis may reflect Crohn's disease or tuberculous or fungal infections spreading from the lungs. Negative stains for infectious agents do not exclude infections.

REFLUX ESOPHAGITIS

- Morphology .... Acute reflux damage consists of superficial epithelial swelling and/or necrosis accompanied by intraepithelial neutrophilic infiltrates. Chronic reflux induces basal cell hyperplasia, epithelial thickening, and elongation of the vascular papillae. To diagnose reflux in endoscopically indeterminate cases, specimens should be taken at least 2.5 cm above the junction of the tubular esophagus and stomach. Oriented specimens that show basal hyperplasia in excess of 15% and papillary elongation in excess of 70% of the epithelial thickness can be used to diagnose reflux in endoscopically indeterminate cases. Reflux is the most common cause of eosinophilic infiltrates in the esophagus. Intraepithelial T cells are typically increased in number. In other situations, some but not all features may be considered sufficient to support a clinical diagnosis of reflux. These alterations are nonspecific and can be seen in other chronic inflammatory conditions.

- Endoscopic features .... Gastroesophageal reflux can be macroscopically graded on a scale of 1 to 4. Mild (grade 1) esophagitis is best characterized by erythematous streaking extending cephalad from the squamocolumnar junction. It is also associated with light contact friability of the mucosa. Erosions with erythematous margins located at and proximal to the squamocolumnar junction typify grade 2 esophagitis. In grade 3 or severe esophagitis, the erosions coalesce and become circumferential. Complicated grade 4 esophagitis presents with large, deep ulcerations. Strictures, bleeding, and Barrett's esophagus are associated with grade 4 esophagitis.

- Clinical features .... Pyrosis, dysphagia, anemia, hematemesis, and/or melena.

- Differential diagnosis ...... Histologic: Any cause of chronic esophagitis, including pill esophagitis, infectious esophagitis, bullous diseases, and idiopathic eosinophilic esophagitis. Epithelial regeneration can simulate squamous cell carcinoma in oblique sections.

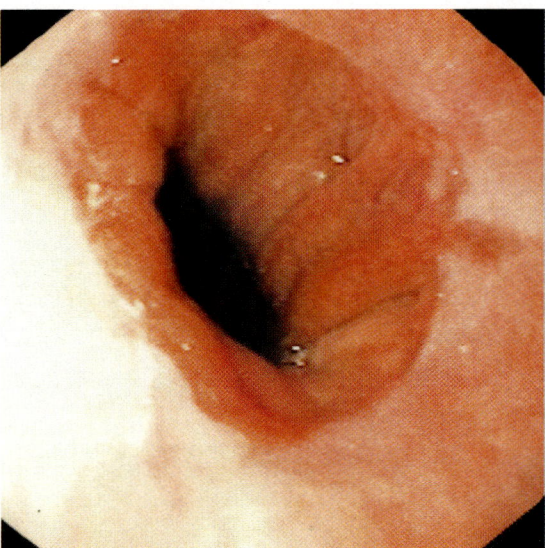

Figure 1-37: **Esophagus. Reflux Esophagitis.** On the right side of the photograph, a small area of mild esophagitis interrupts the well-delineated margin of the squamo-columnar junction.

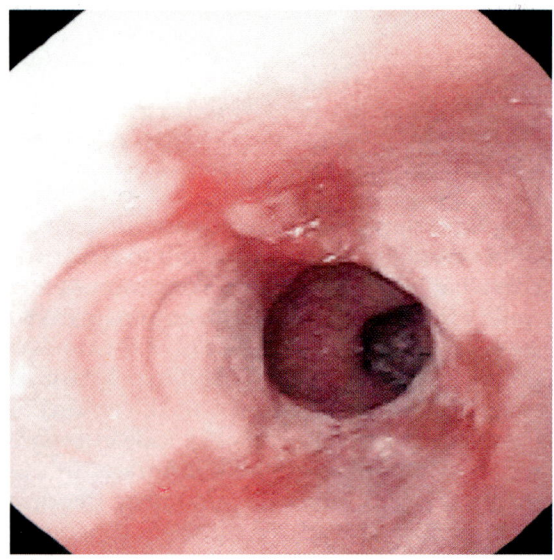

Figure 1-38: **Esophagus. Reflux Esophagitis.** Severe reflux esophagitis with linear ulcers extending up from a stricture.

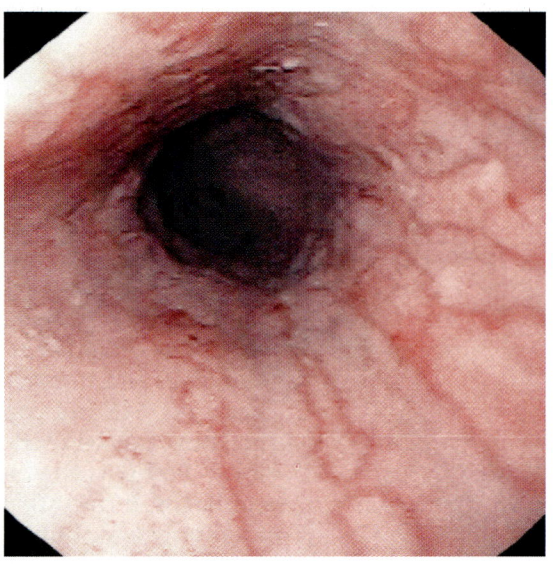

Figure 1-39: **Esophagus. Reflux Esophagitis.** Extensive and coalescing ulceration. The ulcers are long and extend well above the esophagogastric junction.

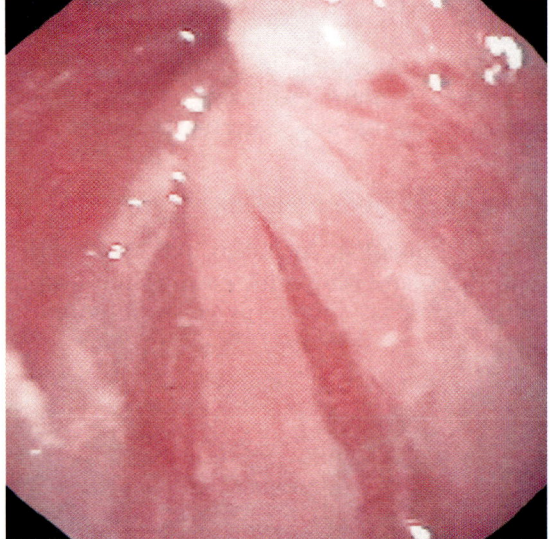

Figure 1-40: **Esophagus. Reflux Esophagitis.** An unusual manifestation of gastroesophageal reflux: the mucosa has become disrupted and appears as linear shreds of tissue.

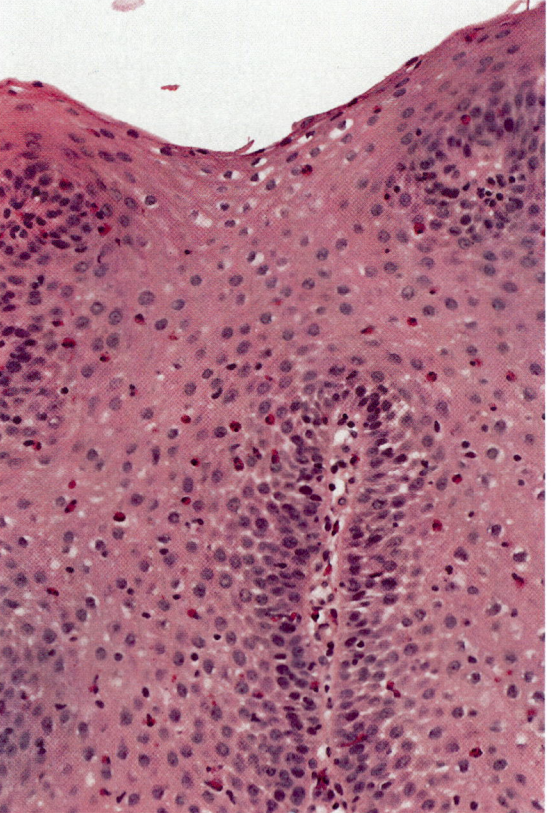

Figure 1-41: **Esophagus. Reflux Esophagitis.** Eosinophils infiltrate the epithelium.

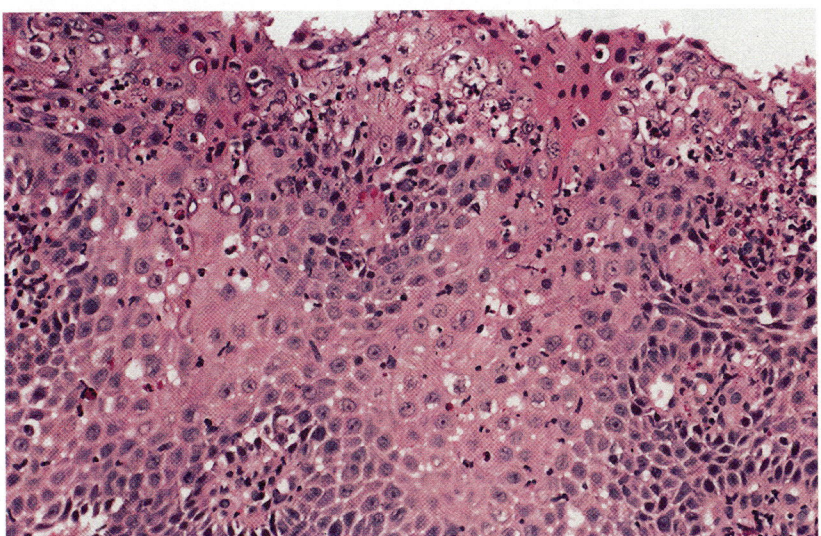

Figure 1-42: **Esophagus. Reflux Esophagitis.** Nonspecific active inflammation and epithelial edema. There is surface epithelial necrosis, infiltrating neutrophils, scattered eosinophils, and increased numbers of twisted intraepithelial T-lymphocytes.

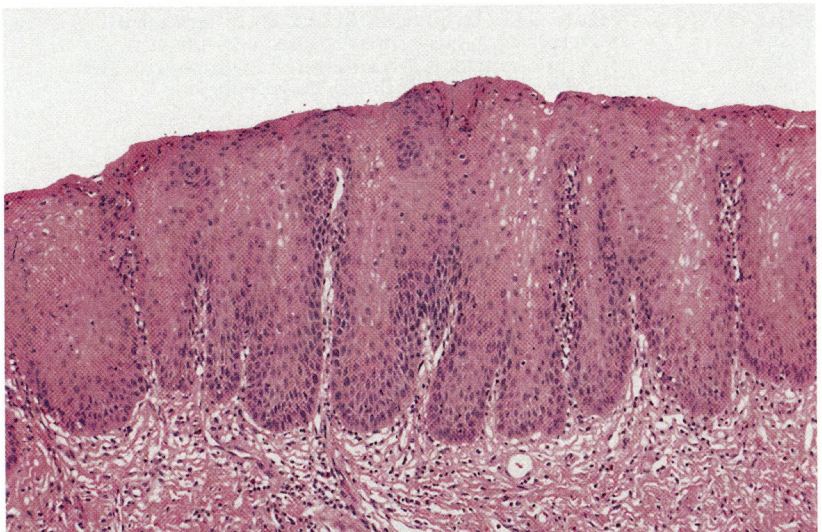

Figure 1-43: **Esophagus. Reflux Esophagitis.** Hyperplastic squamous epithelium. There is basal cell hyperplasia and thickening of the epithelium. Vascular papillae are elongated.

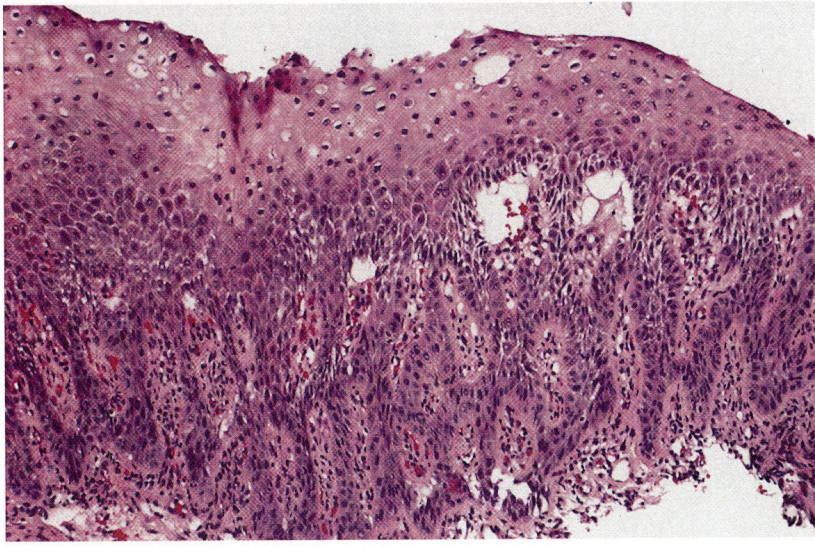

Figure 1-44: **Esophagus. Reflux Esophagitis.** Narrow epithelial extensions into the lamina propria are characteristic of re-epithelialization following ulceration. Individual cells in these extensions show reactive nuclear and cytoplasmic alterations. There is chronic inflammation in the lamina propria.

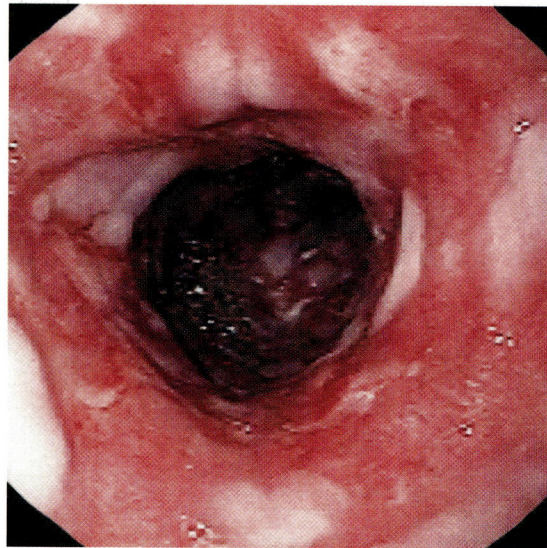

Figure 1-45: **Esophagus. Reflux Esophagitis.** Severe esophagitis in the setting of an esophagogastric anastomosis. Circumferential ulceration with interspersed islands of squamous mucosa. Diffusely mottled esophageal mucosa with areas of hemorrhage. The anastomosis is not stenotic. Centrally, a well-circumscribed gastric-appearing patch with a villiform appearance is in the distal half of the esophagus. The location, several centimeters above the esophagogastric junction, is unusual for both a gastric inlet patch and Barrett's mucosa.

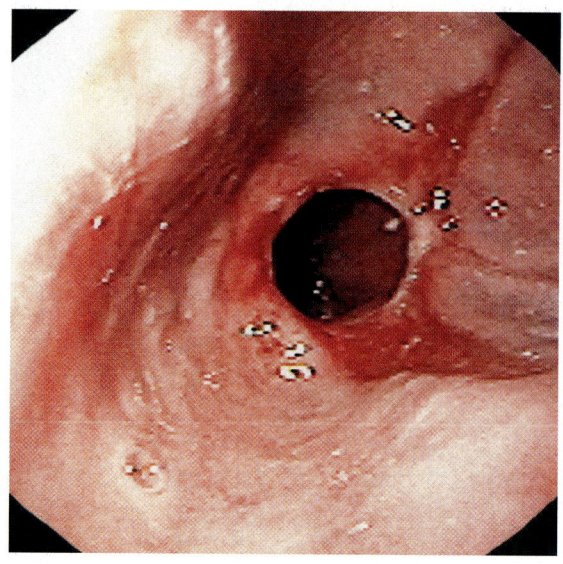

Figure 1-46: **Esophagus. Reflux Esophagitis with Stricture.** A typical-appearing distal esophageal stricture, ringlike with an ulcerating esophagitis that involves the stricture and extends cephalad.

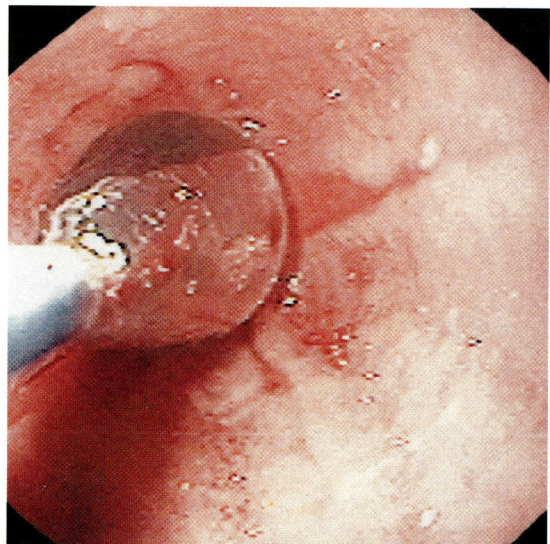

Figure 1-47: **Esophagus. Reflux Esophagitis with Stricture.** A hydrostatic dilating balloon straddled across the stricture. Under direct observation, the stricture is dilated.

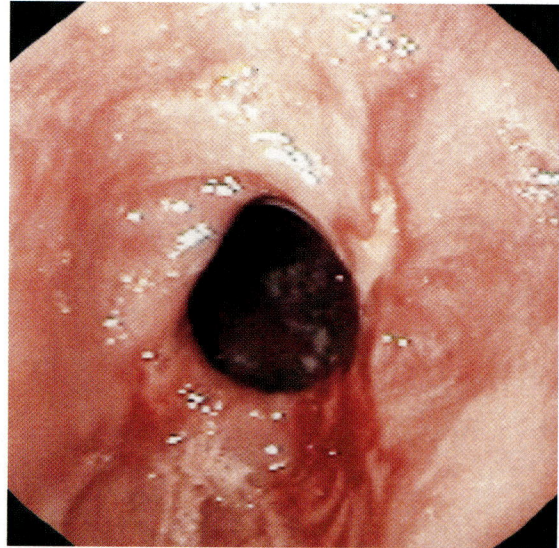

Figure 1-48: **Esophagus. Reflux Esophagitis with Stricture.** A slightly irregular stricture at distal esophagus; scarring due to long-standing reflux and recurrent ulceration. A subtle diverticulum in the lower left portion of the photograph is characteristic of severe esophagitis with stricture and deformity.

INFLAMMATORY POLYPS ASSOCIATED WITH REFLUX

- Morphology .... Inflammatory polyps associated with reflux often occur at or near the squamocolumnar junction and consist of inflamed mucosa of gastric or esophageal type. They have no neoplastic potential. The gastric component is similar to a hyperplastic polyp of the stomach, largely due to foveolar hyperplasia, edema, and inflammation.

- Endoscopic features .... Inflammatory reflux-related polyps vary in size and appearance. These lesions may be diminutive or exceed 1 cm in diameter. The larger polyps often have a villiform surface. They are typically soft, nonulcerated, and nonfriable. These polyps may be associated with a raised fold or ridge leading up to the base of the polyp and arising from the gastric or esophageal side of the polyp. When singular, the polyps are best managed by snare excision, with retrieval of the entire polyp for histology. There are no surface features that distinguish them from a small adenocarcinoma.

- Clinical features .... Chronic gastric esophageal reflux symptoms.

- Differential diagnosis ...... Endoscopic: Gastric hyperplastic polyps, squamous papillomas, adenomas, and small adenocarcinomas of the cardia.

SQUAMOUS PAPILLOMAS ASSOCIATED WITH REFLUX

- Morphology .... Squamous papillomas can resemble inflammatory polyps or, when they are filiform and not associated with obvious endoscopic evidence of reflux, raise the possibility of viral etiology. Recent studies suggest that the majority of these lesions are associated with reflux and do not have a viral etiology.

- Endoscopic features .... Squamous papillomas vary in size from diminutive lesions of several millimeters to more prominent polypoid lesions of up to 1 cm. The polyps are soft, nonfriable, and nonulcerated. They are most often located in the midesophagus.

- Clinical features .... These polyps are incidental findings. Some patients have symptoms of GERD.

- Differential diagnosis ...... Histologic and endoscopic: Rare entities such as viral papillomas and verrucous carcinoma.

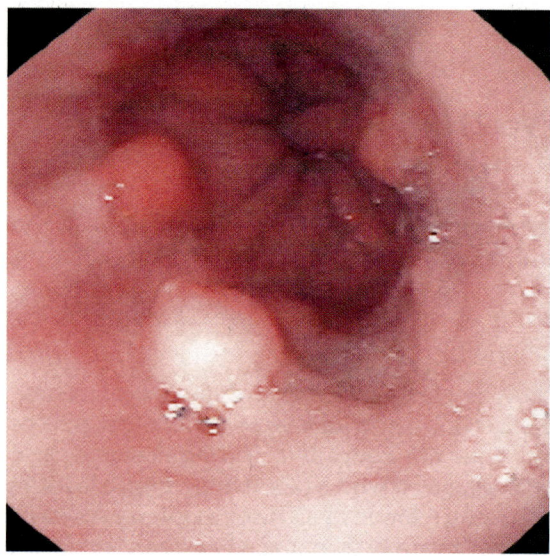

Figure 1-49: **Esophagus. Inflammatory Polyps Associated with Reflux.** At least 3 sessile diminutive polyps at the esophagogastric junction. In the distance, the rosette from a small diaphragmatic hernia. The patient had a long history of GERD.

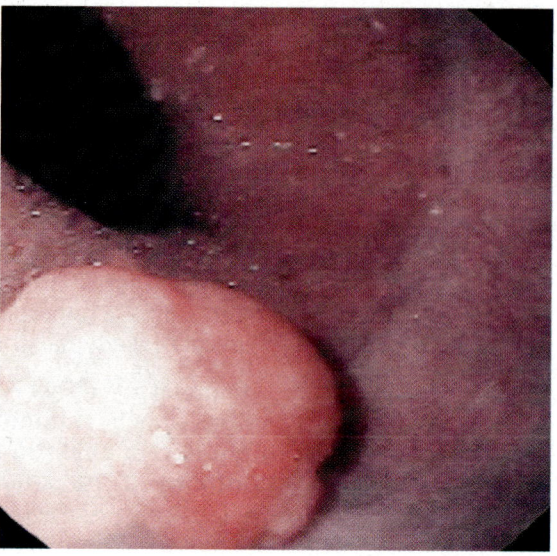

Figure 1-50: **Esophagus. Inflammatory Polyp Associated with Reflux.** Small sessile polyp at the squamocolumnar junction. The surface of the polyp is irregular and without distinguishing features.

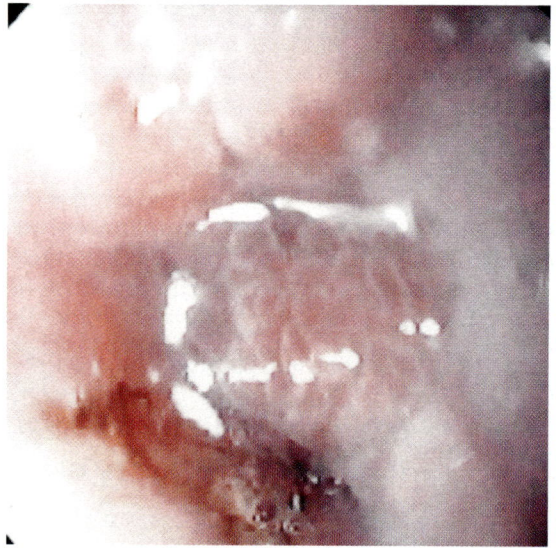

Figure 1-51: **Esophagus. Inflammatory Polyp Associated with Reflux.** Polyp at gastroesophageal junction with a villiform appearance.

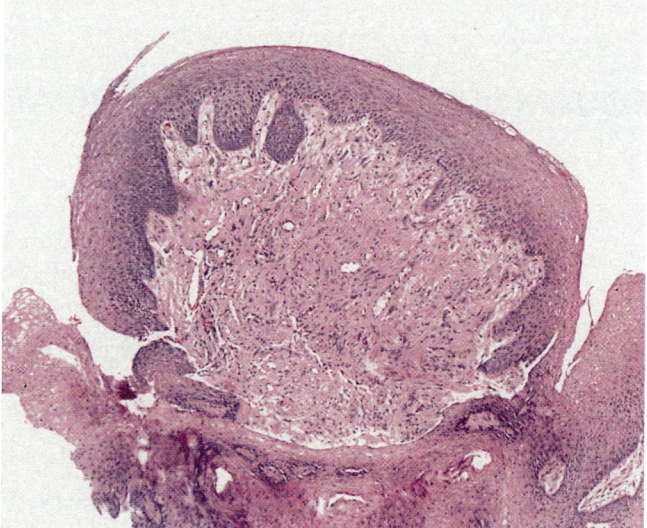

Figure 1-52: **Esophagus. Inflammatory Polyp Associated with Reflux.** This polyp consists of hyperplastic squamous epithelium over fibrovascular stroma (maturing granulation tissue).

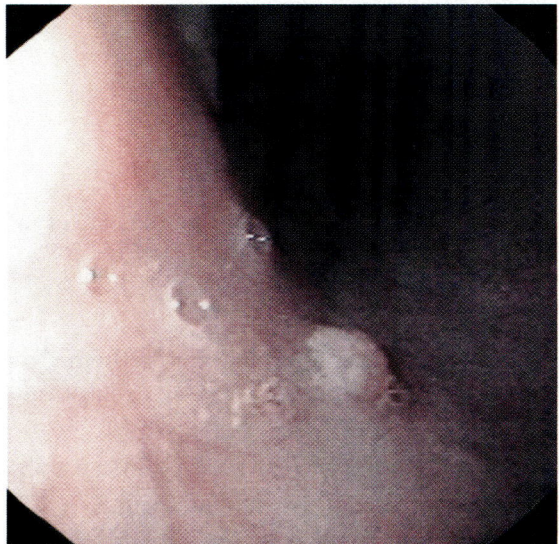

Figure 1-53: **Esophagus. Squamous Papilloma Associated with Reflux.** A minute sessile polyp in the midesophagus.

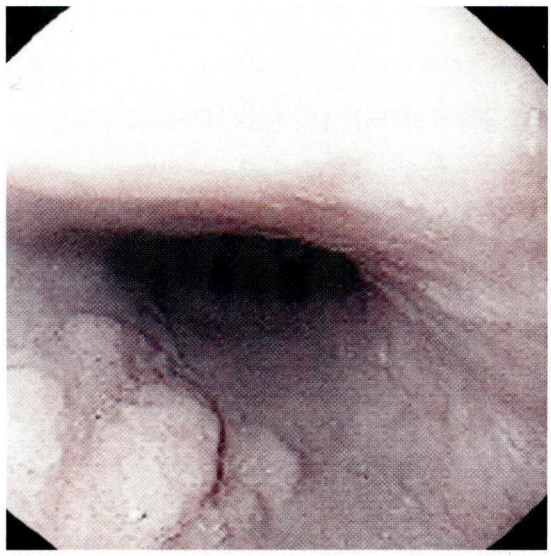

Figure 1-54: **Esophagus. Squamous Papilloma Associated with Reflux.** A sessile polyp with grossly irregular surface features in the distal esophagus. It is not possible to discern whether there is a single polyp or a cluster of diminutive polyps. The surface features are nonspecific.

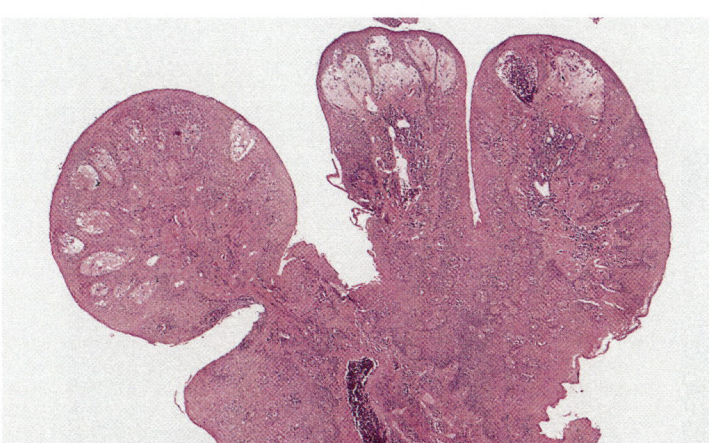

Figure 1-55: **Esophagus. Squamous Papilloma Associated with Reflux.** Multiple broad polypoid excrescences with edema, mild chronic inflammation, and squamous epithelial hyperplasia.

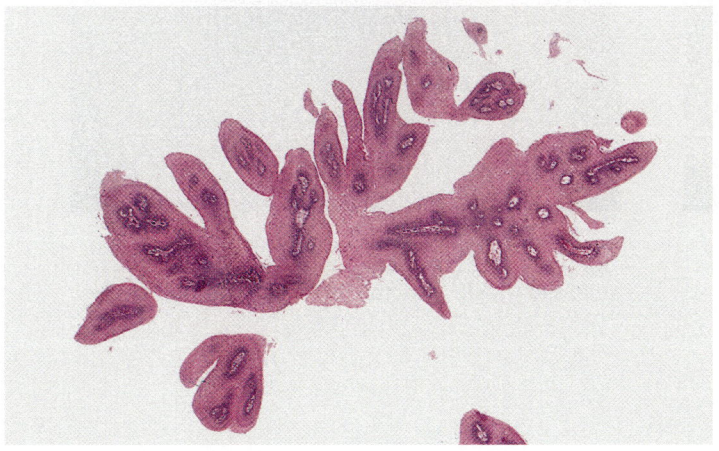

Figure 1-56: **Esophagus. Squamous Papilloma Associated with Reflux.** Delicate squamous papillary excrescences.

EOSINOPHILIC ESOPHAGITIS

- Morphology .... The most common cause of eosinophilic esophagitis is reflux. Sheets of pure eosinophils, but more importantly atypical location, or peripheral eosinophilia suggest other less common clinical conditions. For other causes, see page 18.
- Endoscopic features .... The endoscopic features are nonspecific and range from erythema to ulceration. Ulcers are discrete or diffuse. In the distal esophagus, reflux changes and stricture formation may be present.
- Clinical features .... Dysphagia in young men with midesophageal eosinophilic esophagitis, GERD-related symptoms.
- Differential diagnosis ...... Clinical: Reflux, idiopathic eosinophilic esophagitis, hypersensitivity to drugs and food, pill-induced esophagitis, and parasites.

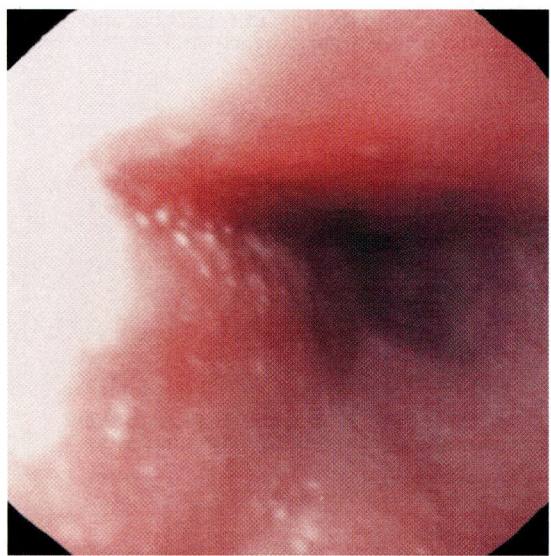

Figure 1-57: **Esophagus. Eosinophilic Esophagitis.** Punctate elevated white lesions dispersed within the proximal esophagus. Remainder of the mucosa is normal.

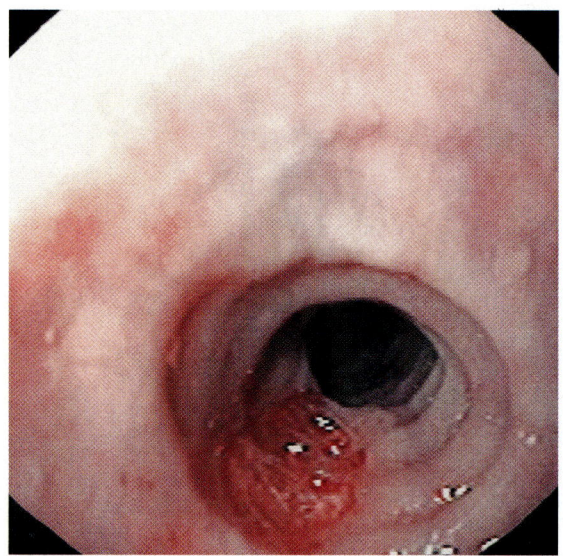

Figure 1-58: **Esophagus. Eosinophilic Esophagitis.** Discrete midesophageal ulcer, nonspecific in appearance and friable. Stricture immediately distal to the ulcer.

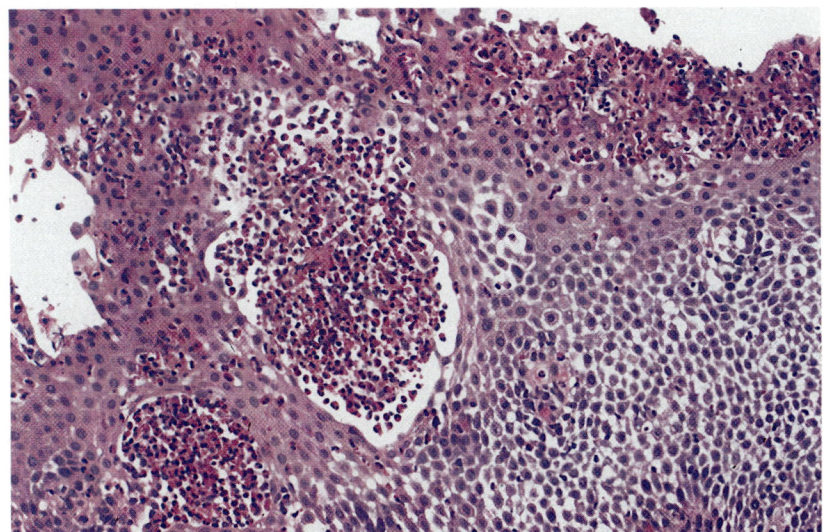

Figure 1-59: **Esophagus. Eosinophilic Esophagitis.** Surface epithelial injury with numerous eosinophils and eosinophilic microabscesses.

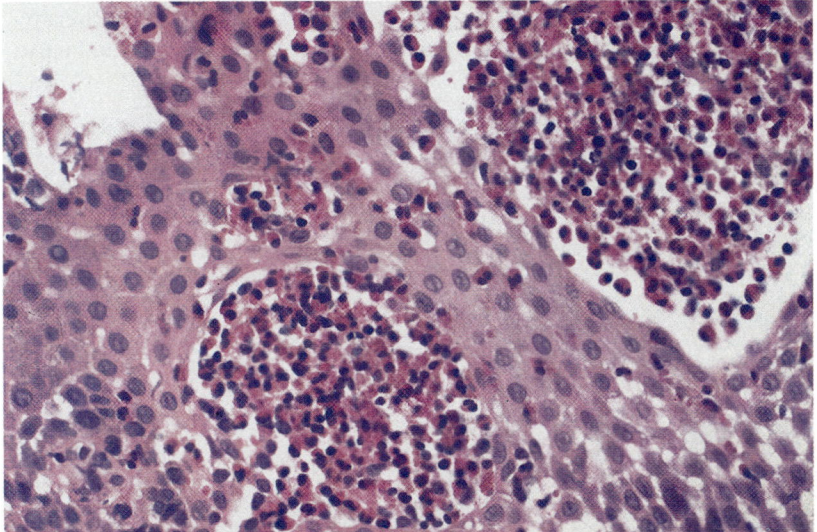

Figure 1-60: **Esophagus. Eosinophilic Esophagitis.** Clusters of eosinophils in squamous epithelium.

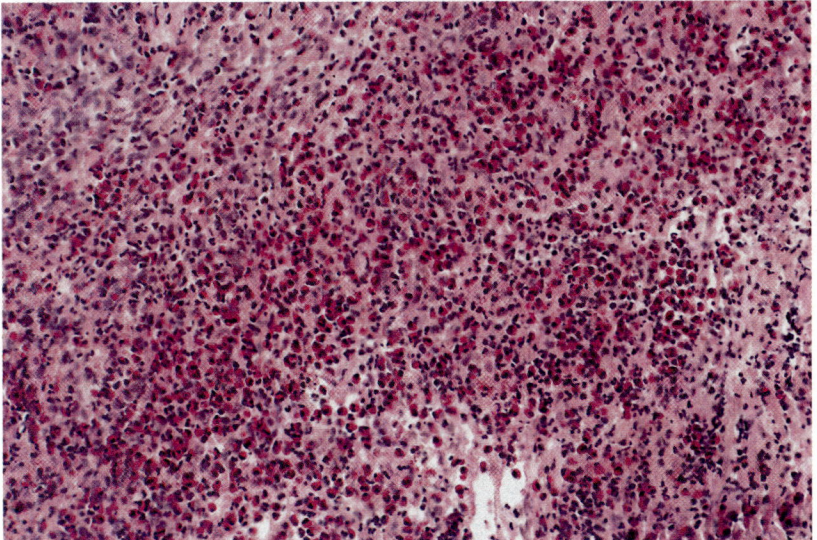

Figure 1-61: **Esophagus. Eosinophilic Esophagitis.** Ulcer base dominated by eosinophils.

CANDIDA ESOPHAGITIS

- Morphology .... *Candida* organisms are found in the superficial epithelial layers and inflammatory exudate, but are not easily seen on H&E-stained sections. Silver or PAS diastase stains are then necessary for identification. Frequently associated with other infectious agents. The squamous epithelium may be normal.

- Endoscopic features .... An exudative esophagitis dominated by patchy coalescing or widespread exudate is present throughout the length of the esophagus. It can taper off or end in the very distal esophagus. The classic exudate is whitish, but it may be yellow or even bile-stained. The mucosa between the exudate appears normal.

- Clinical features .... The patient with *Candida* esophagitis is typically immunosuppressed from a variety of causes, ranging from medication usage such as prednisone, widespread immunosuppressive therapy, e.g., post-transplantation, chemotherapy, AIDS, and a catastrophic illness. The symptoms are those of dysphagia and, more often, odynophagia.

- Differential diagnosis ...... Endoscopic: Swallowed spray topical anesthetic may coalesce within the esophagus to produce focal patches of whitish material that can mimic the appearance and distribution of a *Candida* exudate. The former should be suspected when encountered in any nonimmunosuppressed asymptomatic patient undergoing endoscopy for other indications. The differential diagnosis otherwise lies between other forms of infectious esophagitis and severe reflux esophagitis.

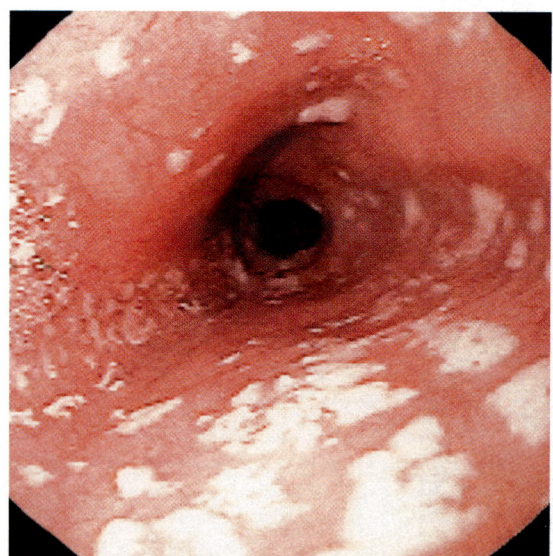

Figure 1-62: **Esophagus. *Candida* Esophagitis.** Patchy white exudate scattered throughout the length of esophagus. In some areas, exudate has coalesced.

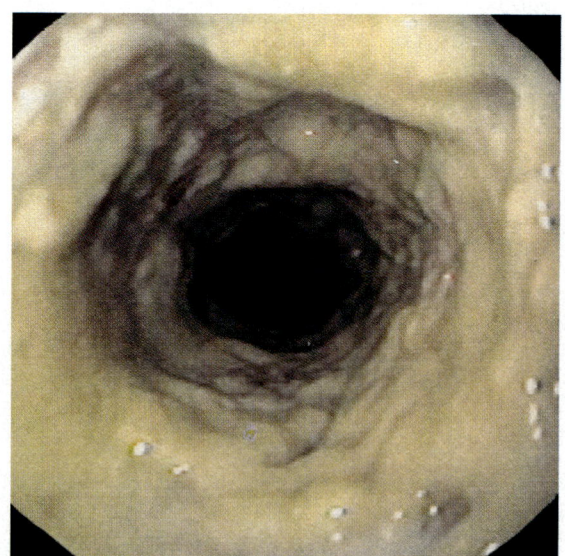

Figure 1-63: **Esophagus. *Candida* Esophagitis.** An extensive exudate covers the mucosa.

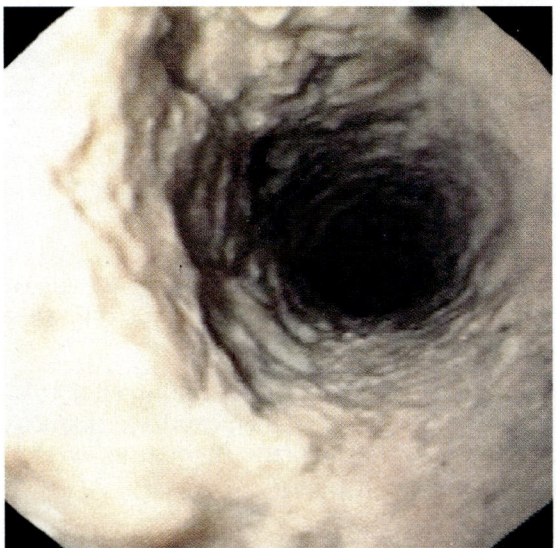

Figure 1-64: **Esophagus.** *Candida* **Esophagitis.** Extensive exudate in a debilitated, hospitalized patient with esophagitis.

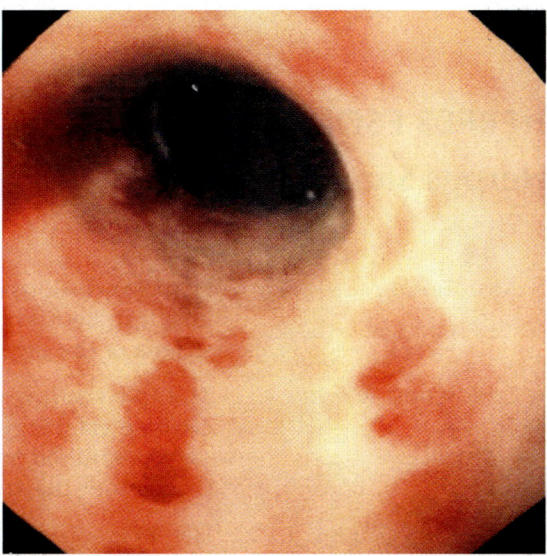

Figure 1-65: **Esophagus.** *Candida* **Esophagitis.** Severe exudative esophagitis with mucosal erythema, friability, and spontaneous bleeding in a bedridden hospitalized patient.

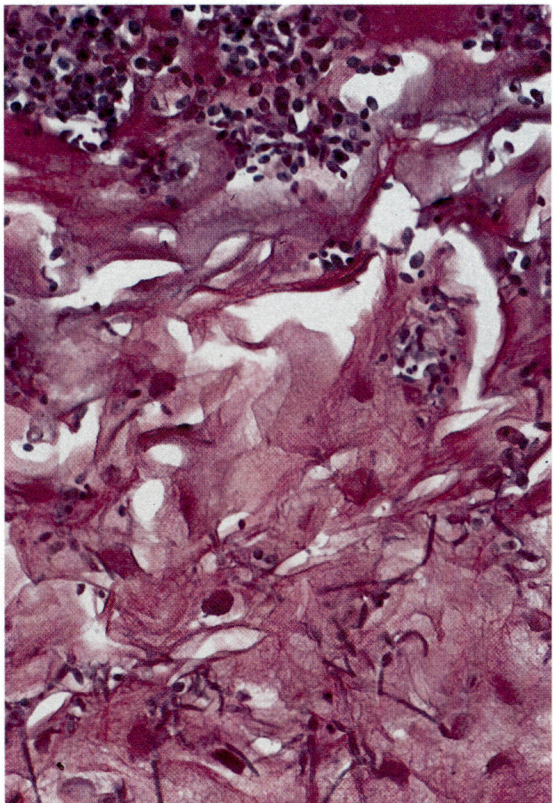

Figure 1-66: **Esophagus.** *Candida* **Esophagitis.** Small budding yeast and pseudohyphae typical of *Candida* species mixed with exfoliating squamous cells.

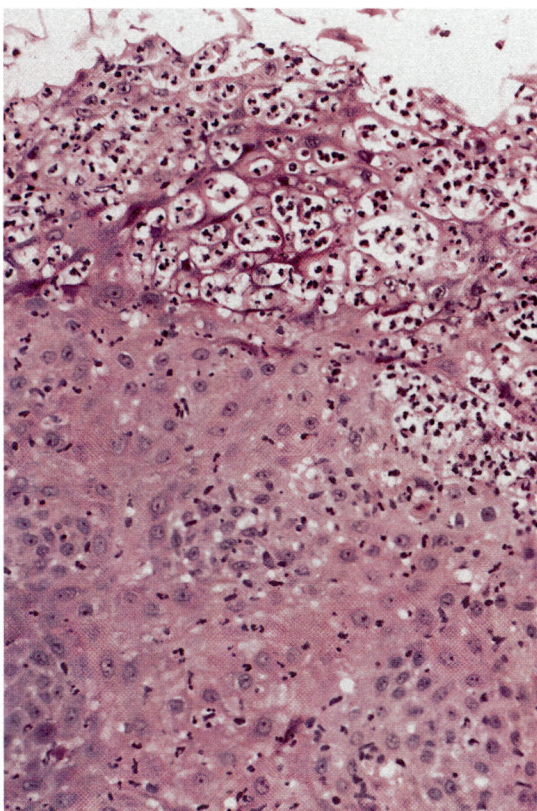

Figure 1-67: **Esophagus.** *Candida* **Esophagitis.** Neutrophilic inflammation and epithelial edema are most prominent in the superficial epithelial layers.

HERPES ESOPHAGITIS
Herpes Simplex Virus

- Morphology .... Herpes inclusions are found in sloughed epithelial cells and in the edges of the ulcers, in contrast to cytomegalovirus, where the diagnostic cells are in the stroma of the ulcer base.

- Endoscopic features .... Multiple shallow ulcers of varying size from several millimeters to several centimeters. Larger ones may be associated with an exudate; smaller ulcers may have raised borders without a central exudate. Herpetic ulcers can occur throughout the entire length of the esophagus.

- Clinical features .... Herpes esophagitis occurs in the nonimmunosuppressed as well as immunosuppressed patient. Healthy young adults may develop a self-limited infection preceded by a viral prodrome with fever and malaise. With extensive ulceration, there may be esophageal spasm with chest pain and dysphagia. Oral and gastric ulcers may occur. The oral lesions may precede the esophageal lesions and the gastric lesions follow the esophageal component. Rarely, GI bleeding occurs when there is gastric ulceration. The predominant clinical feature of herpetic esophagitis is acute odynophagia.

- Differential diagnosis ...... *Candida* esophagitis, CMV esophagitis, and pill esophagitis.

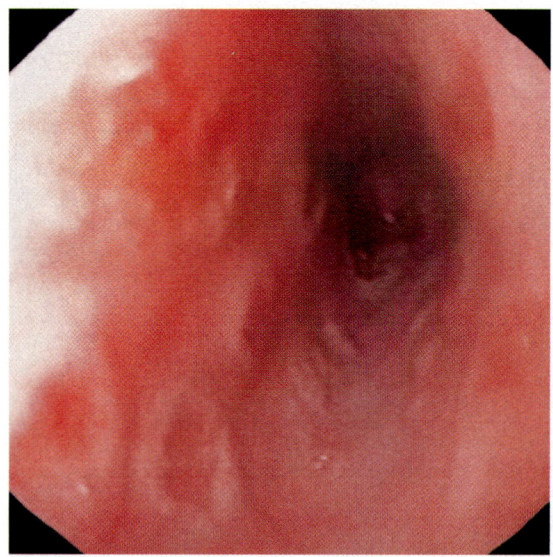

Figure 1-68: **Esophagus. Herpes Esophagitis.** Multiple, round, discrete, inflammatory lesions with slightly raised margins and a nonexudative central area.

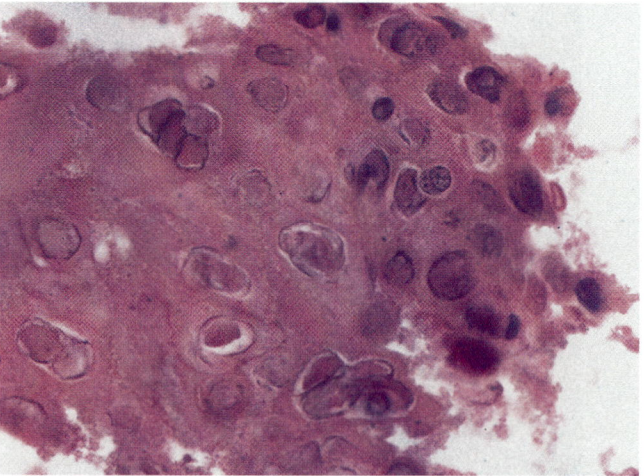

Figure 1-69: **Esophagus. Herpes Esophagitis.** Characteristic nuclear inclusions, some eosinophilic with a halo, some merely a homogenization of the nuclear chromatin (ground-glass nuclei). Multinucleation and molding of one nucleus by another are also characteristic features.

CYTOMEGALOVIRUS ESOPHAGITIS

- Morphology .... Infected endothelial cells clog small vessels and can cause thrombosis. Local ischemia is the likely basis for the large ulcers. Tissue from the ulcer base, especially granulation tissue, is best for diagnosis. When inclusions are few, diagnostic cells are difficult to identify. Immunostains or in situ hybridization for CMV may be necessary to demonstrate the virus.
- Endoscopic features .... The ulceration is typically discrete and focal in the distal esophagus. The size of the ulcers may vary. Chronic ulcers may become large in settings such as transplantation and AIDs. Ulcers can be penetrating and longitudinal, as long as 5 cm.
- Clinical features .... Odynophagia, dysphagia, and bleeding (both acute and indolent).
- Differential diagnosis ...... Herpes esophagitis, AIDS, pill-induced ulceration.

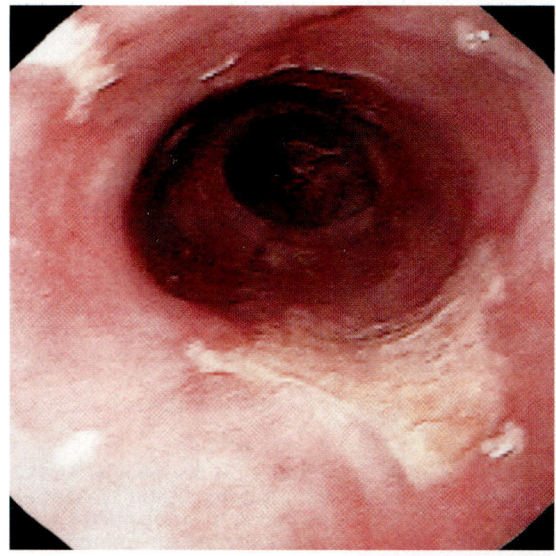

Figure 1-70: **Esophagus. CMV Esophagitis.** Multiple discrete ulcers of varying size, distal esophagus. The ulcer in the foreground is large and irregular, with an overlying exudate.

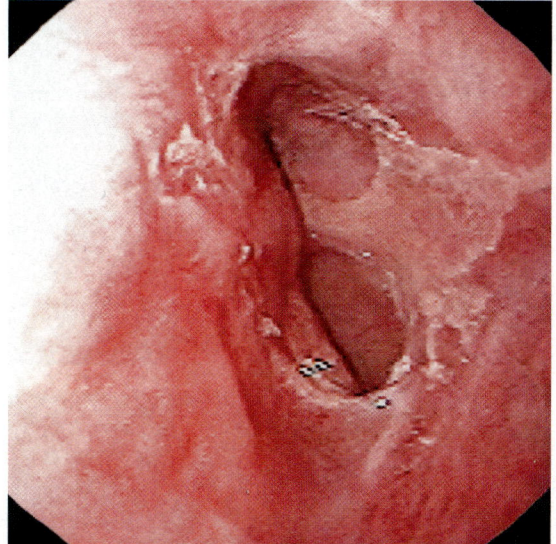

Figure 1-71: **Esophagus. CMV Esophagitis.** A long irregular ulcer in the distal esophagus with luminal deformity and nonspecific exudate.

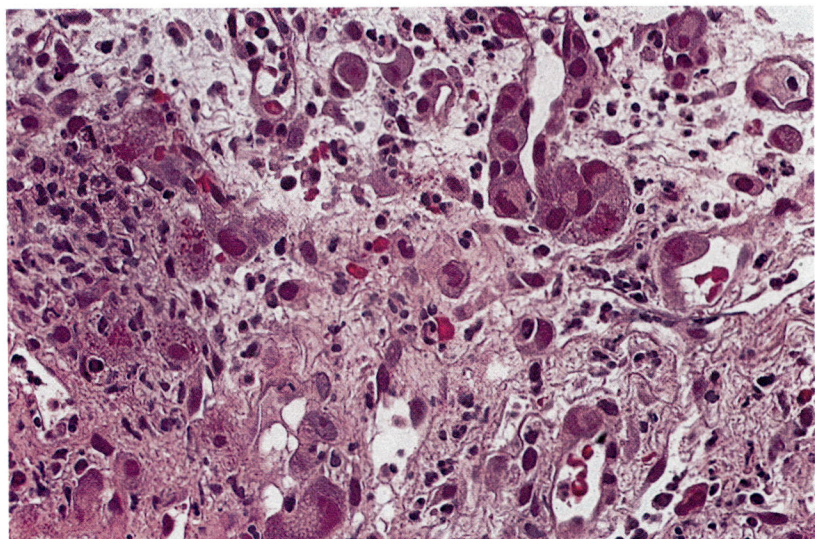

Figure 1-72: **Esophagus. CMV Esophagitis.** Numerous endothelial and occasional isolated stromal cell inclusions. The cells are very large with eosinophilic nuclear and cytoplasmic inclusions. Nuclear inclusions are large, solitary, and often surrounded by a halo. Cytoplasmic inclusions are scattered, multiple, and irregular.

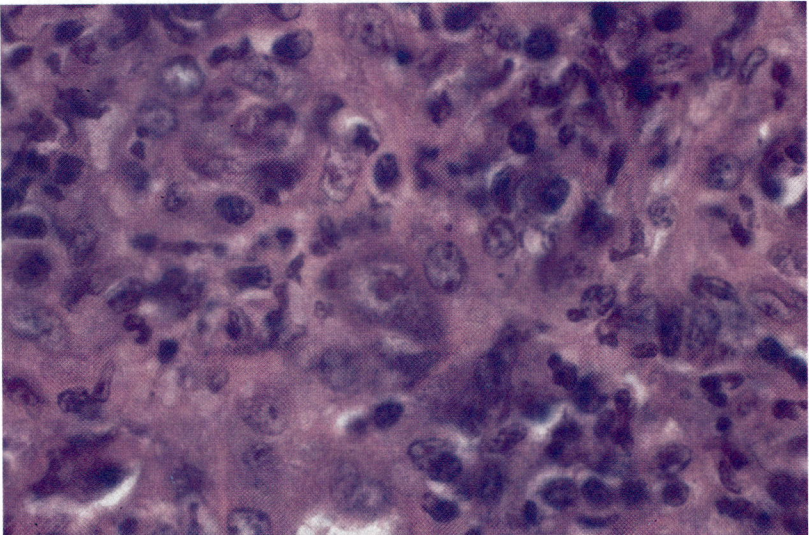

Figure 1-73: **Esophagus. CMV Esophagitis.** Cytomegalovirus inclusion surrounded by inflammation and granulation tissue.

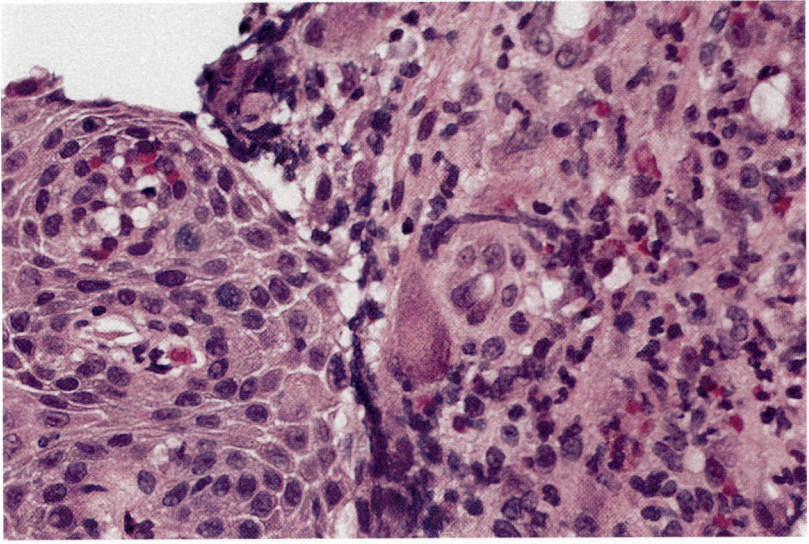

Figure 1-74: **Esophagus. CMV Esophagitis.** Cytomegalovirus inclusion in stroma between glandular and squamous epithelium.

BIZARRE STROMAL CELLS

- Morphology .... Bizarre stromal cells are usually found beneath ulcerated mucosa or within granulation tissue. They may mimic cytomegalovirus and malignant cells, e.g., spindle cell squamous carcinoma and sarcoma. They are negative for cytokeratin and usually positive for vimentin and weakly positive for smooth muscle actin, suggesting a myofibroblastic nature.
- Endoscopic features .... There are no distinctive endoscopic features other than esophagitis with ulceration.
- Clinical features .... None.
- Differential diagnosis ...... Histologic: Cytomegalovirus, spindle cell squamous carcinoma and sarcoma.

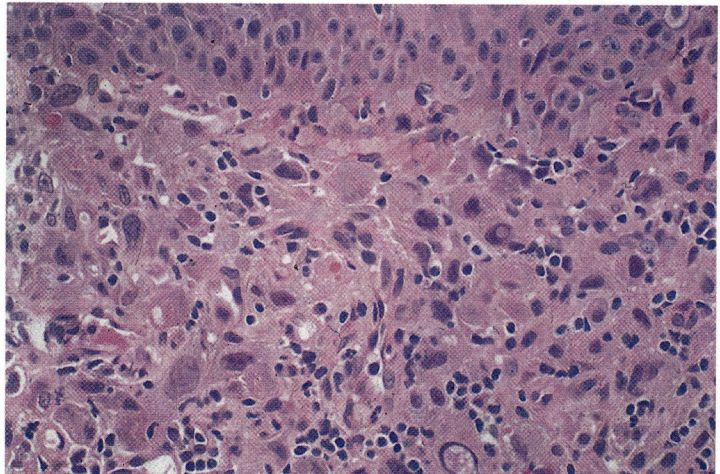

Figure 1-75: **Esophagus. Bizarre Stromal Cells.** Bizarre cells are numerous and mixed with inflammatory elements.

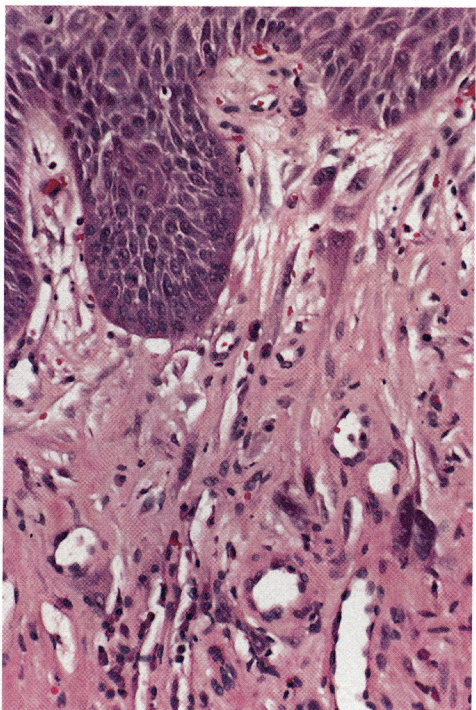

Figure 1-76: **Esophagus. Bizarre Stromal Cells.** A few large, atypical, spindled stromal cells with pleomorphic elongated nuclei and abundant cytoplasm.

CHEMICAL INJURY

- Morphology .... Epithelial necrosis with or without acute or chronic inflammation.

- Endoscopic features .... The endoscopic features vary according to the cause. With acute injury, there is erythema, mucosal edema, friability, bleeding, and ulceration, focal as well as diffuse. With ingestion of caustic agents, there can be frank necrosis with liquefied mucosa and submucosal tissue layers, perforation, and exudate. More indolent injury produces superficial or deep ulcers of varying size with stenosis.

- Clinical features .... Chemical injury typically causes pain. With major acute injury from ingestion of caustic agents, pain is severe and accompanied by severe odynophagia. Less severe injury may result in odynophagia only, with or without some element of constant chest pain. With severe odynophagia, perforation should be suspected. Dysphagia may be present with acute injury due to marked edema and with subacute or indolent injury due to stenosis. Fever after acute chemical injury suggests transmural necrosis with or without perforation.

- Differential diagnosis ...... With acute chemical injury, the major concern is the possibility of transmural necrosis and perforation. With more indolent injury, the differential diagnosis includes reflux, ulceration, and infectious esophagitis such as CMV.

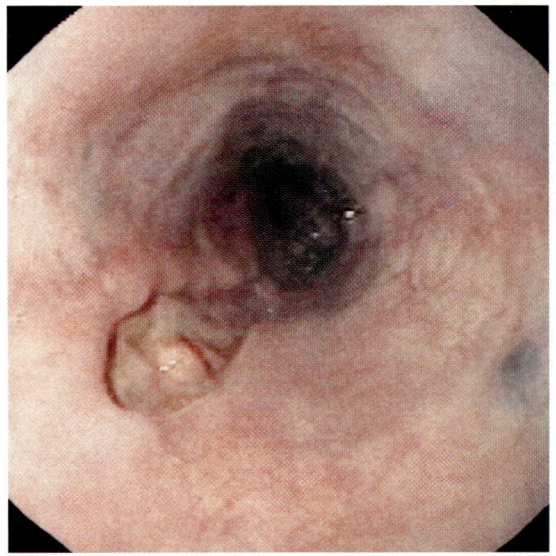

Figure 1–77: **Esophagus. Chemical Injury.** A discrete, chronic-appearing ulcer, the result of mucosal and intramural necrosis from injection sclerotherapy. The undermined edges of the ulcer are typical for sclerosant injury.

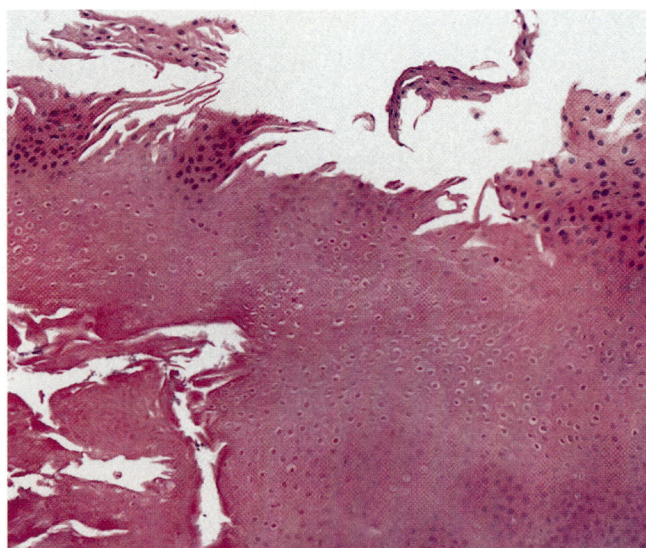

Figure 1-78: **Esophagus. Chemical Injury.** Squamous epithelium with early coagulation necrosis. Epithelial nuclei have disappeared from many cells. Postemetic acute acid injury in an immobilized, debilitated patient.

PILL ESOPHAGITIS

- Morphology .... Histologic alterations are nonspecific and similar to reflux unless foreign material is present. Ulcers may be acute or chronic. Location is key to the diagnosis.

- Endoscopic features .... The lesion is typically a discrete, irregularly shaped, shallow ulcer at the level of the aortic arch (more prevalent in older patients) or in the distal esophagus without any other mucosal abnormalities in the esophagus.

- Clinical features .... Pill-induced esophageal injury usually occurs as a result of taking medications at bedtime with little or no liquid. Reduced esophageal clearance and sensation during sleep facilitate injury. Various medications have been implicated. The most common is tetracycline or one of its derivatives. Other medications include nonsteroidal anti-inflammatory drugs, potassium chloride, iron sulfate, quinidine, corticosteroids, pancreatic enzymes, cloxacillin, dicloxacillin, and oral contraceptives. Odynophagia is the most common symptom, and can be accompanied by retrosternal pain and dysphagia. The diagnosis is made with a careful history. The pill-induced ulcer may become complicated with repetitive injury by stricture formation. Bleeding and perforation are rare.

- Differential diagnosis...... Ulcers due to infections or neoplasms extending into the esophagus from the tracheobronchial tree or regional lymph nodes.

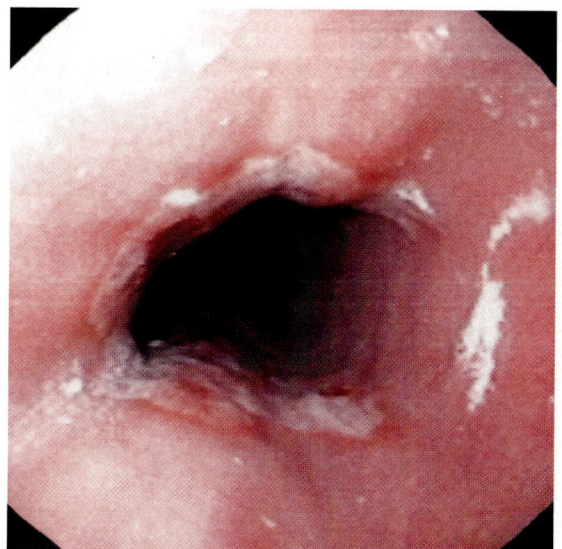

Figure 1-79: **Esophagus. Pill Esophagitis.** Two kissing, shallow, and irregular ulcers in the mid-esophagus.

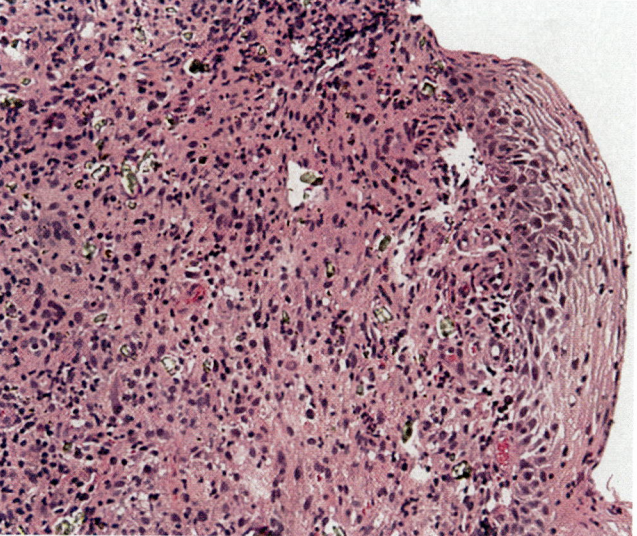

Figure 1-80: **Esophagus. Pill Esophagitis.** Granulation tissue beneath squamous epithelium contains crystalline material. Energy dispersive x-ray analysis revealed iron as a component of the crystals.

RADIATION INJURY

- **Morphology** — Acute radiation produces cell and nuclear enlargement with vacuolar degeneration and necrosis in epithelial and stromal cells. Some of these changes are due to injury; some to repair. Chronic radiation change is due to ischemia. Vessels show intimal concentric fibrosis.

- **Endoscopic features** — Acute radiation injury results in an ulcerating inflammatory condition that includes mucosal edema, diffuse ulceration, friability, spontaneous bleeding, and stricture. Delayed sequelae from radiation may produce stricture, chronic ulceration, and a general mucosal appearance ranging from normal to pale.

- **Clinical features** — Symptoms of acute radiation injury include dysphagia, odynophagia, and chest pain. There may be hematemesis as well as melena. Chronic radiation may result in stricture and dysphagia. Ulcers, when present, contribute to odynophagia. Symptoms are episodic and may be related to extreme temperatures of ingested foods.

- **Differential diagnosis** — Histologic: Bizarre stromal cells, malignant cells, other conditions associated with necrosis or scarring.

    Endoscopic: Acute radiation injury: viral esophagitis and severe ulcerative esophagitis. A segmental and more proximal location of the acute inflammation supports radiation injury. Chronic radiation injury: peptic stricture and recurrent neoplasm.

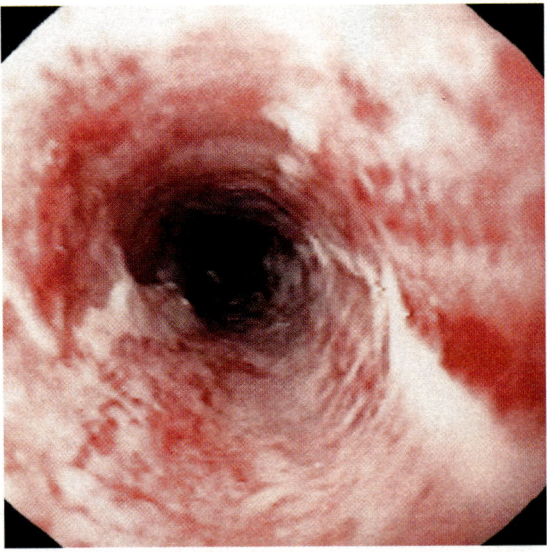

Figure 1-81: **Esophagus. Radiation Injury.** Acute radiation injury with friable ulcerated mucosa and spontaneous bleeding.

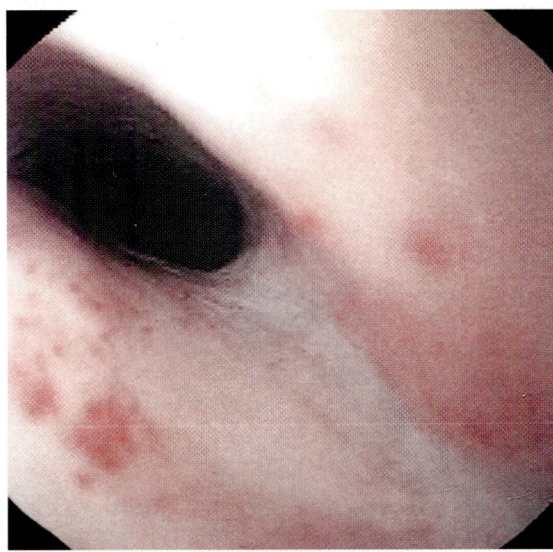

Figure 1-82: **Esophagus. Radiation Injury.** Long-term sequelae from radiation injury with midesophageal stricture and chronic linear ulceration. The involved mucosa is pale with areas of punctate erythema consistent with mucosal hemorrhage.

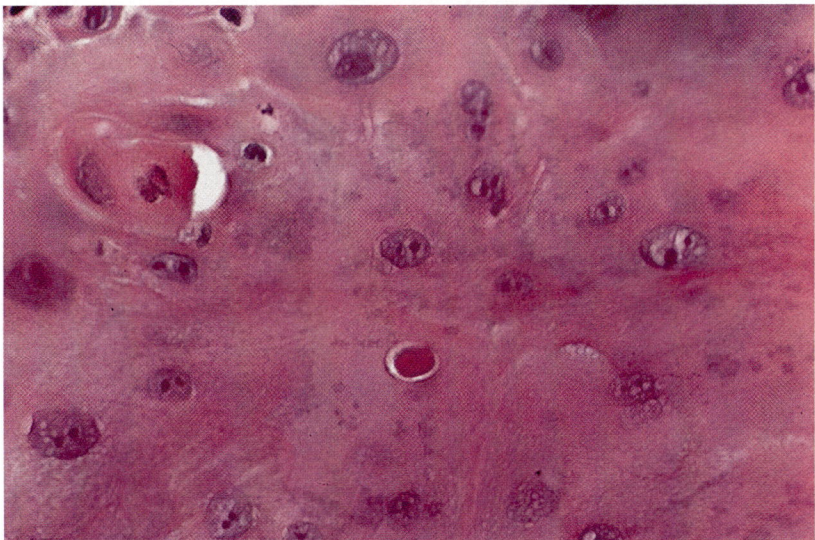

Figure 1-83: **Esophagus. Radiation Injury.** Squamous cells are reactive with ill-defined cytoplasm, obscure cell borders, large vacuolated nuclei, and large macronucleoli. Changes are consistent with, but not diagnostic of, radiation injury.

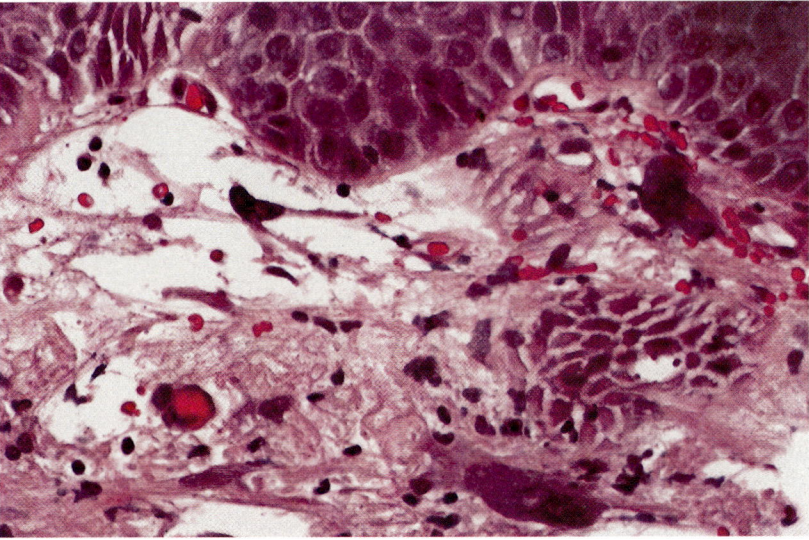

Figure 1-84: **Esophagus. Radiation Injury.** Radiation change in fibroblasts. Cells and nuclei are large and pleomorphic with nuclear and cytoplasmic vacuolization. Morphologically similar to bizarre stromal cells.

GRANULOMATOUS ESOPHAGITIS

- Morphology .... Granulomas may be small, sparse, and poorly defined in superficial biopsies. The presence of intense mononuclear infiltrates should heighten suspicion for granulomatous esophagitis, especially when associated with ulceration, fistula, or nodular lesions in the midesophagus. Tissue should be examined under polarized light for foreign material. Stains for organisms should include PAS and silver stains for fungi and acid-fast stains.
- Endoscopic features .... The endoscopic findings are nonspecific and range from erythema to ulcers of varying size, number, and depth. Crohn's ulcers, as elsewhere, are usually discrete and localized.
- Clinical features .... Chest pain and odynophagia are common. Crohn's ulcers may be deep and transmural, causing chest pain and sometimes perforation.
- Differential diagnosis...... Histologic: Tuberculous and fungal infections, foreign material, Crohn's, sarcoid.

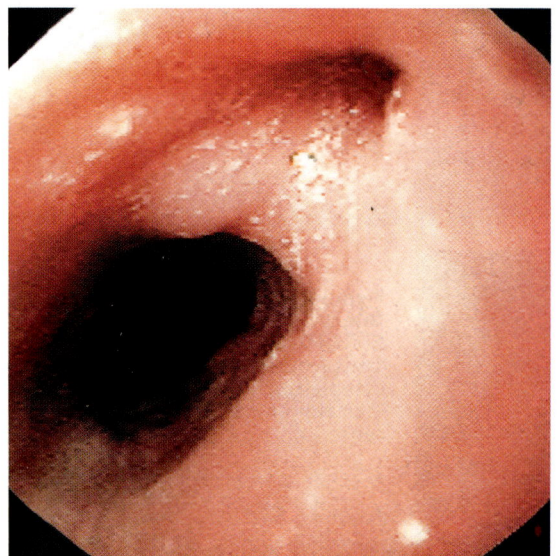

Figure 1-85: **Esophagus. Granulomatous Esophagitis and Fistula.** Two lumens can be seen in this view from within the middle third of the esophagus. The larger lumen represents the true esophageal lumen, the smaller lumen an esophago-bronchial fistula. The mucosa leading up to the fistula opening is intact.

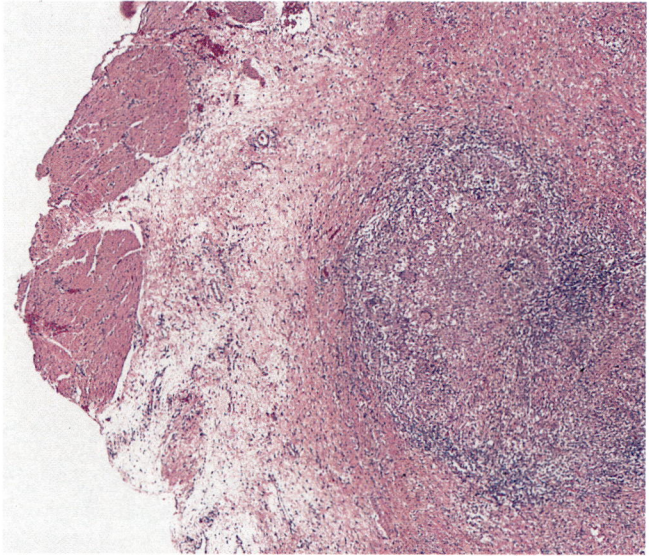

Figure 1-86: **Esophagus. Granulomatous Esophagitis, Tuberculosis.** Caseating granuloma with surrounding inflammation and fibrosis.

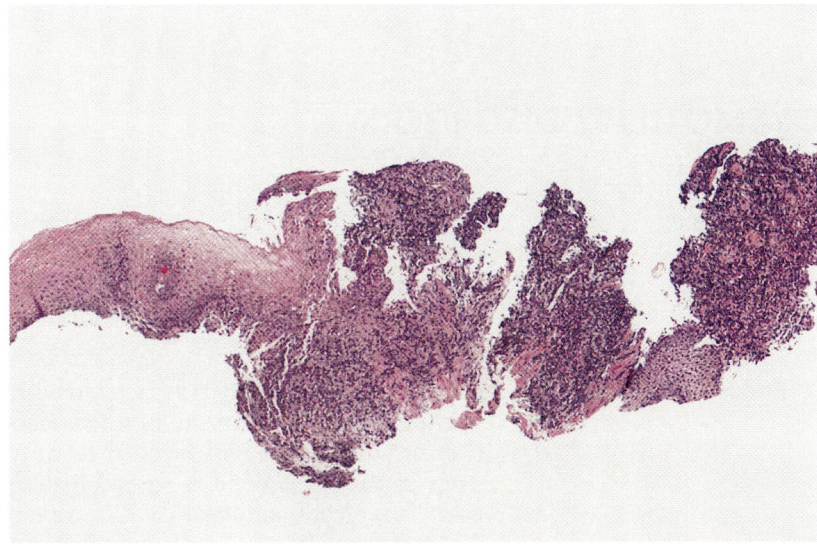

Figure 1-87: **Esophagus. Granulomatous Esophagitis.** Ulcerated esophageal mucosa with a discrete area of chronic inflammation and ulceration. Heavy mononuclear inflammatory infiltrate extends into muscle. Adjacent esophageal mucosa is normal, without the hyperplasia or inflammation of reflux or other topical chemical injury.

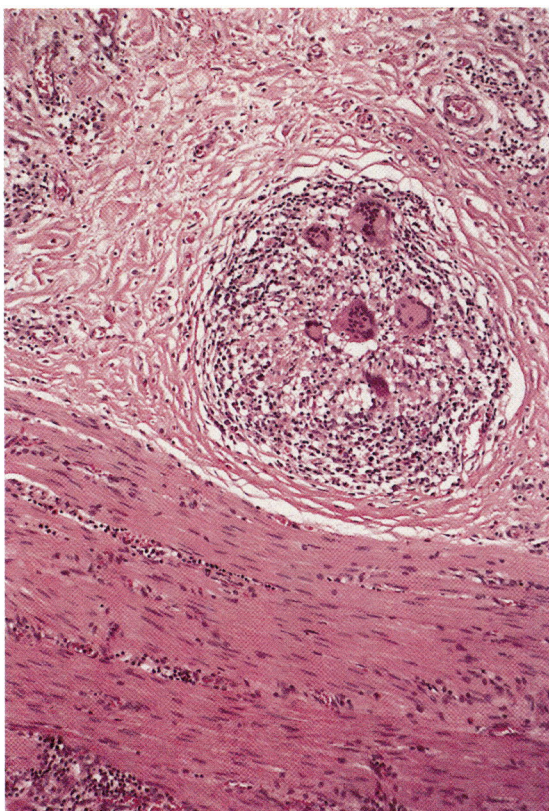

Figure 1-88: **Esophagus. Granulomatous Esophagitis.** Well-developed noncaseating granuloma in the submucosa.

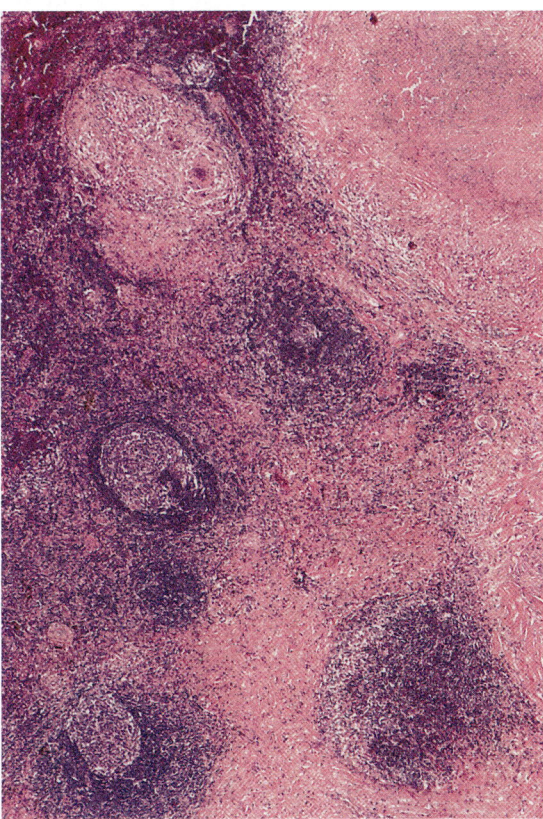

Figure 1-89: **Esophagus. Granulomatous Esophagitis.** Intense chronic lymphoid hyperplasia, and granulomas, the larger with caseous necrosis.

DYSMOTILITY DISORDERS

- Morphology .... Esophageal dysmotility interferes with swallowing and acid clearance, and predisposes to reflux, stasis, ulceration, stricture, and bacterial and fungal overgrowth. May be a cause of overt or occult aspiration. Shallow endoscopic biopsy samples are usually nonspecific and indistinguishable from reflux esophagitis.

- Endoscopic features .... Esophageal dysmotility is associated with several observations. Patients with nonspecific dysmotility involving excessive tertiary contractions and "nutcracker" esophagus will be seen to have multiple spontaneous contractile rings as the endoscope is passed through the esophagus. In scleroderma, there is typically an absence of contractile activity in the distal esophagus. The gastroesophageal junction in flagrant cases is patulous and wide open. In less obvious situations, there may be nonspecific changes of gastroesophageal reflux with varying severity, including peptic-type strictures. In early achalasia, the lumen is normal and the gastroesophageal junction may appear and feel tight as the instrument is passed through this area.

- Clinical features .... In patients with nonspecific dysmotility, including presbyesophagus with excessive tertiary contractions and nutcracker esophagus, the main symptom is that of episodic dysphagia. In patients with achalasia, there is dysphagia and, in advanced cases, regurgitation of collected food and secretions. Patients with scleroderma typically complain of gastroesophageal reflux symptoms, including pyrosis and regurgitation, until there is development of a stricture, at which time the reflux symptoms will improve and the patients will then become symptomatic from the stricture.

- Differential diagnosis ...... Clinical: Causes of dysmotility in achalasia, connective tissue disease such as dermatomyositis and scleroderma, and amyloidosis. Diagnosis is made by direct endoscopic observation, radiologic contrast studies, biopsies of other sites, and additional clinical and serologic parameters.

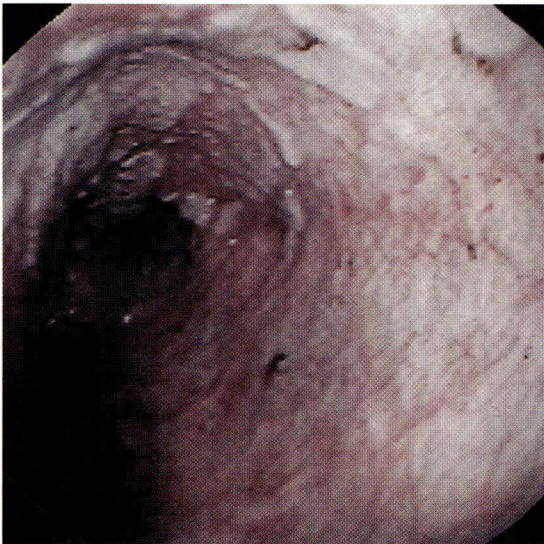

Figure 1-90: **Esophagus. Achalasia.** The lumen is dilated and contains pooled materials as well as adherent debris. Prominent submucosal vascular pattern.

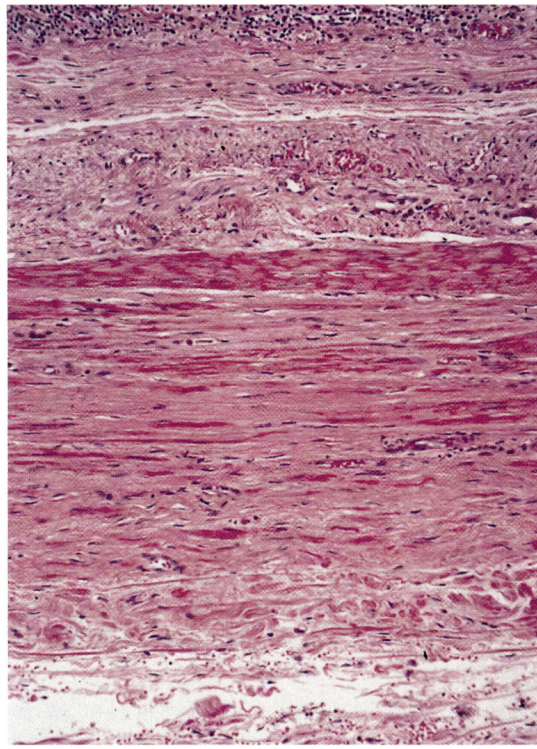

Figure 1-91: **Esophagus. Scleroderma.** Atrophy and fibrosis of muscularis propria.

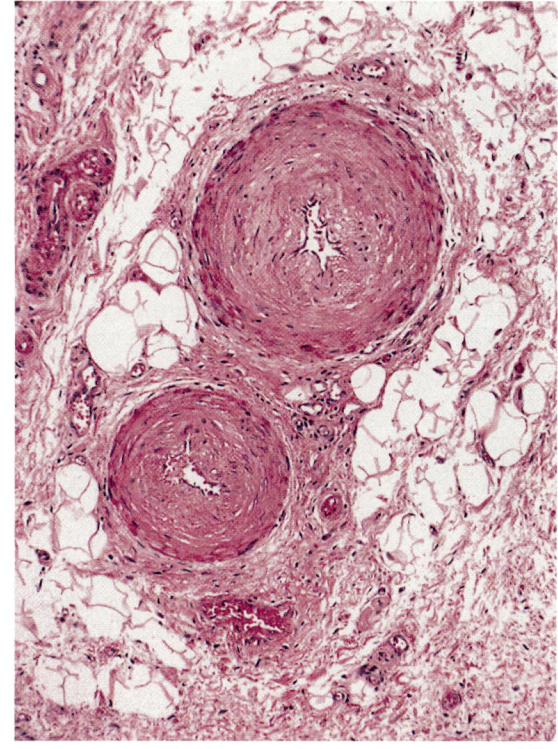

Figure 1-92: **Esophagus. Scleroderma.** Marked arterial concentric intimal fibrosis typical of scleroderma.

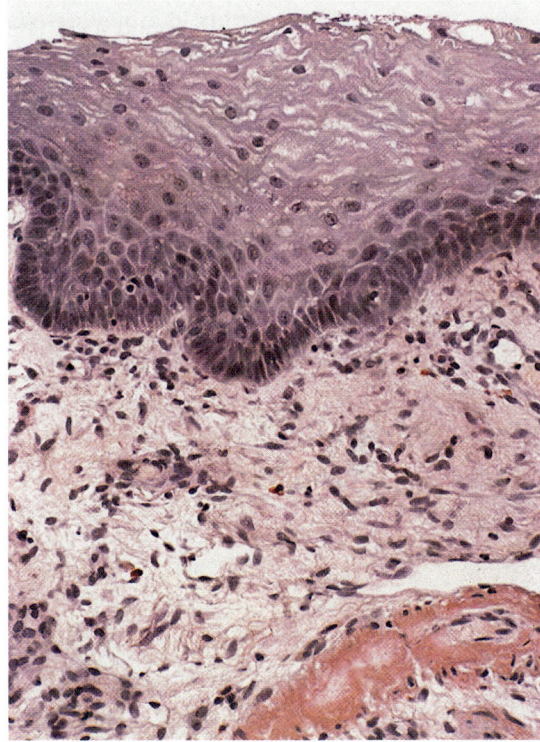

Figure 1-93: **Esophagus. Amyloid.** Congophilic amyloid in an arteriole of the lamina propria.

BARRETT'S ESOPHAGUS

- Morphology .... Barrett's esophagus is defined as: (1) any type of gastric mucosa with or without intestinal metaplasia extending greater than 2 cm into the tubular esophagus (long-segment Barrett's esophagus) and (2) Barrett's metaplastic columnar mucosa anywhere in the tubular esophagus (long- and short-segment Barrett's esophagus). Barrett's metaplastic columnar mucosa is cardia-type gastric mucosa with superimposed incomplete intestinal metaplasia, defined as goblet cell metaplasia without intestinal absorptive cell metaplasia, and resembling colonic mucosa. The presence of intestinal absorptive cells distinguishes complete intestinal metaplasia, which is common in the stomach and less common in the esophagus.

    Although Barrett's esophagus may be lined by any type of gastric epithelium, it is usually cardia-type mucosa with intestinal (goblet cell) metaplasia (Barrett's intestinalized mucosa). Intestinalized mucosa is hyperproliferative, chronically inflamed, and often fibrotic, with glandular architectural distortion and muscular hyperplasia.

- Endoscopic features .... The appearance of short-segment Barrett's esophagus varies from an irregular Z line to 2-cm extensions of gastric-appearing mucosa. Long-segment Barrett's esophagus is in excess of 2 cm. Barrett's mucosa is distinguished by coloration but not by surface features. The squamocolumnar junction in both short- and long-segment Barrett's esophagus may be highly irregular, with cephalad tonguelike extensions and isolated islands of gastric-type mucosa contiguous or close to the new Z line. Reflux changes are common at the squamocolumnar junction (Z line), regardless of location.

- Clinical features .... Reflux symptoms include chronic pyrosis and sour regurgitation. Many patients with Barrett's esophagus have few, if any, symptoms.

- Differential diagnosis ...... Endoscopic: Reflux with erythema and erosions, small hiatal hernia. Irregular Z line.

    Histologic: Normal gastric mucosa in hiatal hernia. Chronic gastritis and intestinal metaplasia in the upper stomach or hiatal hernia. Ectopic gastric mucosa.

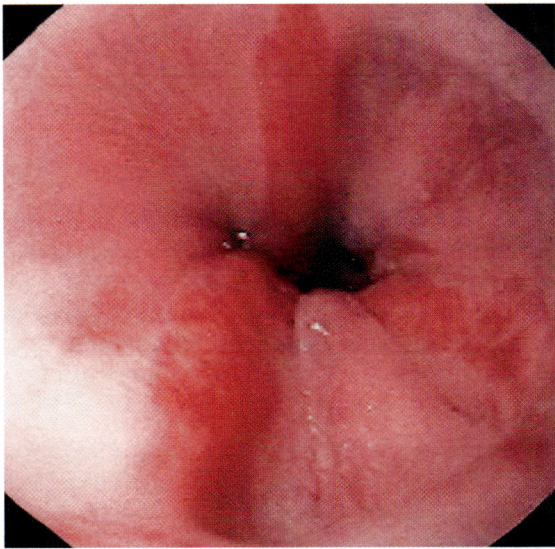

Figure 1-94: **Esophagus. Barrett's Esophagus.** Three tongues of gastric-appearing mucosa extend above the esophagogastric junction into the distal esophagus.

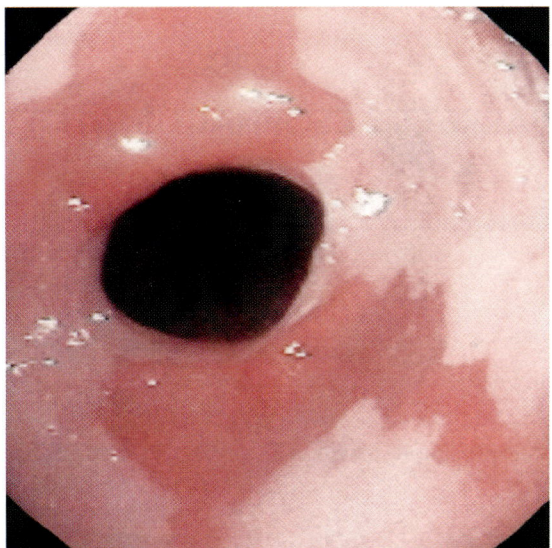

Figure 1-95: **Esophagus. Barrett's Esophagus.** Two large, irregularly shaped tongues of gastric-appearing mucosa extend upward from a circumferential stricture in the distal esophagus. There is no reflux-related inflammatory change such as erythema, ulceration, erosion, or exudate.

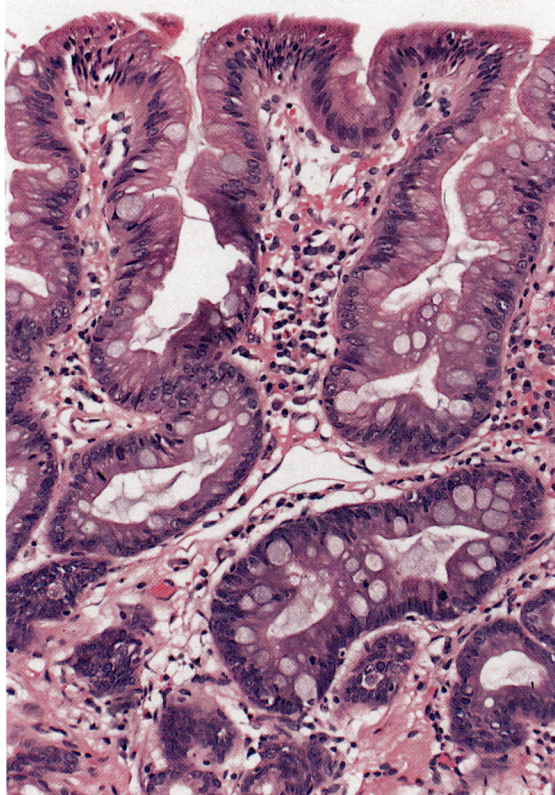

Figure 1-96: **Esophagus. Barrett's Esophagus.** Glandular mucosa with surface gastric foveolar-type epithelium, intestinal metaplasia (goblet cells), and chronic inflammation. Mitotic figures are seen in the basophilic proliferative zone of the pit region.

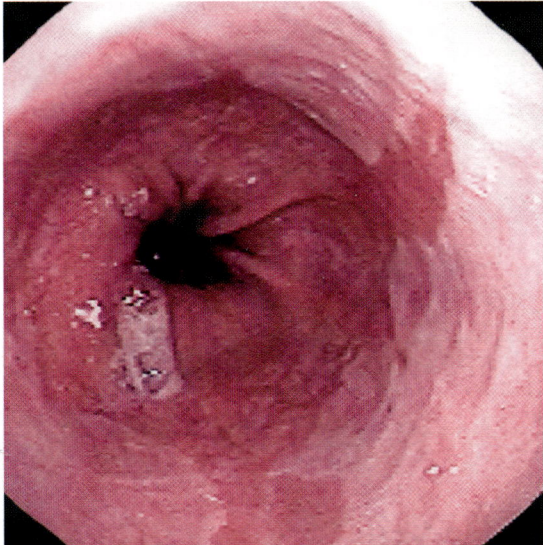

Figure 1-97: **Esophagus. Barrett's Esophagus.** A segment of Barrett's esophagus. The cephalad-migrated Z line is very irregular, with 2 tongues of gastric-type mucosa that contrast with the pale squamous mucosa.

BARRETT'S ESOPHAGUS WITH SQUAMOUS ISLANDS

- Morphology .... Squamous islands may be remnants of squamous mucosa or originate from esophageal gland duct epithelium following injury. Large squamous islands, and the new squamocolumnar junctions, tend to overlie metaplastic glandular epithelium, a potential problem following photodynamic or laser ablation therapy. Dysplastic glands beneath squamous epithelium may simulate invasive adenocarcinoma. Squamous islands may be a source of rare squamous cell carcinoma in Barrett's esophagus.

- Endoscopic features .... Barrett's epithelium contrasts with squamous mucosa and may appear as islands of gastric-type mucosa or be recognized by the presence of white squamous islands in the Barrett's segment close to the new squamocolumnar junction. Squamous islands may follow endoscopic ablation of a Barrett's segment.

- Clinical features .... Reflux symptoms or none.

- Differential diagnosis ...... Histologic: Adenocarcinoma undermining squamous epithelium. Squamous cell carcinoma.

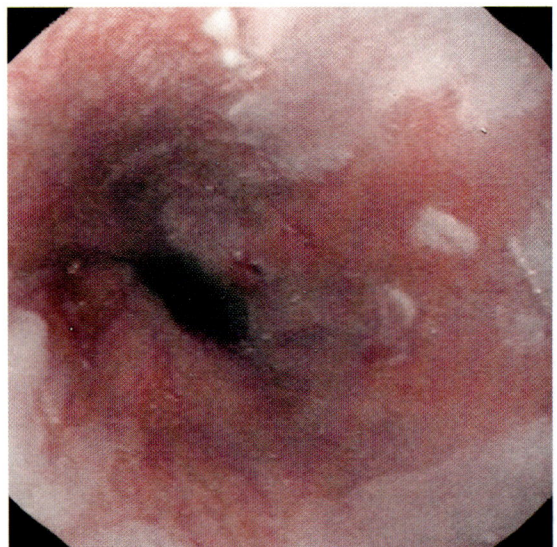

Figure 1-98: **Esophagus. Barrett's Esophagus with Squamous Islands.** Segment of Barrett's esophagus with an irregular Z line. Small islands of esophageal squamous-type mucosa are located just within the gastric mucosa at the Z line.

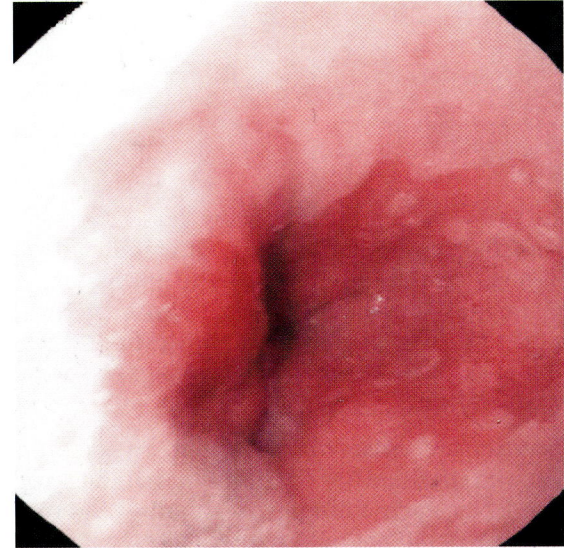

Figure 1-99: **Esophagus. Barrett's Esophagus.** The Z line is irregular. Gastric-type mucosa extends cephalad on the right. There is a small island of squamous mucosa in the lower right portion of the Barrett's segment.

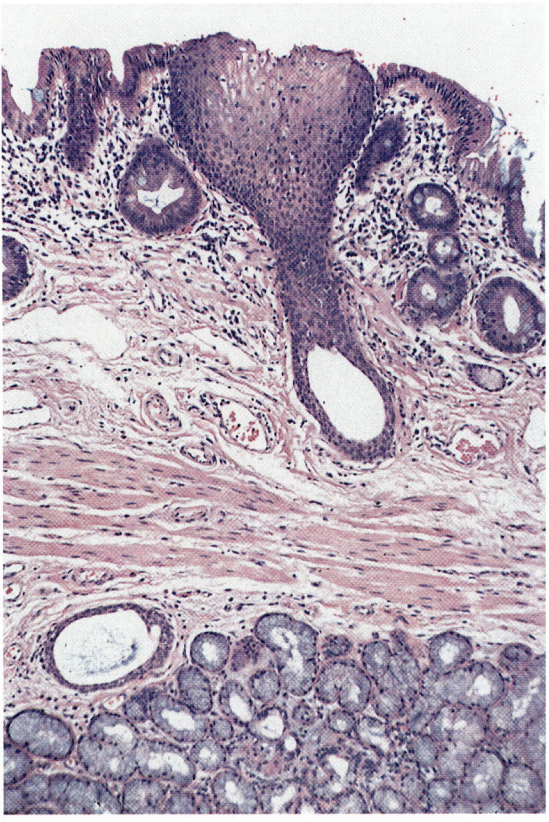

Figure 1-100: **Esophagus. Barrett's Esophagus with Squamous Island.** Squamous metaplasia in an esophageal gland duct, one source of a squamous island.

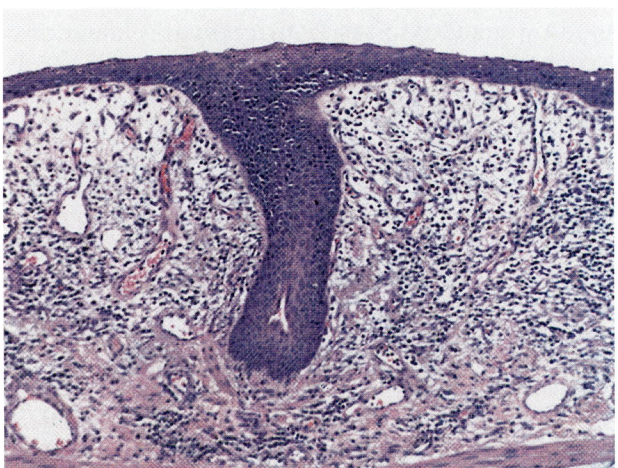

Figure 1-101: **Esophagus. Barrett's Esophagus with Squamous Island.** Re-epithelialized jumbo biopsy site in Barrett's esophagus resected for high-grade dysplasia. Esophageal gland duct epithelium is the source of this squamous island.

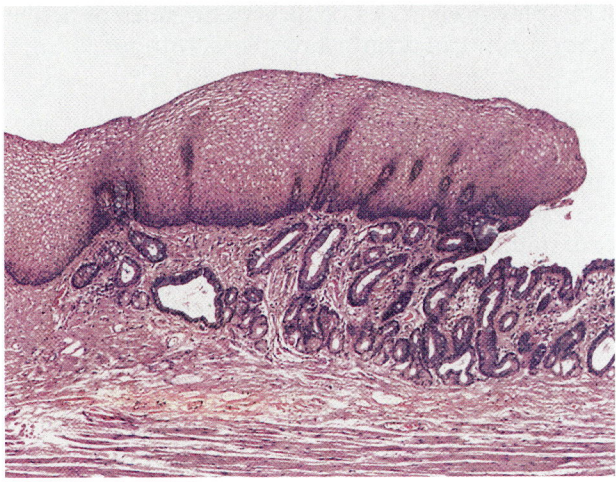

Figure 1-102: **Esophagus. Barrett's Esophagus with Squamous Island.** Squamous epithelium intermingled with and overlying Barrett's epithelium.

DYSPLASIA IN BARRETT'S ESOPHAGUS

- Morphology .... Dysplasia is divided into low- and high-grade. Low-grade dysplasia has cytologic and architectural changes similar to those of colonic adenomas; nuclear stratification is limited to the lower half of the epithelium. High-grade dysplasia has (1) nuclear changes similar to those of low-grade dysplasia, but nuclear stratification extends throughout the full thickness of the epithelium to the luminal surface and/or (2) severe or anaplastic nuclear changes irrespective of stratification.

    In low-grade dysplasia, nuclei are enlarged, elongated, hyperchromatic, mitotically active, crowded, and stratified but not highly variable. Chromatin is coarse but evenly dispersed. Nuclear membrane irregularities and variation in nuclear size, shape, and orientation are mild to moderate. Nucleoli, often multiple and irregular, are small. Moderate architectural and cytologic abnormalities should be mentioned but classified as low-grade dysplasia. High-grade dysplasia is characterized by marked nuclear enlargement and rounding, with significant, marked variation in nuclear size, shape, membrane, and chromatin. Macronucleoli are prominent.

    It may be difficult to separate low-grade dysplasia from reactive proliferations, especially when dysplasia affects only the proliferative zone (gastric pit), as Barrett's epithelium is hyperproliferative. In both, there may be mild nuclear enlargement, stratification, and nuclear overlap, resulting in a basophilic appearance at low magnification. Reactive proliferations, in contrast to dysplasia, are characterized by uniformity between individual cells and amongst adjacent glands. Oblique sections may give the false impression of nuclear stratification or, when through undulations of the proliferating gastric pit, simulate cribriforming, a feature of high-grade dysplasia.

    Regenerative (reparative) reactions, in which the cells are activated to replace denuded epithelium, may have features resembling high-grade dysplasia. Reparative cells have large, round nuclei and prominent macronucleoli. Cytologic uniformity, the hallmark of reactive or reparative proliferation, is the main distinguishing feature. More problematic is a reparative reaction superimposed on low-grade dysplasia. This possibility should be considered when evaluating biopsy samples from edges of ulcers and areas of active inflammation. In this situation, one can diagnose dysplasia without giving a specific grade.

- Endoscopic features .... Dysplasia may be suspected with the use of vital dye stain or chromoscopy. After washing the Barrett's segment with 10% acetyl cysteine, methylene blue is applied to the Barrett's mucosa. Removal of the mucous layer will facilitate the uptake of methylene blue stain. An inhomogeneous staining pattern and, even more so, the absence of staining implies the probability of dysplasia and helps direct biopsies. There is little experience with this method at present. Dysplasia may otherwise present as a subtle and focal roughened or polypoid appearance to the mucosal surface.

- Differential diagnosis ...... Histologic: It can be difficult to distinguish dysplasia from reactive/regenerative change or from invasive adenocarcinoma in biopsy samples.

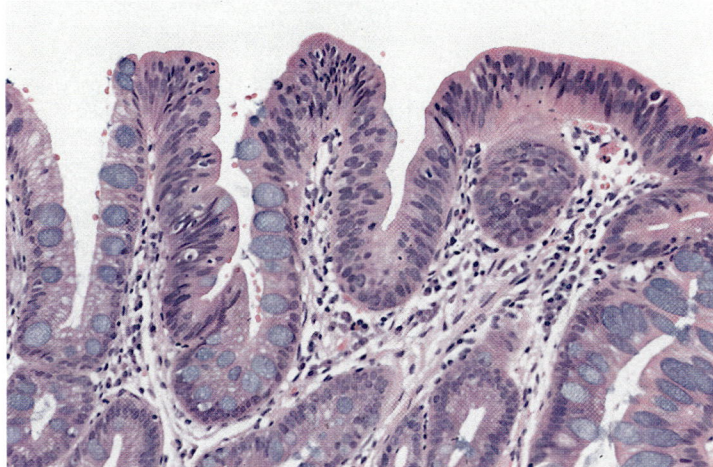

Figure 1-103: **Esophagus. Low-Grade Dysplasia in Barrett's Esophagus.** Mild nuclear enlargement, elongation, hyperchromasia, and stratification mainly in the lower half of the epithelium support a diagnosis of low-grade dysplasia. Dysplasia extends to the esophageal luminal surface. The contrast between dysplastic areas and nondysplastic areas provides the basis for an unequivocal diagnosis. Goblet cells are diminished in areas of dysplasia.

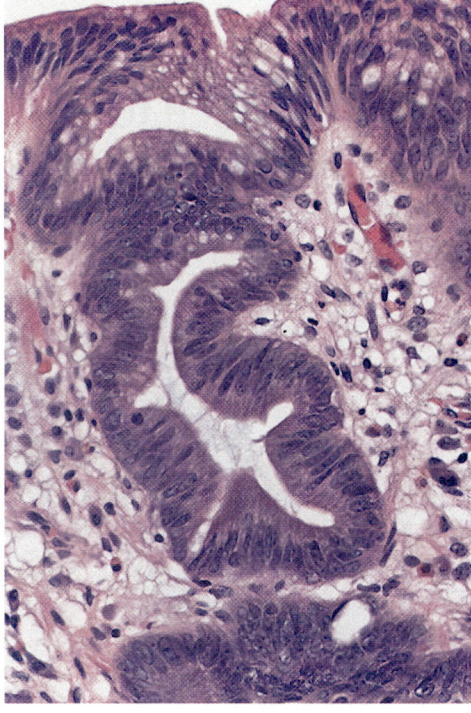

Figure 1-104: **Esophagus. Low-Grade Dysplasia in Barrett's Esophagus.** Enlarged, elongated, hyperchromatic and stratified nuclei, with slightly irregular nuclear membranes, cell-to-cell cytologic variability, i.e., nuclear size, shape, and orientation. Nuclear stratification does not reach the gland lumen, and cytologic abnormalities are equivalent to those of an ordinary adenoma of the colon.

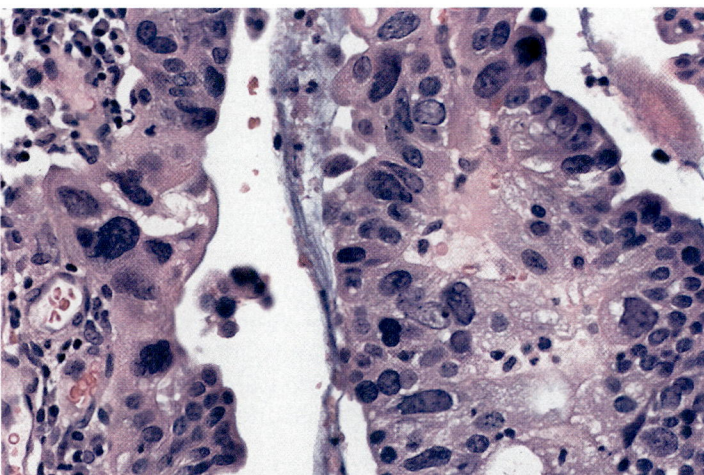

Figure 1-105: **Esophagus. High-Grade Dysplasia in Barrett's Esophagus.** Architecturally high-grade as judged by nuclear stratification, crowding, and overlap. Cytologically high-grade with large pleomorphic nuclei.

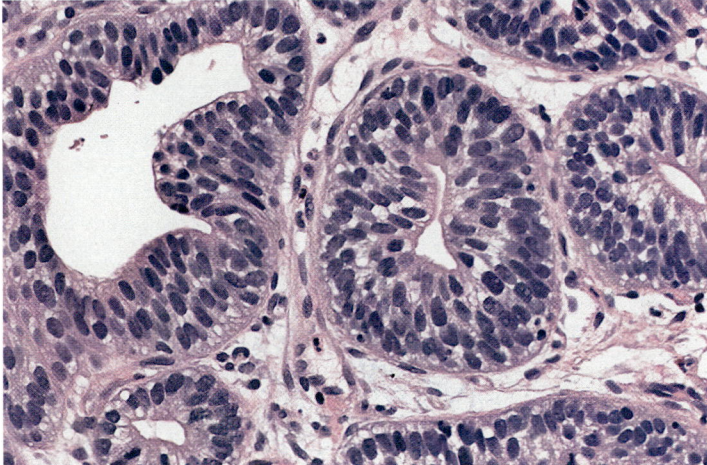

Figure 1-106: **Esophagus. High-Grade Dysplasia in Barrett's Esophagus.** Nuclear abnormalities no different from those seen in low-grade dysplasia, but nuclear stratification extends throughout the full thickness of the epithelium.

BARRETT'S ESOPHAGUS, DYSPLASIA VARIATIONS

- Morphology .... Dysplasia intermediate between low- and high-grade, by virtue of cytologic changes or nuclear stratification, is best classified as low-grade. Intermediate grades of dysplasia (i.e., moderate dysplasia) should be mentioned as clinicians may wish to increase surveillance frequency.

    Dysplasia in Barrett's esophagus is usually multifocal and may involve large or small areas. When high-grade dysplasia is identified in biopsy samples, low-grade dysplasia is usually extensive. Dysplasia may be confined to the pits or the glands, with apparent sparing of the surface epithelium.

- Endoscopic features .... Without chromoendoscopy, several endoscopic observations suggest the presence of focal dysplasia in Barrett's esophagus, including localized surface irregularity, nodularity, and polypoid change.
- Clinical features .... None.
- Differential diagnosis ...... Histologic: High- versus low-grade dysplasia.

BARRETT'S ESOPHAGUS, HIGH-GRADE DYSPLASIA

- Morphology .... Biopsy material with high-grade dysplasia is sometimes suspicious for invasive adenocarcinoma. Features that raise suspicion include glands occluded by highly dysplastic cells, crowded dysplastic glands, and necrotic cells in gland lumens. Without evidence of single cell infiltration, irregular infiltrating small glands, solid sheets, or desmoplasia, a definite diagnosis of adenocarcinoma should not be made.
- Endoscopic features .... Focal surface nodularity and polypoid change suggest the possibility of high-grade dysplasia.
- Clinical features .... None. Typically few, if any, symptoms.
- Differential diagnosis ...... Histologic: Adenocarcinoma.

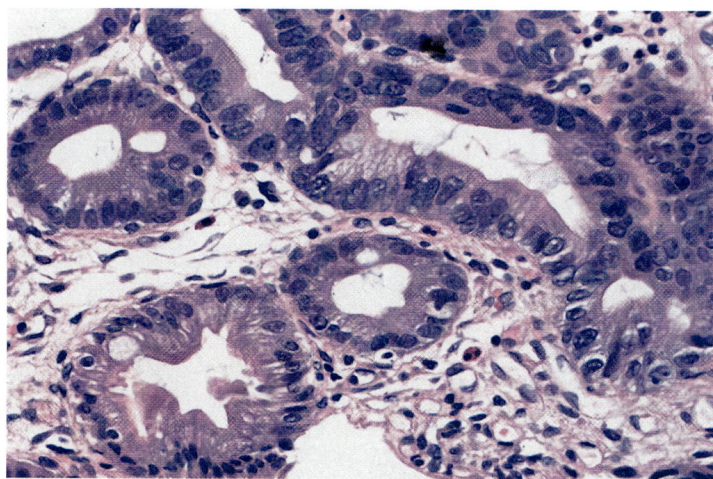

Figure 1-107: **Esophagus. Dysplasia in Barrett's Esophagus, Intermediate between Low- and High-Grade (Moderate Dysplasia).** Nuclear enlargement, irregularity, and cell-to-cell variability are greater than average for low-grade dysplasia. Nuclei are somewhat round, and nuclear chromatin is irregularly dispersed. Since nuclear pleomorphism is only borderline for high-grade dysplasia and nuclear stratification is within the limits for low-grade dysplasia, this lesion is best classified as low-grade dysplasia.

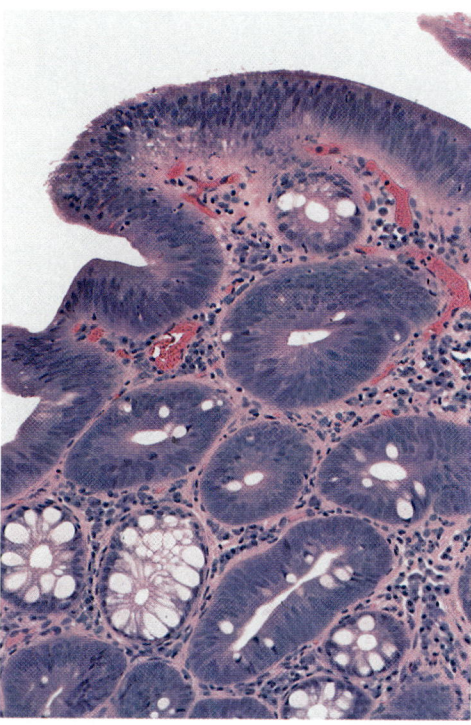

Figure 1-108: **Esophagus. Dysplasia in Barrett's Esophagus, Intermediate between Low- and High-Grade (Moderate Dysplasia).** Nuclear cytology is low-grade, but nuclear stratification approaches the epithelial surface. Because of the extent of nuclear stratification, this lesion approaches high-grade dysplasia but is best classified as low-grade dysplasia.

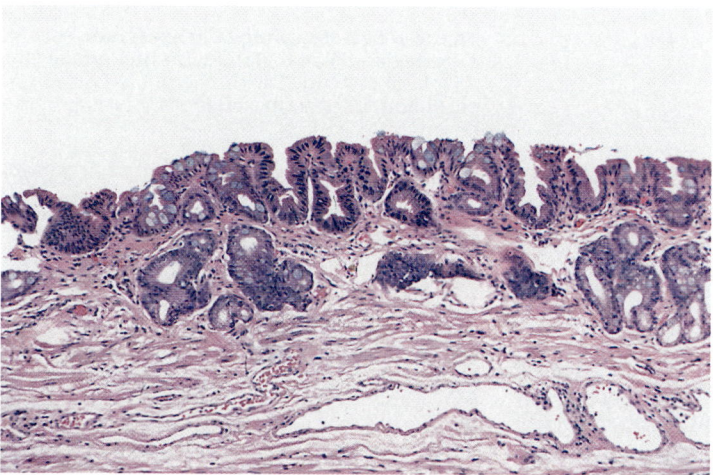

Figure 1-109: **Esophagus. Dysplasia in Barrett's Esophagus.** Spotty distribution of dysplasia in glandular pits and surface, intermingled with nondysplastic Barrett's epithelium.

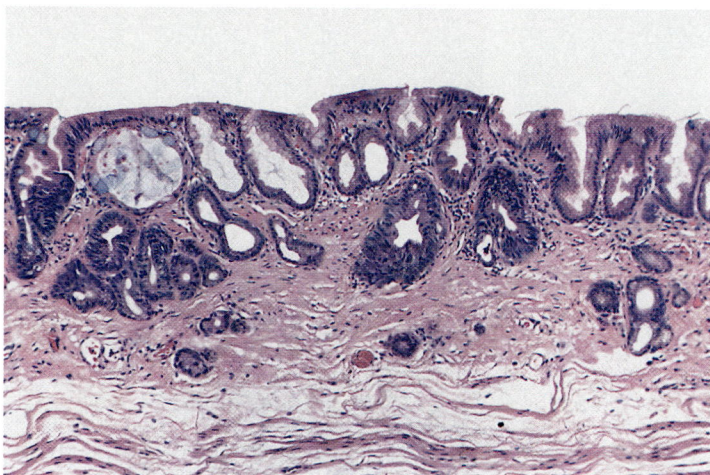

Figure 1-110: **Esophagus. Dysplasia in Barrett's Esophagus.** Dysplasia in pits and glands, with only minimal focal surface involvement.

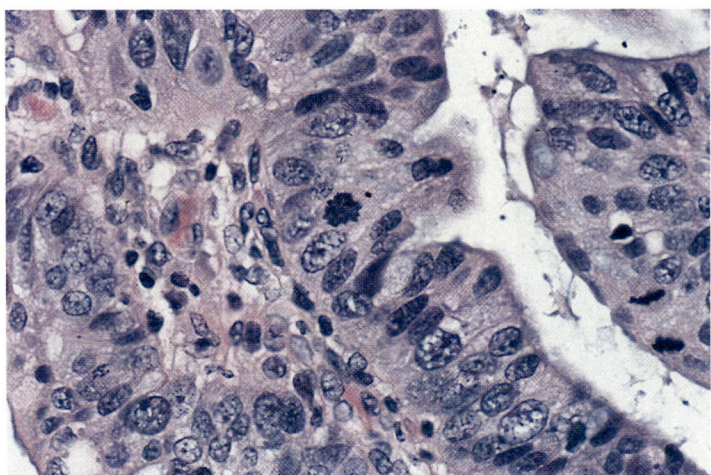

Figure 1-111: **Esophagus. High-Grade Dysplasia in Barrett's Esophagus.** Dysplasia with both high-grade nuclear changes and full-thickness epithelial stratification. Large nuclear size (compared to stromal lymphocytes and endothelial cells), irregular chromatin, irregular nucleoli, and frequent mitotic figures.

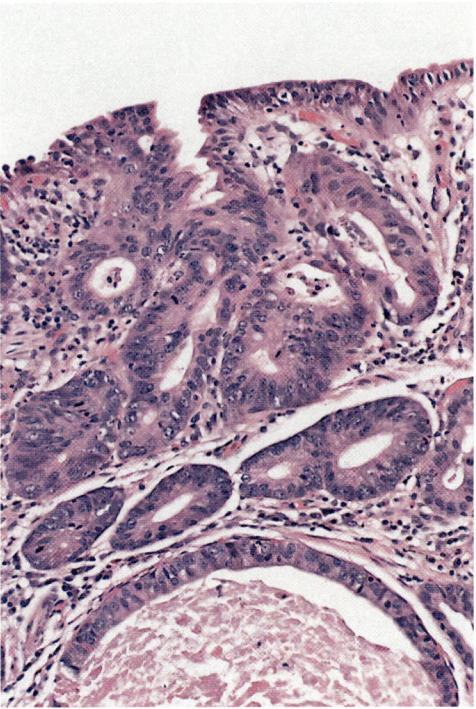

Figure 1-112: **Esophagus. High-Grade Dysplasia.** Dilated gland with high-grade dysplasia distended with necrotic debris raises suspicion for invasive adenocarcinoma.

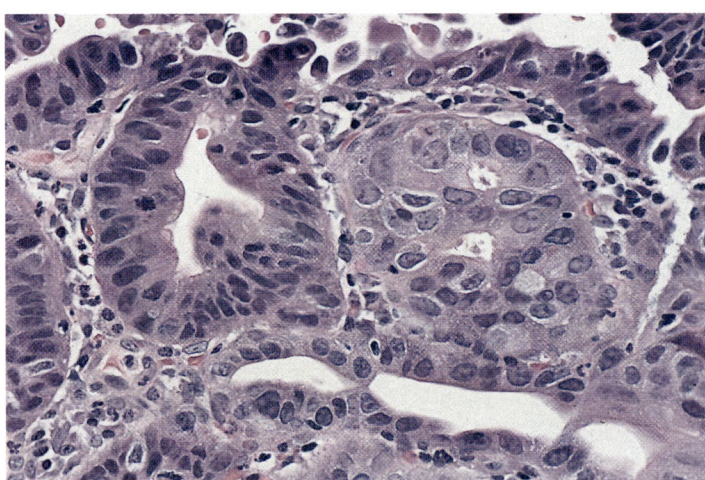

Figure 1-113: **Esophagus. High-Grade Dysplasia in Barrett's Esophagus.** Cells are large with increased nuclear-to-cytoplasmic ratio. Cribriform structure and irregular contours in the glands.

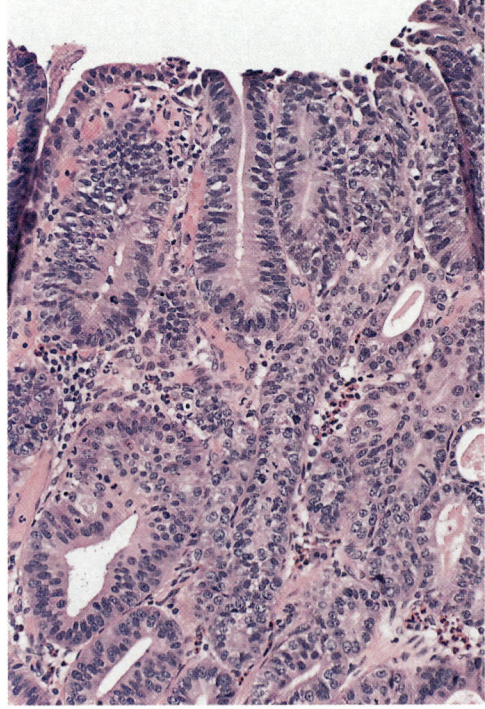

Figure 1-114: **Esophagus. High-Grade Dysplasia in Barrett's Esophagus.** Crowded glands with high-grade dysplasia suggestive of invasive adenocarcinoma.

BARRETT'S ESOPHAGUS, REACTIVE ATYPIA VERSUS DYSPLASIA

- Morphology .... Low magnification is important in distinguishing reactive/regenerative changes from dysplasia. Reactive/regenerative changes are uniformly distributed in the mucosa and tend not to stand out at low magnification. It is helpful to compare the nuclear size and appearance in questionably dysplastic areas to that of clearly normal epithelium elsewhere in the specimen. The distinction between reactive changes, atypia indefinite for dysplasia, and low-grade dysplasia is difficult, despite defined criteria.

- Endoscopic features .... None, or if chromoendoscopy is used (vital dye staining with methylene blue), the staining pattern may be inhomogeneous.

- Clinical features .... None.

- Differential diagnosis ...... Histologic: Low-grade dysplasia.

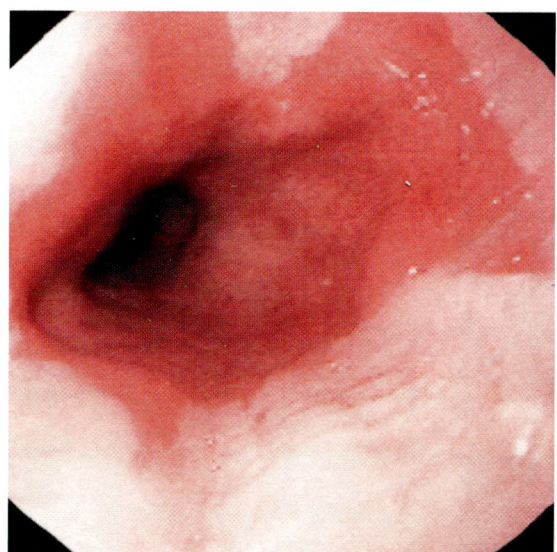

Figure 1-115: **Esophagus. Barrett's Esophagus.** Barrett's segment with a focal mucosal abnormality which is suspicious for dysplasia.

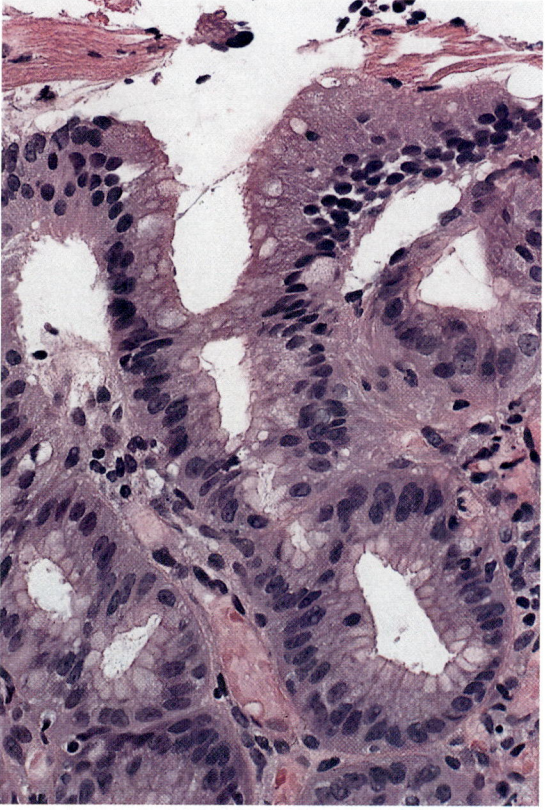

Figure 1-116: **Esophagus. Barrett's Esophagus, Atypia Indefinite for Dysplasia.** Focus with nuclear enlargement and overlap near mucosal surface.

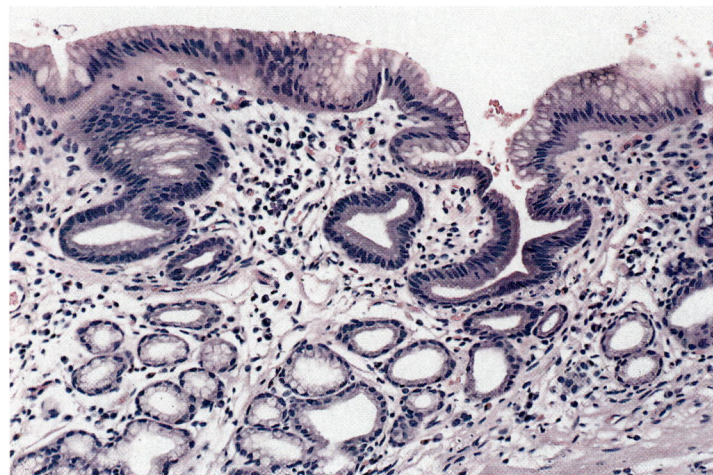

Figure 1-117: **Esophagus. Barrett's Esophagus, Regenerative Atypia.** Nuclear enlargement, slight stratification, and mitotic figures in the regenerative zone. The nuclear uniformity, regular nuclear separation, cytoplasmic basophilia, and identical appearance of the adjacent pits support the regenerative nature of the process. Oblique section of the surface epithelium (left) simulates nuclear stratification.

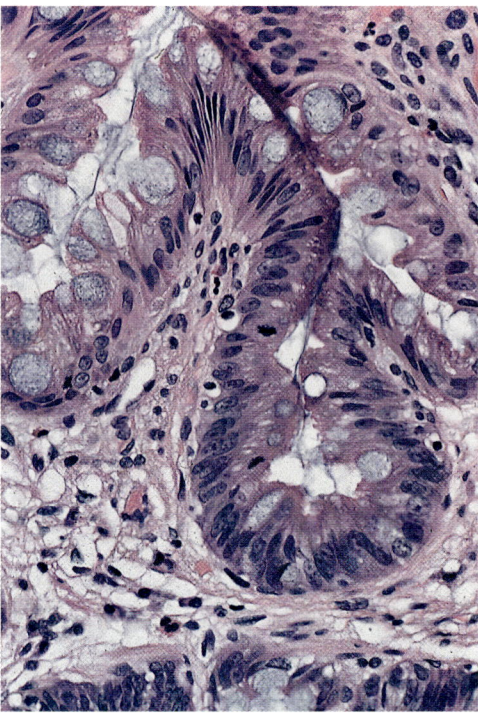

Figure 1-118: **Esophagus. Barrett's Esophagus, Low-Grade Dysplasia.** The degree of nuclear irregularity, enlargement, crowding, stratification, and reduction in mucus are diagnostic of low-grade dysplasia.

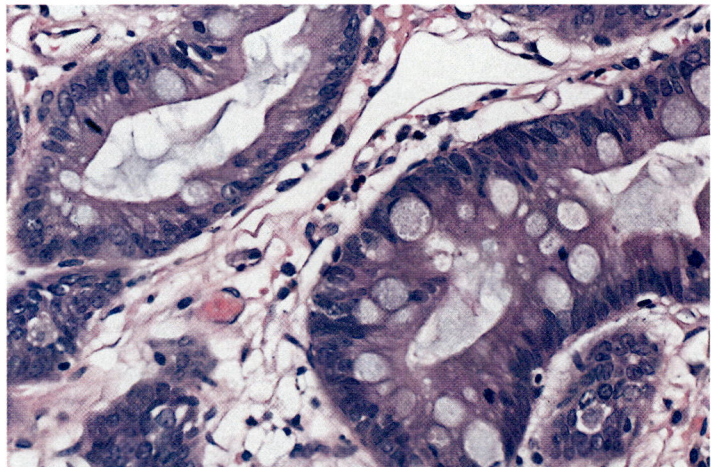

Figure 1-119: **Esophagus. Barrett's Esophagus, Regenerative Atypia.** Slight nuclear enlargement, mild stratification, relatively uniform nuclei, and preservation of mucin support a diagnosis of regenerative atypia.

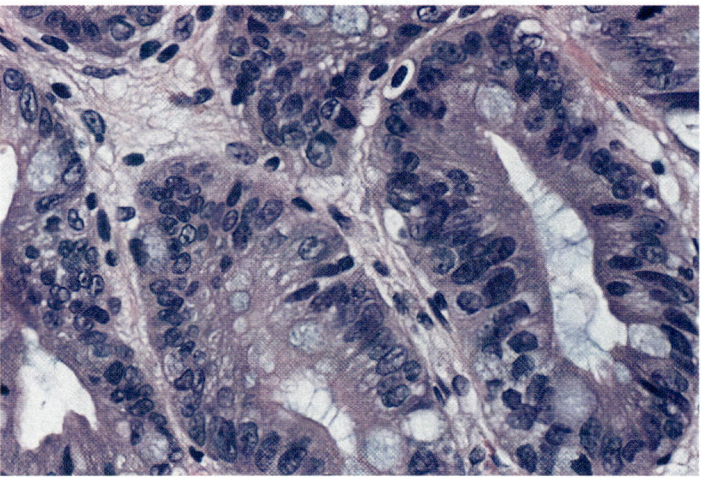

Figure 1-120: **Esophagus. Barrett's Esophagus, Atypia Indefinite for Dysplasia.** Nuclear enlargement and irregularity favor dysplasia; however, the preservation of mucin in some of the cells raises the possibility of regenerative change. Best classified as atypia indefinite for dysplasia.

BARRETT'S ESOPHAGUS, DYSPLASIA, STRICTURE, ULCER, MASS

- Morphology .... When high-grade dysplasia is detected on biopsy, invasive adenocarcinoma may already be present. The risk is related to the clinical circumstance at the time of detection. When found in surveillance samples from otherwise normal Barrett's esophagus, the risk is on the order of 10% or less. This holds true when ulcers are present. However, the risk of carcinoma is much greater, up to 50%, when samples are random from patients who are not under surveillance (and probably symptomatic) or when there are visible nodules, plaques, or strictures.

- Endoscopic features .... Complications of Barrett's esophagus include stricture located either at the new squamocolumnar junction or within the Barrett's segment. In the latter location, a malignancy should be suspected. Strictures at the new squamocolumnar junction are due to active reflux esophagitis. Discrete ulcers can develop in any location within a Barrett's segment and may cause dyspepsia. Ulcers may bleed and cause either occult GI blood loss anemia or acute bleeding when a vessel in the ulcer base becomes exposed. Carcinoma can present as nodules, polyps, or circumferential masses.

- Clinical features .... Ulcers may be associated with dyspepsia and mild dysphagia. Strictures typically cause dysphagia. High-grade dysplasia in flat, nodular, or polypoid mucosa is usually asymptomatic. Masses may cause dysphagia. Reflux strictures at the upper margin of the Barrett's segment cause dysphagia with or without associated reflux symptoms.

- Differential diagnosis ...... Endoscopic: Localized mucosal nodules, polyps, ulcers, strictures, or masses are all suspect for adenocarcinoma.

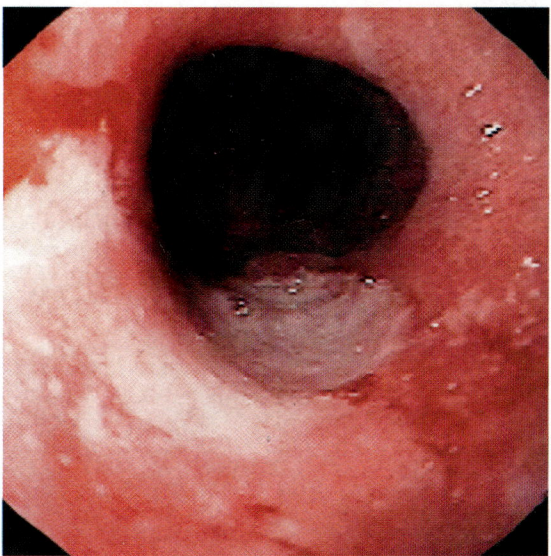

Figure 1-121: **Esophagus. Barrett's Esophagus, Ulcer.** Discrete clean-based ulcer with smooth margins within the distal portion of a long Barrett's segment. High-grade dysplasia was present.

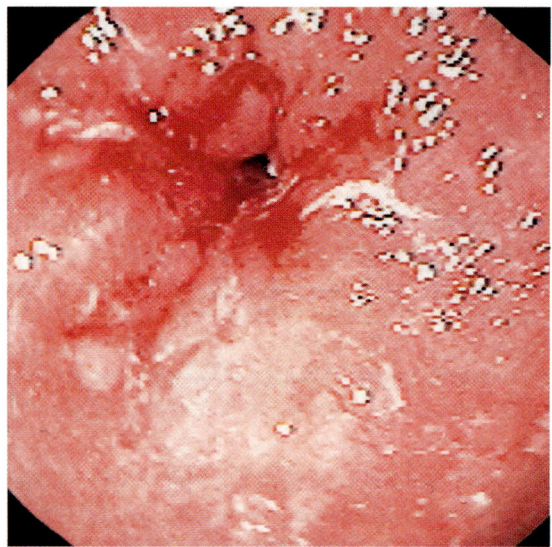

Figure 1-122: **Esophagus. Barrett's Esophagus, Stricture.** High-grade stricture at the distal end of a Barrett's segment. The surrounding mucosa appears thickened and nodular. The blood is due to contact trauma from the endoscope tip. High-grade dysplasia was present.

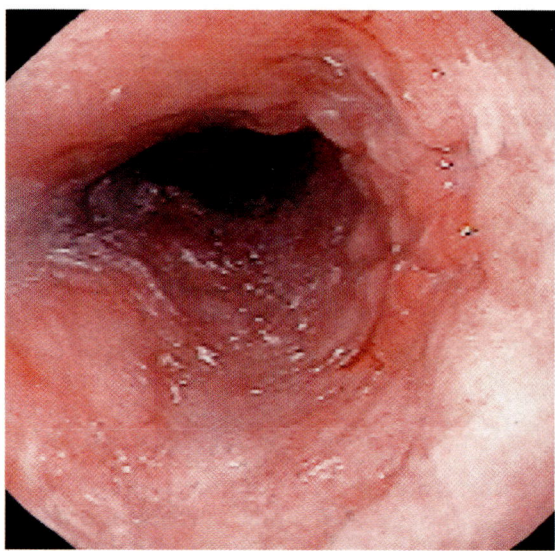

Figure 1-123: **Esophagus. Barrett's Esophagus, Nodules.** Long-segment Barrett's esophagus with a localized area of nodular mucosa on the right side of the lumen in the central portion of the photo, suspicious for carcinoma.

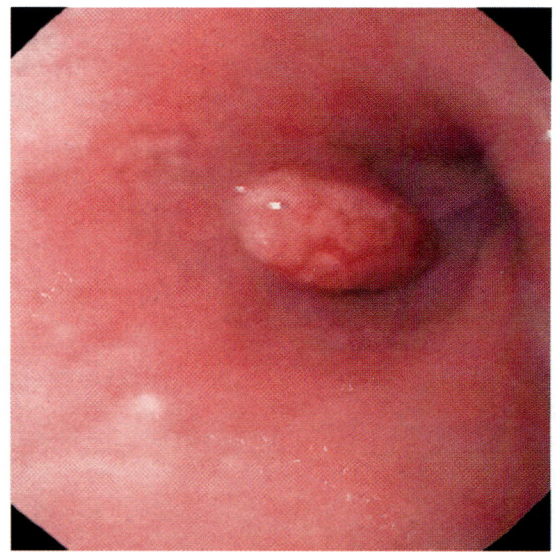

Figure 1-124: **Esophagus. Barrett's Esophagus, Polyp.** Small polyp with irregular surface within Barrett's esophagus. High-grade dysplasia was present.

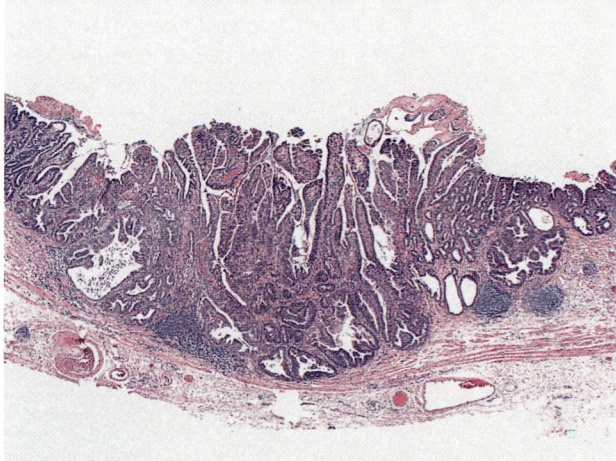

Figure 1-125: **Esophagus. Barrett's Esophagus, Nodule.** High-grade dysplasia with villous architecture forming a macroscopic nodule. Dysplastic glands push the muscularis mucosae downward. Glands are variably crowded, irregular, and distended.

ADENOCARCINOMA

- Morphology .... Adenocarcinomas in Barrett's esophagus are similar to gastric adenocarcinomas. Growth patterns commonly vary within the tumor. Some adenocarcinomas are so well-differentiated on the surface that histologic diagnosis by biopsy is impossible, even in widely invasive and metastatic neoplasms. Signet-ring cell carcinomas may be difficult to detect because of their ability to undermine normal mucosa. Poorly differentiated tumors or tumor samples containing few cells occasionally require immunostains for diagnosis.

- Endoscopic features .... Tumors encountered in the absence of known Barrett's esophagus become symptomatic and are detected when they obstruct the esophagus. Obvious malignancies are usually exophytic, friable, and ulcerated, and bleed spontaneously. Carcinomas detected during surveillance may be inapparent or may present as small masses, nodules, or irregular mucosa.

- Clinical features .... Obstruction and weight loss with advanced malignancy.

- Differential diagnosis ...... Histologic: Dysplasia versus well-differentiated adenocarcinoma.

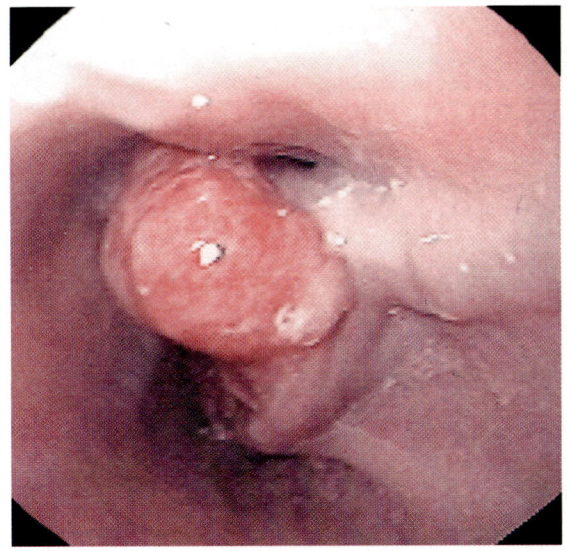

Figure 1-126: **Esophagus. Adenocarcinoma.** Barrett's segment with discrete, large nodule protruding into the lumen. Elevated cords of mucosa extend laterally and cephalad from the nodule, suspicious for submucosal extension of a carcinoma.

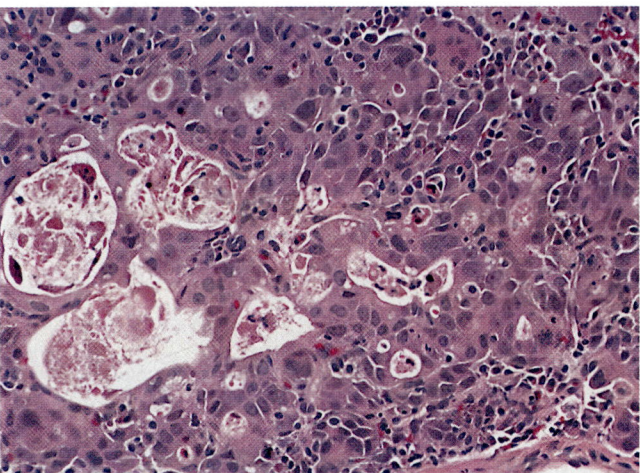

Figure 1-127: **Esophagus. Adenocarcinoma.** Poorly formed, infiltrating, neoplastic glands.

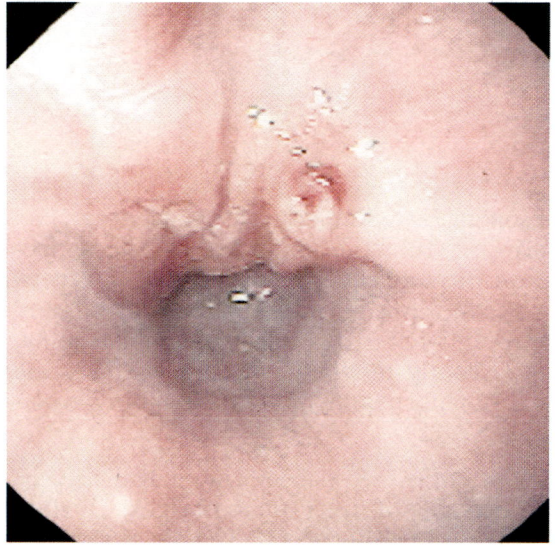 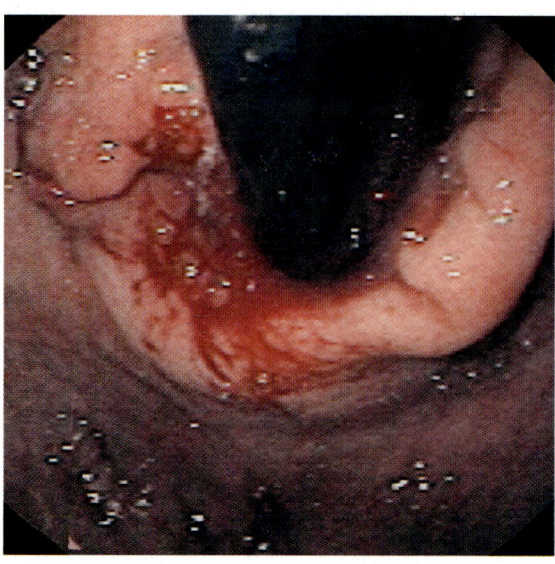

Figure 1-128: **Esophagus. Signet-Ring Cell Carcinoma.** A small, highly irregular mass with a bleeding, ulcerated area in a Barrett's segment. The lumen is narrowed. There appears to be submucosal cephalad extension of the mass in the upper left portion of the photo and a cicatricial contraction of the esophagus in the region of this mass.

Figure 1-129: **Esophagus, Distal. Adenocarcinoma.** Retroflexed view. Thickened, ulcerated, bleeding polypoid mass at cardia/gastroesophageal junction.

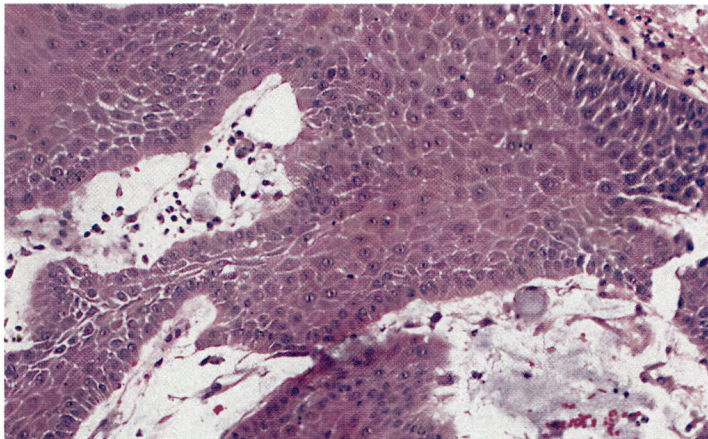

Figure 1-130: **Esophagus. Signet-Ring Cell Carcinoma.** A few mucin-filled signet-ring cells lie beneath obliquely sectioned squamous epithelium.

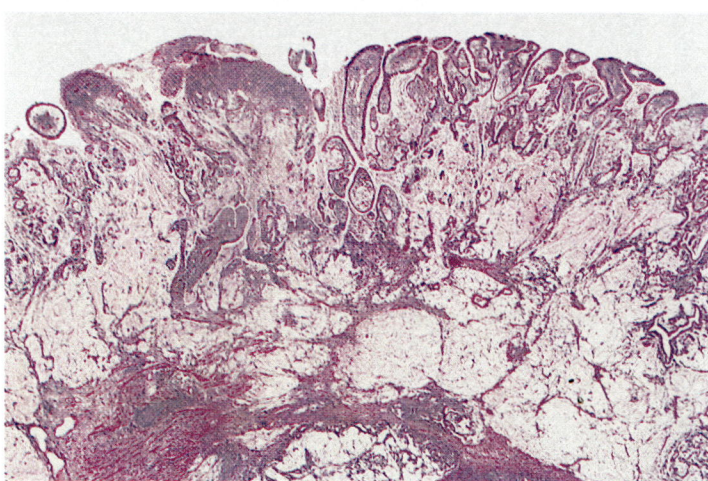

Figure 1-131: **Esophagus. Adenocarcinoma, Mucinous.** Villous projections of neoplastic cells overlie pools of mucin.

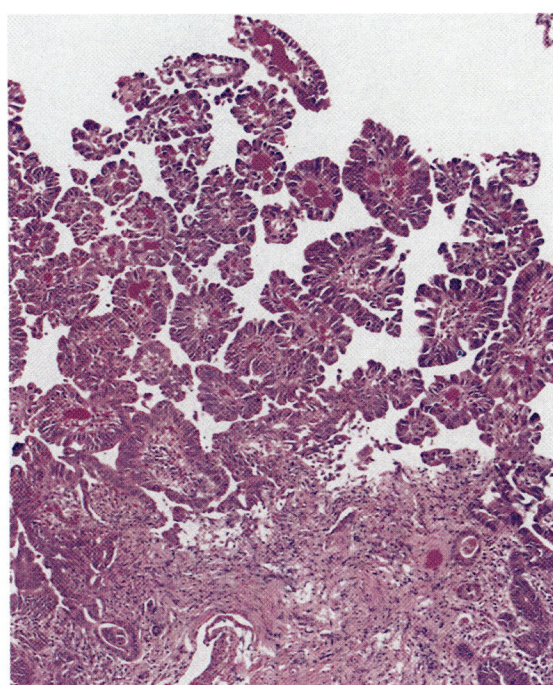

Figure 1-132: **Esophagus. Adenocarcinoma, Papillary.** Neoplastic papillary fronds and infiltrating glands.

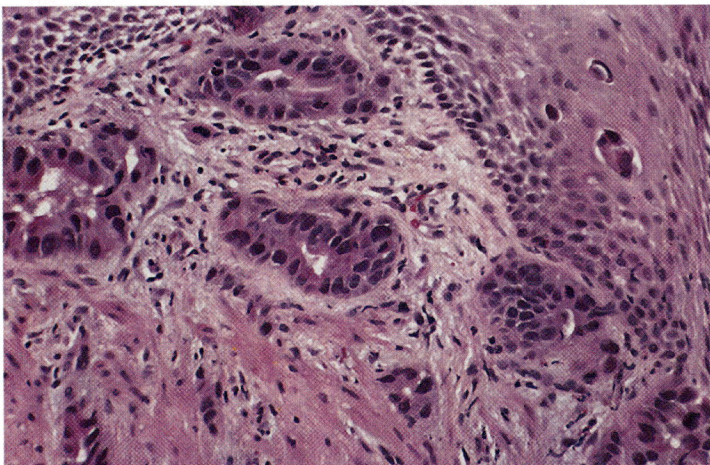

Figure 1-133: **Esophagus. Adenocarcinoma.** Well-differentiated glands and small clusters of tumor cells undermine and infiltrate squamous epithelium.

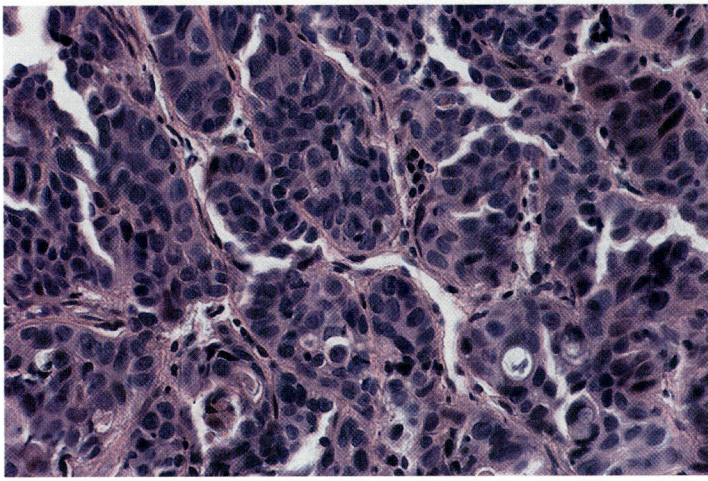

Figure 1-134: **Esophagus. Adenocarcinoma.** Tightly packed nests and trabeculae of tumor cells, some with mucin.

SQUAMOUS DYSPLASIA

- Morphology .... Squamous dysplasia is characterized by cells with increased nuclear-to-cytoplasmic ratio, hyperchromatic irregular nuclei, and loss of orientation. Regenerative epithelium and dysplasia share decreased maturation. Unlike dysplasia, cytologic uniformity, lack of nuclear overlap, and maintenance of polarity are features of regeneration.

- Endoscopic features .... Both focal dysplasia and carcinoma may coexist with erosions, plaque-like abnormalities, nodules, or circumferential obstructing tumors. The endoscopist looks for subtle mucosal changes and carefully examines the proximal cardia just beyond the squamocolumnar junction, both from antegrade and retroflexed viewing perspectives, especially when performing surveillance endoscopy in high-risk populations. A biopsy should be performed on any abnormality, no matter how subtle.

    Chromoendoscopy (vital dye staining) of the epithelial surface has been used in the esophagus (as well as in the colon and rectum) to highlight dysplastic tissue. Lugol's iodine and methylene blue are used in the esophagus, the latter in Barrett's esophagus. Normal esophageal squamous mucosa takes on a darkly stained appearance with iodine, whereas dysplastic tissue and malignancies do not pick up the stain and appear as yellow (unstained) areas.

- Clinical features .... None.

- Differential diagnosis ...... Endoscopic: Ectopic gastric mucosa. Iodine will not stain ectopic mucosa.

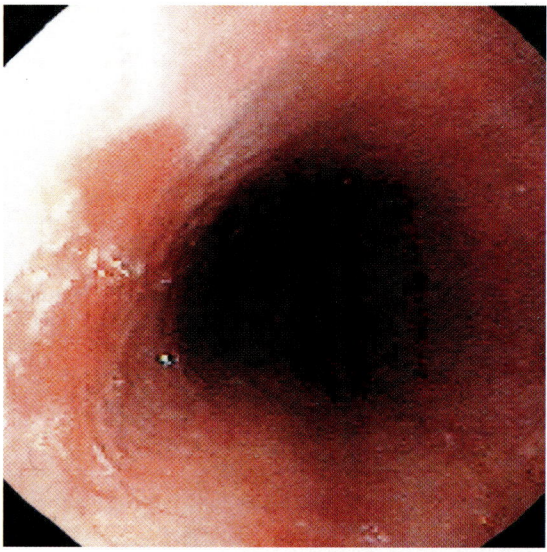

Figure 1-135: **Esophagus. Squamous Dysplasia.** A discrete atypical patch of erythematous mucosa in the proximal esophagus on the left side of the photo.

Figure 1-136: **Esophagus. Squamous Dysplasia.** The same segment of esophagus seen in the previous figure stained with Lugol's iodine. The normal squamous mucosa is stained darkly while the atypical erythematous area is unstained, consistent with dysplasia.

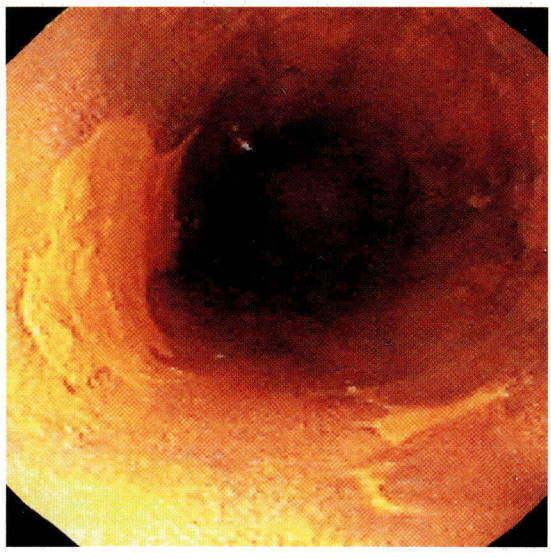

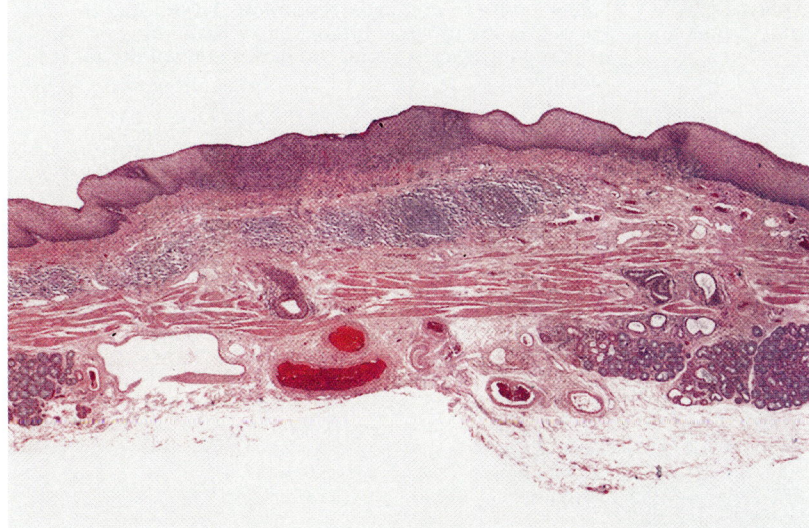

Figure 1-137: **Esophagus. Squamous Dysplasia.** A well-defined basophilic area in an architecturally normal squamous epithelium. Underlying band of chronic inflammation.

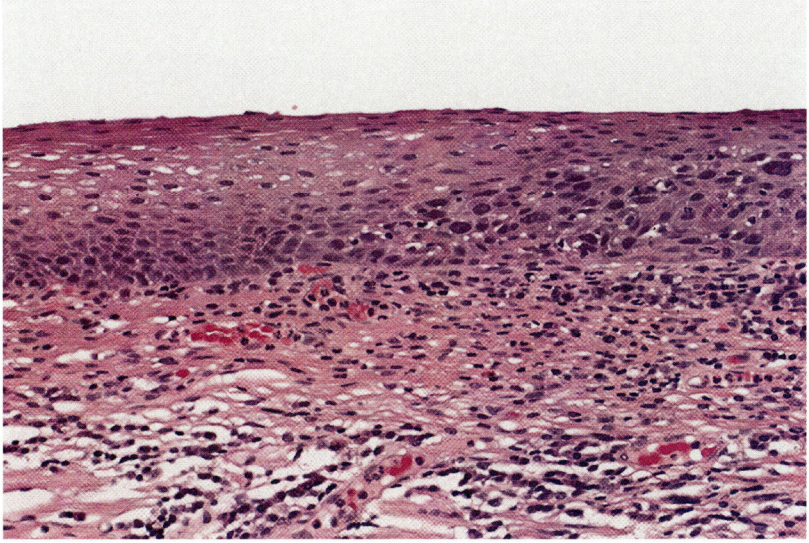

Figure 1-138: **Esophagus. Squamous Dysplasia.** Abrupt transition between normal (left) and dysplastic (right) epithelium. Enlarged, irregular, hyperchromatic nuclei with loss of maturation.

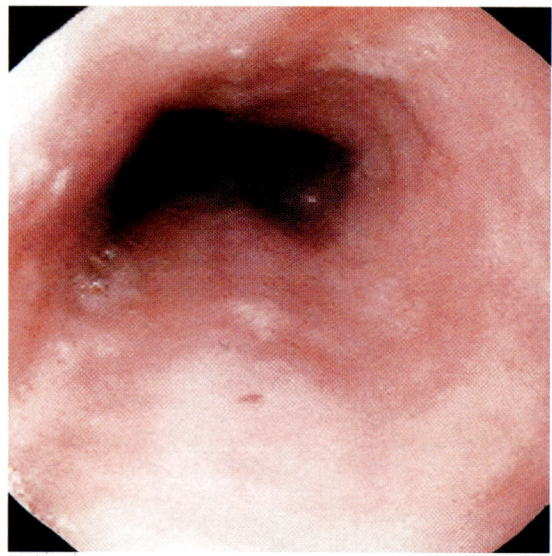

Figure 1-139: **Esophagus. Squamous Dysplasia.** A normal-appearing midesophagus of homogeneous color and appearance.

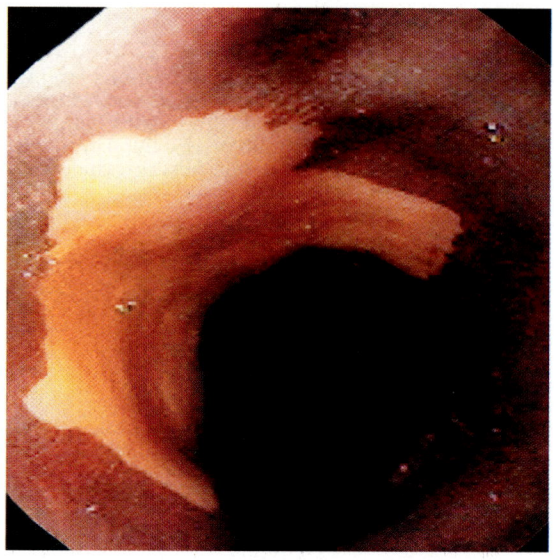

Figure 1-140: **Esophagus. Squamous Dysplasia.** Lugol's iodine reveals a bright yellow island of unstained dysplastic tissue and darkly stained normal mucosa.

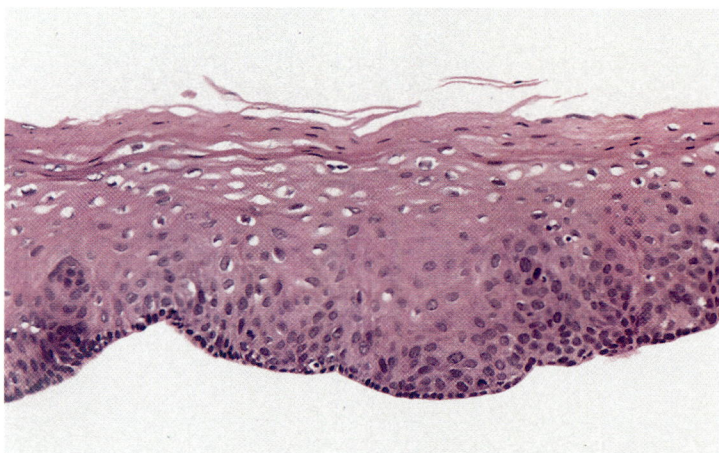

Figure 1-141: **Esophagus. Squamous Dysplasia, Low-Grade.** Large hyperchromatic nuclei and loss of normal nuclear orientation, limited to the lower layers of the epithelium.

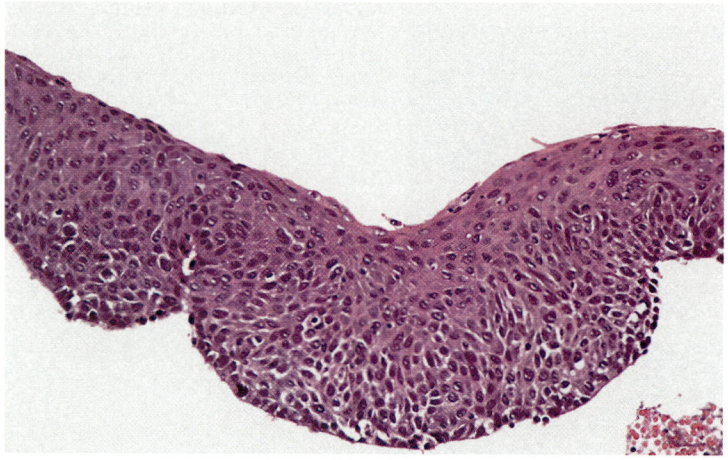

Figure 1-142: **Esophagus. Squamous Dysplasia, High-Grade.** Dysplastic cells extend from base to surface.

SQUAMOUS CELL CARCINOMA

- Morphology .... Esophageal squamous cell carcinomas are similar to those at other sites in the upper aerodigestive tract. Uncommon morphologic variants of squamous cell carcinoma may confound the diagnosis. The small cell variant is more aggressive, while the verrucous variant is indolent. In squamous cell carcinoma, multifocality in the oropharynx, larynx, and esophagus occurs. Invasive squamous cell carcinoma originating in adjacent structures, e.g., bronchus, may mimic primary esophageal carcinoma. Endoscopic biopsies from well-differentiated tumors may be too superficial to demonstrate stromal invasion. Oblique sections of reactive squamous lesions (pseudoepitheliomatous hyperplasia) may simulate invasive squamous cell carcinoma.

- Endoscopic features .... In early stages of squamous cell carcinoma, local areas of salmon-colored, gastric-appearing mucosa are seen, often associated with erosion and ulceration. There may be plaques of roughened or "cobblestoned" mucosa. In more advanced stages, there are nodules and mass lesions that are exophytic, ulcerated, necrotic, and friable, and that bleed spontaneously.

- Clinical features .... Asymptomatic lesions in high-risk populations (Asians, smokers, and drinkers), dysphagia.

- Differential diagnosis ...... Endoscopic: Ectopic gastric mucosa. Plaques can be confused with infectious esophagitis with exudate. Mass lesion in the distal esophagus: adenocarcinoma in Barrett's. Mass in proximal esophagus: nonpigmented malignant melanoma.

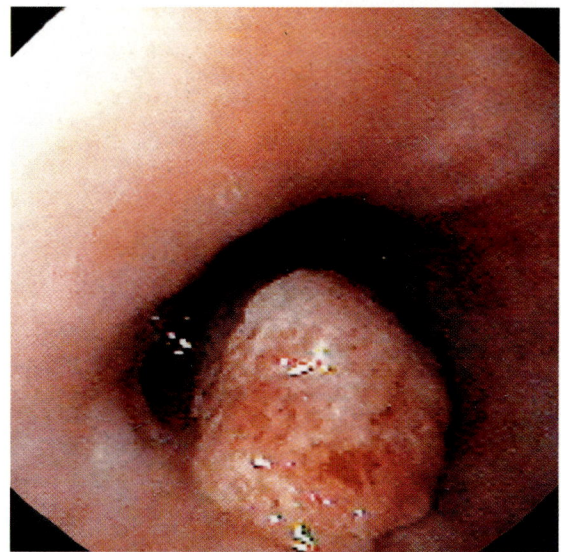

Figure 1-143: **Esophagus, Distal. Squamous Cell Carcinoma.** A discrete, irregularly shaped, friable, neoplastic-appearing nodule with foci of spontaneous hemorrhage.

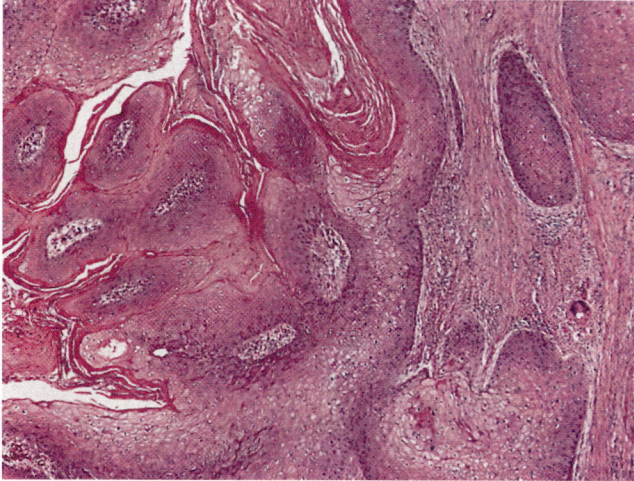

Figure 1-144: **Esophagus. Squamous Cell Carcinoma, Verrucous Type.** Well-differentiated squamous cell proliferation. Cellular atypia is minimal. Invasion is subtle. Lower border appears to be pushing into the stroma with minimal response. Surface is villiform and hyperkeratotic. Resembles a wart and may be impossible to diagnose on biopsy due to high degree of differentiation. Diagnosis requires clinicopathologic correlation.

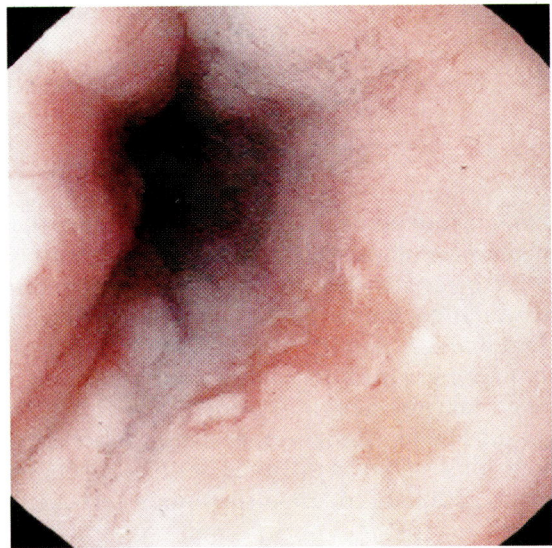

Figure 1-145: **Esophagus, Distal. Squamous Cell Carcinoma.** A small patch of irregularly shaped, salmon-colored mucosa is in the foreground. A small erosion with white exudate is at the left of this atypical patch.

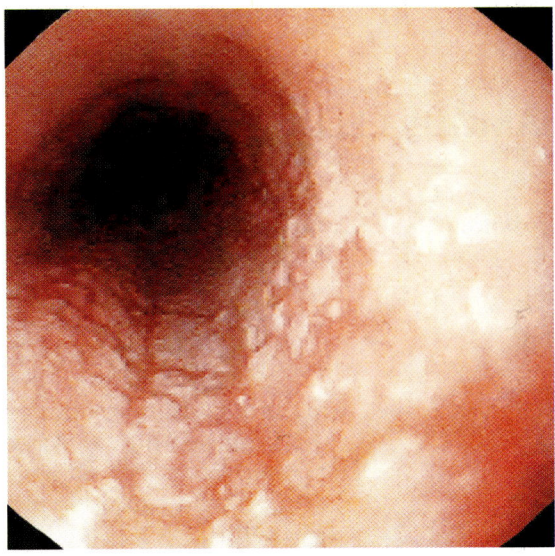

Figure 1-146: **Esophagus, Distal. Squamous Cell Carcinoma.** Coarsely roughened mucosa with multiple mucosal plaques.

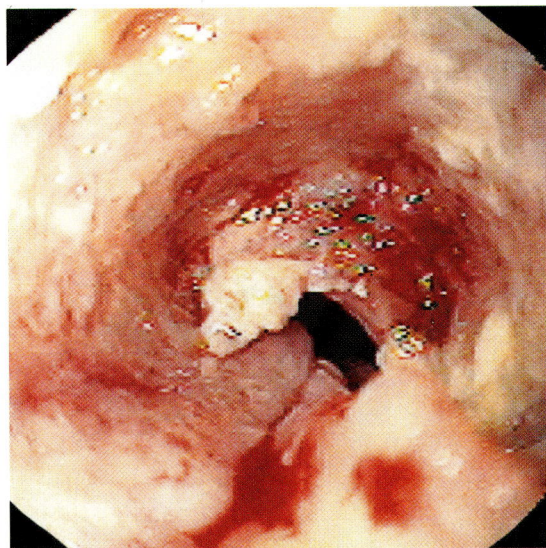

Figure 1-147: **Esophagus, Distal. Squamous Cell Carcinoma.** Circumferential, obstructing, necrotic, ulcerated, and spontaneously bleeding neoplasm in the distal esophagus.

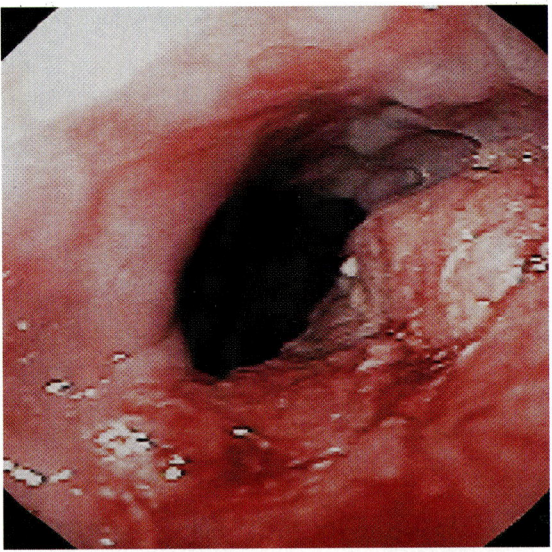

Figure 1-148: **Esophagus, Middle. Squamous Cell Carcinoma.** Ulcerating mass compromises lumen and extends over 4 cm. The proximal location is suggestive of squamous cell carcinoma.

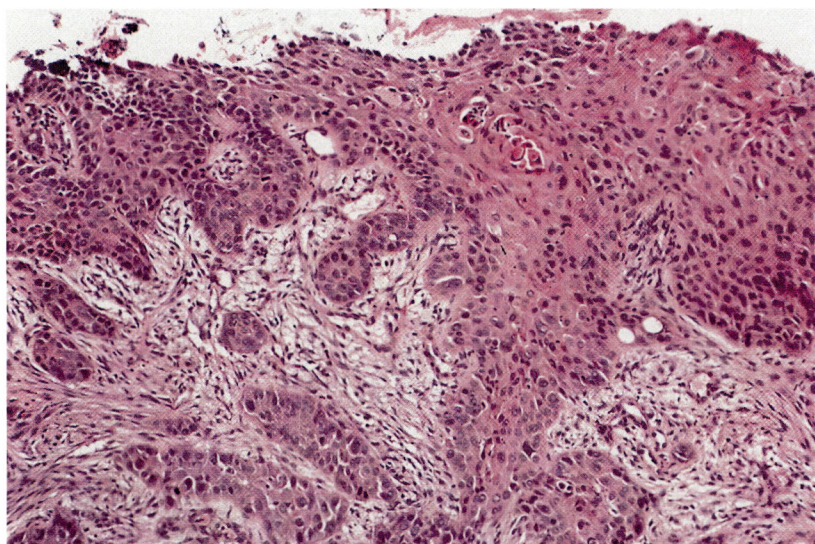

Figure 1-149: **Esophagus. Squamous Cell Carcinoma.** Atypical surface epithelium and invasive nests with stromal proliferation (desmoplastic response); the most common pattern.

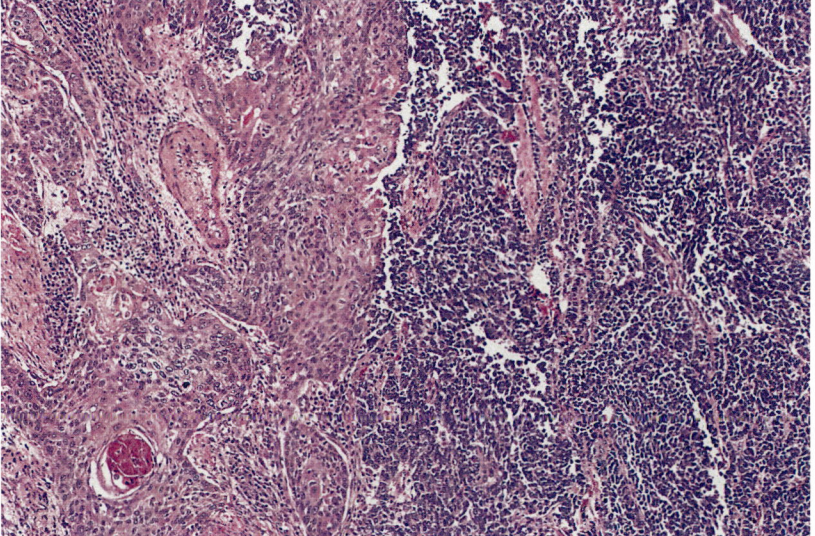

Figure 1-150: **Esophagus. Squamous Cell Carcinoma with Small Cell Component.** Invasive squamous cell carcinoma (left). Small cell component (right). Small cells have minimal cytoplasm and grow diffusely in sheets.

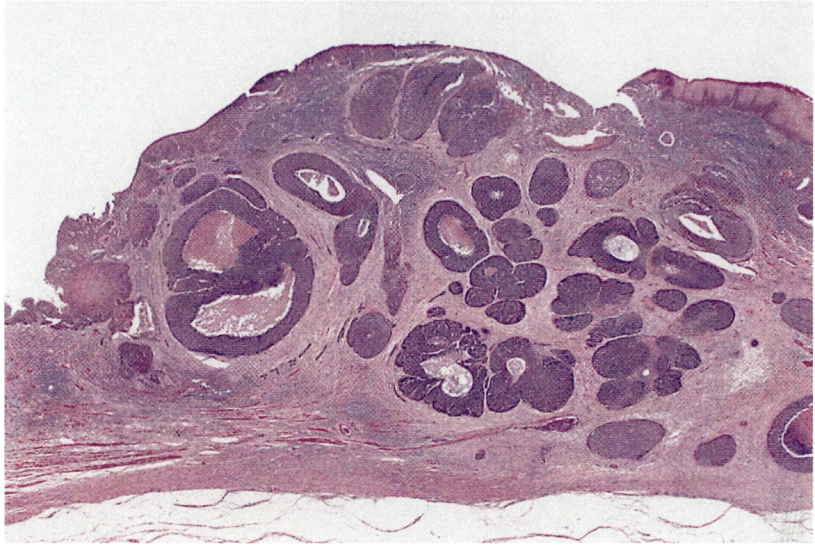

Figure 1-151: **Esophagus. Squamous Cell Carcinoma, Basaloid Variant.** Small squamous cells with scant cytoplasm grow in cohesive, centrally necrotic nests. Resembles basal cell carcinoma, but is aggressive.

MALIGNANT MELANOMA

- Morphology .... Melanoma can masquerade as carcinoma, lymphoma, and sarcoma. The cells may be large, small, spindled, nested, dispersed, or ballooned. Melanin pigment may not be present. Immunostains (S-100, HMB-45) are often necessary for diagnosis. Premalignant melanocytic lesions confirm a primary.
- Endoscopic features .... Malignant melanoma of the esophagus appears as an advanced exophytic, ulcerated, friable neoplasm with spontaneous bleeding. The lesions are more often discretely localized, even pedunculated, rather than circumferential. Advanced lesions typically obstruct.
- Clinical features .... Dysphagia, in a person with known metastatic disease or history of primary melanoma. Although most melanomas are metastatic, primary melanomas occur.
- Differential diagnosis ...... Endoscopic: Carcinoma, metastatic disease.

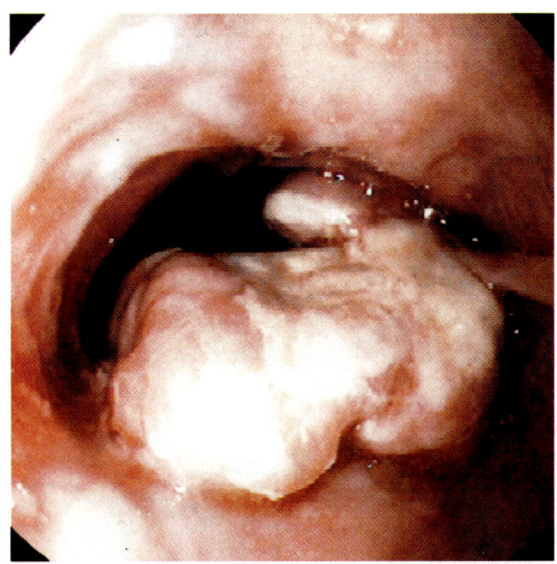

Figure 1-152: **Esophagus. Melanoma.** Obstructing, ulcerated, proximal esophageal neoplasm. The mass is a large sessile polyp.

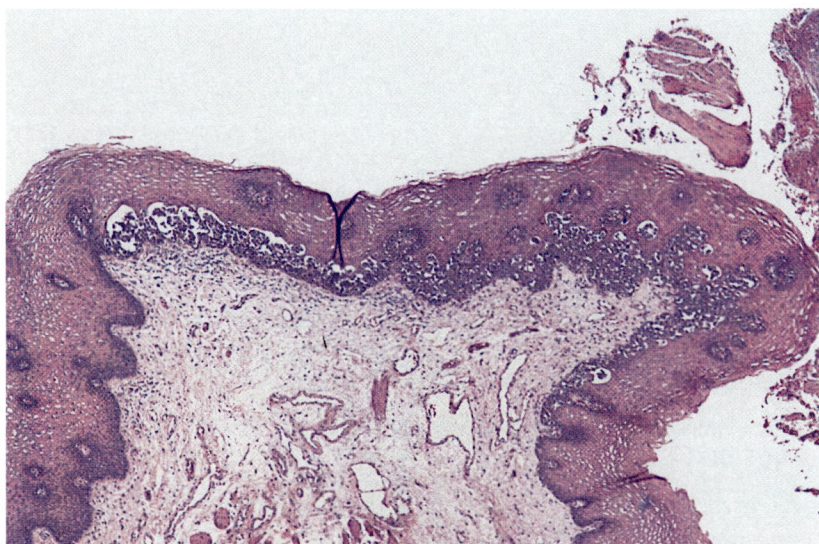

Figure 1-153: **Esophagus. Melanoma.** Melanocytic activity in the squamous epithelium (adjacent to an invasive melanoma).

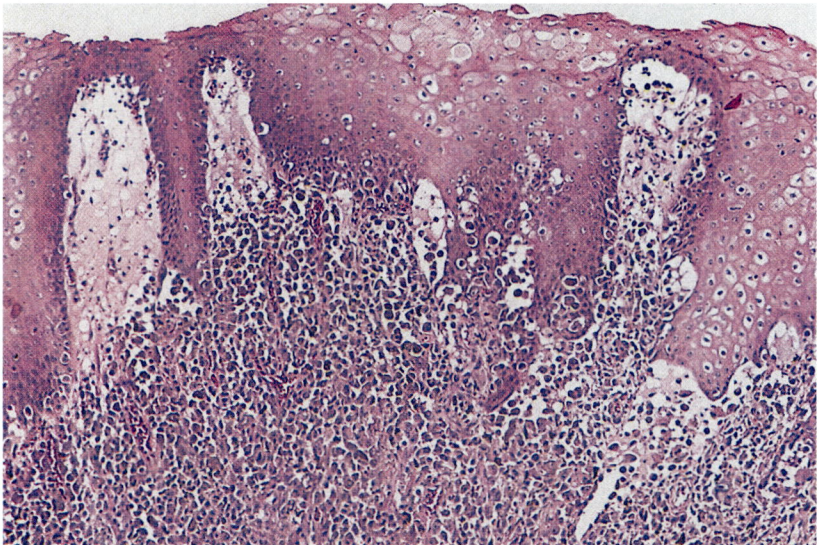

Figure 1-154: **Esophagus. Melanoma.** Large, polygonal, noncohesive cells in sheets, apparently originating from the base of the hyperplastic squamous epithelium.

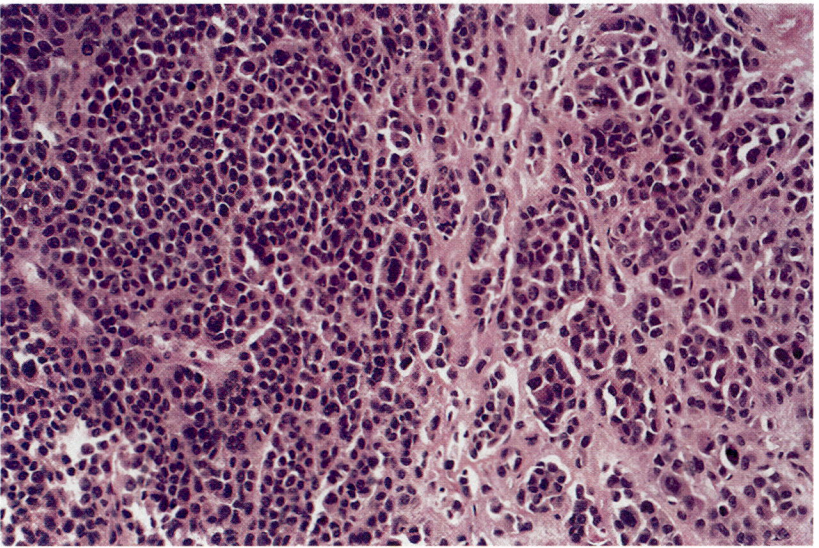

Figure 1-155: **Esophagus. Melanoma.** This alveolar nest pattern is common in melanoma, but not sufficiently distinctive for definitive diagnosis. No melanin pigment.

METASTATIC TUMORS

- Morphology .... Metastases are generally covered by normal, reactive, or focally ulcerated squamous mucosa. A midesophageal location may indicate extension from paratracheal or parabronchial lymph nodes. Often the primary site cannot be determined from morphology, even when supplemented with immunostains. Large cell lymphoma can mimic carcinoma, sarcoma, and melanoma. Immunohistochemistry is required for distinction.
- Endoscopic features .... Nonspecific mucosal nodularity with or without coloration change, ulcerated mass, or nodule.
- Clinical features .... Known metastatic disease, dysphagia, absence of symptoms.
- Differential diagnosis ...... Endoscopic: Primary esophageal cancer, pill-induced ulcer, and phlebectasia.

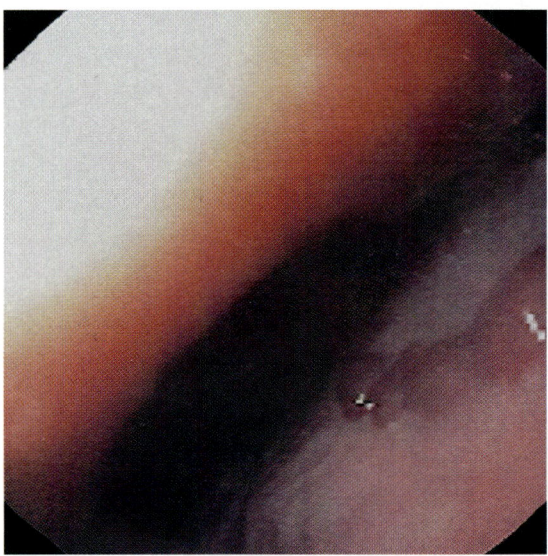

Figure 1-156: **Esophagus. Metastatic Carcinoma.** There is a dark red, raised linear nodularity of the proximal esophagus seen at right.

ESOPHAGUS

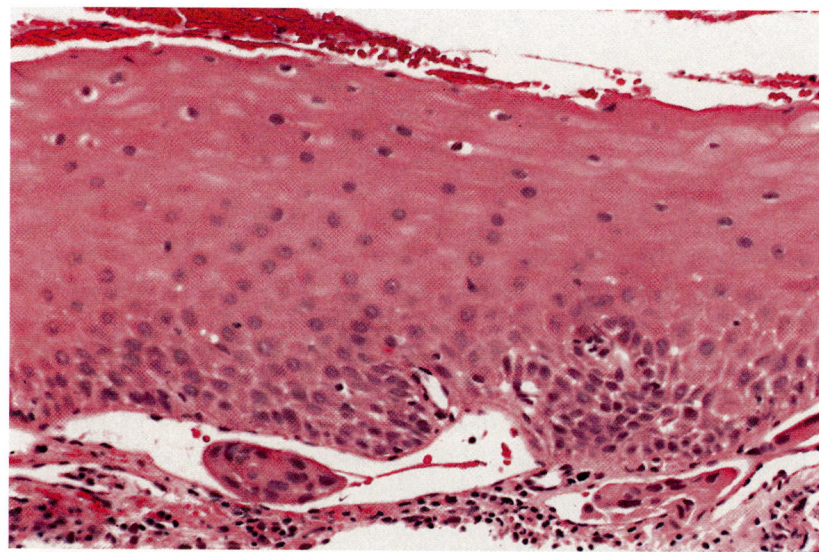

Figure 1-157: **Esophagus. Metastatic Breast Carcinoma.** Clusters of carcinoma cells in vascular spaces. Overlying squamous epithelium is normal.

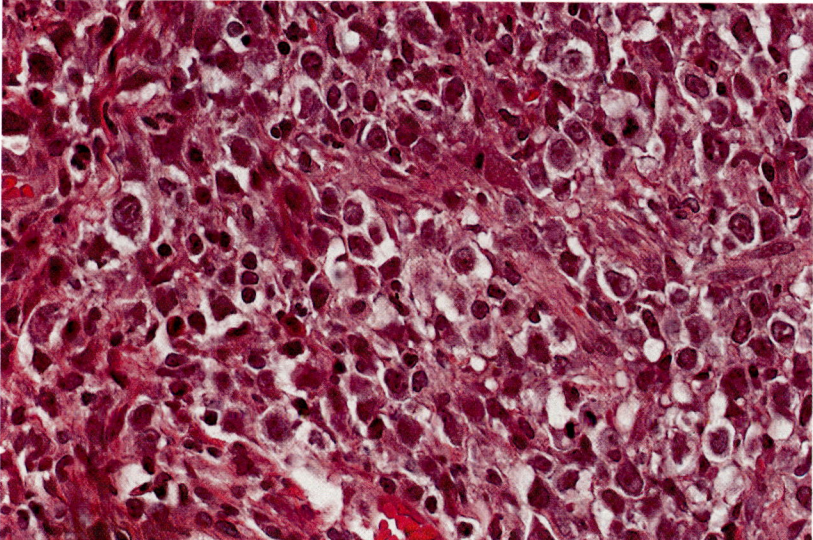

Figure 1-158: **Esophagus. Metastatic Breast Carcinoma.** Biopsy specimen with fragment of squamous epithelium and clusters of atypical cells.

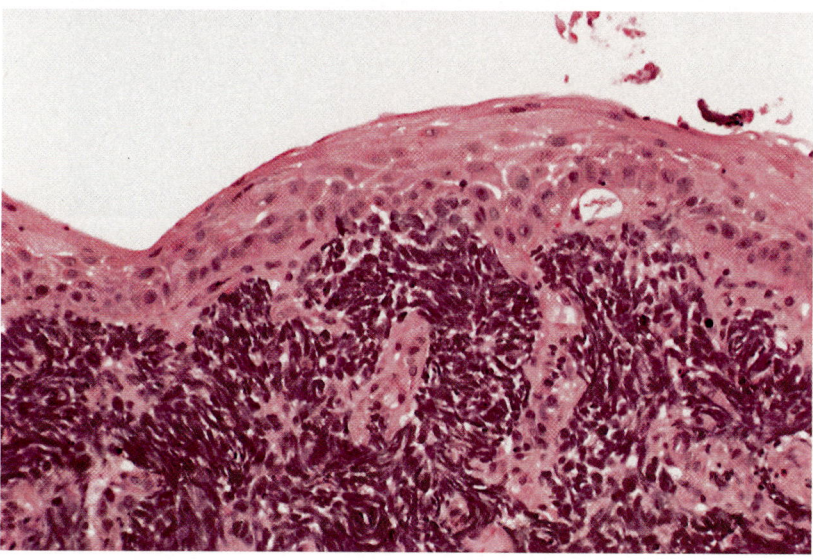

Figure 1-159: **Esophagus. Metastatic Small Cell Carcinoma.** Sheets of dark, small, crushed cells without visible cytoplasm undermine reactive squamous epithelium.

VASCULAR LESIONS

- Morphology .... Hemangiomas and other vascular lesions in the esophagus are rare. Granulation tissue may mimic a hemangioma. The plump appearance of the endothelial cells and proliferating vascular channels typical of granulation tissue are helpful in distinguishing it from a hemangioma. Any vascular-appearing lesion in HIV-positive individuals, no matter how benign in appearance, is likely Kaposi sarcoma.
- Endoscopic features .... Prominent vascular abnormality; size and configuration vary. Lesions are blue or purple and elevated, with either a smooth or nodular surface.
- Clinical features .... Chronic blood loss anemia, hemoptysis; known diffuse hemangiomatosis.
- Differential diagnosis ...... Endoscopic: Phlebectasia, metastatic nodule.

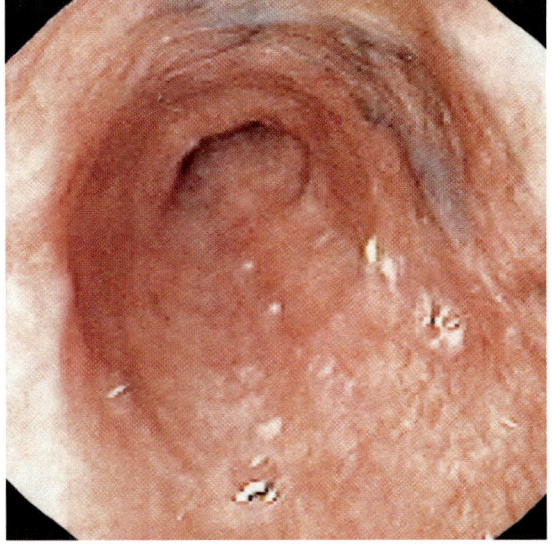

Figure 1-160: **Esophagus. Hemangioma.** A sprawling, slightly elevated, blue-hued vascular lesion is in the upper portion of the photo, located in the midesophagus.

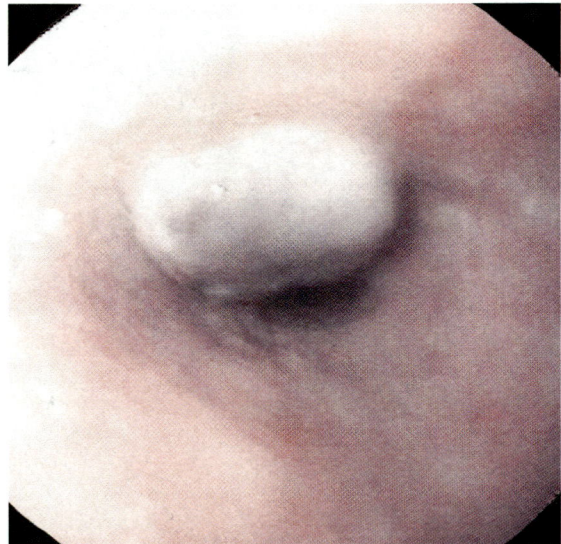

Figure 1-161: **Esophagus. Vascular Abnormality.** Soft, pliable, smooth, blue, 2-cm mass in midesophagus.

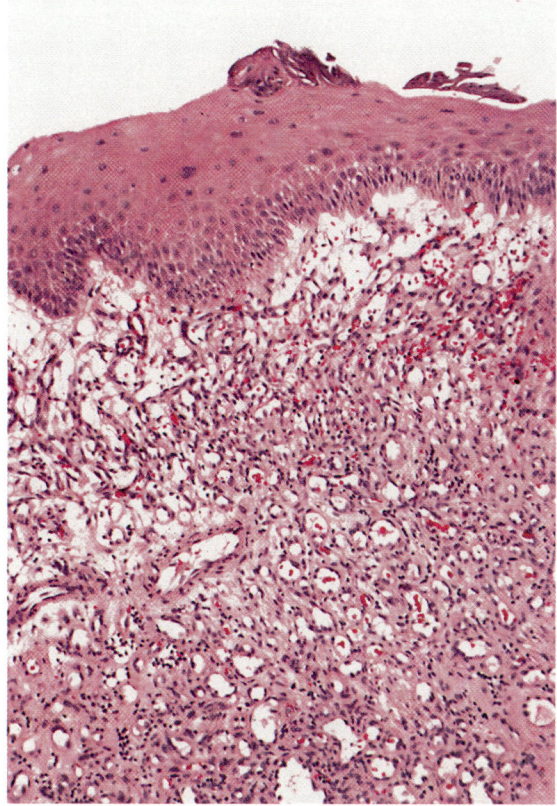

Figure 1-162: **Esophagus. Capillary Hemangioma.** Proliferating capillaries in the lamina propria. Slightly reactive squamous epithelium.

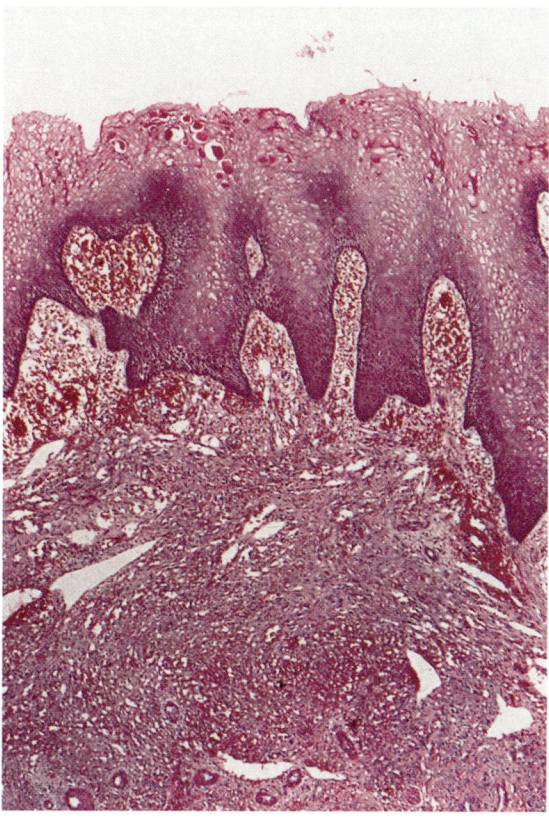

Figure 1-163: **Esophagus. Kaposi Sarcoma.** Tight spindle cell proliferation and small, poorly formed vascular spaces. Squamous epithelium is hyperplastic with prominent downgrowths.

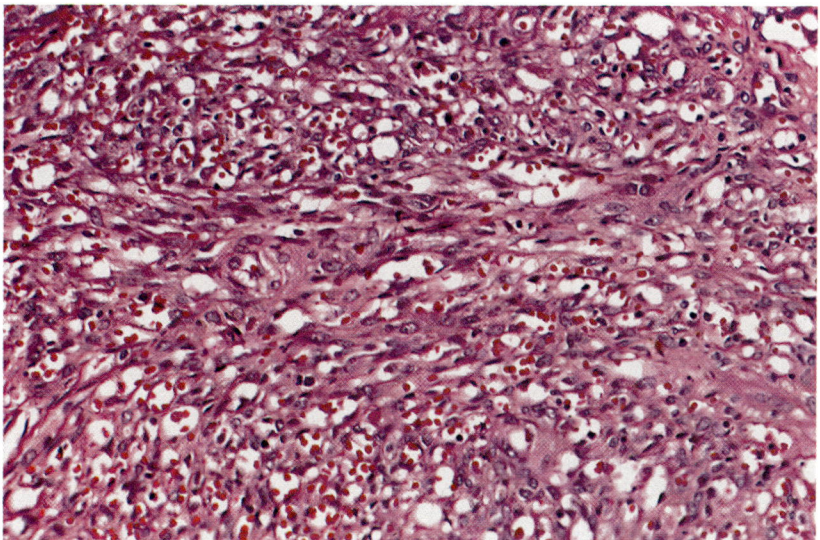

Figure 1-164: **Esophagus. Kaposi Sarcoma.** Red cells scattered between spindle cells and in poorly formed vascular spaces.

FIBROVASCULAR POLYP

- Morphology .... These soft polyps are usually elongated and may grow to incredible lengths, fill the esophagus, and even be regurgitated. They are composed of a loose, well-vascularized stroma covered by squamous epithelium.
- Endoscopic features .... The polyps are typically large, long, fingerlike lesions. They may attain considerable size and obstruct the lumen.
- Clinical features .... None or dysphagia.
- Differential diagnosis ...... Endoscopic: Isolated esophageal varix, leiomyoma, or other submucosal polypoid mass.

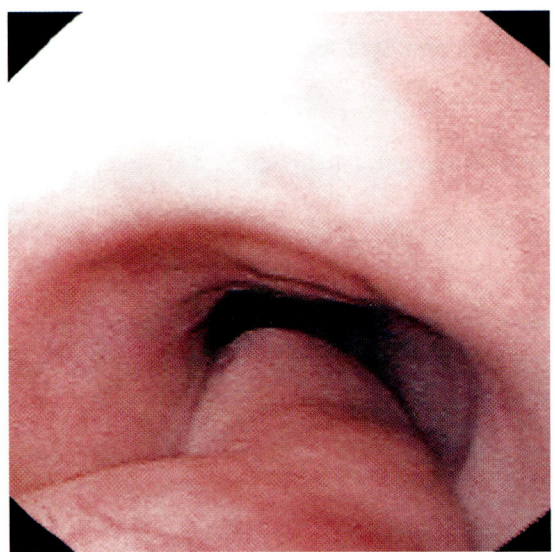

Figure 1-165: **Esophagus. Fibrovascular Polyp.** Smooth, elongated polyp with intact overlying mucosa.

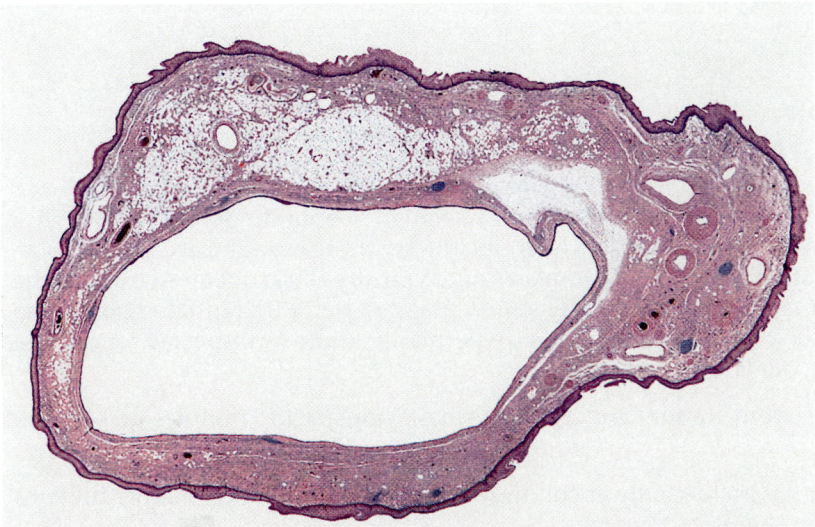

Figure 1-166: **Esophagus. Fibrovascular Polyp.** Cross section of a fibrovascular polyp with a central cyst.

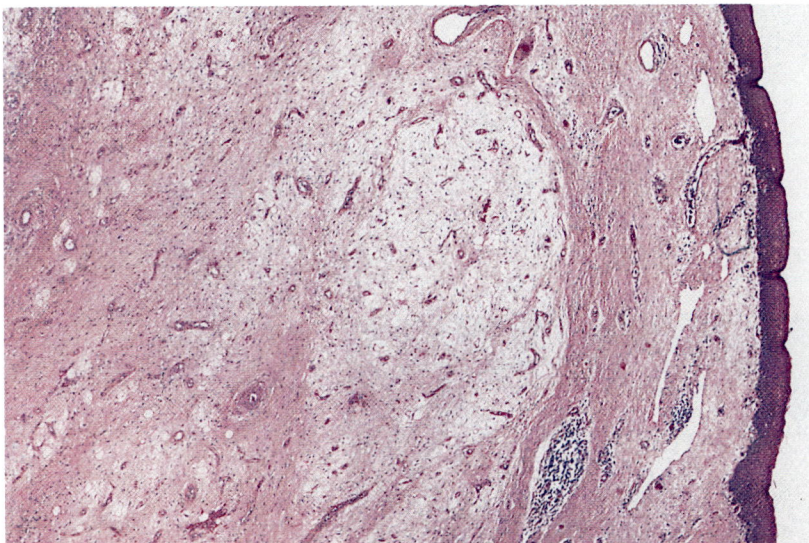

Figure 1-167: **Esophagus. Fibrovascular Polyp.** Loose, well-vascularized connective tissue covered by normal esophageal squamous epithelium.

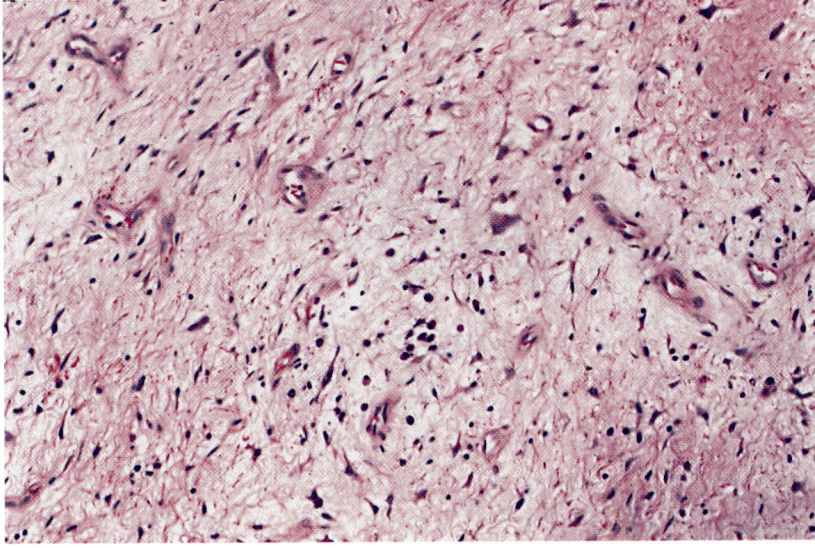

Figure 1-168: **Esophagus. Fibrovascular Polyp.** Edematous connective tissue with fibroblasts, capillaries, and scattered inflammatory cells.

GRANULAR CELL TUMOR

- Morphology .... Granular cell tumors are uncommon, benign neoplasms of neural type (S-100 protein-positive) found throughout the gastrointestinal tract. The cells are large with pink granular cytoplasm and typically elicit squamous hyperplasia. This can mask the granular cells and simulate a well-differentiated carcinoma. A biopsy with marked squamous hyperplasia should be inspected for granular cells in the lamina propria.
- Endoscopic features .... Granular cell tumors are typically small, nonspecific nodules or polypoid lesions.
- Clinical features .... Most often incidentally encountered. The esophagus and anus are the most frequent digestive tract sites.
- Differential diagnosis ...... Endoscopic: Squamous cell carcinoma, submucosal or mucosal neoplasm of any variety.

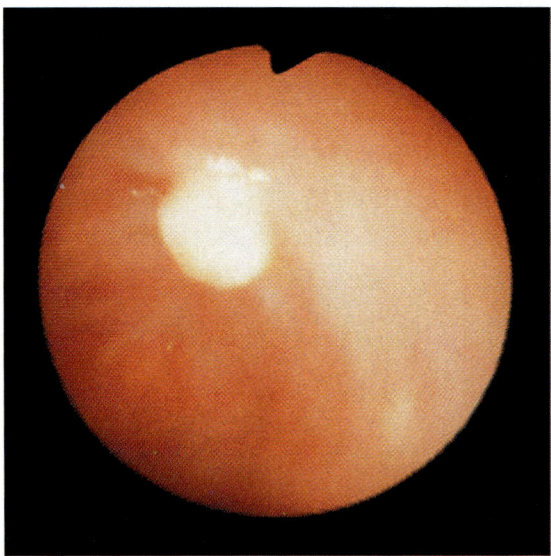

Figure 1-169: **Esophagus. Granular Cell Tumor.** Small, midesophageal, yellow polyp without ulceration or exudate.

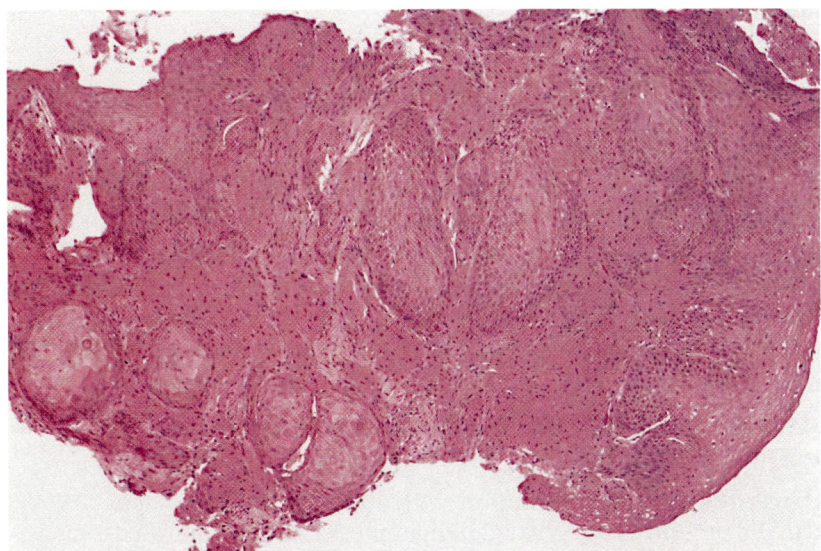

Figure 1-170: **Esophagus. Granular Cell Tumor.** Focal, small polypoid nodule with prominent mature squamous nests.

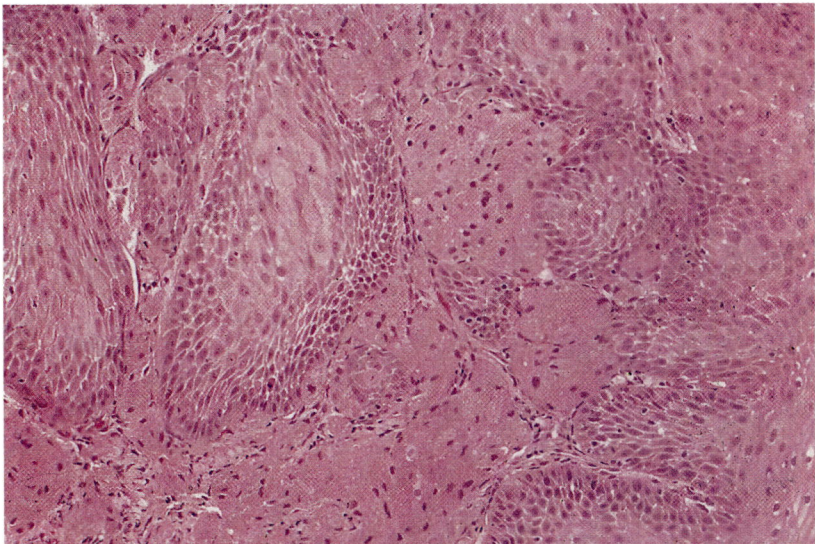

Figure 1-171: **Esophagus. Granular Cell Tumor.** Pale cells in the lamina propria, between the squamous nests, have voluminous pink granular cytoplasm and small round nuclei.

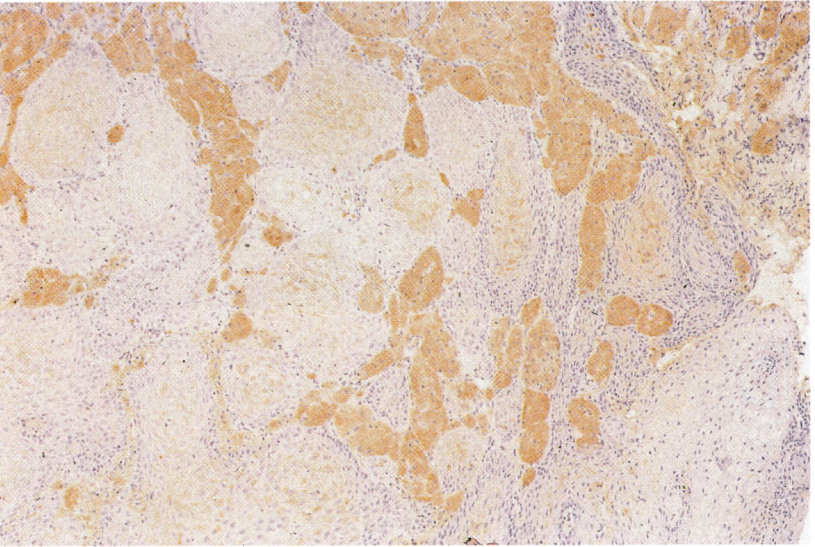

Figure 1-172: **Esophagus. Granular Cell Tumor.** Positive immunoreactivity for S-100 protein in the granular cells. The latter are dwarfed by the unstained hyperplastic squamous proliferation.

STROMAL TUMORS

- Morphology .... Stromal tumors are a group of neoplasms that may be of smooth muscle (leiomyomas, leiomyosarcomas), neural (schwannomas), or adipose (lipoma) type. Smooth muscle tumors are generally small and arise from the muscularis mucosae or muscularis propria. The majority are benign. Diagnosis is based on mitotic rate and size. Schwannomas and lipomas are rare, and their behavior is benign.

- Endoscopic features .... Stromal tumors are submucosal, vary in size, and typically have uninvolved overlying mucosa if benign.

- Clinical features .... When large, they create obstruction with intermittent dysphagia. When ulcerated, the presentation is that of hematemesis, melena, or iron deficiency anemia.

- Differential diagnosis ...... Endoscopic: Any submucosal tumor, e.g., leiomyoma, leiomyosarcoma, lipoma, schwannoma, metastatic cancer, and granular cell tumor.

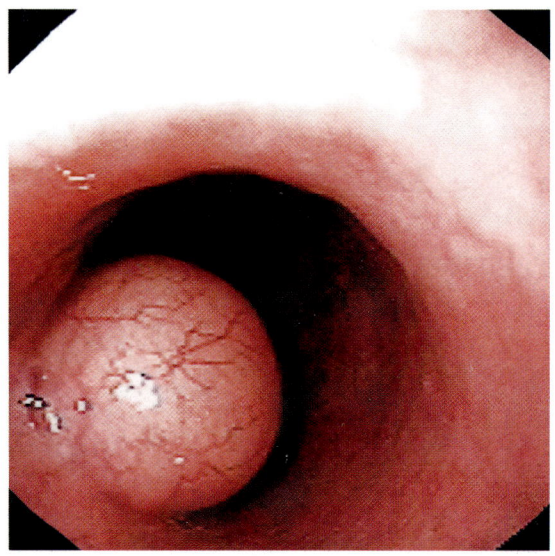

Figure 1-173: **Esophagus. Leiomyosarcoma.** Discrete midesophageal submucosal nodule with prominent mucosal vasculature overlying the nodule. The well-rounded appearance and projection into the lumen are more suspicious for a lipoma.

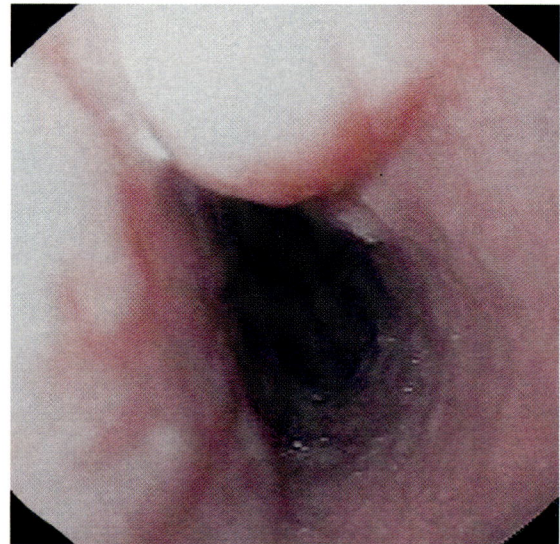

Figure 1-174: **Esophagus. Lipoma.** Proximal esophageal submucosal mass with intact overlying mucosa and minimal encroachment of the lumen.

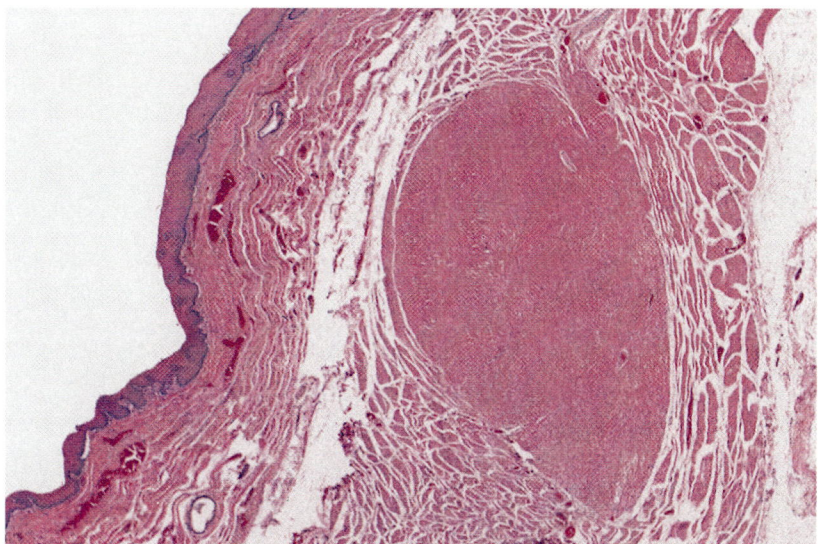

Figure 1-175: **Esophagus. Leiomyoma.** Small, round, well-circumscribed leiomyoma in muscularis propria.

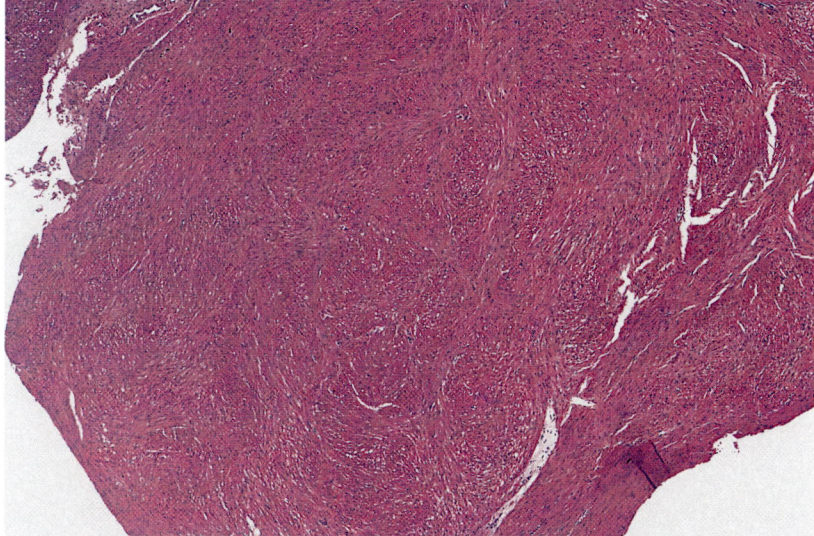

Figure 1-176: **Esophagus. Leiomyoma.** Proliferation of spindle cells arranged in interlacing fascicles.

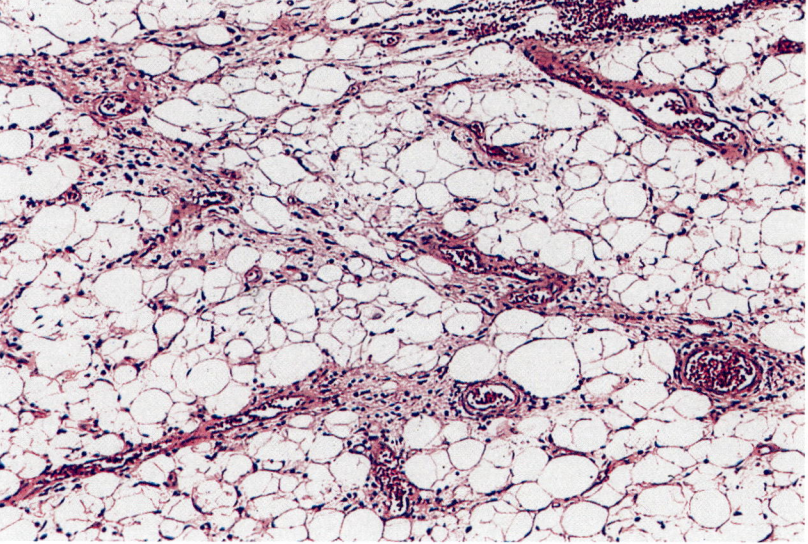

Figure 1-177: **Esophagus. Lipoma.** Well-vascularized mature adipose tissue.

CHAPTER 2

STOMACH

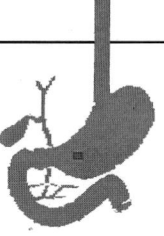

Endoscopic examination 78	Benign ulcers 125
Histology 79	Cameron erosion 129
Normal stomach 80	Dieulafoy lesion 131
Patterns of injury: gastritis and gastropathy 84	Varices and vascular malformations 132
Acute gastritis 87	Atrophic gastritis with carcinoid tumors 135
Active chronic gastritis 88	Carcinoid tumor 137
Focal atrophy/metaplasia and chronic atrophic gastritis 92	Pancreatic heterotopia and metaplasia 139
Lymphocytic gastritis 95	Fundic gland polyp 141
Eosinophilic gastritis 95	Hyperplastic polyp 143
Granulomatous gastritis 98	Juvenile polyp and Peutz-Jeghers polyp 145
Acute erosive gastropathy 101	Inflammatory fibroid polyp 147
Reactive gastropathy 103	Dysplasia 149
Reactive gastropathy, bile reflux 108	Adenoma 151
Xanthelasma 111	Malignant ulcer 153
Gastropathy, radiation/chemotherapy 113	Adenocarcinoma 155
Portal hypertensive gastropathy 115	Signet-ring cell carcinoma 159
Watermelon stomach 117	Malignant lymphoma 161
Hypertrophic gastropathy and gastritis 119	Stromal tumors (smooth muscle/stromal, neurogenic, lipomatous) 165
Cytomegalovirus gastropathy 122	Metastatic tumors 171
Miscellaneous infections 122	

ENDOSCOPIC EXAMINATION

A complete examination requires direct and retroflexed viewing, utilizing insufflation to separate the rugae. Pooled materials are evacuated to allow mucosal inspection in each anatomic region, noting landmarks and distensibility. Normal gastric mucosa is salmon-colored, in contrast to the pale esophageal mucosa. Its surface is uniform, without a distinctive pattern, and the grooves that define the areae gastricae (mosaic, snakeskin, or fishnet pattern) are usually not visible. The mucosa is assessed for nodules, masses, erythema, hemorrhage, erosions, and friability. Friability may be an indicator of a bleeding disorder or amyloidosis. A pale mucosa that reveals the submucosal vasculature suggests mucosal atrophy.

Upon completion of the antegrade examination of the stomach and duodenum, the retroflexed exam is performed. The distal rosette of any hiatal hernia is examined for Cameron erosions or ulcers, or the linear scars from these.

Biopsy is necessary to determine if the mucosa is normal, inflamed, affected by a chemical injury, gastropathy, or malignancy. A normal-appearing mucosa may be inflamed, while an erythematous mucosa may be merely congested.

Erythema may be focal or diffuse. Focal erythema may represent hemorrhage, congestion, or angiectasias. *Hemorrhagic erythema* due to trauma or stress is punctate and more vividly red than erythema due to congestion. *Congestive erythema* may or may not be associated with inflammation (gastritis or gastropathy) and may be focal or diffuse. *Portal hypertensive gastropathy* presents with diffuse, congestive erythema and a mucosal mosaic pattern, or with fine red miliary or speckled angiectasias, especially in the fundus. *Watermelon stomach* is characterized by angiectasias arrayed linearly along the crests of the antral folds but may be speckled and diffusely distributed, indistinguishable from antral angiectasias sometimes encountered in portal hypertensive gastropathy. *Radiation angiectasias* are usually antral and variable in size and shape. The angiectasias of *angiodysplasia* are usually discrete and distributed throughout the stomach. These lesions may be surrounded by a characteristic pale rim of mucosa referred to as the "halo sign." High-resolution video endoscopes may reveal the characteristics of angiectasias.

Ulcer size, location, and relative depth are noted. Smooth margins with orderly, radiating folds are features of peptic ulcers. In contrast, mucosal malignancies are irregular, raised, and nodular, with firm or friable margins. Peptic ulcers should be assessed for active or recent bleeding. In the absence of active bleeding, important observations include the presence of altered blood, a visible vessel (pigmented or nonpigmented protuberance), or a focally attached, dense, adherent clot over an exposed vessel.

Rugal folds are assessed by size and distensibility with air insufflation. Large firm folds suggest infiltrating malignant neoplasm, carcinoma or lymphoma. In these conditions the mucosal areae gastricae may be prominent. Loss of gastric distensibility may be the only indication of a diffusely infiltrating malignancy, typically signet-ring cell carcinoma. Endoscopic ultrasound, which images the composite layers of the gastric wall, is useful in identifying malignant infiltration that disrupts these layers.

Biopsies are taken using the same techniques as in the esophagus. Mucosectomy is more easily performed and is the preferred method for complete removal of focal lesions and for sampling enlarged folds. Biopsy texture gives added information. Malignant lesions are firm and tend to fragment when biopsied. Biopsy specimens should be taken from the edges of ulcers and also from the surrounding mucosa to determine whether gastritis is present.

HISTOLOGY

The gastric mucosa is composed of foveolar and glandular compartments. The superficial mucosa contains the foveolar compartment, characterized by tall columnar cells with abundant eosinophilic cytoplasm. The deep mucosa contains the glandular compartment composed of mucous, parietal, chief, and endocrine cells.

The foveolae are widely separated, sometimes having a villous architecture. The portion of the foveolar compartment that dips down to the glandular compartment, is termed the gastric pit. Undifferentiated stem cells are located at the junction of the foveolar and glandular compartments at the base of the gastric pit. These undifferentiated cells turn over every 3 to 6 days and differentiate into foveolar cells and specialized glandular cells, e.g., mucous, parietal, chief, and endocrine cells. Mucosal injury causes proliferation of these undifferentiated cells, which results in elongation of the proliferative zone, i.e., foveolar hyperplasia.

The glandular compartments of the antrum and cardia are similar, being composed of coiled glands lined by cuboidal mucous cells, occasional parietal (oxyntic) cells, and endocrine cells. The glands in the cardia are widely spaced and often cystic, but are otherwise indistinguishable from the antrum. The glands of the body/fundus are straight, tubular, and composed of mucous neck, parietal (oxyntic), chief, and endocrine cells. The mucous neck cells are located in the upper third near the junction of the glands and gastric pits; parietal cells predominate at the midgland region; and chief cells are concentrated in the lower third of the glands. The foveolar/glandular ratio of the antrum/cardia is about 1:1 and that of the body/fundus is about 1:4. In atrophic gastritis, there may be loss of glands and/or the glands of the fundus and body are replaced with goblet cells or mucin-secreting cells similar to antral/pyloric glands.

At regular intervals, the surface epithelium dips to the muscularis mucosae, where it forms a mosaic of grooves defining the areae gastricae (Fig. 2-6). These grooves accommodate gastric expansion. In portal hypertension and other congestive conditions, the grooves may appear as a mosaic (fishnet or snakeskin) pattern of white lines.

The lamina propria contains widely scattered inflammatory cells (plasma cells, lymphocytes, and eosinophils). They are more numerous toward the mucosal surface and in the antrum. Isolated lymphoid aggregates are sparsely dispersed along the muscularis mucosae (Fig. 2-6). Neutrophils outside of the vascular compartment are abnormal.

The microvascular system consists of arterioles, which penetrate the muscularis mucosae and give rise to a capillary network beneath the surface epithelial basement membrane (Fig. 2-8). The capillaries collect into venules, which descend to the submucosa. Following an inflammatory stimulus, neutrophils and mononuclear cells are released just beneath the surface epithelium, forming a superficial band of gastritis, which, with time, extends to the deep mucosa. In chronic venous hypertension, the superficial venules and capillaries become ectatic and their walls sclerotic.

The muscularis mucosae consists of a double layer of smooth muscle cells separating the mucosa from the submucosa. Individual smooth muscle fibers course perpendicularly through the lamina propria and attach to the sides of the glands and the surface epithelium to anchor and order the mucosa (Fig. 2-10). The smooth muscle fibers are more prominent in the antrum than in the body, presumably due to forceful antral contractions and mucosal prolapse common to this area.

NORMAL STOMACH

- Morphology .... The gastric mucosa is composed of a superficial foveolar and a deep glandular compartment. The latter consists of mucous glands in the cardia and antrum and oxyntic glands in the fundus and body. The cardia resembles the antrum, except that the glands are more widely spaced and often cystic. Scattered inflammatory cells (plasma cells, eosinophils, and lymphocytes) and isolated lymphoid nodules are normal components. Neutrophils outside of the vascular compartment are abnormal. Individual smooth muscle cells are more prominent in the antrum than in the body/fundus.

- Endoscopic features .... The gastric mucosa is examined with attention to distensibility, anatomic landmarks (the squamocolumnar junction, lesser curvature, incisura, and pylorus), and the anatomic regions of the stomach (antrum, body, fundus, and cardia). The examination includes retroflexion to visualize the proximal stomach.

    Prior to air insufflation, rugal folds are easily seen within the body of the stomach (Fig. 2-2). In between antral contractions, the antrum fills out well and the pylorus is seen at various stages of patency, depending on motile activity. The normal stomach should distend well, and a flattening of the rugal folds (Figs. 2-3 and 2-4) can be expected. Secretions are commonly encountered along the greater curvature within the more proximal body and fundus.

- Differential diagnosis ...... Endoscopic: Normal mucosa may be histologically abnormal. Erythematous mucosa may be histologically normal or show only mild congestion.

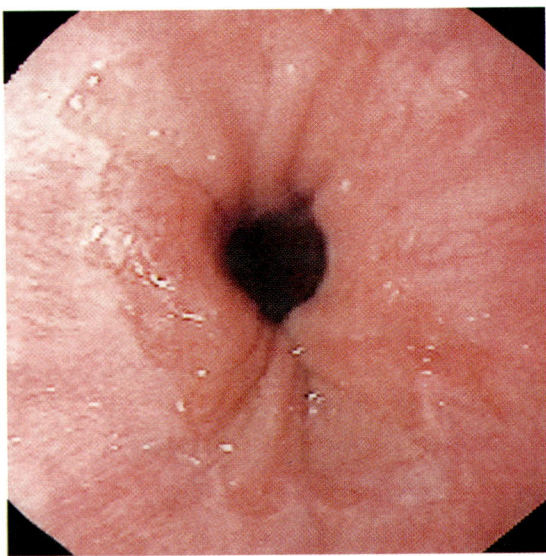

Figure 2-1: **Stomach. Normal Gastroesophageal Junction.** Pale squamous mucosa contrasts with the pink, glistening gastric mucosa.

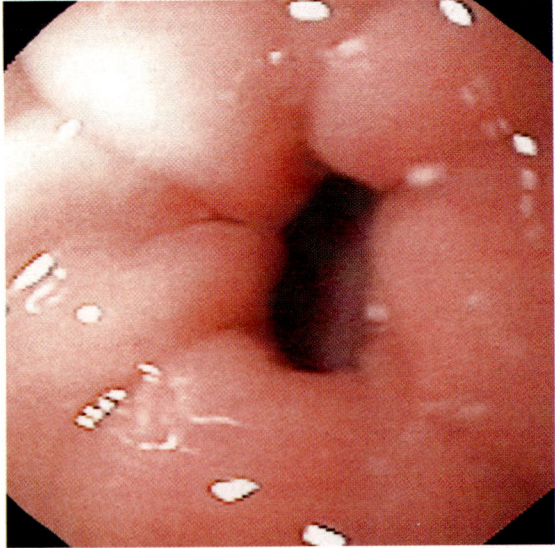

Figure 2-2: **Stomach. Normal.** Rugal folds prior to air insufflation.

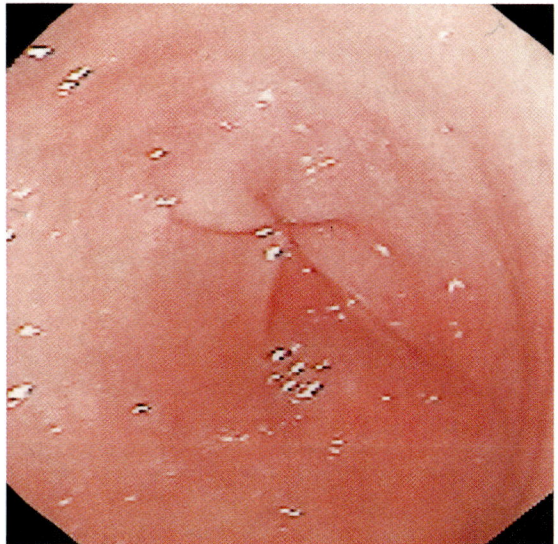

Figure 2-3: **Stomach. Normal.** Pink, glistening, flattened antral mucosa following air insufflation.

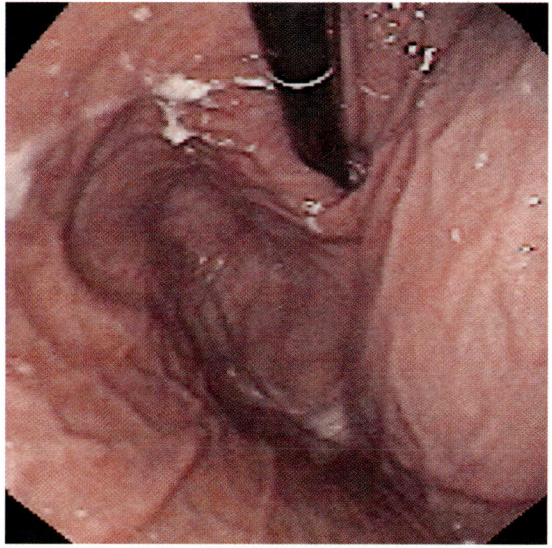

Figure 2-4: **Stomach. Normal.** Retroflexed view of fundus and cardia illustrates flattened rugal folds in a well-distended stomach. Cardia is snug around the insertion tube of the endoscope.

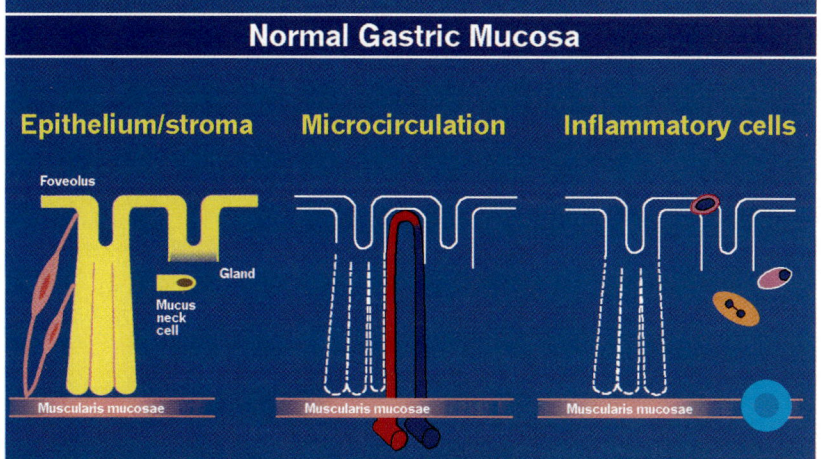

Figure 2-5: **Stomach. Normal.** Diagram depicts features of normal gastric mucosa, specifically the foveolar, neck, and glandular compartments and their support structures; the microvascular compartment; and the distribution of inflammatory cells.

Figure 2-6: **Stomach, Body/Fundus. Normal.** The mucosa consists of a superficial foveolar and a deep glandular compartment. At regular intervals the surface epithelium dips to the muscularis mucosae, forming grooves defining the areae gastricae. The foveolar/glandular ratio is about 1:4. An isolated lymphoid nodule is at the muscularis mucosae.

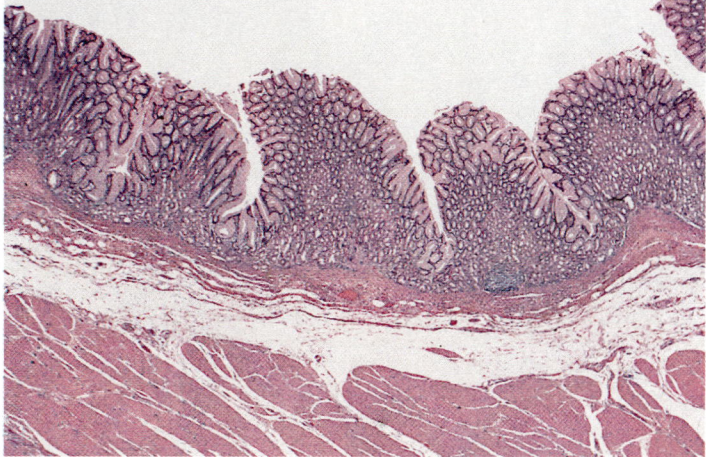

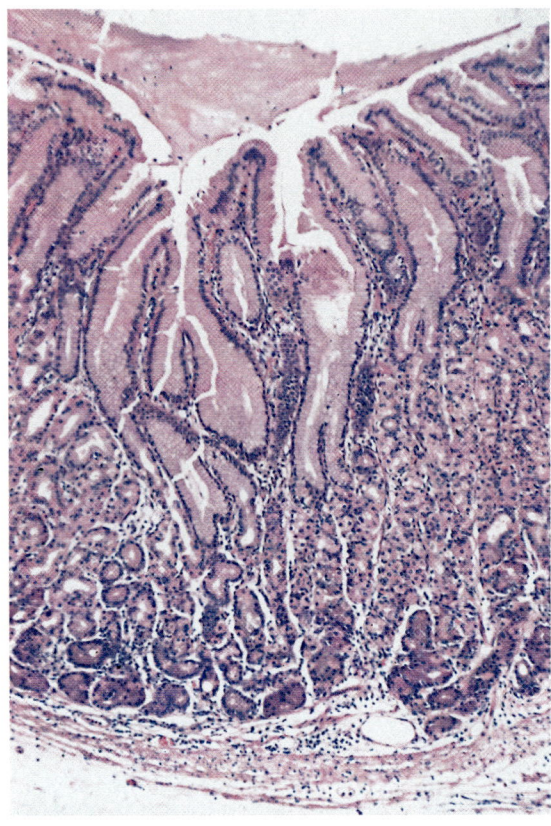

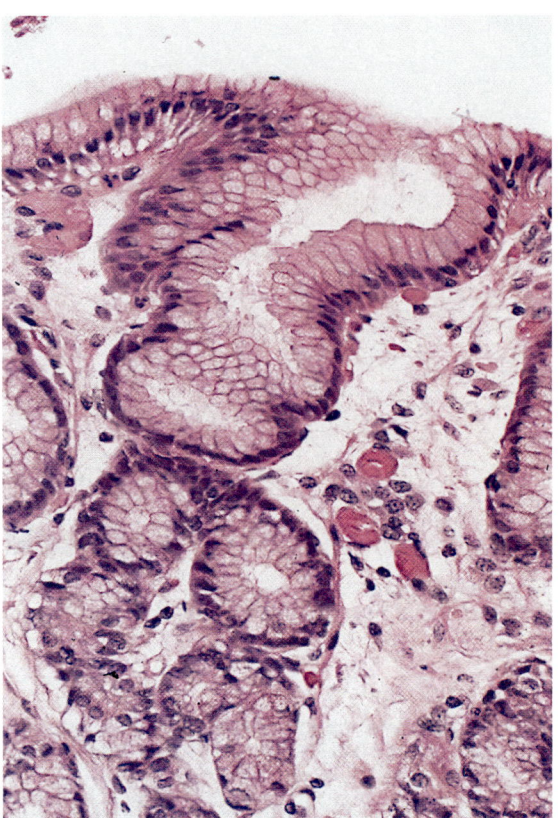

Figure 2-7: **Stomach. Normal Body/Fundus.** The foveolar compartment contains the foveolae/gastric pits and is covered by a layer of insoluble mucin. The pits are lined by columnar cells with abundant pale, eosinophilic cytoplasm containing mucin. Straight, parallel, evenly spaced tubular glands extend from the bases of the pits. Mucous neck cells are concentrated near the neck, parietal cells in the midportion, and chief cells in the base of the glands. Occasional inflammatory cells are in the lamina propria. A dilated lymphatic channel is above the muscularis mucosae.

Figure 2-8: **Stomach. Normal Foveolar Compartment.** The cellular components in the lamina propria include stromal cells and rare plasma cells. The capillary network located directly beneath the surface epithelium contains occasional circulating neutrophils. Foveolar cell cytoplasm is abundant and clear/eosinophilic, and the nuclei are small, round, regular, and basally oriented. Mitotic figures are absent. The cells in the proliferative zone (junction of the foveolae and glands) have less cytoplasm, and the nuclei appear more basophilic.

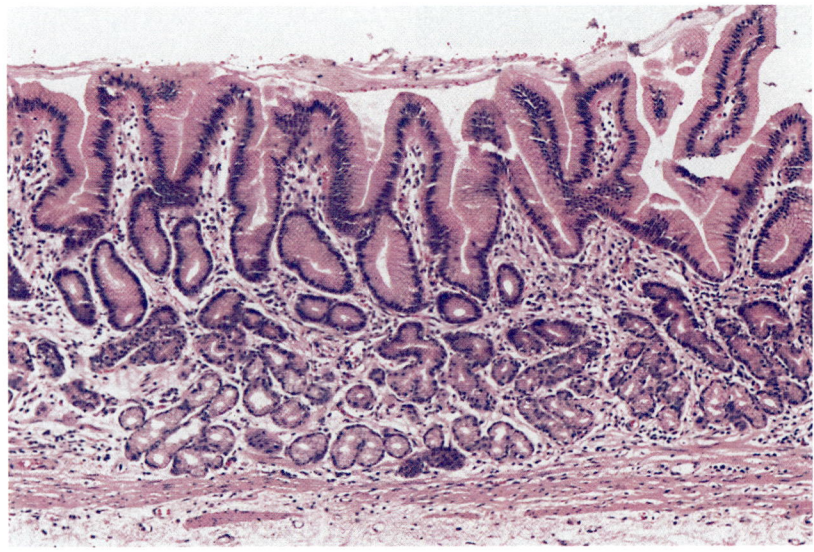

Figure 2-9: **Stomach. Normal Antrum.** The foveolar/glandular ratio is about 1:1. The glandular compartment consists of coiled, irregularly spaced, mucin-secreting glands. Plasma cells, lymphocytes, and eosinophils are more frequent in the antrum than in the body.

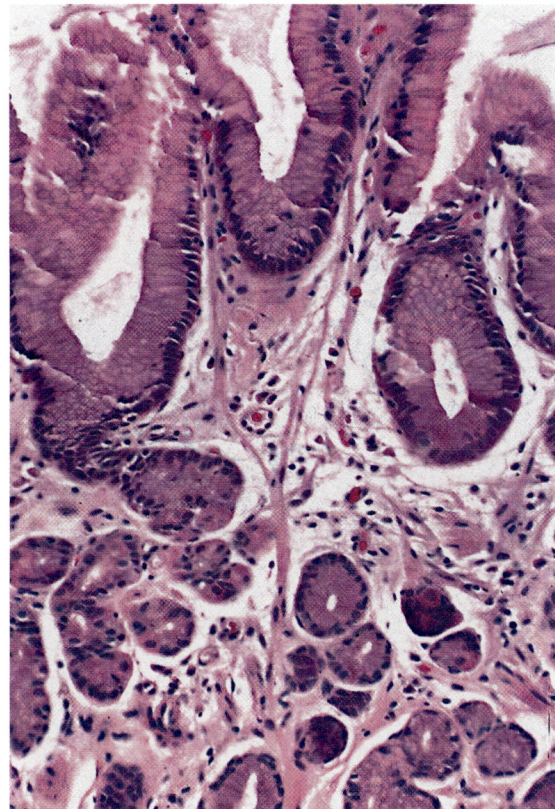

Figure 2-10: **Stomach. Normal Antrum.** Individual muscle fibers from muscularis mucosae extend vertically through the lamina propria to attach to the sides of the glands, foveolae, and surface epithelium.

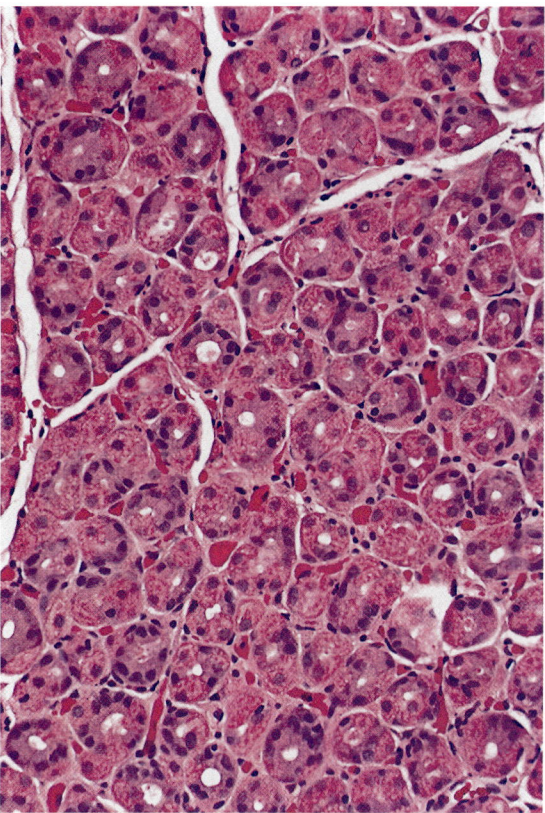

Figure 2-11: **Stomach. Normal Body/Fundus.** Oblique section demonstrates closely packed, evenly spaced glands of uniform diameter. Parietal cells are abundant in this midgland cross section.

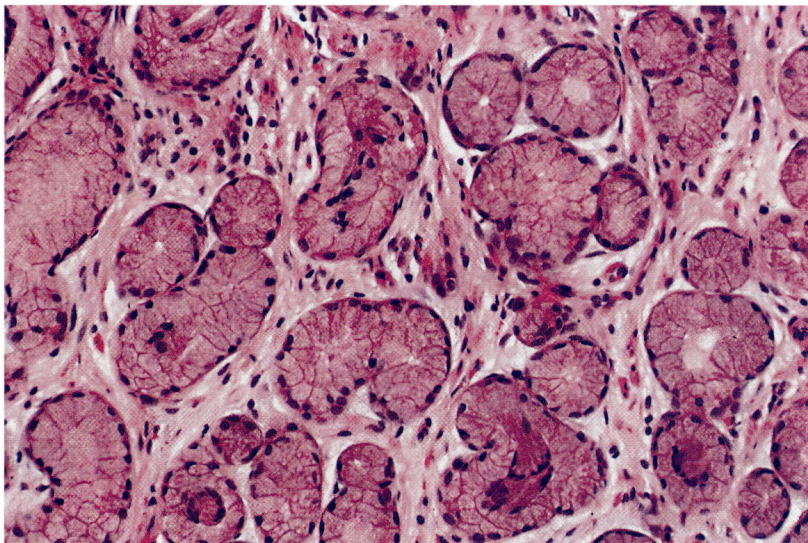

Figure 2-12: **Stomach. Normal Antrum.** Oblique section shows irregularly shaped and spaced glands lined by mucous cells. Most of the cells in the lamina propria are stromal (fibrocytes, endothelial cells, and smooth muscle cells).

PATTERNS OF INJURY: GASTRITIS AND GASTROPATHY

Some agents that injure the gastric mucosa elicit inflammation; some do not. In our opinion, the term *gastritis* is best reserved for conditions characterized by inflammation, and *gastropathy* for those with evidence of injury to the epithelium or endothelium in the absence of inflammation.

Both gastritis and gastropathy can be divided into a limited number of reaction patterns, each with a different set of potential etiologies and clinical associations. Patterns of gastritis and gastropathy, exclusive of specific infections, are described in Tables 2-1 and 2-2.

Table 2-1. Patterns of gastritis

Pathologic Diagnosis	Pathologic Findings	Etiology	Possible Endoscopic Findings	Probable Clinical Associations
Acute gastritis	Neutrophilic inflammation	*H pylori*	Normal; large folds, erosions	Acute gastroenteritis
		Streptococcal species, other bacteria	Erythema, distended stomach, exudate	Perforation, gangrene
Chronic and active chronic gastritis, common pattern	Mixed inflammation +/- foveolar hyperplasia, erosion/ulcer, intestinal metaplasia, atrophy	*H pylori*, *H heilmanii*, autoimmune	Normal erythema, nodularity, and friability; thin body folds with prominent vessels. Prominent mosaic mucosal surface pattern.	None, dyspepsia, duodenal or gastric ulcer, adenocarcinoma, MALT lymphoma, pernicious anemia
Distinctive patterns				
Lymphocytic gastritis	Common pattern and increased intraepithelial lymphocytes	Hypersensitivity to gliaden, other proteins; autoimmune	Chronic erosive gastritis (nodules with central ulceration), giant body folds	Celiac sprue, Menetrier disease, autoimmunity, *H pylori*
Granulomatous gastritis	Multifocal active chronic inflammation/ulcers/fissures/granulomas	Crohn's, sarcoid, idiopathic, fungi, mycobacteria, spirochetes, parasites, drugs, vasculitis; foreign body	Variable; thickened folds, ulceration	Depends on underlying disease
Eosinophilic gastritis	Sheets of eosinophils	Idiopathic, food and drug allergy, parasites	Prominent antral folds, hyperemia, nodularity, ulcer; normal	Pain, nausea, vomiting, early satiety, weight loss, anemia
Hypertrophic lymphocytic gastritis	Lymphocytic gastritis with extreme foveolar hyperplasia	Menetrier disease	Giant body folds	Pain, weight loss, vomiting, +/- protein loss

Adapted from *Gastroenterology*, 1995;108:917-924.

Table 2-2. Patterns of gastropathy

Pathologic Diagnosis	Pathologic Findings	Etiology	Possible Endoscopic Findings	Probable Clinical Associations
Acute erosive gastropathy	Microvascular ischemia (erosions), minimal focal inflammation	Alcohol, NSAIDs, other drugs, hypovolemia, stress, uremia, etc.	Erosions, subepithelial hemorrhages	Bleeding
Reactive gastropathy, common pattern	Foveolar hyperplasia +/- erosion/ulcer. No inflammation except near ulcer.	NSAIDs, bile reflux, uremia	Same as acute erosive gastropathy	
Reactive gastropathy with features suggestive of bile reflux	Common pattern with subnuclear vacuoles	Bile reflux	Erythema, friability, bleeding	Vomiting bile, pain, usually post-Billroth I or II
Reactive gastropathy with features suggestive of radiation or chemotherapy	Common pattern with cellular and nuclear enlargement, vacuolization, macronucleoli	Radiation, chemotherapy	Ulcers, predominantly antral	Perforation, pain
Congestive gastropathy	Common pattern with superficial vascular ectasia +/- microthrombi	Portal hypertension	Antral erythema, red spots, mosaic pattern	Cirrhosis, bleeding, splenic vein thrombosis
		Watermelon stomach	Linear erythema on folds radiating from pylorus	Proximal gastric atrophy/ anemia
		Scleroderma		Sclerodactaly, CREST syndrome
Hypertrophic gastropathy	Massive foveolar hyperplasia with little or no inflammation	Menetrier disease	Giant body folds	Pain, weight loss, vomiting, +/- protein loss

Adapted from *Gastroenterology*, 1995;108:917-924.

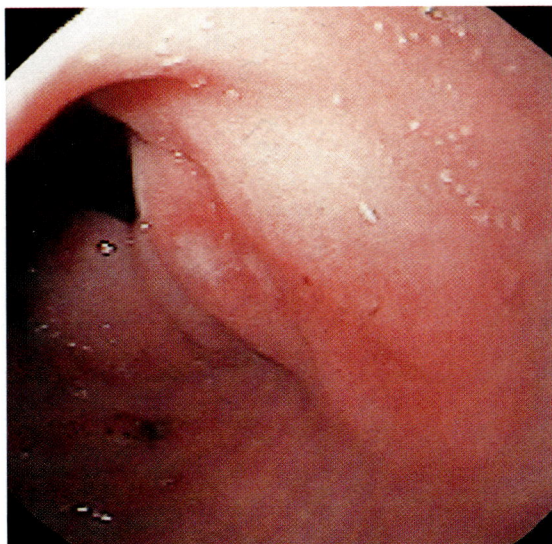

Figure 2-13: **Stomach. Gastric Erythema and Erosion.** Two small, shallow erosions in the prepyloric antrum. Etiology is unclear; NSAID injury or *H pylori* infection may have this endoscopic appearance.

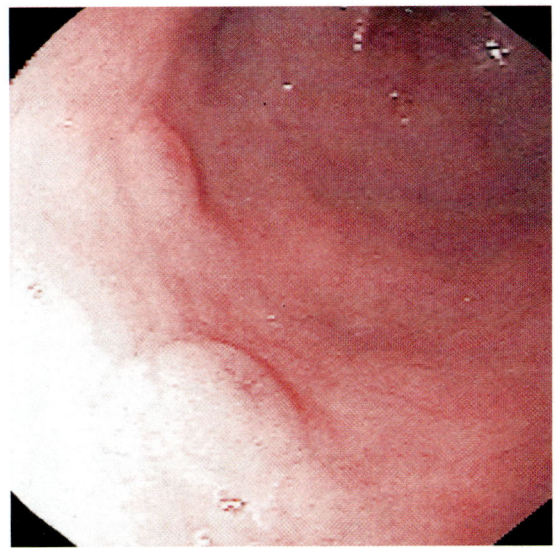

Figure 2-14: **Stomach. Gastric Nodules with Erosion.** Mild erythema and small, raised nodules with surface erosions. Biopsy revealed reactive gastropathy with erosions.

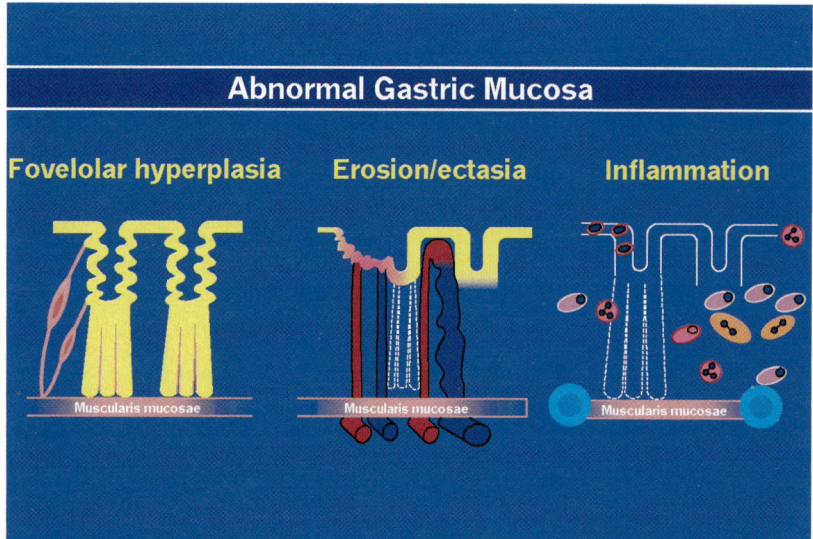

Figure 2-15: **Stomach. Patterns of Injury.** Diagram illustrates tortuosity of the gastric pits, vascular abnormalities with associated erosions and ectasia, and inflammation—all features of mucosal injury from a variety of causes.

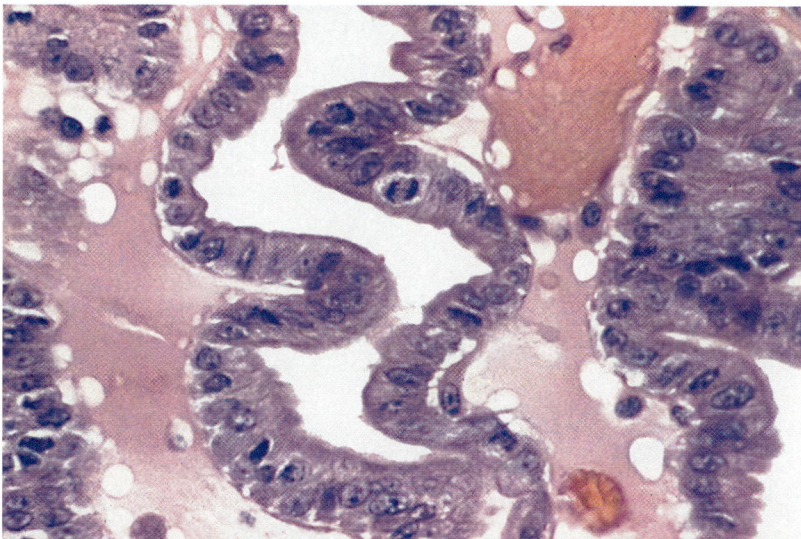

Figure 2-16: **Stomach. Foveolar Hyperplasia in Reactive Gastropathy.** In addition to foveolar hyperplasia, the lamina propria is edematous. Capillaries and venules are dilated. No inflammatory exudate.

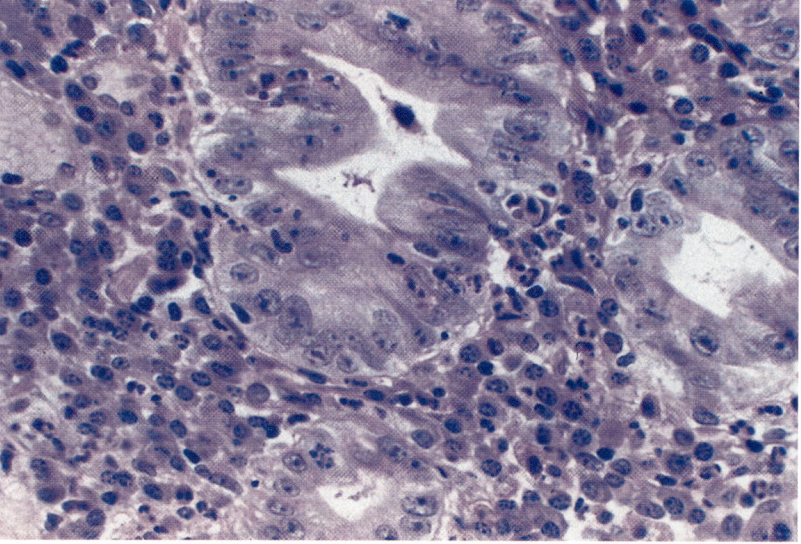

Figure 2-17: **Stomach. Foveolar Hyperplasia in Active Chronic Gastritis.** Inflammation expands the lamina propria. Neutrophils infiltrate the epithelium. Foveolae are tortuous, and epithelial cells show reactive/regenerative change.

ACUTE GASTRITIS

- Morphology .... Neutrophilic inflammation without increased mononuclear inflammatory cells.
- Endoscopic features .... May be normal or enlarged mucosal folds, erythema, and erosions.
- Clinical features .... Acute gastroenteritislike illness.
- Differential diagnosis ...... Etiologic: *H pylori* (acute), streptococcus, other bacteria. (See Table 2-1.)

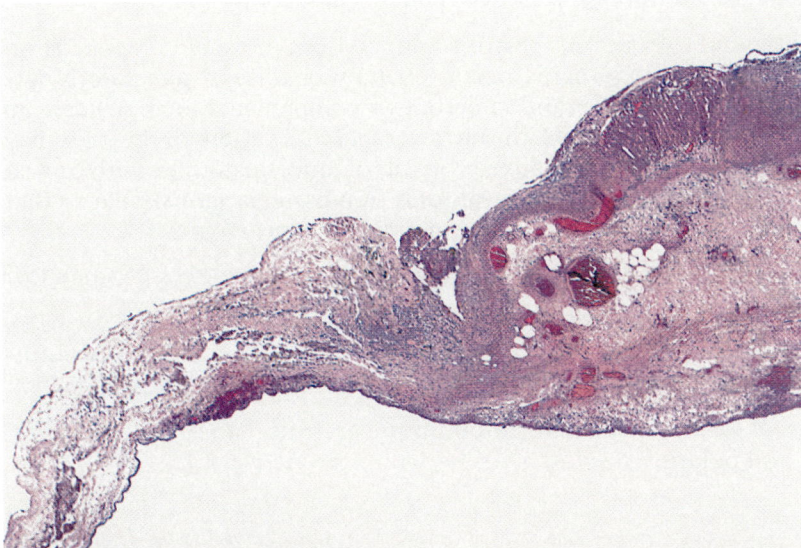

Figure 2-18: **Stomach. Acute Gastric Ulcer.** Deep, penetrating ulcer with near dissolution of the wall and serositis. Minimal chronic inflammation or fibrosis indicates an acute process.

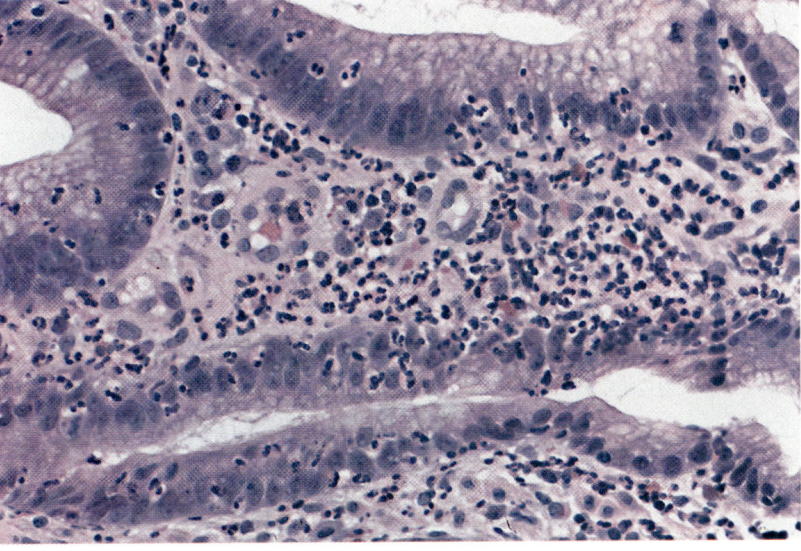

Figure 2-19: **Stomach. Acute Gastritis.** Neutrophils fill lamina propria and infiltrate epithelium. Few plasma cells present. Swollen endothelial cells with prominent nuclei may be confused with mononuclear inflammatory cells.

ACTIVE CHRONIC GASTRITIS

- Morphology .... See Table 2-1. A significant mononuclear cell infiltrate is the hallmark of chronic gastritis. In active chronic gastritis, there are also neutrophils in the lamina propria and infiltrating the gastric epithelium. *H pylori* is the cause of over 90% of cases of active chronic gastritis. Other causes include Crohn's disease, autoimmune gastritis, and rare infectious agents such as *H heilmanii*. The topography of active chronic gastritis varies with etiology. *H pylori* gastritis is generally a diffuse, antral-predominant infection; however, the organisms may shift proximally with antisecretory therapy or bile reflux. Autoimmune gastritis predominates in the body. Crohn's disease is usually patchy, antral-predominant, and occasionally associated with granulomas. In *H pylori* gastritis, when the organism is eliminated, neutrophils disappear in a few weeks, but mononuclear cells may persist for up to a year.

- Endoscopic features .... The appearance of chronic gastritis ranges from normal to varioliform gastritis (Fig. 2-22). Erythema may be patchy or diffuse, punctate, finely speckled or in linear streaks, and sometimes accompanied by hemorrhages up to 5 mm. The mucosa may lack the normal rugal fold pattern or the folds may be enlarged. The varioliform pattern consists of mucosal nodules with central erosions, often on the crests of rugal folds. A mosaic pattern similar to that seen in portal hypertension is sometimes due to *H pylori* gastritis.

- Clinical features .... Asymptomatic, dyspepsia, ulcer symptoms.

- Differential diagnosis ...... Histologic: Artifactual strands of tenacious mucus may mimic *H pylori*. Additional stains, e.g., Wenger-Angritt, Genta, and Giemsa, and immunohistochemical reactions are useful as ancillary procedures to identify *H pylori*.

    Etiologic: *H pylori*, *H heilmanii*, autoimmune gastritis, Crohn's disease, lymphoma, and polyps.

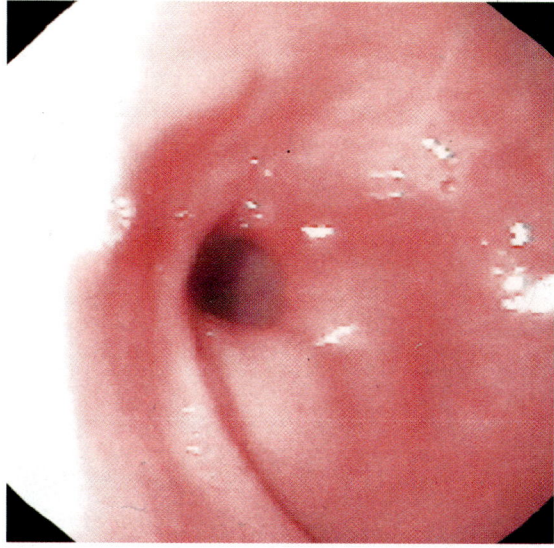

Figure 2-20: **Stomach, Antrum. Active Chronic Gastritis.** Stenotic pylorus. Rimlike fold may represent scar from previous ulcer. Mottled erythema in antrum suggests active inflammation.

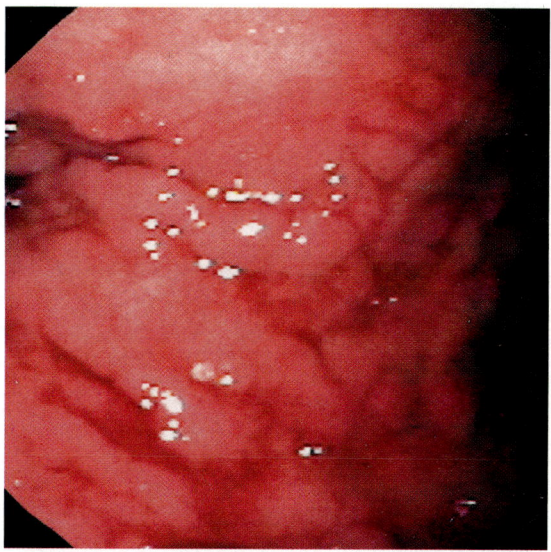

Figure 2-21: **Stomach, Fundus. Active Chronic Gastritis.** Prominent erythematous, friable rugal folds in body of stomach. Friability correlates with active inflammation.

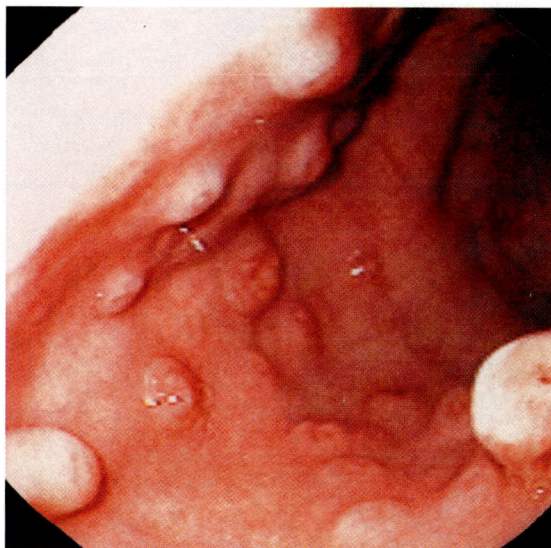

Figure 2-22: **Stomach, Antrum. Active Chronic Gastritis with Erosions.** Multiple nodules with erosions in body of stomach. This has been referred to as varioliform gastritis and reflects a chronic erosive inflammatory process.

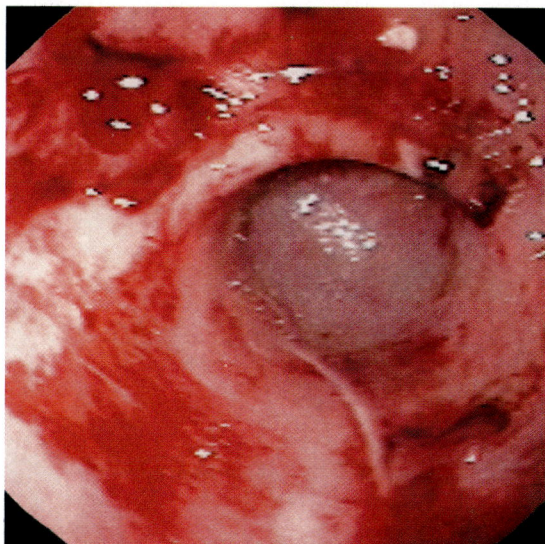

Figure 2-23: **Stomach, Antrum. Active Chronic Gastritis with Hemorrhage.** Florid hemorrhagic gastritis. Patchy erythema and mucosal hemorrhage without obvious erosions or ulceration.

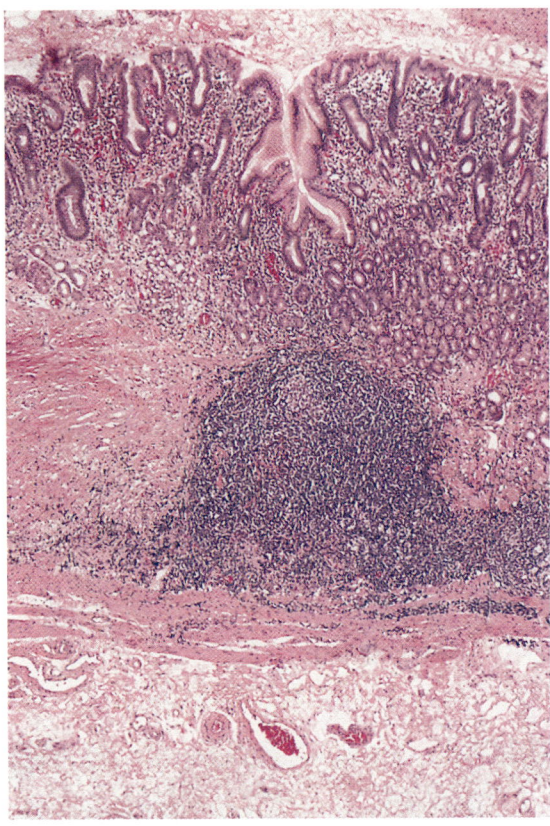

Figure 2-24: **Stomach, Antrum. Active Chronic Gastritis with Lymphoid Hyperplasia.** Lymphoid nodule in chronic gastritis beneath groove on edge of areae gastricae.

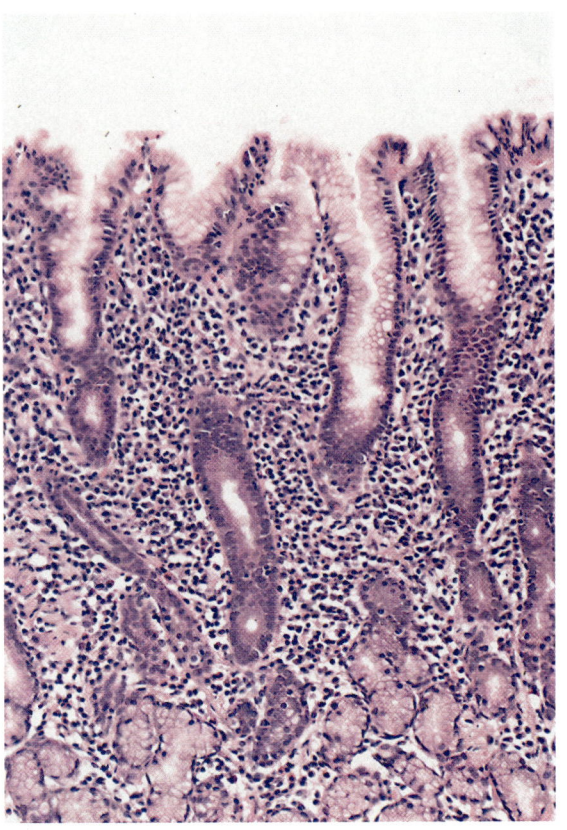

Figure 2-25: **Stomach, Antrum. Active Chronic Gastritis.** Chronic inflammatory infiltrate expands upper lamina propria. Rare neutrophils infiltrate gastric pits.

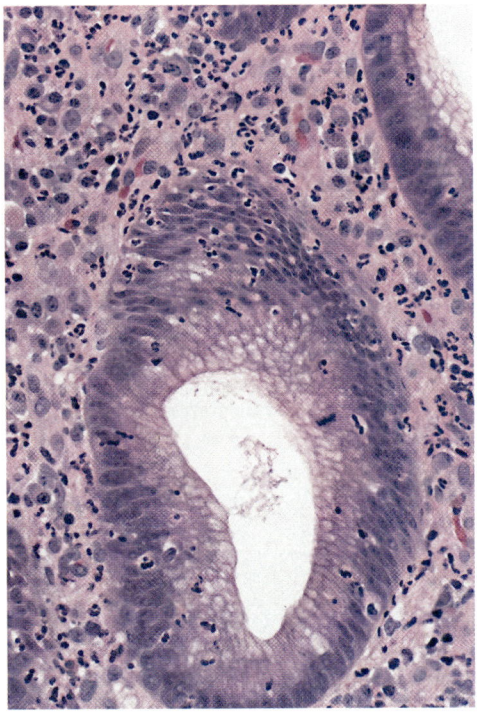

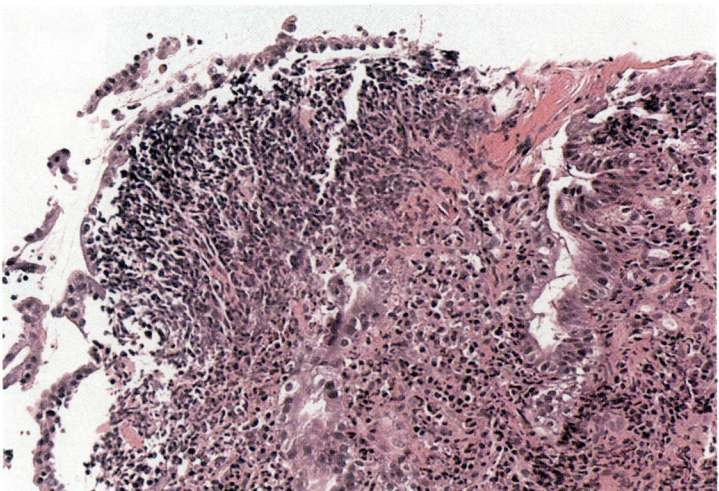

Figure 2-26: **Stomach, Antrum. Active Chronic Gastritis with Erosion.** Edge of erosion. Necrotic inflammatory cells suggest pre-existing intense inflammation.

Figure 2-27: **Stomach, Antrum. Active Chronic Gastritis.** Neutrophils associated with reactive/regenerative epithelium.

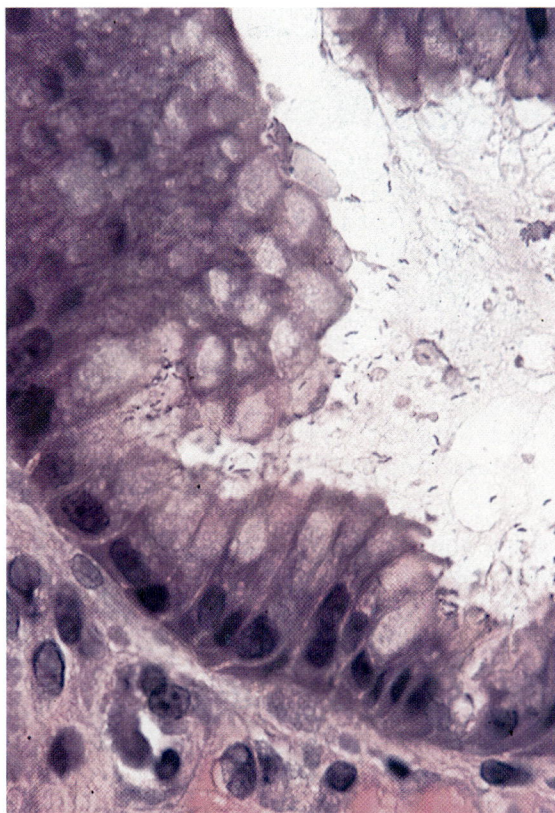

Figure 2-28: **Stomach. *H pylori*.** Numerous curved bacteria in overlying mucus.

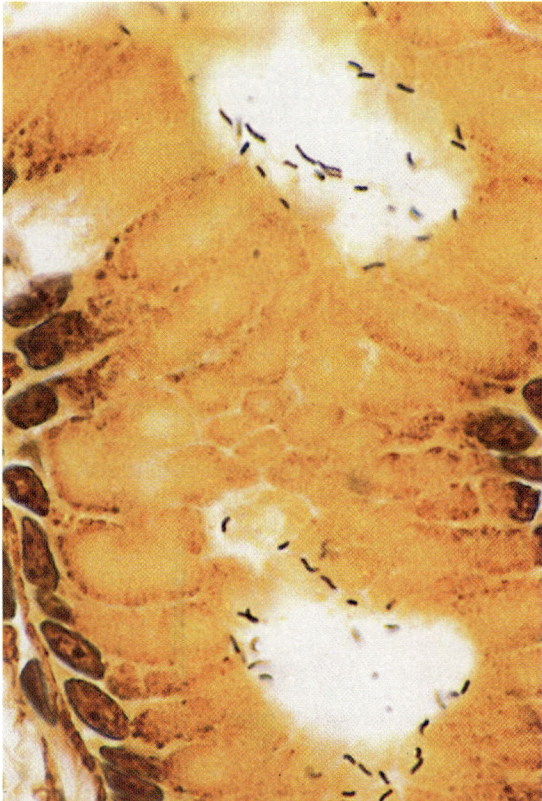

Figure 2-29: **Stomach. *H pylori*.** Wenger-Angritt stain demonstrates *H pylori* (4 to 8 microns).

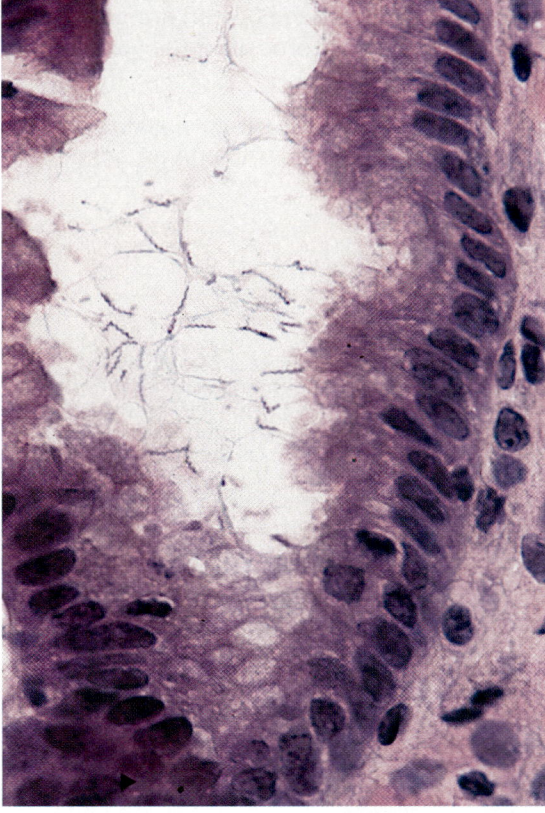

Figure 2-30: **Stomach. *H heilmanii*.** Long, tightly coiled bacteria in mucus. Length (10 to 15 microns) and coiled appearance distinguish *H heilmanii* from *H pylori*.

FOCAL ATROPHY/METAPLASIA AND CHRONIC ATROPHIC GASTRITIS

- Morphology .... Gastric atrophy means loss of gastric glands or a significant loss of functional glandular mucosa (e.g., by intestinal metaplasia). The histologic criteria for atrophy are not clearly defined and are somewhat controversial. Intestinal metaplasia may evolve from a variety of chronic injuries, most often chronic gastritis. Isolated foci of goblet cells are not equivalent with atrophy. Body glands are often replaced by pyloric/antral glands; occasionally, this is the only change. Pyloric metaplasia alone can only be recognized if the biopsy location is known. Atrophy may occur as a focal or multifocal process throughout the stomach, or as a generalized process affecting the body of the stomach.

- Endoscopic features .... If atrophy is extensive and involves the body, the characteristic findings are loss of rugal folds and a prominent visible submucosal vascular network. Intestinal metaplasia in the body may appear as pink or white, raised or nodular islands surrounded by pale mucosa and a prominent network of submucosal vessels. In the antrum, intestinal metaplasia is recognized as small, irregular, white, or salmon-colored plaques.

- Clinical features .... Focal or multifocal atrophy is asymptomatic and usually does not produce significant loss of function. It is important because intestinal metaplasia heralds increased risk for neoplasia. The clinicopathologic entity of atrophic gastritis is associated with loss of acid secretion, B_{12} deficiency, and ultimately pernicious anemia. Chronic atrophic gastritis of the body is common in the watermelon stomach syndrome. Findings of chronic atrophic gastritis can support the diagnosis.

- Differential diagnosis ...... Endoscopic: Nodular intestinal metaplasia must be distinguished from sessile polyps that occur in the same setting, e.g., hyperplastic polyps, adenomas, and carcinoids.

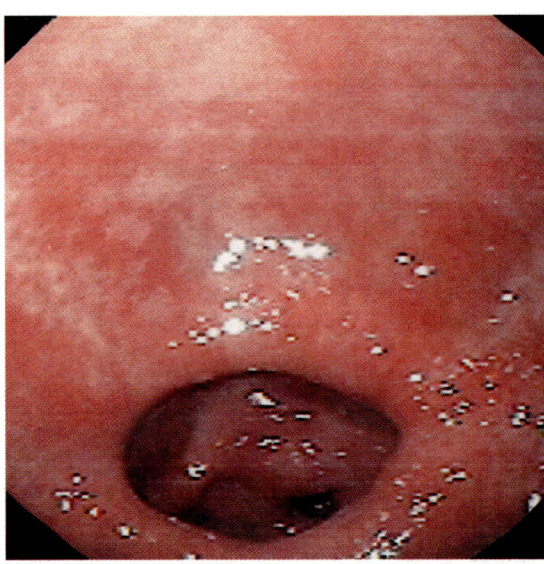

Figure 2-31: **Stomach, Antrum. Active Chronic Gastritis with Intestinal Metaplasia.** Mucosa mottled and erythematous, with slightly raised pale areas suggestive of intestinal metaplasia.

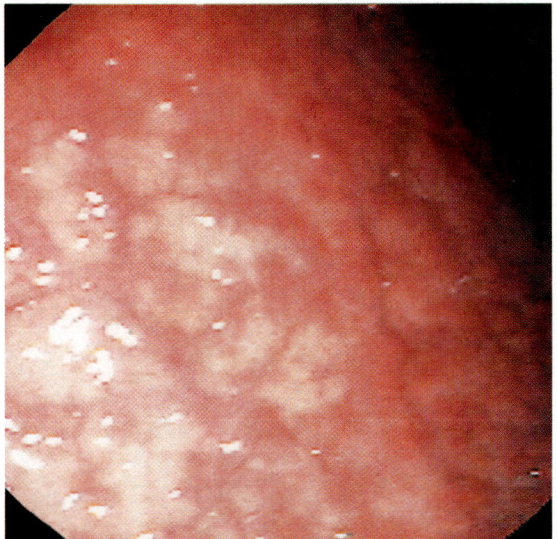

Figure 2-32: **Stomach, Body. Active Chronic Gastritis, Intestinal Metaplasia, *H pylori*.** Pale mucosa with prominent submucosal vascular patterns and raised nodular white patches of intestinal metaplasia.

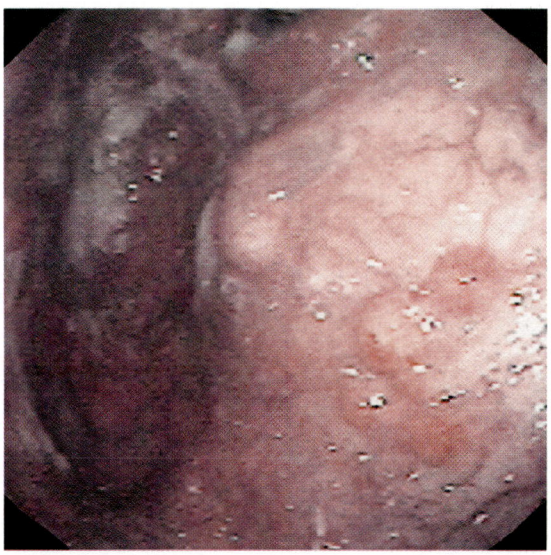

Figure 2-33: **Stomach. Chronic Atrophic Gastritis.** Small nodular islands of intestinal metaplasia in the background of a thin mucosa with prominent submucosal vasculature.

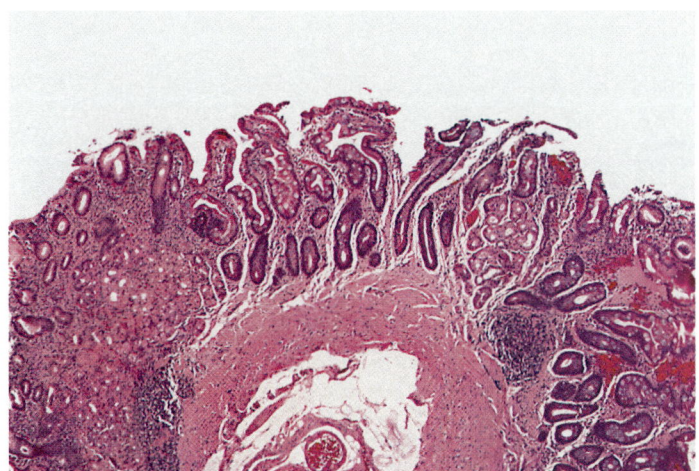

Figure 2-34: **Stomach, Body. Chronic Atrophic Gastritis.** Residual inflamed body-type mucosa (left); extensive intestinal and focal pyloric metaplasia (right).

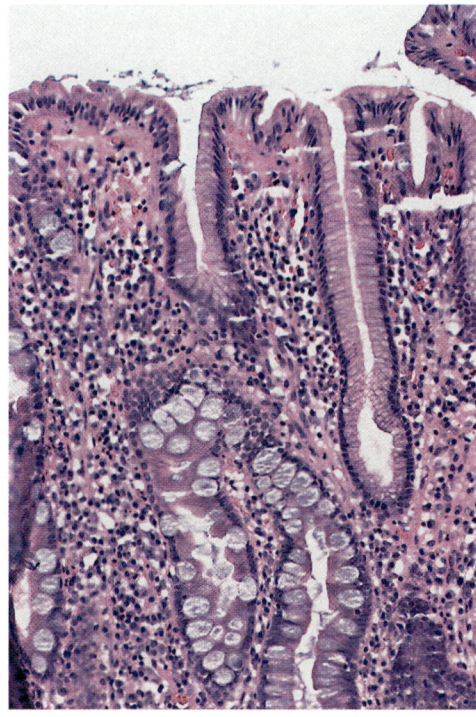

Figure 2-35: **Stomach. Chronic Gastritis, Intestinal Metaplasia.** Goblet and intestinal absorptive cells partially replace foveolar epithelium.

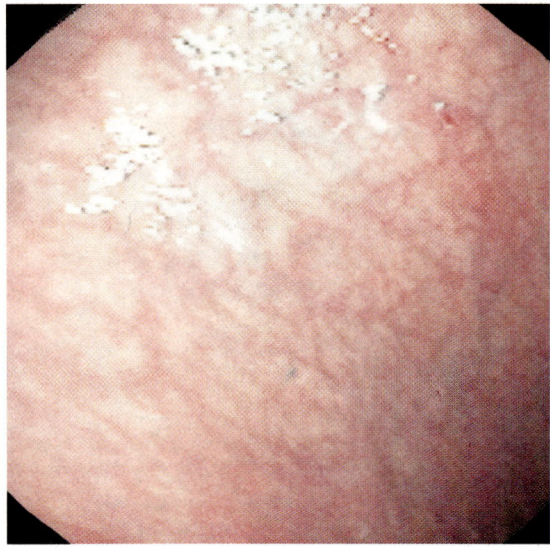

Figure 2-36: **Stomach, Body. Chronic Atrophic Gastritis.** Classic appearance of atrophic gastritis with dropout of rugal folds and thin mucosa. The submucosal vascular network is readily apparent.

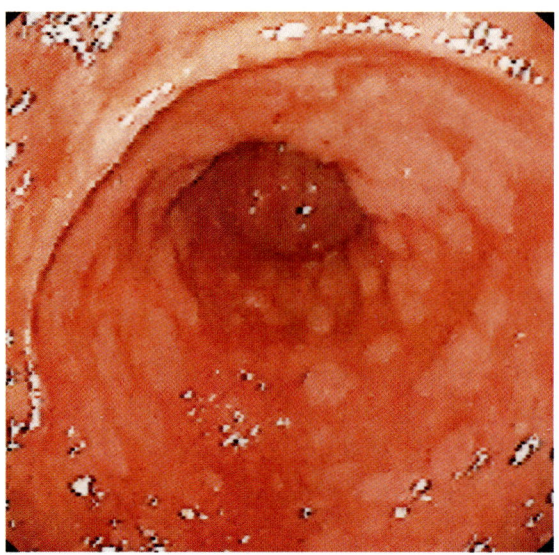

Figure 2-37: **Stomach, Antrum. Chronic Atrophic Gastritis.** Multiple irregular islands of intestinal metaplasia in the immediate prepyloric area. The mucosa surrounding the islands of metaplasia shows submucosal vasculature, consistent with atrophy.

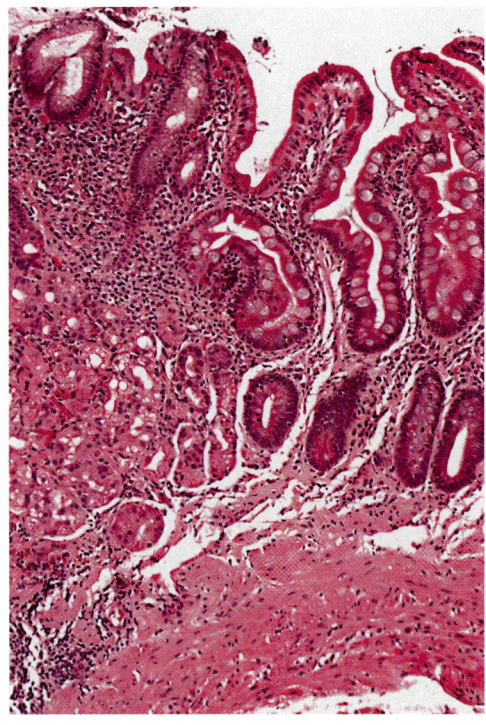

Figure 2-38: **Stomach, Body. Chronic Atrophic Gastritis.** Body mucosa replaced by intestinalized epithelium with goblet, absorptive, and Paneth cells. Residual body-type glands (left).

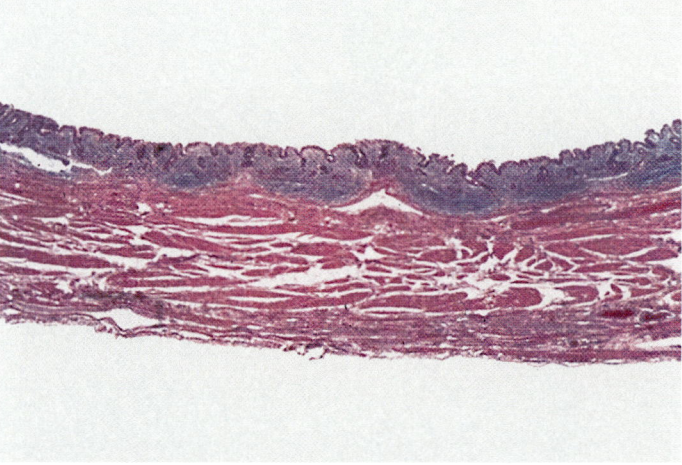

Figure 2-39: **Stomach, Body. Chronic Atrophic Gastritis.** Body mucosa is chronically inflamed and completely replaced by a thin, intestinalized mucosa with lymphoid hyperplasia.

LYMPHOCYTIC GASTRITIS

- Morphology .... Indistinguishable from the common pattern of active chronic gastritis, except for increased numbers of intraepithelial T-lymphocytes, which characterize the lesion. Lymphocytic gastritis is a pangastritis that is often body-predominant, but antrum is more involved in celiac sprue.

- Endoscopic features .... The mucosa may be normal or have focal or diffuse erythema, granularity, friability with or without ulcers, varioliform features or focal hypertrophic changes.

- Clinical features .... Dyspepsia, malabsorption syndrome or Menetrier syndrome.

- Differential diagnosis ...... Histologic: Active chronic gastritis.

    Endoscopic: Any gastritis, gastropathy.

    Etiologic: Celiac sprue, hypersensitivity to other antigens, Menetrier, and *H pylori*.

EOSINOPHILIC GASTRITIS

- Morphology .... The antrum is most frequently involved. Infiltrates affect any layer(s), most commonly submucosa and muscularis propria. Submucosal edema is frequently severe. Mucosal involvement is typically patchy, necessitating multiple biopsies.

- Endoscopic features .... Normal or nonspecific findings include erythema with a variety of patterns and distribution. Diagnosis is dependent upon random mucosal biopsies.

- Clinical features .... Symptoms reflect layer involved: mucosa—diarrhea; submucosa and muscularis propria—obstruction; subserosa—ascites.

- Differential diagnosis ...... Histologic: Active chronic gastritis, common pattern.

    Endoscopic: Any gastritis, gastropathy.

    Clinical: Eosinophilic gastritis resulting from allergic reactions to foods, drugs, or parasites; hypereosinophilic syndromes; Churg-Strauss vasculitis; and the idiopathic form.

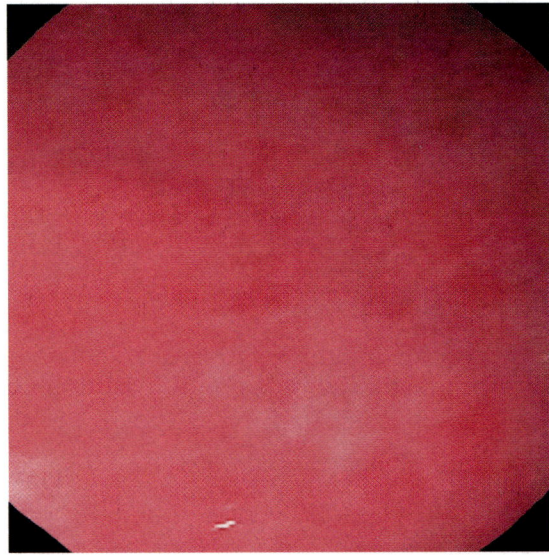

Figure 2-40: **Stomach, Antrum. Lymphocytic Gastritis.** There is an irregular pattern of erythema that is nonspecific but suggestive of gastritis.

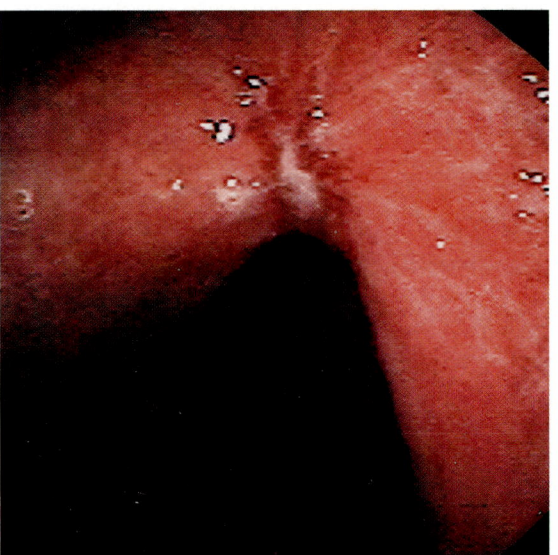

Figure 2-41: **Stomach. Lymphocytic Gastritis.** Shallow ulcer, not raised above the mucosal level, favors benign etiology. Radiating folds toward ulcer suggest healing.

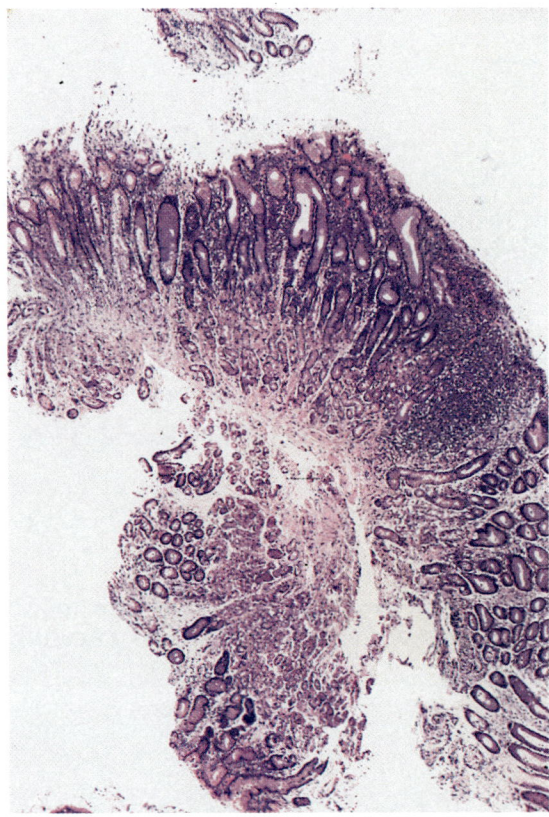

Figure 2-42: **Stomach, Body. Lymphocytic Gastritis.** Eroded nodule on the crest of a large fold in body (varioliform gastritis). The nodule consists of localized lymphocytic gastritis.

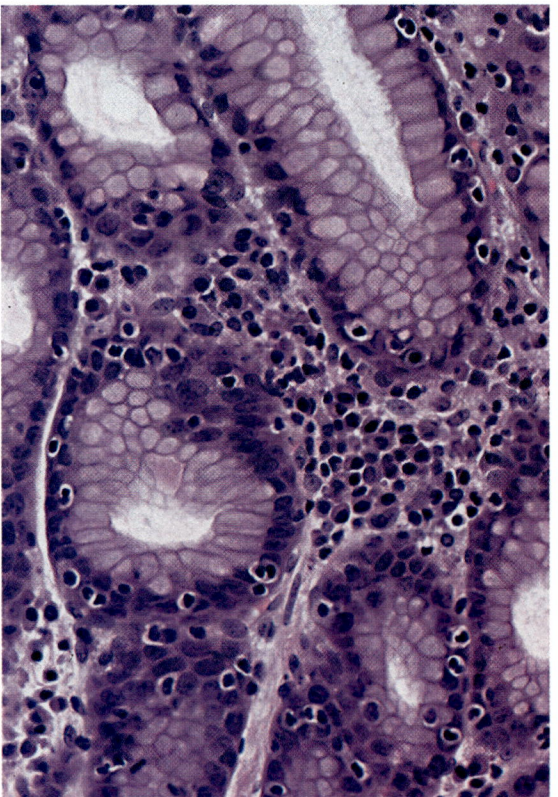

Figure 2-43: **Stomach, Body. Lymphocytic Gastritis.** Increased intraepithelial lymphocytes without evidence of epithelial damage contrast with lymphoepithelial lesions of MALT lymphoma (Fig. 2-216). Lymphocytes have twisted nuclei characteristic of T cells.

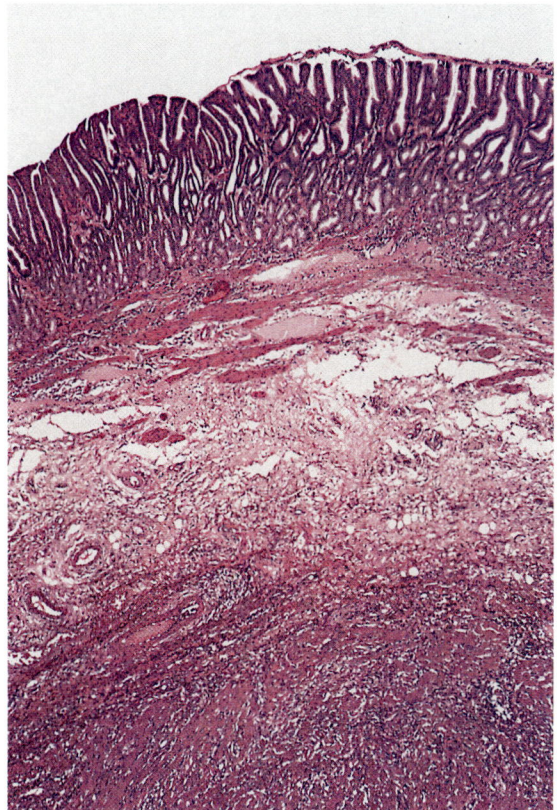

Figure 2-44: **Stomach, Antrum. Eosinophilic Gastritis.** Muscularis propria heavily infiltrated by eosinophils. Marked submucosal edema with splayed muscularis mucosae. Mucosa largely uninvolved. Biopsy in this area would miss the lesion. Mucosal involvement typically patchy, requiring multiple biopsies.

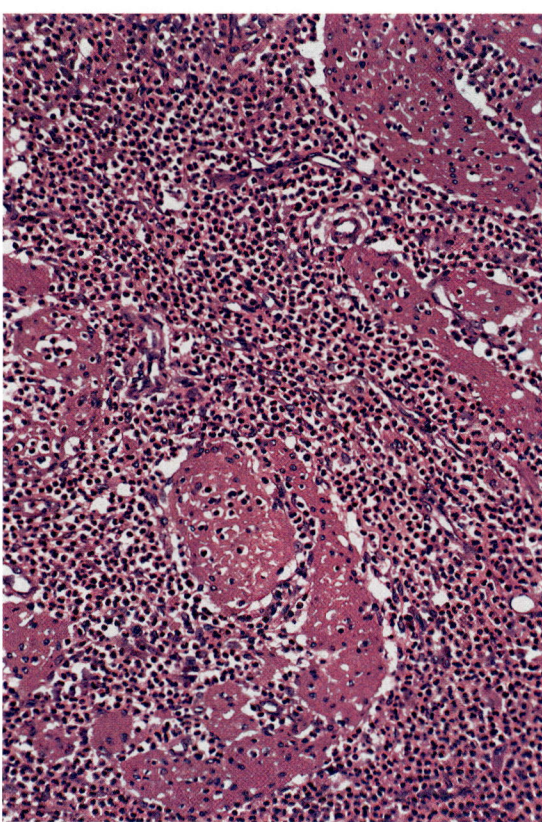

Figure 2-45: **Stomach, Antrum. Eosinophilic Gastritis.** High magnification of muscularis propria of Fig. 2-44. Sheets of eosinophils infiltrate and disperse muscle bundles. Muscle cells show typical degenerative myocytolysis.

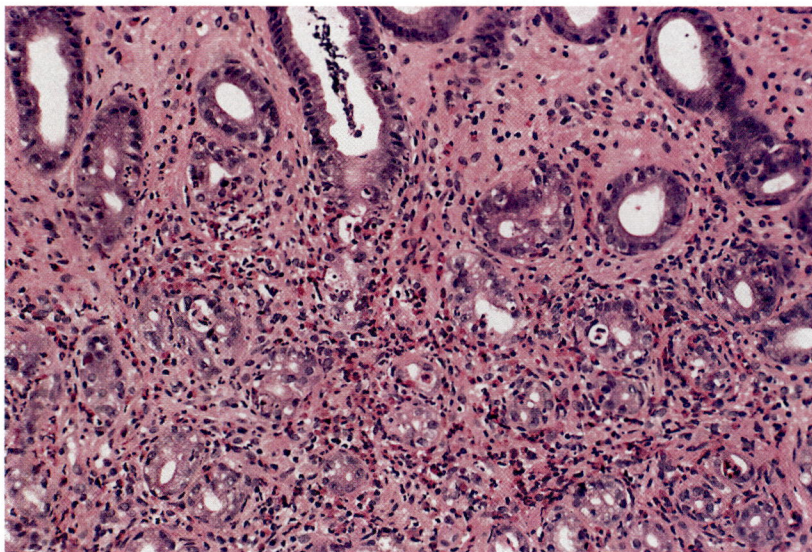

Figure 2-46: **Stomach, Antrum. Eosinophilic Gastritis.** Large numbers of eosinophils infiltrate the lamina propria. Characteristically, the deep mucosa is affected. Glands are infiltrated but not destroyed. Lamina propria is expanded by edema.

GRANULOMATOUS GASTRITIS

- Morphology .... Histologic features vary according to etiology, but rarely point to a specific cause. Special stains for organisms and examination with polarized light for foreign material are needed. Negative stains do not exclude an infectious etiology. In *sarcoid*, typically there are numerous compact epithelioid granulomas and little or no inflammation. *Crohn's* disease is usually antral-predominant. Sharply defined erosions or, in advanced cases, fissuring ulcers are characteristic. The inflammatory process is often chronic and patchy. In early or mild cases, foci of active chronic inflammation may be small and discrete and granulomas subtle and infrequent.

- Endoscopic features .... The appearance of the mucosa may be normal, or there may be erythema, punctate erosions, fissuring ulcers, large folds, or gastric wall thickening visualized by endoscopic ultrasound.

- Clinical features .... Nonspecific dyspepsia, nausea with or without vomiting, or complete absence of symptoms. *Sarcoid* is usually asymptomatic. *Crohn's* patients usually have duodenal or other intestinal involvement at time of diagnosis.

- Differential diagnosis ...... Endoscopic: Peptic ulcer disease, lymphoma.

    Etiologic: Crohn's, sarcoid, infections including tuberculosis, fungal, spirochetal, parasitic, idiopathic (isolated granulomatous gastritis), vasculitis, drug reaction, collagen vascular disorder.

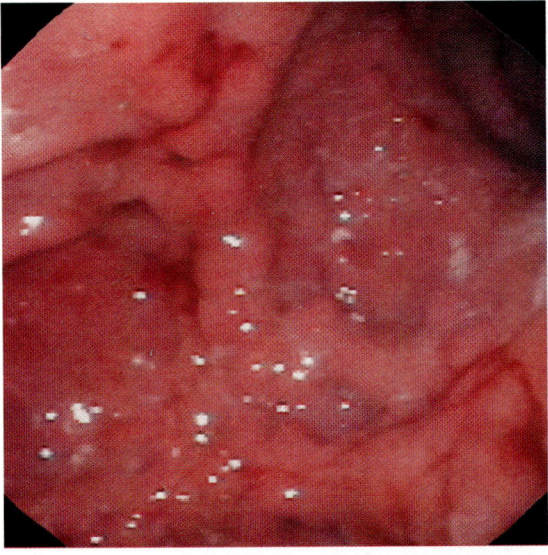

Figure 2-47: **Stomach. Granulomatous Gastritis, Crohn's.** The gastric mucosa is thickened and the usual linear rugal folds replaced by transverse nodular folds and multiple irregular ulcers. These findings suggest either an infiltrative disorder such as lymphoma or, in this patient with a known history, Crohn's disease.

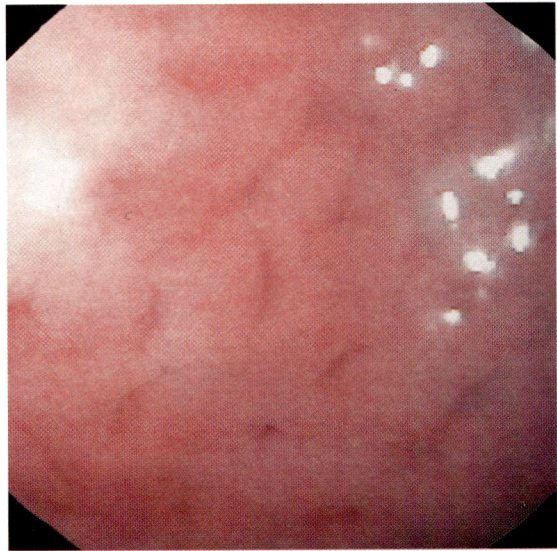

Figure 2-48: **Stomach. Crohn's Disease.** Thickened mucosa with superficial linear erosions.

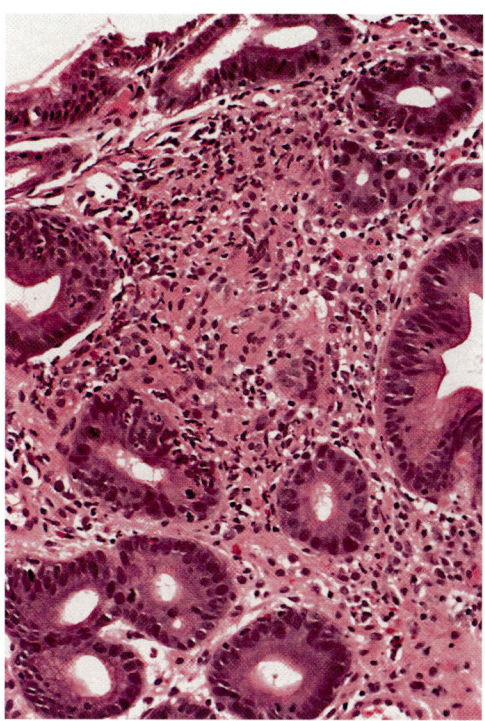

Figure 2-49: **Stomach. Granulomatous Gastritis.** Patchy, focal, active chronic inflammation and an epithelioid granuloma.

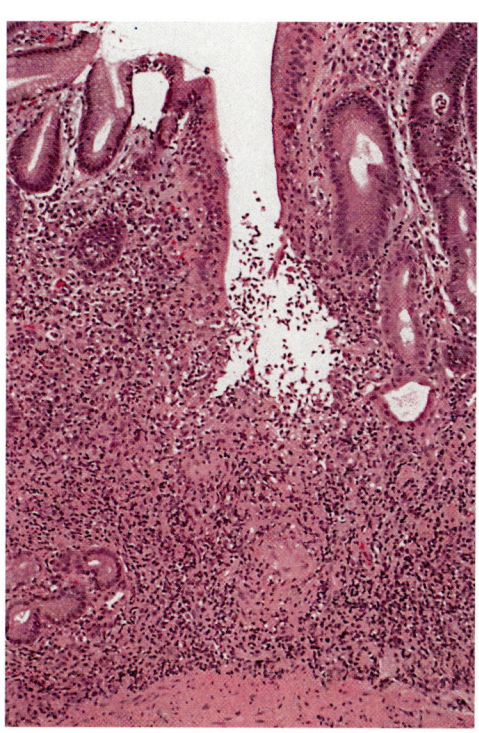

Figure 2-50: **Stomach. Granulomatous Gastritis, Crohn's.** Sharply punched-out aphthous erosion with active chronic inflammation and an epithelioid granuloma.

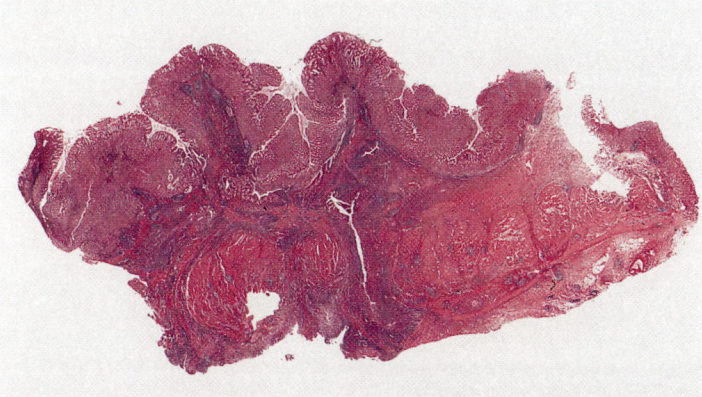

Figure 2-51: **Stomach. Granulomatous Gastritis, Crohn's.** Full-thickness section with transmural fissure and inflammation characteristic of Crohn's disease.

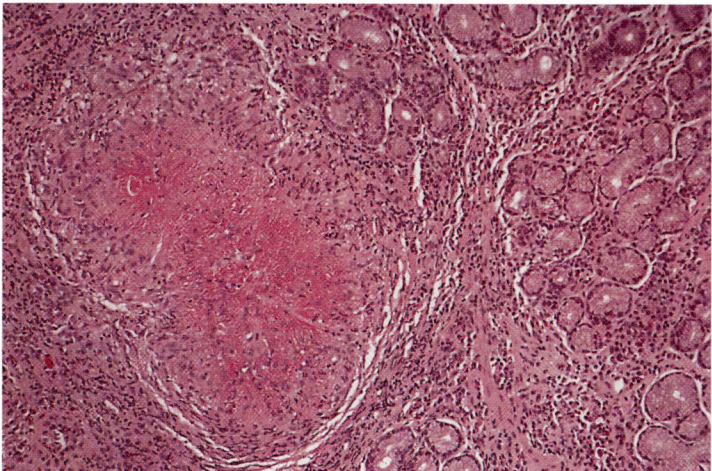

Figure 2-52: **Stomach, Antrum. Granulomatous Gastritis.** Caseous granuloma and active chronic inflammation rich in eosinophils. Necrosis favors infection.

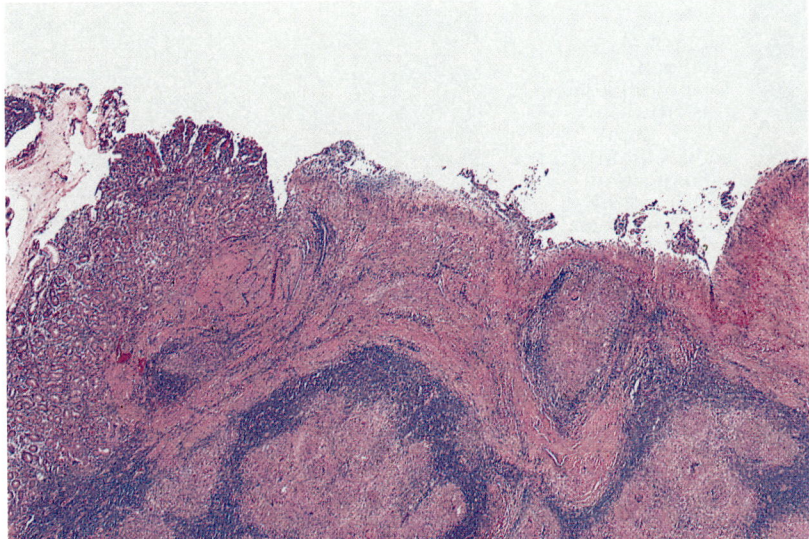

Figure 2-53: **Stomach. Granulomatous Gastritis, Tuberculosis.** Large shallow ulcer with confluent necrotizing granulomas.

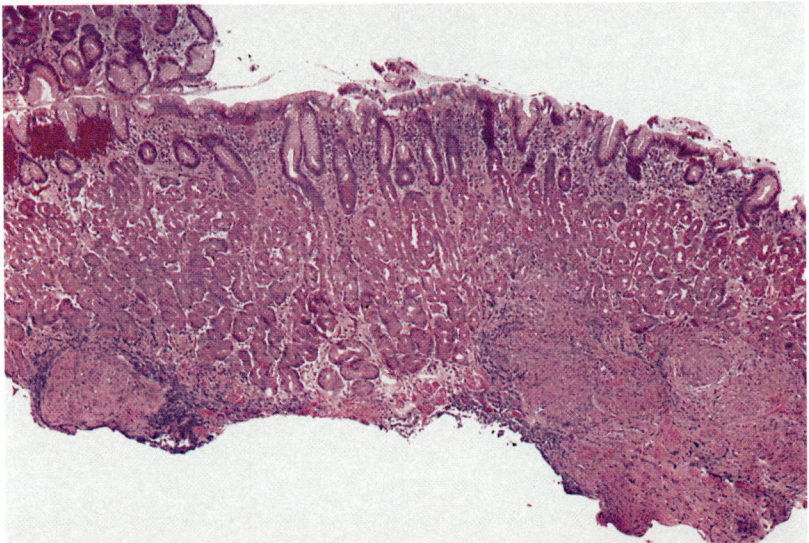

Figure 2-54: **Stomach. Granulomatous Gastritis, Sarcoid.** Multiple epithelioid granulomas; no other significant inflammation.

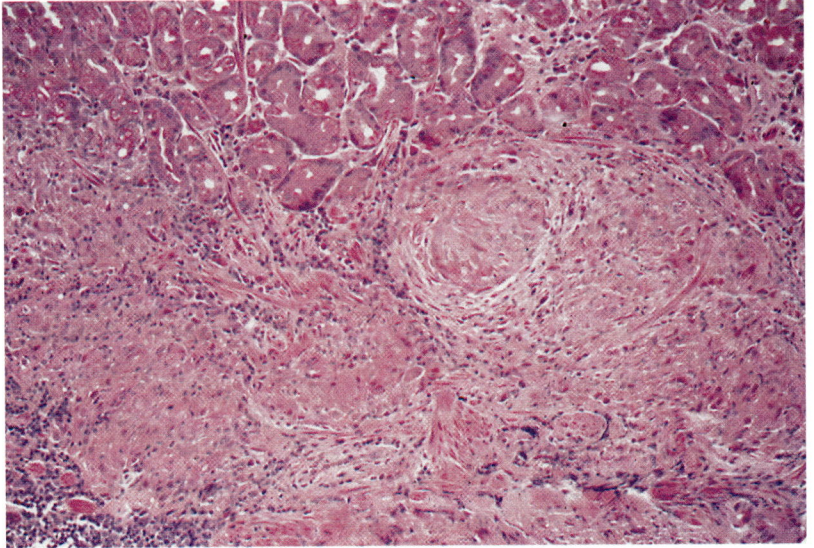

Figure 2-55: **Stomach. Granulomatous Gastritis, Sarcoid.** Gastric mucosa with compact epithelioid granulomas.

ACUTE EROSIVE GASTROPATHY

- Morphology .... Biopsies of early erosions may show only hemorrhage. In the absence of epithelial reactive/regenerative change, this cannot be distinguished from endoscope-induced trauma. Acute erosive gastropathy is defined by the absence of epithelial regenerative change (acute) and inflammation (gastropathy).
- Endoscopic features .... Range from punctate erythema with mucosal friability, erosions, and shallow ulcers, to large linear and irregularly shaped ulcers.
- Clinical features .... Bleeding.
- Differential diagnosis ...... Etiologic: Alcohol, NSAIDs, other drugs, hypovolemia, stress, uremia.

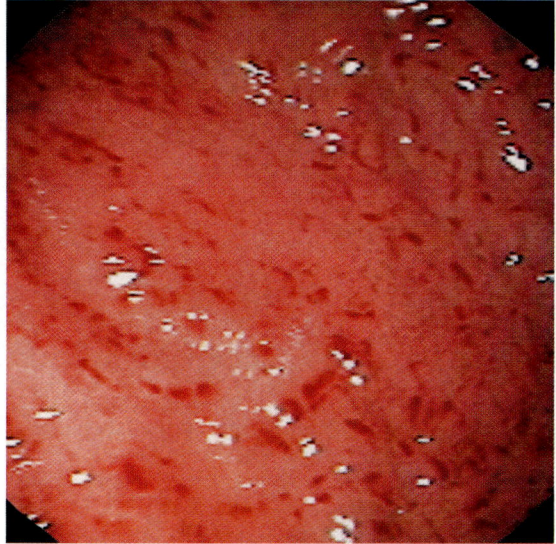

Figure 2-56: **Stomach. Hemorrhagic Gastropathy.** Body of stomach along greater curvature. Innumerable punctate areas of erythema could represent mucosal hemorrhage or areas of mucosal vascular ectasia. Friable mucosa.

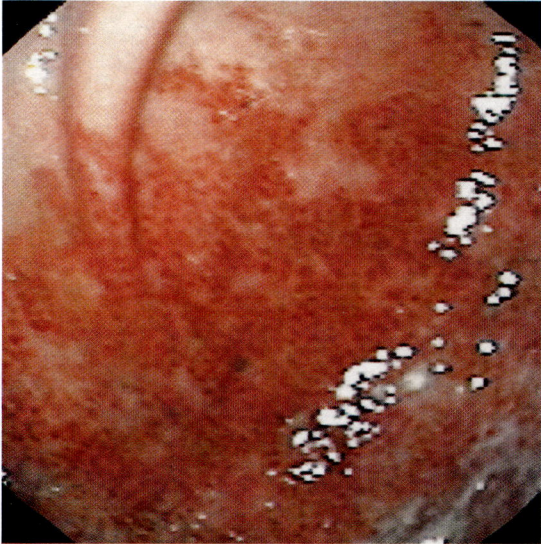

Figure 2-57: **Stomach. Hemorrhagic Gastropathy.** Mucosal hemorrhage in antrum secondary to stress (i.e., postsurgical).

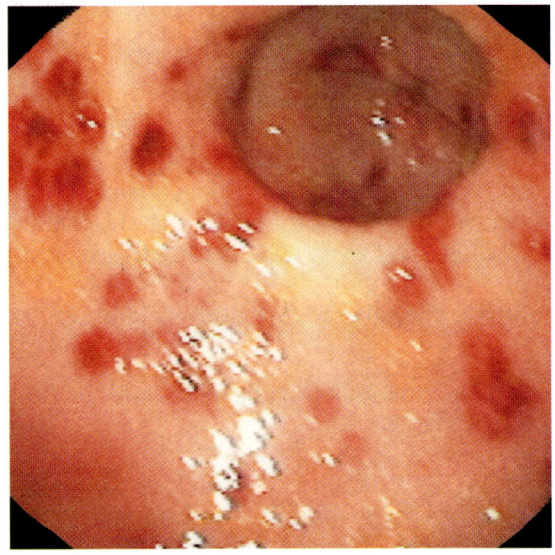

Figure 2-58: **Stomach. Hemorrhagic Gastropathy.** Multiple mucosal hemorrhages due to nasogastric tube trauma.

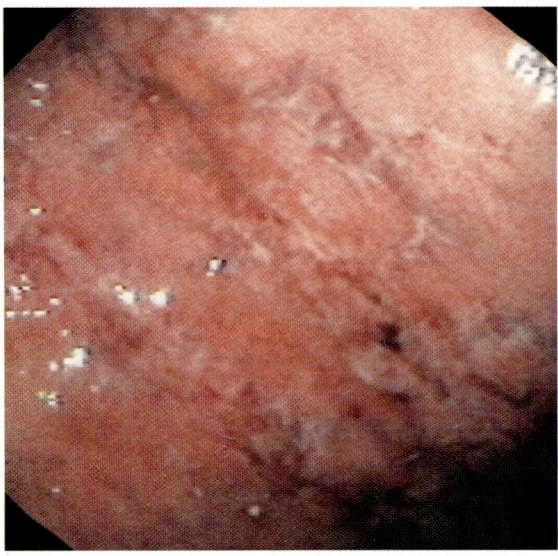

Figure 2-59: **Stomach. Hemorrhagic Gastropathy.** Mucosal erosions and hemorrhage due to stress.

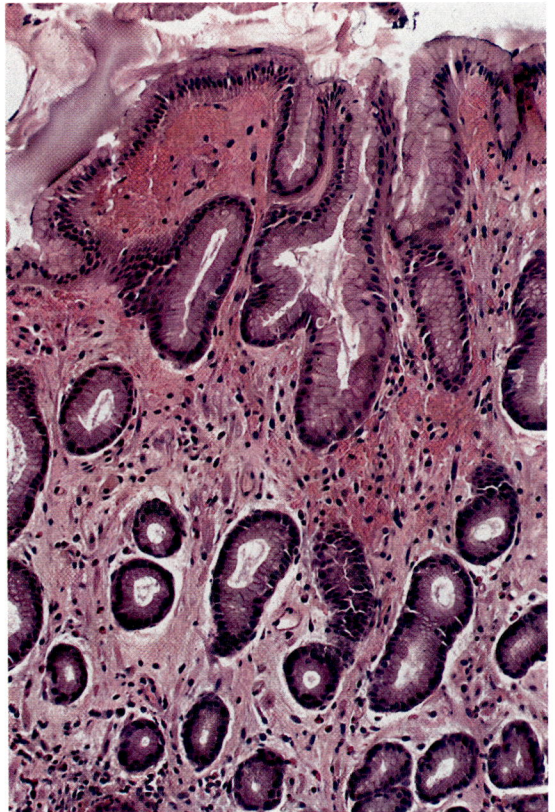

Figure 2-60: **Stomach. Hemorrhage.** Hemorrhage in the lamina propria without degenerative or regenerative epithelial changes.

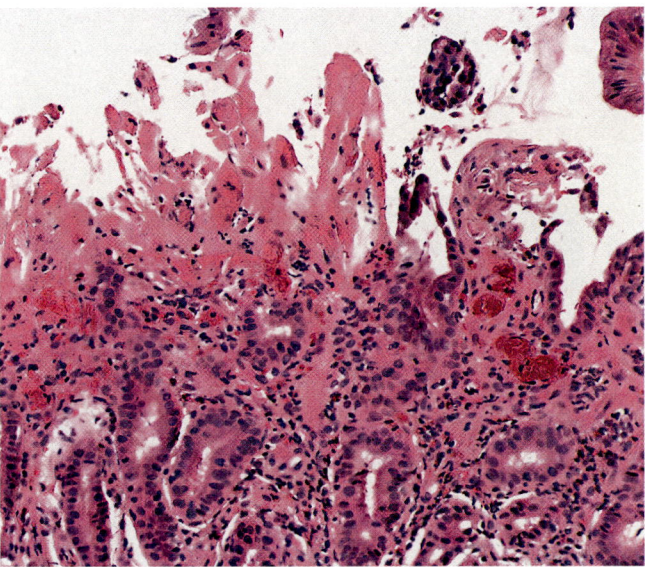

Figure 2-61: **Stomach. Erosion.** Congestion, necrosis, fibrinous exudate, with early reactive epithelial change and minimal inflammation on the edge.

REACTIVE GASTROPATHY

- Morphology .... Reactive gastropathy is characterized by foveolar hyperplasia, few inflammatory cells in the lamina propria, pink stromal cell cytoplasm, and edema. Foveolar hyperplasia is a nonspecific reactive epithelial proliferation, the result of mucosal damage of various causes including gastritis. Regenerative epithelial changes and increased numbers of mitotic figures in the proliferative zone help to distinguish mild hyperplasia from normal antral foveolae, which can be slightly tortuous. Foveolar hyperplasia, when accompanied by intense cellular reactive/regenerative change, may resemble dysplasia. An overall uniform appearance of the changes suggests a reactive process.

    Microvascular ischemia results in erosions. Precise pathogenic mechanisms may differ, depending on etiology. The initial injury produces erosion followed by a healing phase. Healing results from regenerative proliferation (foveolar hyperplasia) in adjacent gastric pits and can be exuberant. Erosions are limited to the mucosa; ulcers extend into the submucosa, a feature that cannot be determined on superficial biopsy samples. In gastropathy, the inflammation is limited to the edge or base of the erosion; in gastritis, inflammation is diffuse in the lamina propria.

    Changes of reactive gastropathy occur over submucosal mass lesions, especially stromal tumors.

- Endoscopic features .... Lesions are typically confined to the antrum but occur elsewhere, especially the distal rosette of a hiatal hernia and the pylorus. Depending on the cause and duration of injury, the endoscopic appearance may range from patchy antral erythema, punctate spots, and erosions often radiating from the pylorus, to polyps and stomal polypoid hyperplasia (following enterostomy). If there is erosion or ulcer, the adjacent foveolar hyperplasia can appear as a polyp. Since gastritis and gastropathy can be identical endoscopically, it is important to sample both abnormal and normal areas.

- Clinical features .... Symptoms, when present, are nonspecific and include dyspepsia, nausea, and bloating.

- Differential diagnosis ...... Etiologic: NSAIDs and other drugs, alcohol, bile reflux, uremia, portal hypertension, radiation, chemotherapy, and underlying mass.

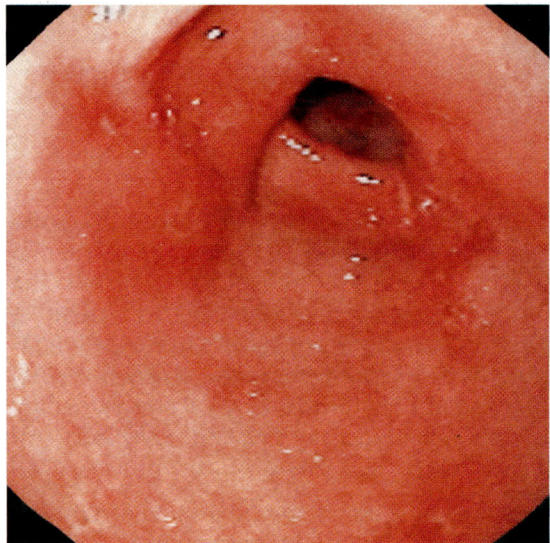

Figure 2-62: **Stomach. Reactive Gastropathy.** Several small, shallow erosions in antrum. There is intense erythema surrounding the erosions and patchy erythema with coalescence. Appearance consistent with NSAID injury.

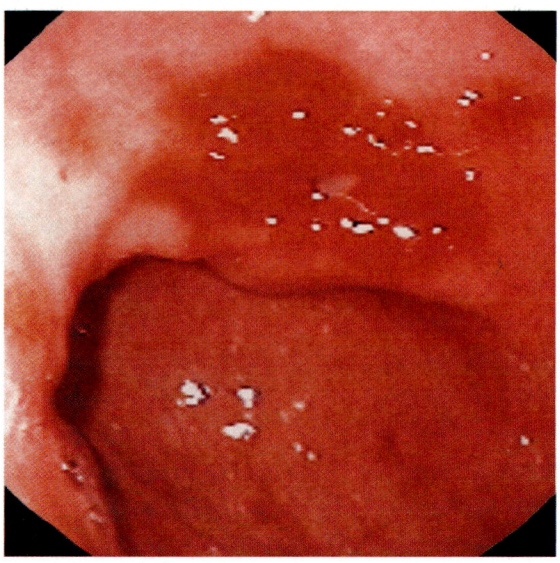

Figure 2-63: **Stomach. Reactive Gastropathy.** Small, penetrating ulcer/erosion with surrounding intense mucosal erythema in distal body along lesser curvature. The intensity of the erythema suggests that the ulcer may be related to chemical injury, as with NSAIDs.

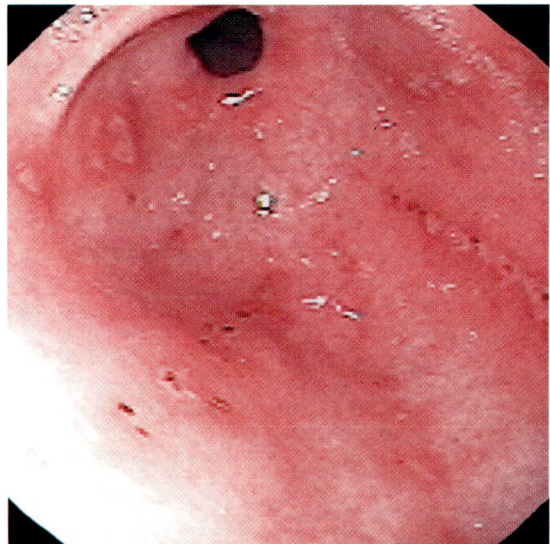

Figure 2-64: **Stomach. Reactive Gastropathy.** Multiple superficial erosions in linear array from the pylorus through the length of the antrum. The appearance and distribution of these erosions favor chemical or medication-induced injury. The extremely shallow depth and narrow width of these erosions suggest they are resolving.

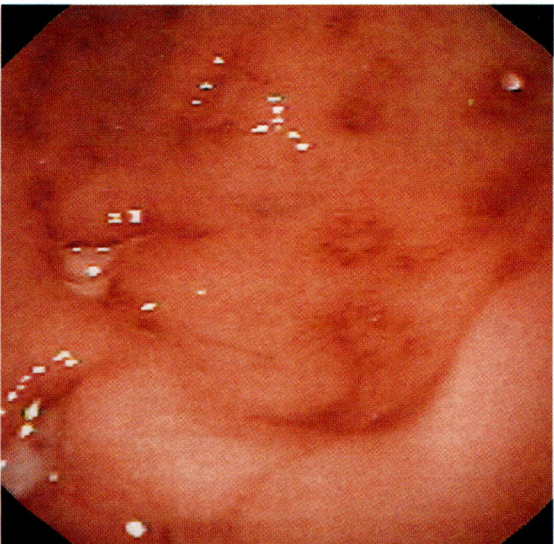

Figure 2-65: **Stomach. Reactive Gastropathy.** Two small ulcers with surrounding edema and erythema, within the antrum along the greater curvature. The intense erythema favors chemical or drug injury as opposed to *H pylori* infection.

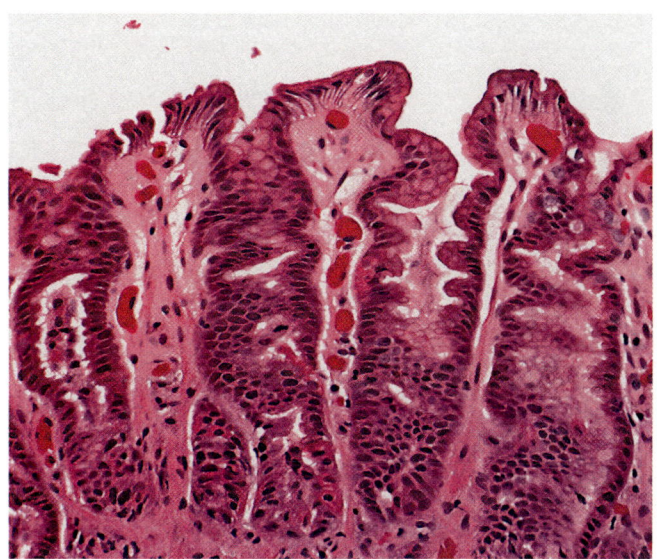

Figure 2-66: **Stomach, Antrum. Reactive Gastropathy.** Foveolar hyperplasia in the absence of significant inflammation. The capillaries and venules are congested but not ectatic.

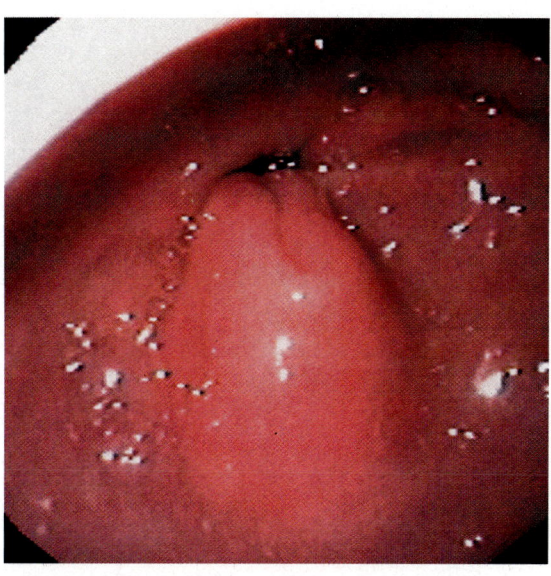

Figure 2-67: **Stomach, Antrum. Submucosal Mass with Superficial Reactive Gastropathy.** Small submucosal mass with central depression. Superficial biopsy showed reactive gastropathy.

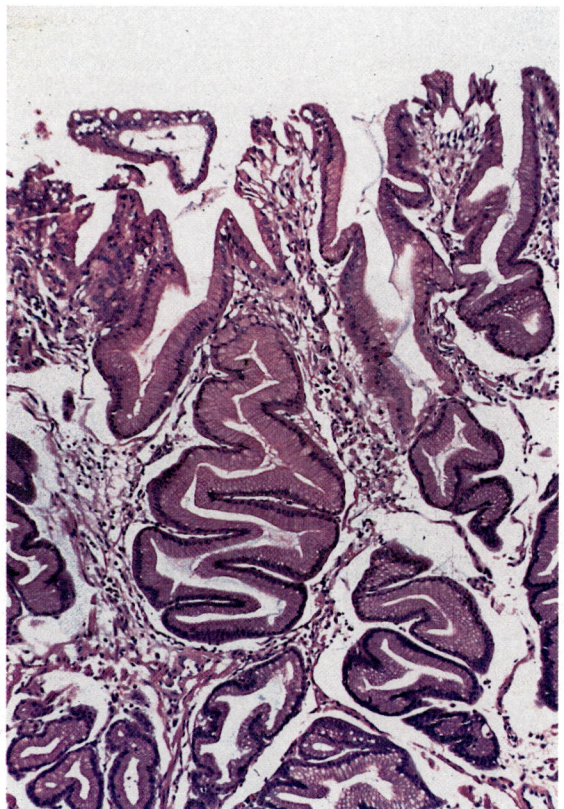

Figure 2-68: **Stomach. Reactive Gastropathy, Common Pattern.** Marked foveolar hyperplasia. Empty, pink lamina propria. No features to suggest etiology.

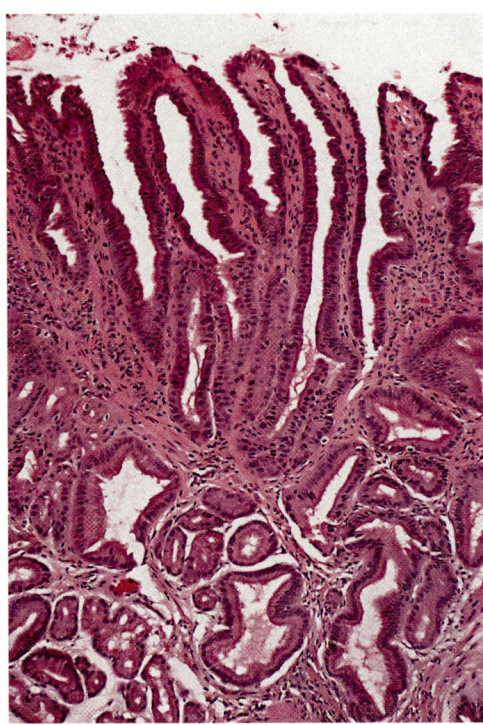

Figure 2-69: **Stomach. Reactive Gastropathy. Common Pattern.** Epithelial regenerative changes include loss of foveolar cell mucin. Nuclei enlarged, hyperchromatic, and crowded; mitoses frequent. Marked foveolar elongation results in villous or papillary appearance. These features mimic dysplasia. Cytologic detail and uniformity help in the distinction.

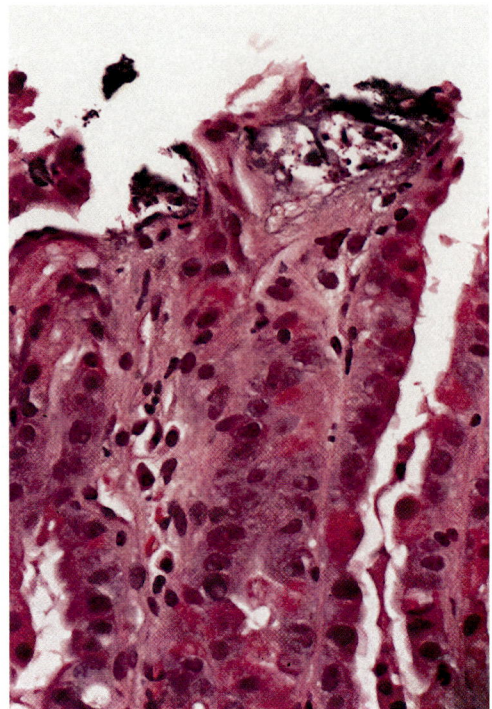

Figure 2-70: **Stomach. Reactive Gastropathy. Common Pattern.** Higher magnification shows the reactive/regenerative foveolar cell changes: nuclei enlarged, rounded, and hyperchromatic, with large macronucleoli. Uniformity between cells distinguishes this reaction from dysplasia. Bluish purple cytoplasm obscures nuclear chromatin detail, characteristic of regenerative atypia. Black pigment at the surface is an aluminum compound related to dialysis in uremic patient.

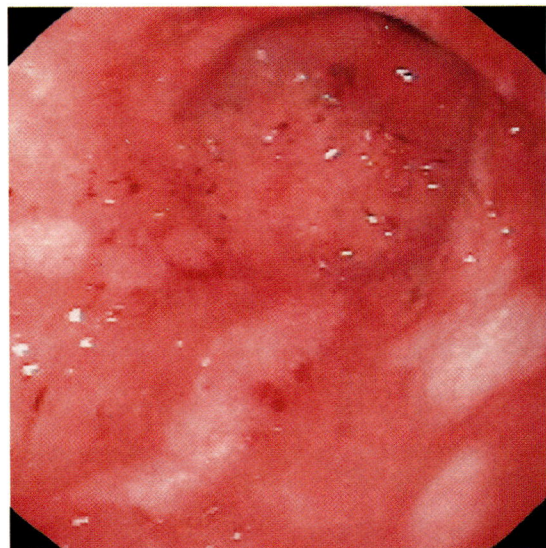

Figure 2-71: **Stomach, Antrum. Reactive Gastropathy with Erosions.** Intense erythema and large superficial ulcerations in antrum, consistent with an acute process such as stress or chemical injury.

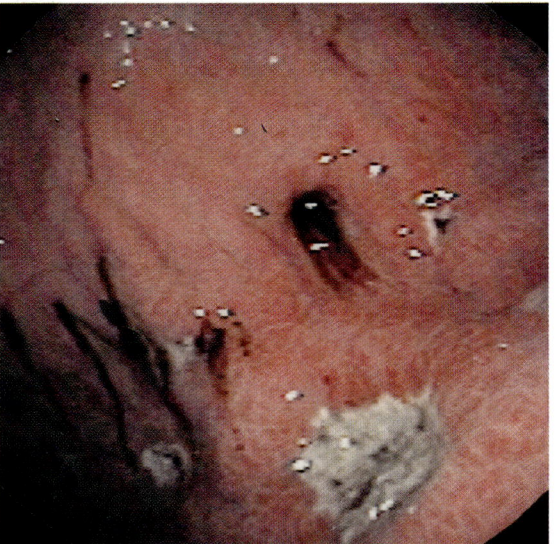

Figure 2-72: **Stomach, Distal Body. Reactive Gastropathy with Erosion.** Mucosal mosaic pattern and erythema. Shallow ulceration contains altered blood.

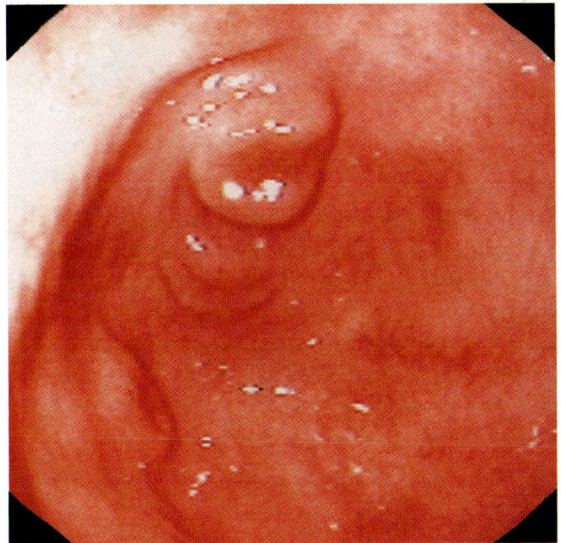

Figure 2-73: **Stomach, Antrum. Reactive Gastropathy, Healing Erosion.** Mucosal nodule with central erosion and heaped-up edges.

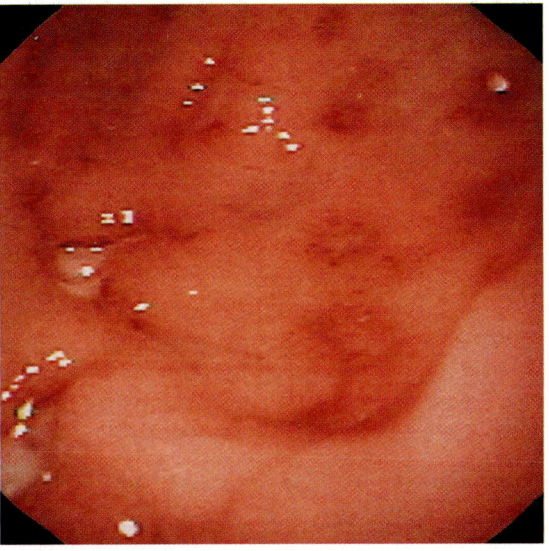

Figure 2-74: **Stomach, Antrum. Reactive Gastropathy.** Erosions with edema, erythema, and friability. Intense erythema suggests a chemical or drug injury.

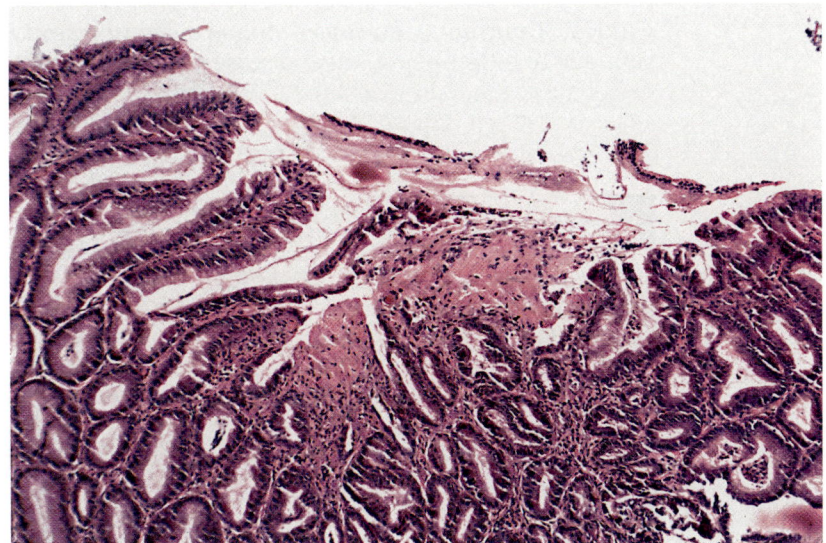

Figure 2-75: **Stomach, Antrum. Reactive Gastropathy, Healing Erosion.** Focal superficial necrosis with fibrinous exudate. Foveolar hyperplasia at periphery of erosion corresponds to raised edges seen endoscopically (Fig. 2-73). Minimal inflammation.

REACTIVE GASTROPATHY, BILE REFLUX

- Morphology .... Bile reflux commonly occurs after Billroth enterostomies, usually done for peptic disease caused by *H pylori*. Bile stimulates foveolar proliferation and also suppresses (and may eliminate) *H pylori*. If *H pylori* are eliminated, inflammation recedes and disappears with time, leaving only foveolar hyperplasia. Epithelial subnuclear vacuoles are infrequently seen, but are characteristic of bile reflux. Foveolar hyperplasia due to bile reflux proximal to enterostomies may be massive, i.e., stomal polypoid hyperplasia. The polyps are sessile but variable in size, shape, and configuration.

- Endoscopic features .... Erythema, edema, friability, enlarged folds, and stomal polyps.

- Clinical features .... Dyspepsia, nausea, and emesis. Patients who have undergone vagotomy, antrectomy, and gastroenterostomy may have symptoms of gastric retention. Complicating bezoars can exacerbate gastric retention symptoms and induce gastroesophageal reflux symptoms. Peristomal polyps may lead to chronic occult GI blood loss.

- Differential diagnosis ...... Endoscopic: Enlarged gastric folds due to bile reflux may mimic lymphoma or infiltrative diseases. Stomal polyps require biopsy to exclude dysplasia.

    Clinical: Recurrent peptic ulcer, stomal ulceration, and gastric outlet obstruction due to either peptic ulcer disease or recurrent malignancy.

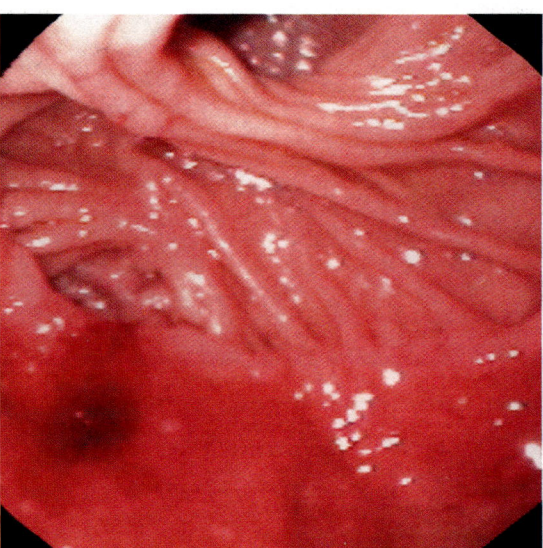

Figure 2-76: **Stomach, Anastomosis. Reactive Gastropathy, Bile Reflux.** A partial view of a Billroth II gastroenteric anastomosis. The gastric side of the mucosa (lower third of figure) is diffusely erythematous and friable. These findings are consistent with bile reflux injury.

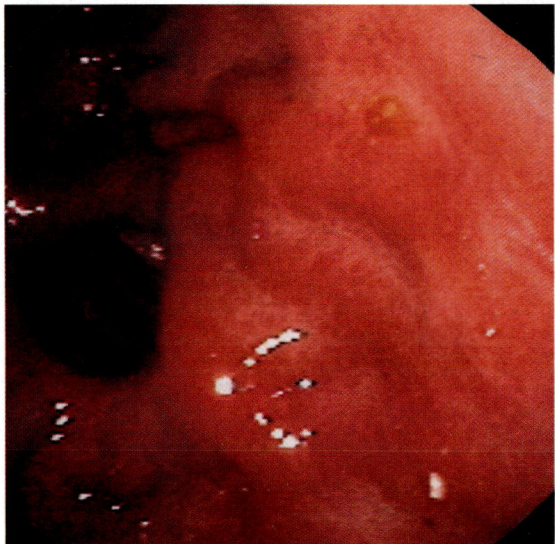

Figure 2-77: **Stomach. Reactive Gastropathy, Bile Reflux.** Erythematous gastric mucosa due to bile reflux; proximal to enterostomy.

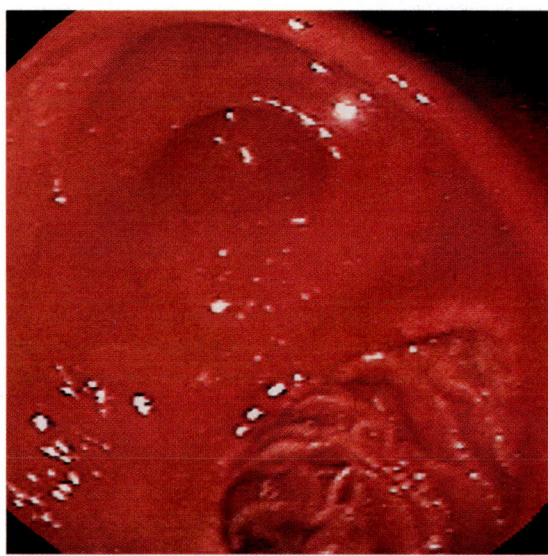

Figure 2-78: **Stomach. Reactive Gastropathy, Bile Reflux.** Gastric mucosa surrounding a gastroenterostomy; anastomosis is erythematous and friable, possibly due to bile reflux.

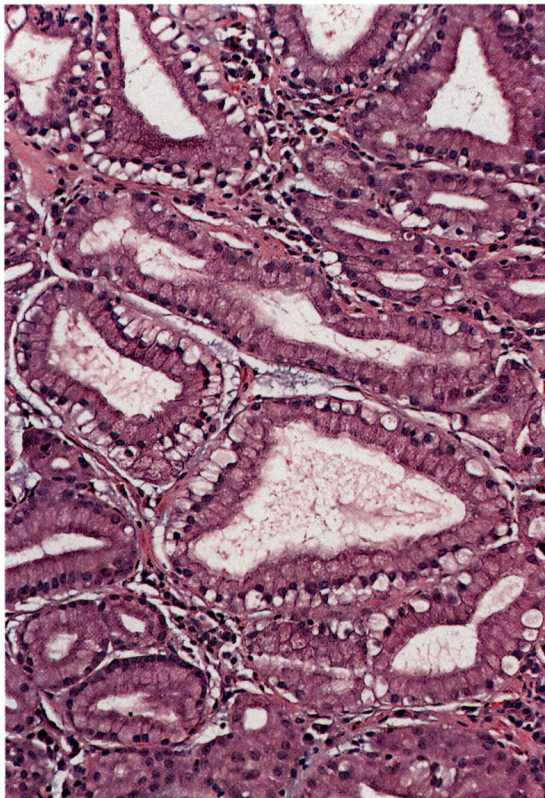

Figure 2-79: **Stomach Proximal to Enterostomy. Reactive Gastropathy, Subnuclear Vacuoles Due to Bile Reflux.** Large subnuclear vacuoles in foveolar epithelial cells. Minimal inflammation.

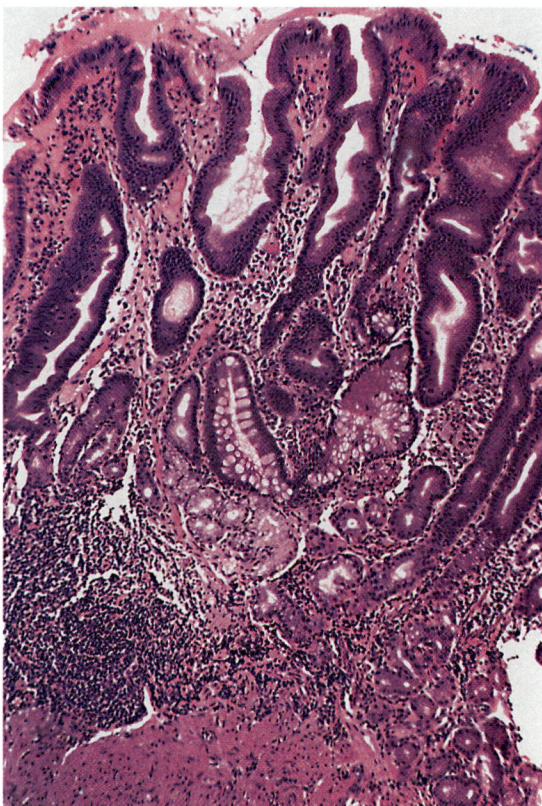

Figure 2-80: **Stomach Proximal to Enterostomy. Reactive Gastropathy Due to Bile Reflux Superimposed on Chronic *H pylori* Gastritis.** Marked foveolar hyperplasia superimposed on chronic atrophic gastritis (due to *H pylori*), characterized by a lack of fundic glands, pyloric and intestinal metaplasia, and lymphoid hyperplasia near the muscularis mucosae.

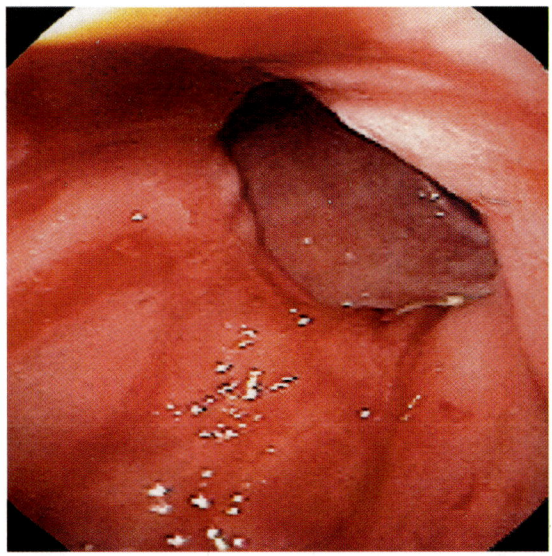

Figure 2-81: **Stomach, Anastomosis, Billroth II. Bile Reflux Gastropathy.** Linear streaks of erythema proximal to the Billroth II anastomotic line and ulcer.

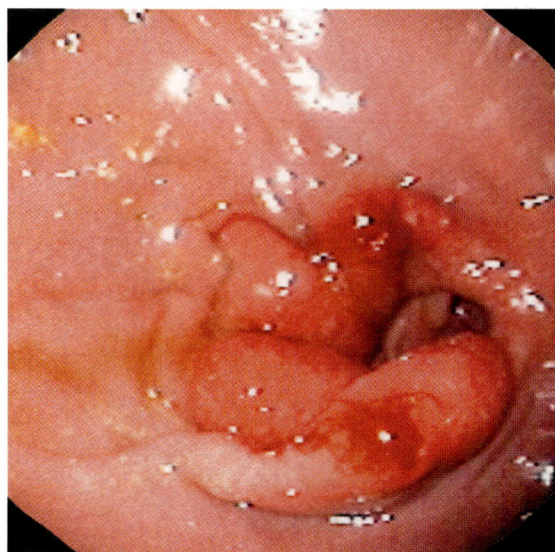

Figure 2-82: **Stomach, Anastomosis, Billroth II. Stomal Polypoid Hyperplasia, Bile Reflux.** Large polypoid folds proximal to the anastomosis. Bile staining.

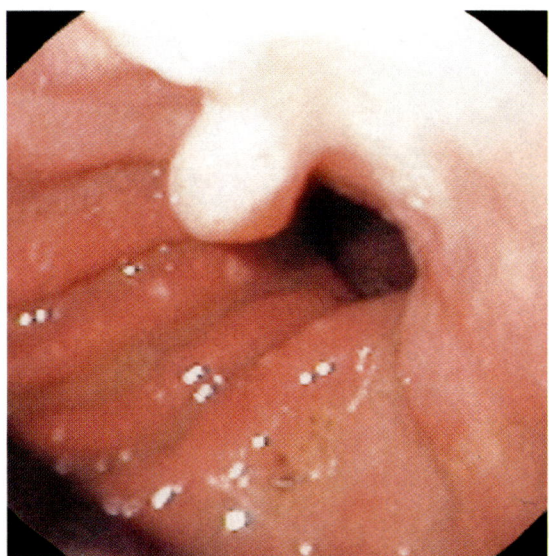

Figure 2-83: **Stomach, Anastomosis, Billroth II. Stomal Polypoid Hyperplasia, Bile Reflux.** Mucosal swelling, erythema, tiny erosions, and a single large polyp proximal to the anastomosis.

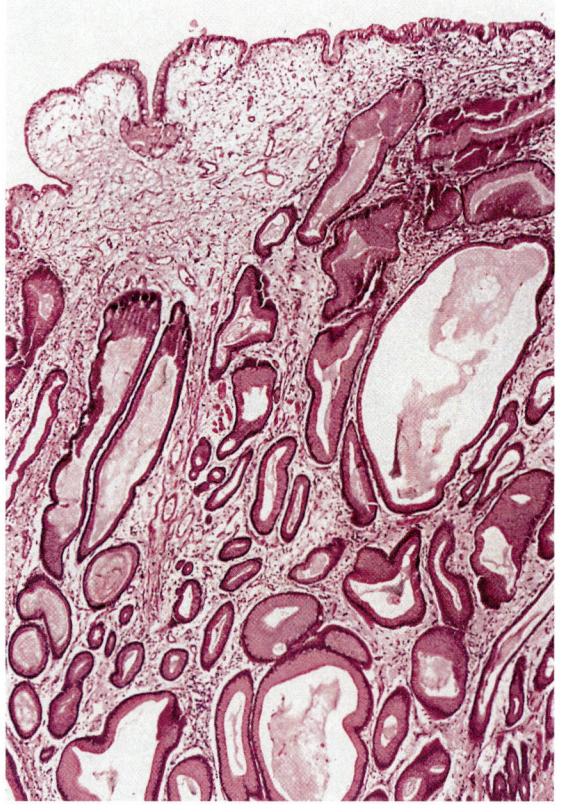

Figure 2-84: **Stomach, Anastomosis, Billroth II. Stomal Polypoid Hyperplasia.** Foveolar hyperplasia and massive edema, indistinguishable from a hyperplastic polyp.

XANTHELASMA

- Morphology .... Xanthelasmas are common in chronic gastritis and in patients with bile reflux following antrectomy and gastroenteric anastomosis. They are related to lipid accumulation following cellular breakdown. Cytoplasm is negative for mucin, unlike signet-ring cells.
- Endoscopic features .... Raised, yellow-white mucosal plaques or nodules with discrete margins.
- Clinical features .... Incidental finding.
- Differential diagnosis ...... Histologic: Signet-ring cell carcinoma.

    Endoscopic: Islands of intestinal metaplasia.

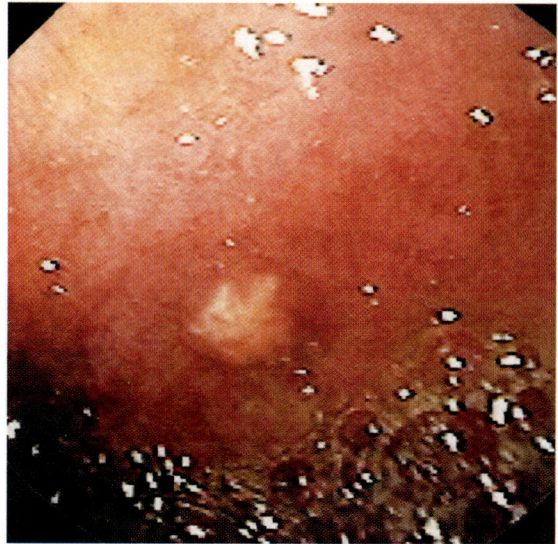

Figure 2-85: **Stomach, Body. Xanthelasma.** Multiple yellow-white nodules/plaques with irregular borders located on gastric folds. The yellow, plaquelike appearance is distinctive.

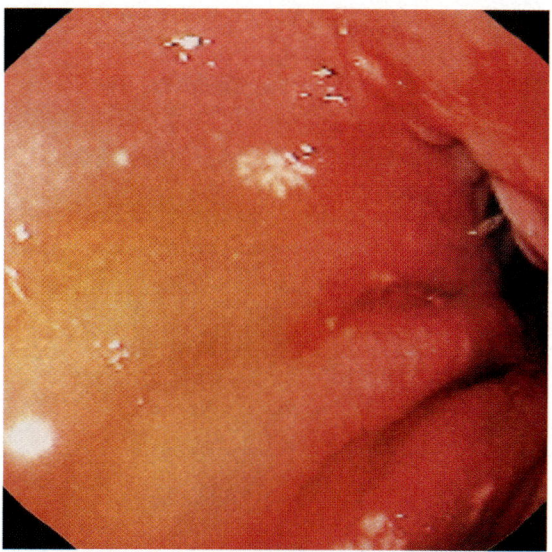

Figure 2-86: **Stomach, Body. Xanthelasma.** Multiple stellate, yellow patches and bile staining.

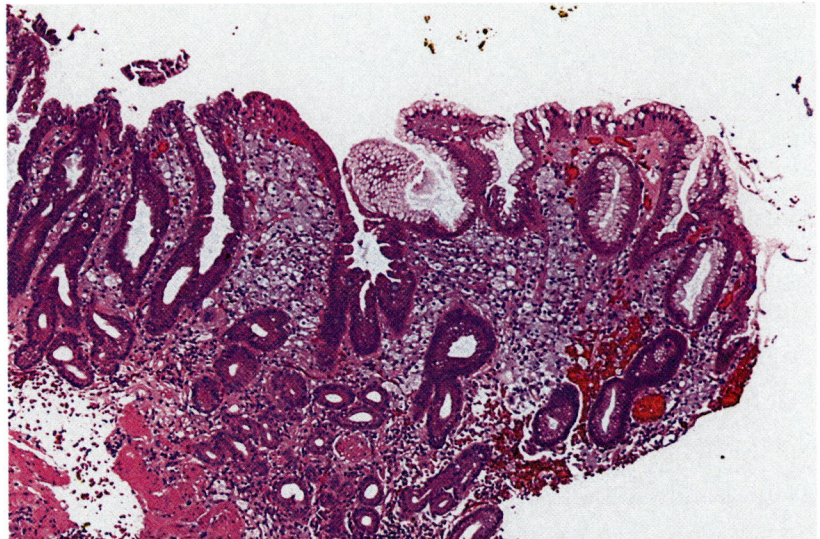

Figure 2-87: **Stomach, Body. Xanthelasma.** Focal expansion of lamina propria by clear cells. Regenerative epithelial change and chronic inflammation (left).

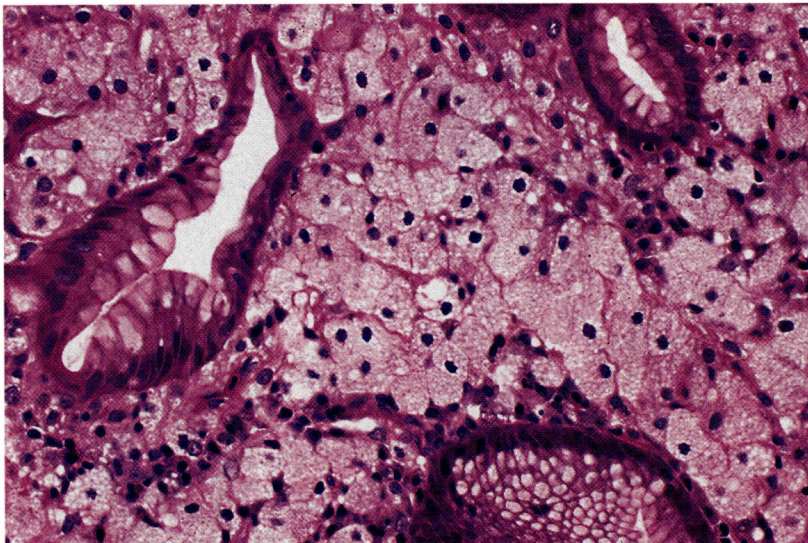

Figure 2-88: **Stomach, Body. Xanthelasma.** Foamy histiocytes expand the lamina propria. Nuclei are small, round, regular, and centrally located.

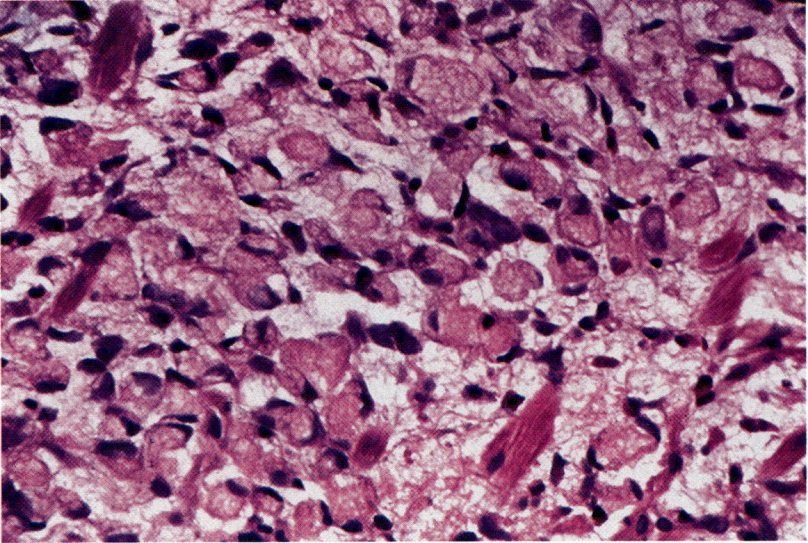

Figure 2-89: **Stomach. Signet-Ring Cell Carcinoma.** Nuclear enlargement and peripheral displacement by cytoplasmic mucin distinguish this from xanthelasma.

GASTROPATHY, RADIATION/CHEMOTHERAPY

- Morphology .... Cytologic changes, although not specific, help to distinguish radiation/chemotherapy gastropathy from other etiologies. Cytologic atypia is easily confused with dysplasia, emphasizing the need for a complete clinical history.

- Endoscopic features .... The delayed sequelae of radiation injury present as pale, friable mucosa with numerous angiectasias that vary in size and shape, and bleed spontaneously. Chemotherapy may cause nonspecific mucosal erythema, shallow ulcers, and erosions of variable size and configuration.

- Clinical features .... Radiation angiectasias can cause chronic GI blood loss. Chemotherapy may be associated with dyspepsia and nausea.

- Differential diagnosis ...... Endoscopic: *Radiation*-induced mucosal angiectasias in the absence of any history cannot be differentiated from the antral angiectasias of watermelon stomach and those associated with severe portal hypertensive gastropathy. The endoscopic differential diagnosis of *chemotherapy*-induced changes is that of peptic ulcer disease and acute injury from drugs, chemicals, acute radiation, and dysplasia.

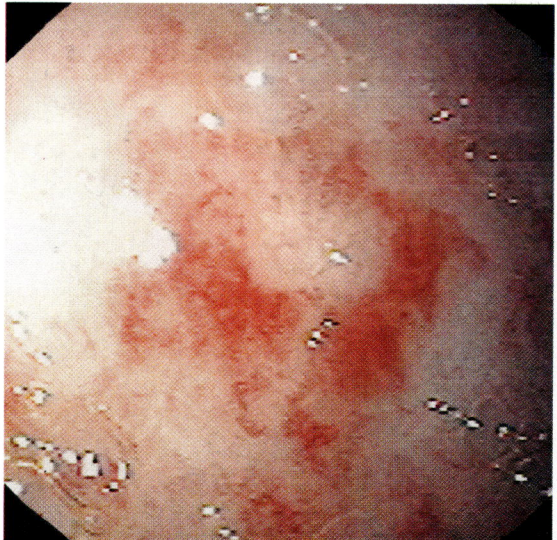 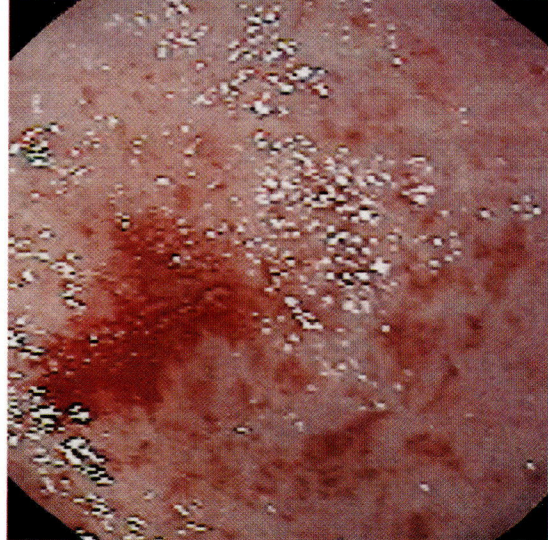

Figures 2-90 and 2-91: **Stomach. Radiation Injury.** Multiple minute, antral, mucosal angiectasias from prior radiation. A scant amount of fresh blood is overlying the small vascular lesions.

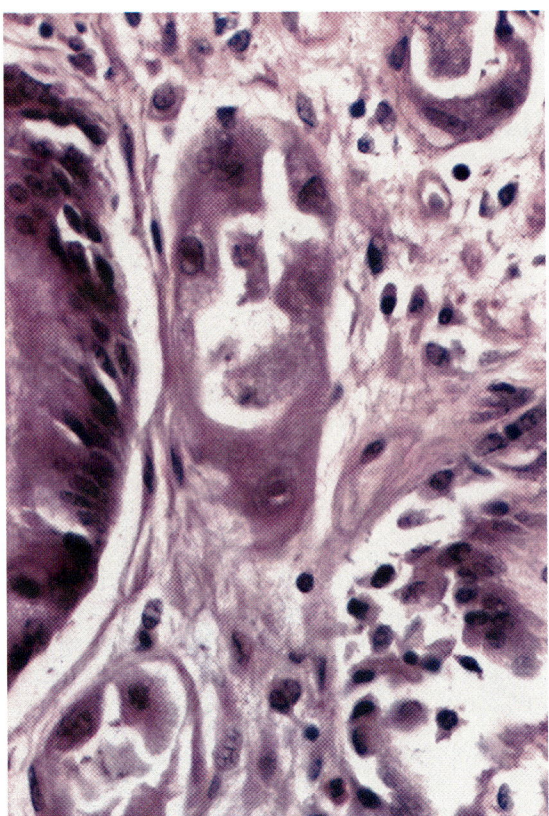

Figure 2-92: **Stomach. Radiation Effect.** Acute radiation changes include cellular and nuclear enlargement, cytoplasmic vacuolization, and large macronucleoli.

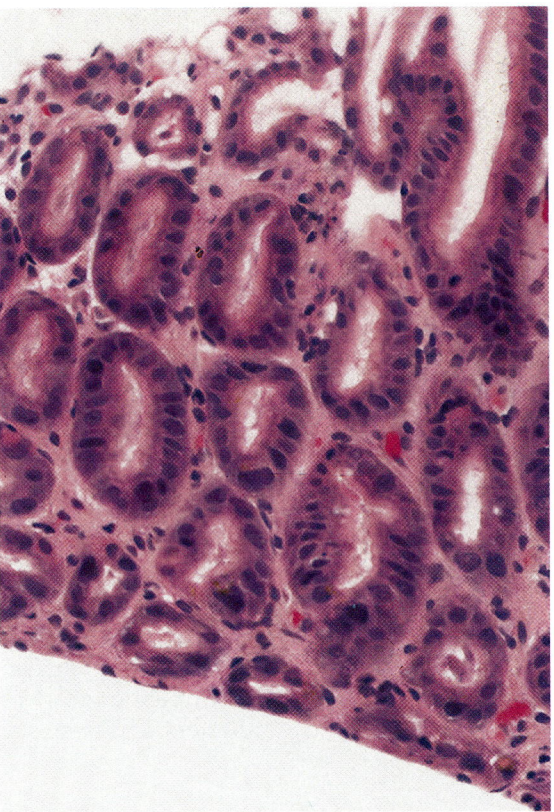

Figure 2-93: **Stomach. Chemotherapy Effect.** Nuclear enlargement and atypia resemble dysplasia.

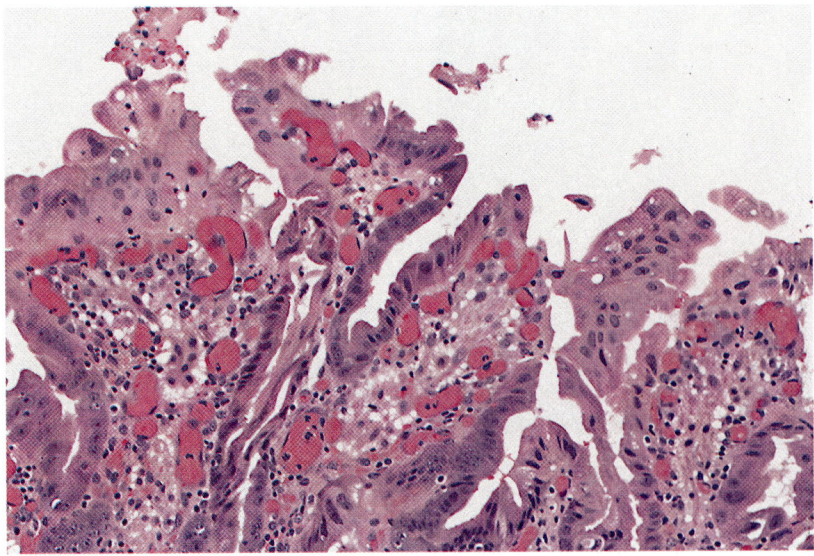

Figure 2-94: **Stomach. Chemotherapy Effect.** Congestion, foveolar regeneration and elongation, cellular and nuclear enlargement, and atypia.

PORTAL HYPERTENSIVE GASTROPATHY

- Morphology .... Chronic venous hypertension and/or increased blood flow cause ectasia and sclerosis of the walls of superficial mucosal capillaries and venules. Obstruction of venous outflow may be intermittent, as in prolapse, or chronic due to portal vein thrombosis, obstruction by tumor, or cirrhosis of the liver. The histology is the same whatever the etiology. The distribution depends on specific factors, e.g., location of obstruction and pattern of collaterals.

- Endoscopic features .... The prominent mosaic pattern, typically pronounced in the body, is the most characteristic endoscopic finding of portal hypertensive gastropathy. More advanced forms also have punctate erythematous lesions that occur in the proximal stomach, especially within the fundus. Milder forms of the gastropathy may present with a fine red-pink miliary or speckled pattern. The antrum may be nodular with raised folds radiating from the pylorus, sometimes punctuated with erosions. Mucosal vascular ectasias may be distributed throughout the antrum in a random fashion or form discrete stripes, often on top of the raised folds. They may extend into the body as well. The folds may contain varices that are typically deeper than superficial esophageal varices and can only be confirmed by endoscopic ultrasound.

- Clinical features .... Usually incidental. In the presence of mucosal vascular ectasias and severe portal hypertensive gastropathy, patients may experience chronic GI blood loss anemia, either occult or accompanied by the episodic passage of melena.

- Differential diagnosis ...... Endoscopic: Punctate erythematous spots, especially in the proximal stomach, cannot be distinguished from those associated with *H pylori*. The prominent mosaic pattern and accompanying prominent folds may be seen in any infiltrative disorder such as lymphoma and leukemia, and also with *H pylori* infection. Antral angiectasias are not distinguishable from those associated with watermelon stomach (gastric antral vascular ectasia (GAVE)).

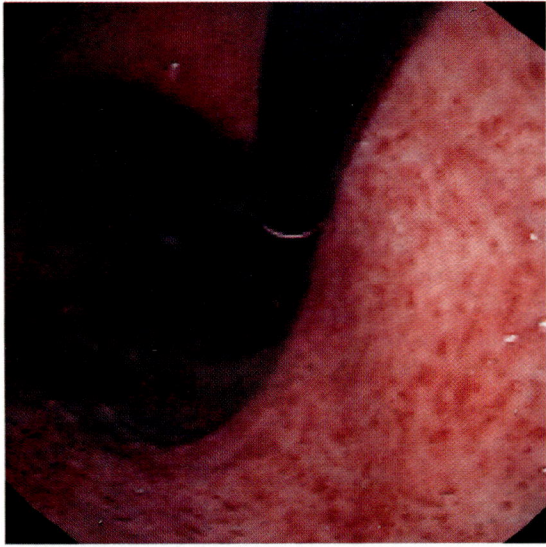

Figure 2-95: **Stomach. Portal Hypertensive Gastropathy, Portal Hypertension.** Diffuse punctate erythema. Scarlatina-type rash pattern involves nearly all of the mucosa, except the antrum.

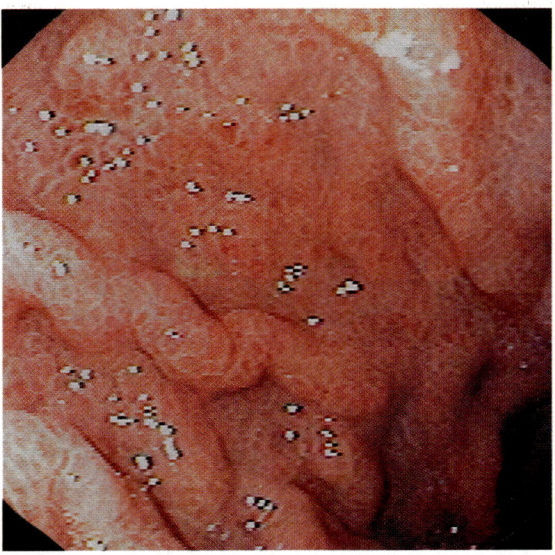

Figure 2-96: **Stomach. Portal Hypertensive Gastropathy, Portal Hypertension.** Typical appearance of severe portal hypertensive gastropathy. Prominent mosaic pattern, diffuse erythema along with more focal and intense punctate erythema.

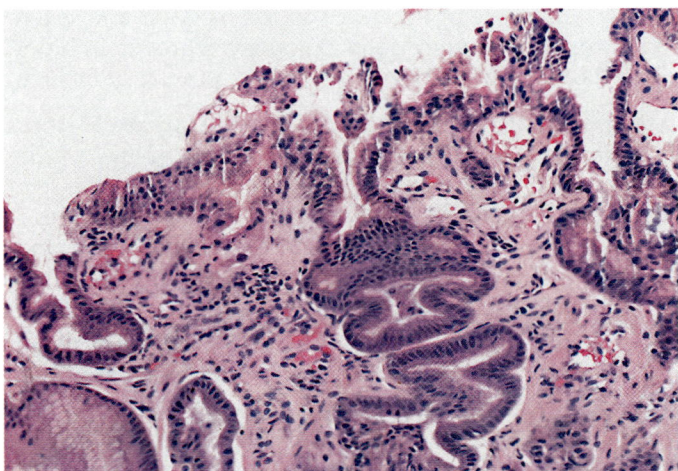

Figure 2-97: **Stomach. Portal Hypertensive Gastropathy, Portal Hypertension.** Vascular ectasia and sclerosis beneath surface epithelium. Foveolar hyperplasia.

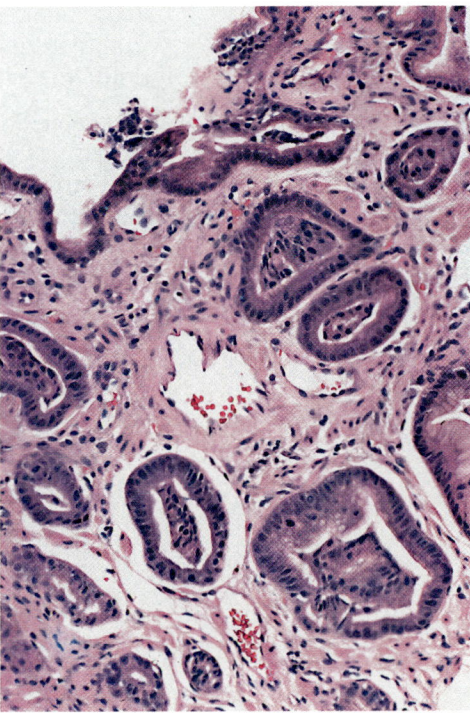

Figure 2-98: **Stomach. Portal Hypertensive Gastropathy, Portal Hypertension.** Sclerotic, ectatic capillaries in the lamina propria.

WATERMELON STOMACH

- Morphology .... Whatever the etiology, the histologic features of congestive gastropathy are similar. Organizing fibrin microthrombi are more commonly seen in watermelon stomach. Patients with watermelon stomach (striped pattern) frequently have a proximal chronic atrophic gastritis, often with pernicious anemia.

- Endoscopic features .... While the angiectasias of watermelon stomach are characteristically linear along the crests of antral folds radiating from the pylorus, they may be diffusely distributed in the antrum, a pattern more commonly seen with portal hypertension. Angiectasias of portal hypertension wax and wane, while those of watermelon stomach tend to be fixed. In watermelon stomach, hyperplastic polyps develop at sites of previous deep thermal coagulation injury, (e.g., laser). The proximal stomach may appear atrophic, with loss of rugal folds and prominent submucosal vessels.

- Clinical features .... Patients are usually female. The main clinical finding is chronic occult bleeding. Many patients have Raynaud phenomenon or connective tissue disorders such as scleroderma, mixed connective tissue disease, and primary biliary cirrhosis. Patients with chronic atrophic gastritis may have pernicious anemia. These clinical features are characteristic of watermelon stomach.

- Differential diagnosis ...... Endoscopic: Portal hypertension and sequelae of radiation injury. It is important to distinguish watermelon stomach without portal hypertension (includes scleroderma) from portal hypertensive gastropathy, as watermelon stomach may be controlled by endoscopic therapy while portal hypertensive gastropathy does not respond.

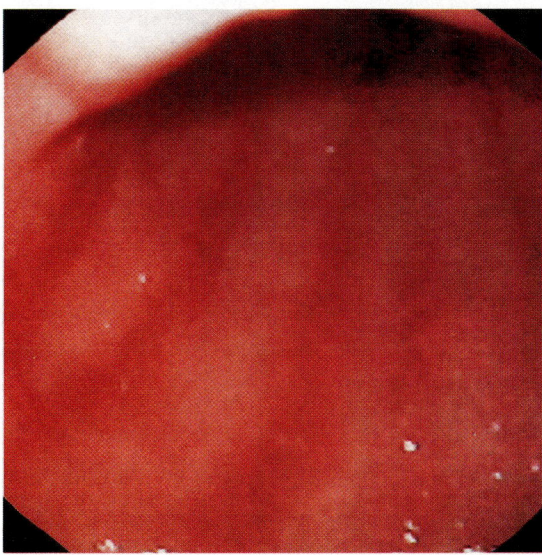

Figure 2-99: **Stomach, Antrum. Watermelon Stomach.** Characteristic linear mucosal vascular lesions in the antrum, located on the tops of raised and convoluted folds.

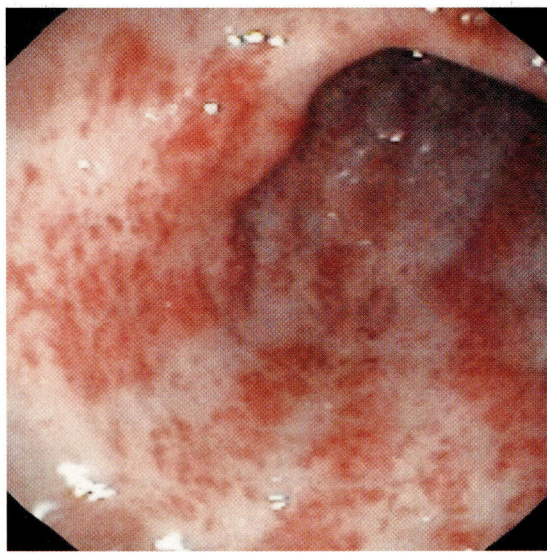

Figure 2-100: **Stomach, Antrum. Watermelon Stomach.** Numerous mucosal vascular lesions. The majority are in a linear array, consistent with watermelon stomach. Polypoid lesions in the upper portion of the photograph may be hyperplastic polyps.

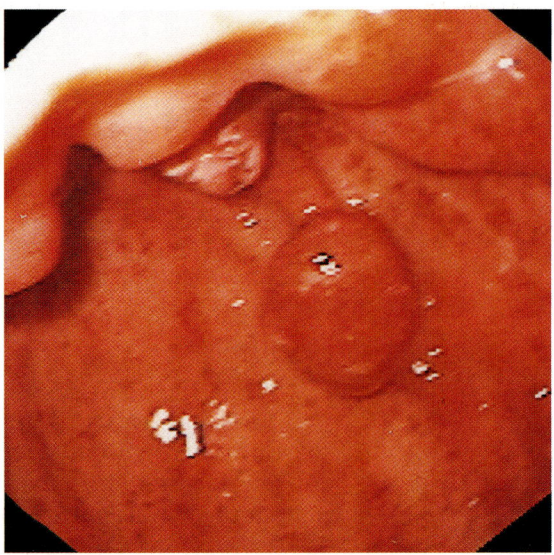

Figure 2-101: **Stomach, Antrum. Hyperplastic Polyp, Watermelon Stomach.** Several polyps in antrum of patient previously treated with laser therapy for watermelon stomach. Linear erythema suggests persistent vascular ectasia.

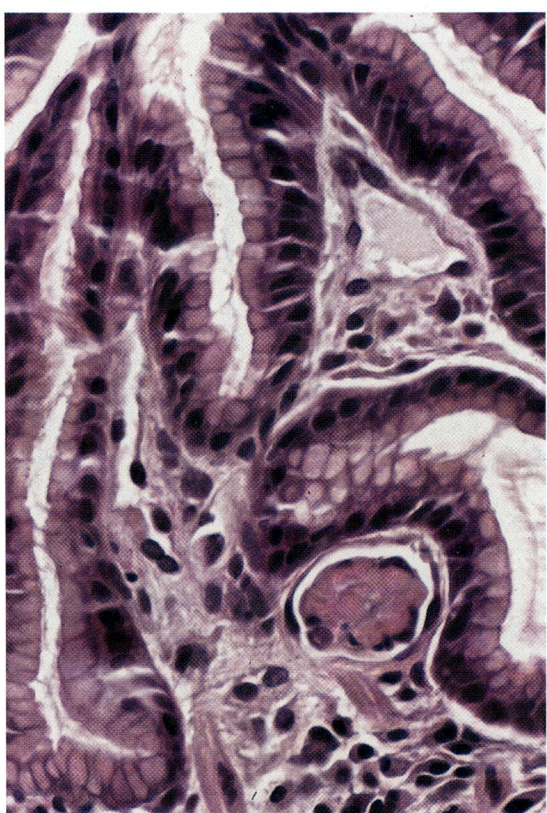

Figure 2-102: **Stomach, Antrum. Congestive Gastropathy, Watermelon Stomach.** Thick-walled, ectatic vessels in the foveolar compartment, with an organizing fibrin microthrombus. Foveolar hyperplasia.

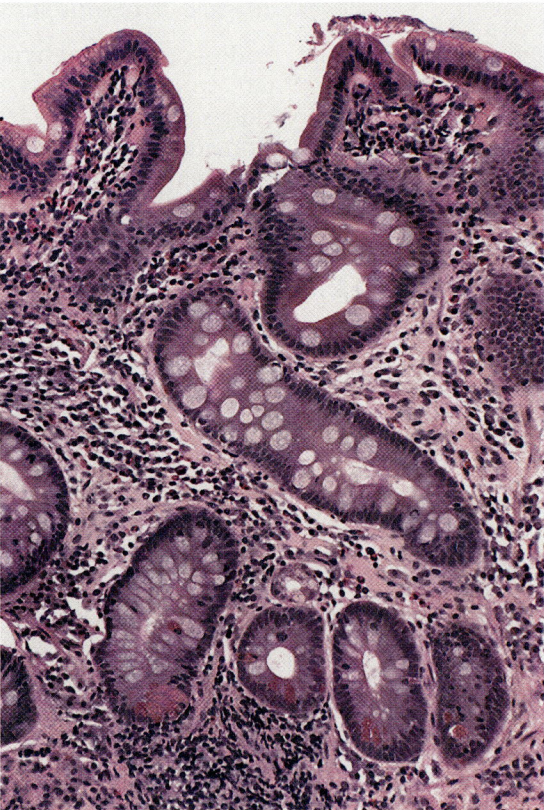

Figure 2-103: **Stomach, Antrum. Chronic Atrophic Gastritis and Watermelon Stomach.** Chronically inflamed body-type mucosa replaced by intestinal (goblet cell) epithelium.

HYPERTROPHIC GASTROPATHY AND GASTRITIS

- Morphology .... Giant mucosal folds in the body may be due to gastritis or gastropathy. In Zollinger-Ellison (ZE) syndrome, the thick mucosa and large folds are produced by an increased parietal cell mass due to the trophic effect of gastrin from an endocrine cell tumor. Hypertrophic gastropathy causing Menetrier syndrome is the result of massive foveolar hyperplasia and deeper glandular atrophy. There is little or no inflammation, unless the folds become eroded. Inflammation, when present, tends to consist largely of eosinophils, suggesting a possible allergic mechanism. Hypertrophic gastritis causing Menetrier syndrome is a hypertrophic variant of lymphocytic gastritis. The pattern of inflammation is similar to that seen in celiac sprue and lymphocytic colitis, suggesting either a hypersensitivity or autoimmune mechanism. Large body folds can be seen in *H pylori* gastritis.

- Endoscopic features .... The dominant feature is enlarged rugal folds. A common finding is a prominent mucosal cobblestone pattern due to the accentuation of the areae gastricae. There may be a large amount of pooled, nonbilious secretions.

- Clinical features .... Symptoms may be nonspecific in all forms. In ZE syndrome, patients have hypergastrinemia, hyperchlorhydria, and atypical or uncontrollable peptic ulceration frequently involving the second portion of the duodenum. Patients with hypertrophic gastropathy or gastritis may have abdominal pain, hyperchlorhydria or hypochlorhydria, depending on the stage of disease, and protein loss (Menetrier syndrome). Children with Menetrier syndrome have been described as having hypertrophic gastropathy with increased eosinophils, which may be self-limited.

- Differential diagnosis ...... Endoscopic: Zollinger-Ellison, Menetrier hypertrophic gastropathy, portal hypertensive gastropathy, hypertrophic lymphocytic gastritis, *H pylori* gastritis, infiltrative disorders, e.g., lymphoma, leukemia, diffusely infiltrating carcinomas, and metastatic carcinoma.

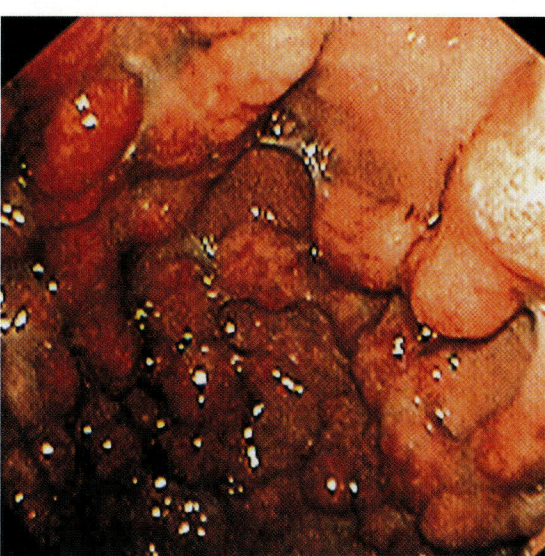

Figure 2-104: **Stomach. Hypertrophic Gastropathy.** Enlarged rugal folds with prominent cobblestone pattern.

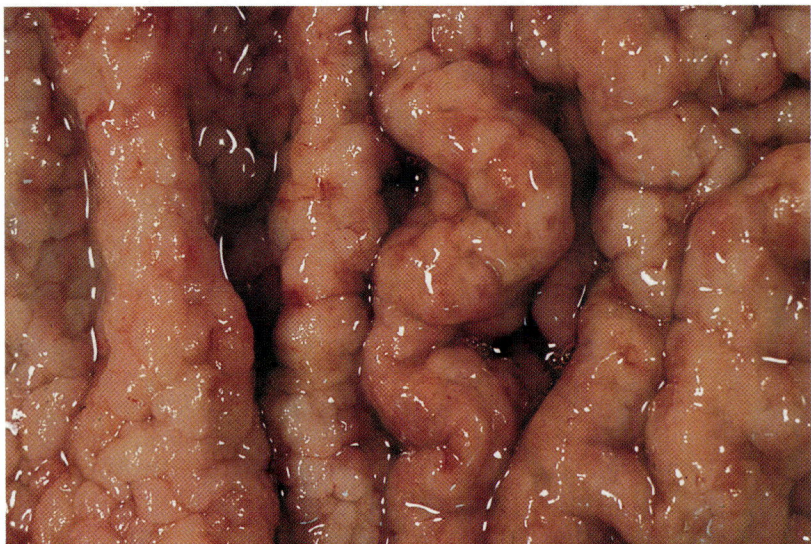

Figure 2-105: **Stomach, Body. Hypertrophic Gastropathy.** Large folds with accentuated areae gastricae producing a cobblestone pattern. Gross photo.

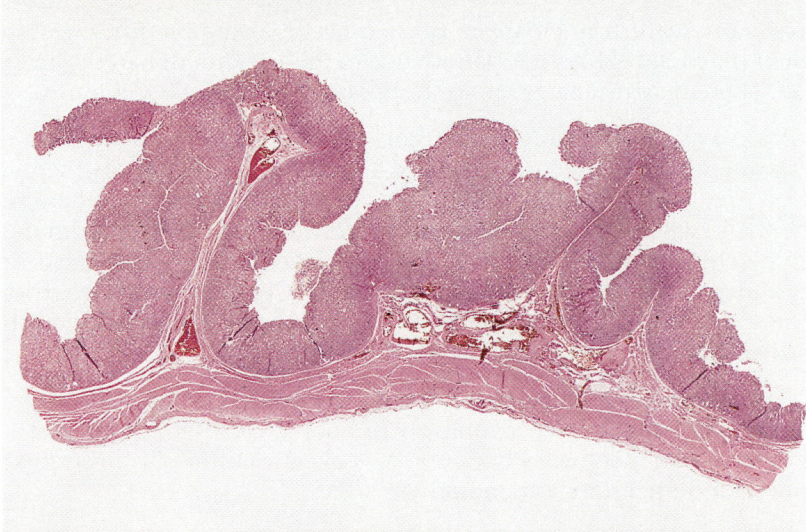

Figure 2-106: **Stomach, Body. Hypertrophic Gastropathy. Zollinger-Ellison Syndrome.** Full-thickness section showing thick mucosa and large folds.

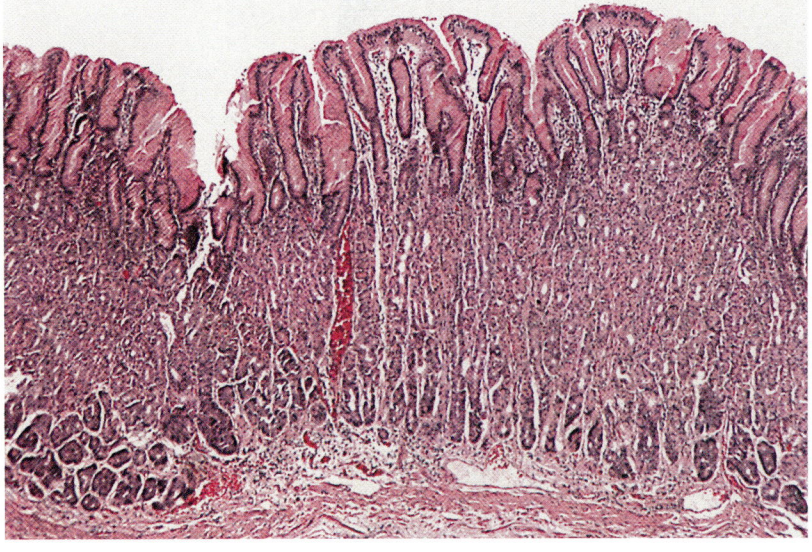

Figure 2-107: **Stomach, Body. Hypertrophic Gastropathy. Zollinger-Ellison Syndrome.** Increased mucosal thickness due to increased parietal cell mass. Gastric pits normal, glands elongated.

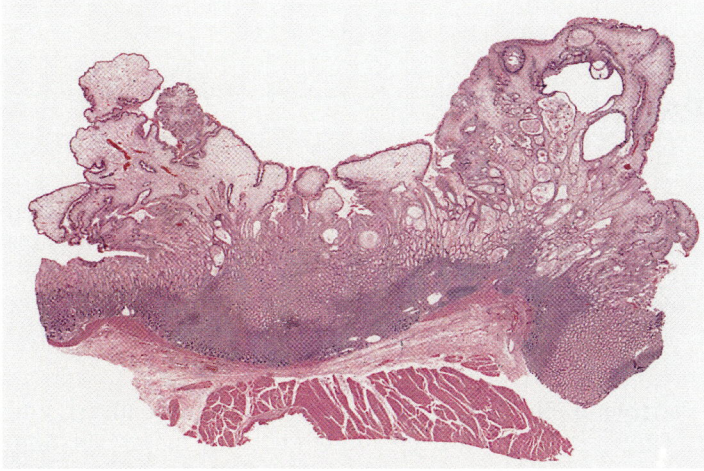

Figure 2-108: **Stomach, Body. Hypertrophic Gastropathy.** Full-thickness section shows massive mucosal thickening due to foveolar hyperplasia and edema.

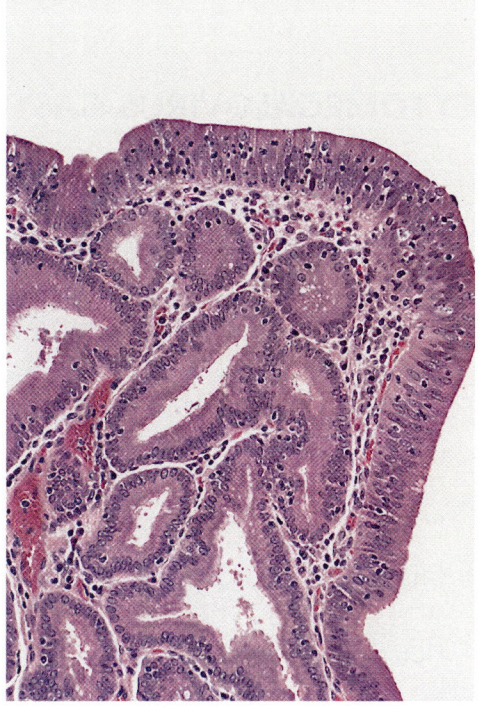

Figure 2-109: **Stomach, Body. Hypertrophic Lymphocytic Gastritis.** Foveolar hyperplasia, active chronic inflammation in the lamina propria, and marked increase in intra-epithelial lymphocytes, particularly in surface epithelium.

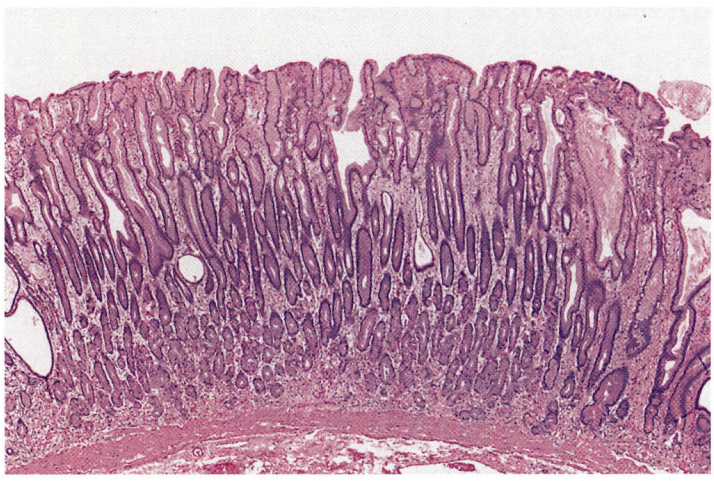

Figure 2-110: **Stomach, Body. Hypertrophic Gastropathy.** Foveolar hyperplasia with cysts and glandular atrophy; no inflammation.

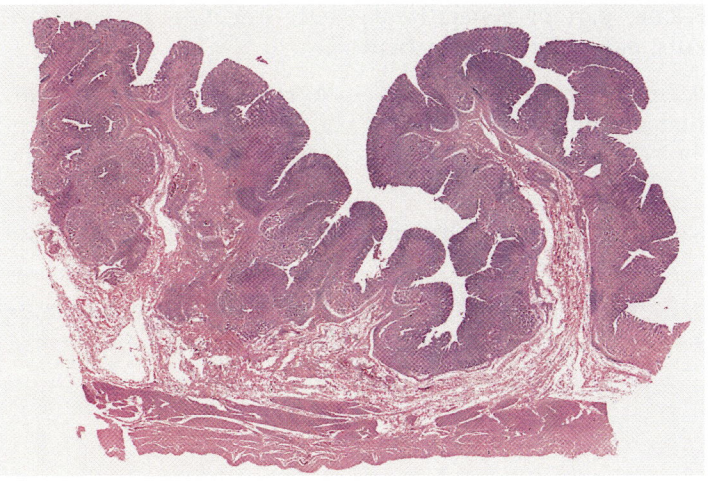

Figure 2-111: **Stomach, Body. Hypertrophic Lymphocytic Gastritis.** Full-thickness section with thick mucosa, accentuated areae gastricae, large folds, and submucosal edema.

CYTOMEGALOVIRUS GASTROPATHY

- Morphology .... CMV infects epithelial, endothelial, and stromal cells. Gastric CMV often shows foveolar hyperplasia with minimal inflammation, but may produce gastritis. Ulcer edges are frequently inflamed. CMV inclusions can be difficult to identify in granulation tissue. Endothelial inclusions may occlude vascular lumens and cause secondary thromboses resulting in localized ischemia and ulceration.

- Endoscopic features .... The features are variable, including punctate erosions, multiple ulcers, and large single ulcers. Large ulcers can be deep enough to cause major bleeding. Other findings include mucosal hemorrhages and thickened folds. Overall endoscopic features can suggest an acute inflammatory process or a chronic and indolent ulcerating process.

- Clinical features .... CMV is relatively common, but symptomatic involvement of the GI tract is generally limited to immunosuppressed individuals.

- Differential diagnosis ...... Histologic: Atypical reactive stromal cells may mimic CMV-infected cells. The inclusions are usually characteristic, but can be easily missed when sparse and unaccompanied by inflammation.

    Endoscopic: Erosions and ulcers in gastropathy and gastritis.

MISCELLANEOUS INFECTIONS

- Morphology .... *Candida* species: Commonly colonize chronic ulcers. Colonization, in contrast to invasive candidiasis, does not prolong healing or require antifungal therapy. Silver or PAS stains are needed to exclude invasion. May be a primary pathogen in immunosuppressed patients. Stomach is the second most common site of infection after esophagus. In colonization, there are white plaques in the ulcer base. In immunosuppressed patients, there may be multiple small ulcers and plaques.

    Cryptosporidium: Rare; part of generalized enteric infection in immunocompromised hosts, particularly HIV patients.

    Strongyloides: Extremely rare and seen only in overwhelming infestations. Must be differentiated from other nematodes, e.g., *Anisakis*. Cause of eosinophilic gastritis, but eosinophils are usually confined to the region of the parasite.

    Tuberculosis: Uncommon but increasing in prevalence. Produces a granulomatous gastritis.

- Comment .... *H pylori* is common, but all other infections are rare in the stomach because of the acid environment.

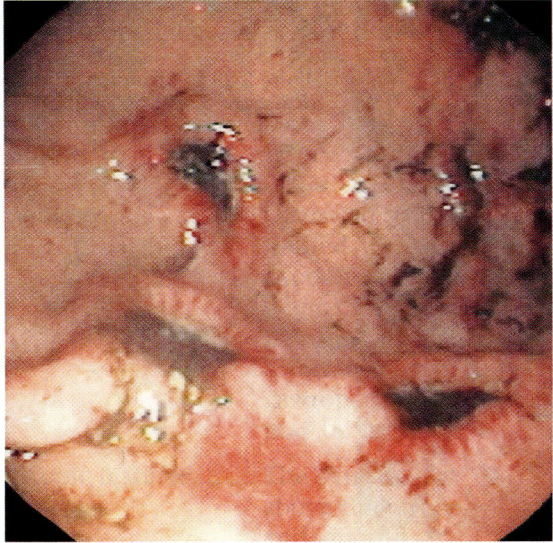

Figure 2-112: **Stomach. CMV Ulcers.** Three shallow ulcers with elevated margins contain dark material in the bases, presumably altered blood. Spotty erythema at ulcer margins.

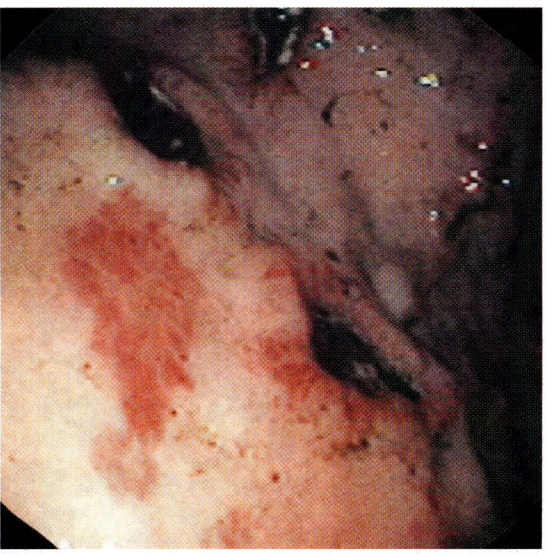

Figure 2-113: **Stomach. CMV Ulcers.** Large patch of erythema between two ulcers. The elevated margins and erythema favor an inflammatory process and mottled erythema suggests mucosal hemorrhage.

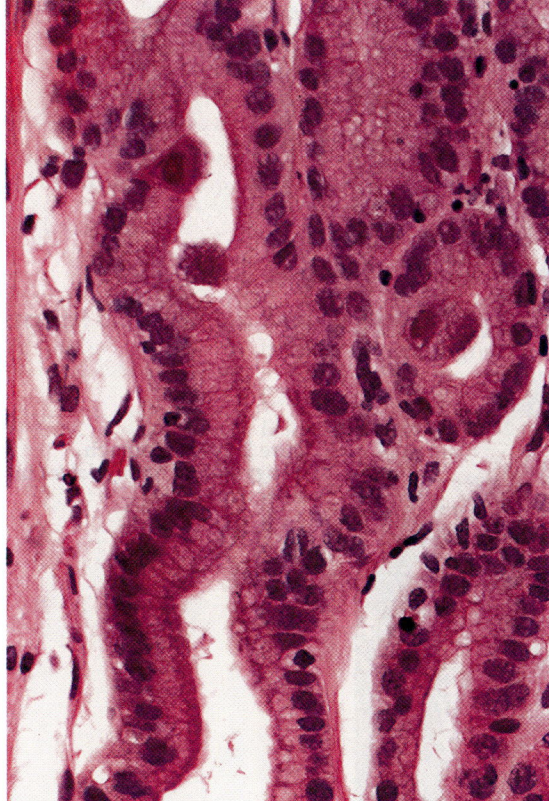

Figure 2-114: **Stomach. CMV Gastropathy.** CMV inclusions in foveolar epithelium. Cellular enlargement and large nuclear inclusions are characteristic.

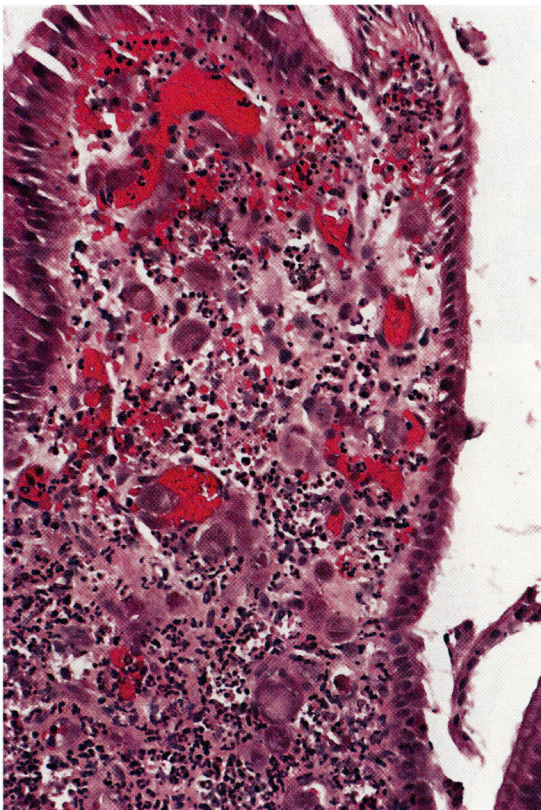

Figure 2-115: **Stomach. CMV Gastropathy.** Inclusions in large stromal and endothelial cells and acute inflammation from edge of ulcer.

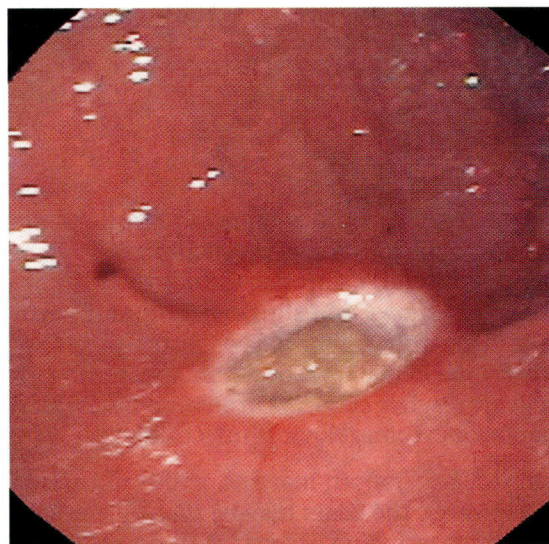

Figure 2-119: **Stomach. Peptic Ulcer.** Sharply defined ulcer with smooth, erythematous margins and fibrinopurulent exudate at the base.

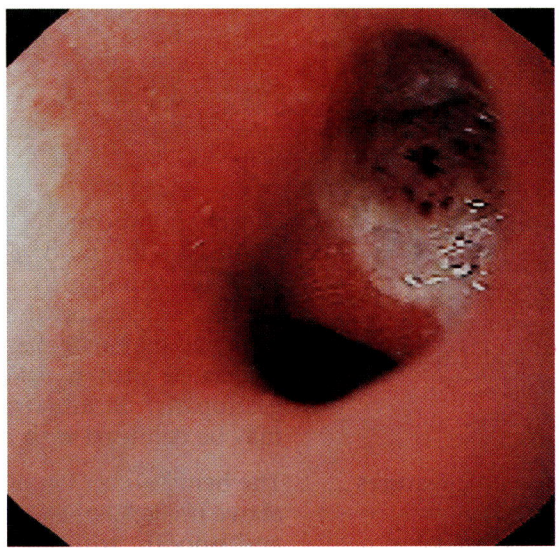

Figure 2-120: **Stomach. Peptic Ulcer.** Erythematous mucosa surrounds penetrating ulcer. Black eschar (altered blood) partially covers the ulcer base.

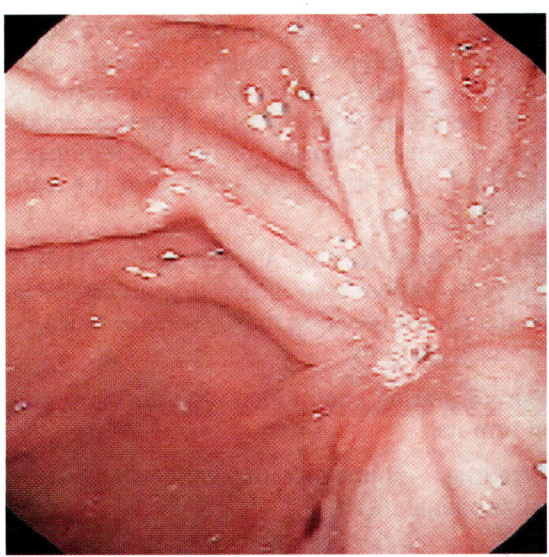

Figure 2-121: **Stomach. Healing Peptic Ulcer.** Radiating folds toward ulcer with smooth margins and clean base. Stellate scar indicates healing.

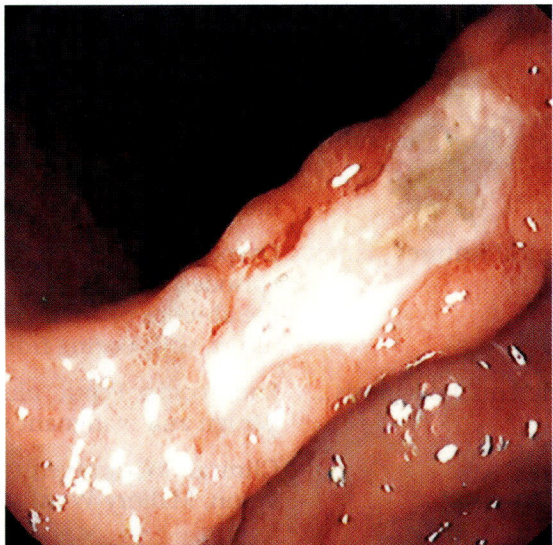

Figure 2-122: **Stomach. Peptic Ulcer.** Incisura ulcer. Although the margin of the ulcer is irregular, it is well-defined. Erythema and a minor amount of blood at the interface of the ulcer base and margins, a typical area for oozing. No visible vessel in the ulcer base.

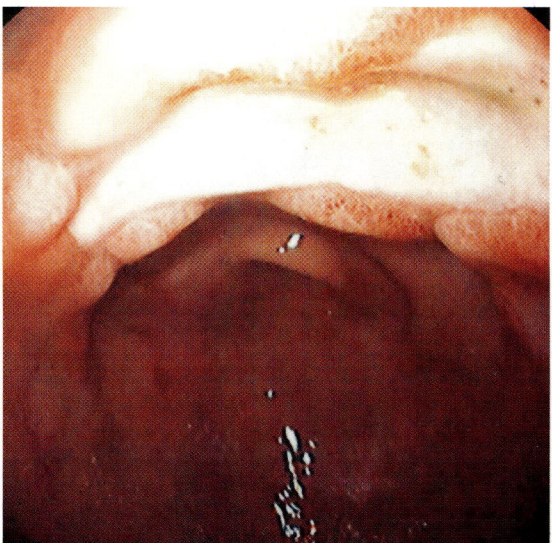

Figure 2-123: **Stomach. Peptic Ulcer.** Despite the raised margins, the well-defined edge of the ulcer base and lack of apparent elevation or mass effect favor a benign ulcer. Biopsies nevertheless are indicated.

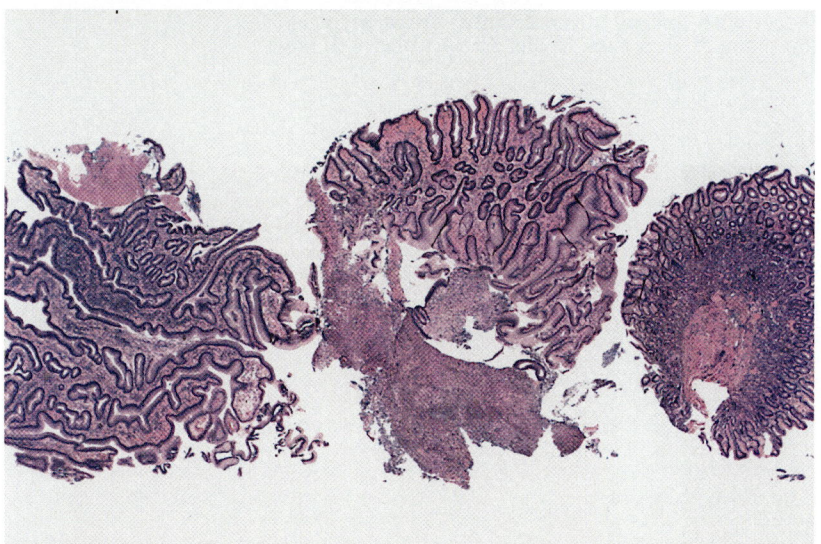

Figure 2-124: **Stomach. Peptic Ulcer.** Typical biopsy specimen: fragments of ulcer base (lower center), normal mucosa (right), and elongated and tortuous foveolae of reactive gastropathy (top center and left).

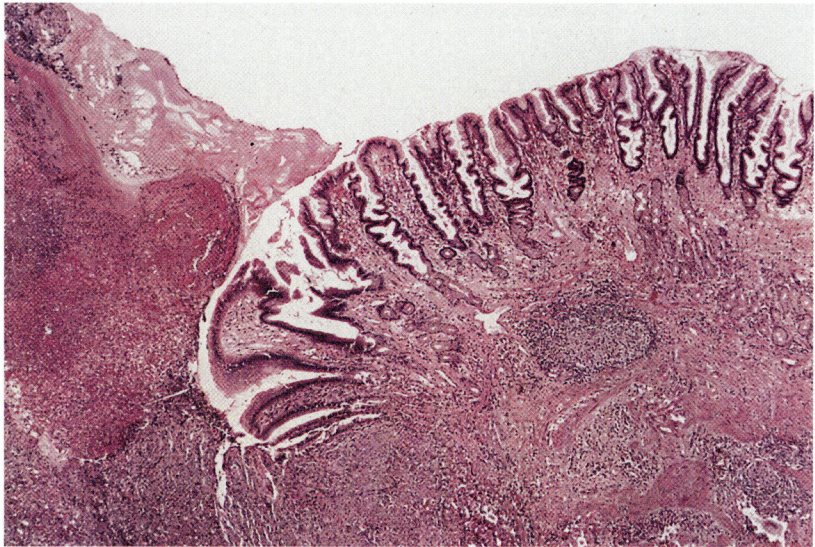

Figure 2-125: **Stomach. Chronic Peptic Ulcer.** Inflammation restricted to the base and edge of the ulcer. In this case, despite lymphoid hyperplasia, there is no background of diffuse gastritis.

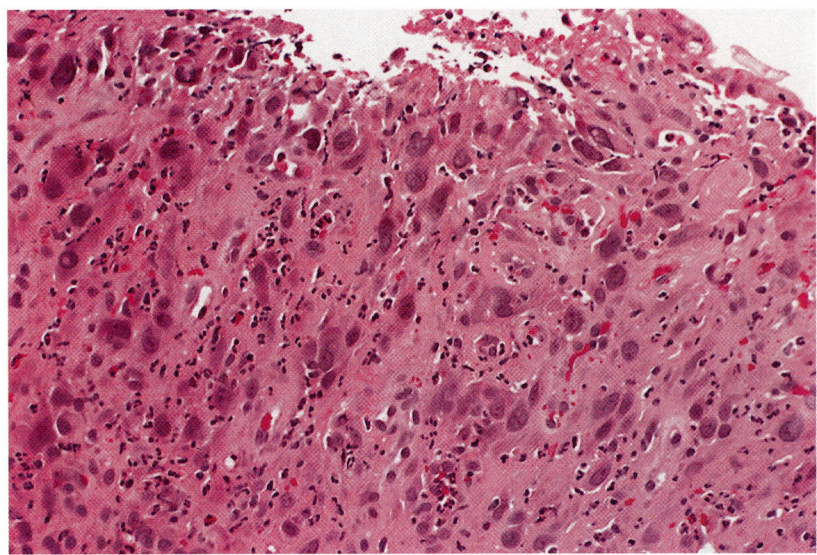

Figure 2-126: **Stomach. Ulcer with Bizarre Stromal Cells.** Large, atypical spindle cells in granulation tissue of ulcer base. Nuclei are vesicular with large nucleoli.

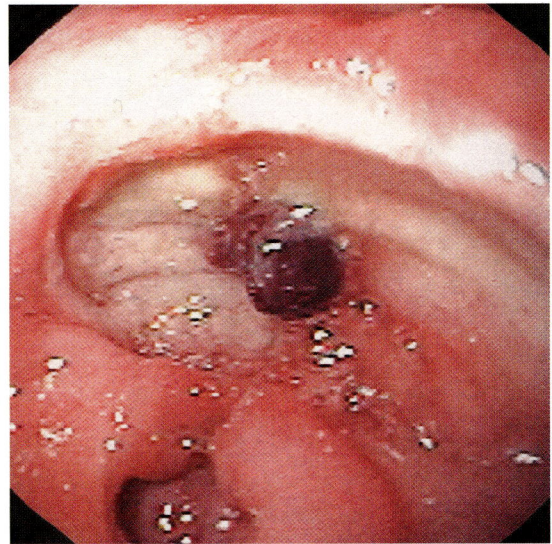

Figure 2-127: **Stomach. Peptic Ulcer with Visible Vessel and Clot.** Penetrating, prepyloric gastric ulcer with densely adherent focal blood clot.

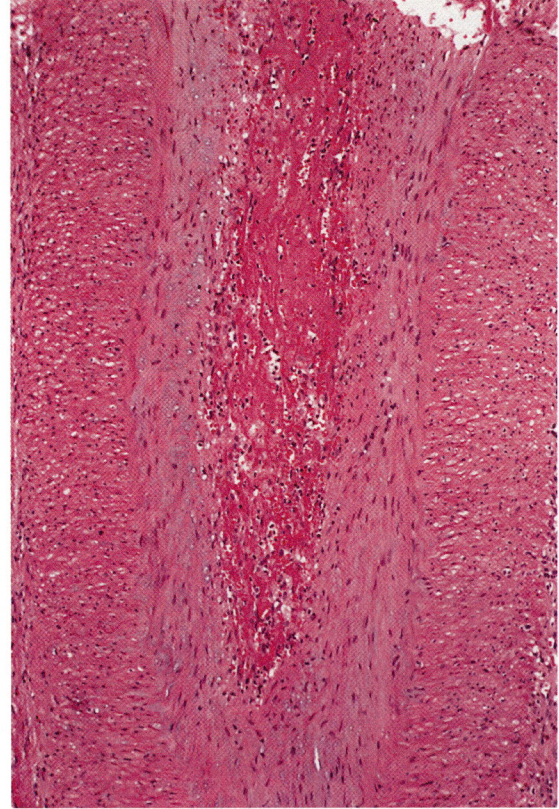

Figure 2-128: **Stomach. Visible Vessel, Ulcer Base.** Thrombosed artery in base of large ulcer.

CAMERON EROSION

- Morphology .... The Cameron erosion, no different histologically than other erosions (or ulcers), is located on the tops of the mucosal folds of sliding hiatal hernias, and presumably is due to pressure ischemia. The association of the large hiatal hernia with this lesion was made by Dr. Alan Cameron at the Mayo Clinic.

- Endoscopic features .... The Cameron erosion is unique to large hiatal hernias. The lesion may appear as a linear ulceration or a more shallow erosion distinctively located on the tops of the rugal folds comprising the distal rosette of a hiatal hernia. In some patients, the ulcers are round and deep. They may be found in various stages ranging from frank ulceration to thin, linear, healed scars surrounded by slightly erythematous, prominent mucosa.

- Clinical features .... The Cameron lesion gives rise to chronic GI blood loss. Rarely, a large ulceration produces overt bleeding with hematemesis or melena. Patients otherwise have typical symptoms of hiatal hernias, with meal-induced mechanical discomfort as well as gastroesophageal reflux-type symptoms. The ulcers are suspected to arise from mechanical irritation of the gastric mucosa at the passage point through the diaphragmatic hiatus. NSAIDs may contribute to the formation of these ulcers. There is no definitive evidence to suggest that *H pylori* is a contributing factor.

- Differential diagnosis ...... Endoscopic: Erosions of other cause such as NSAIDs, alcohol, stress-induced erosions.

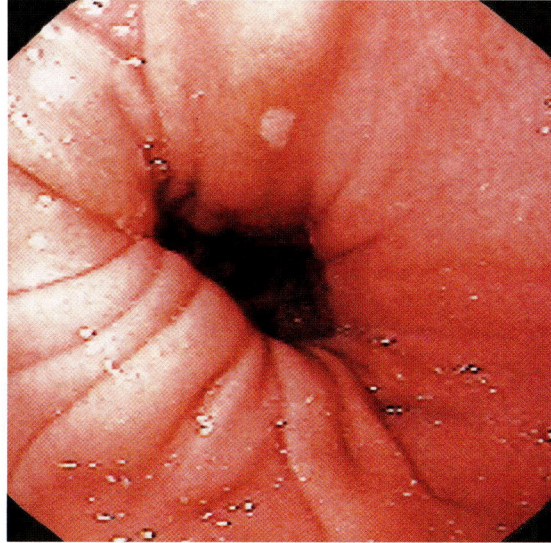

Figure 2-129: **Stomach. Cameron Erosion.** Large hiatal hernia with superficial erosion on gastric folds.

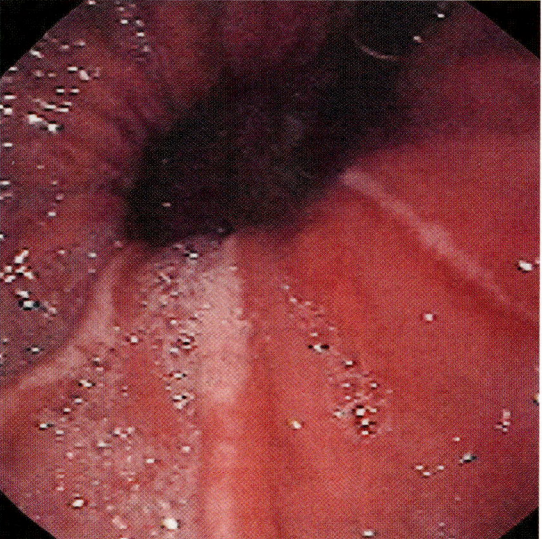

Figure 2-130: **Stomach. Cameron Erosion.** Three linear erythematous streaks with white clean-based shallow ulcers on the surface of the gastric folds.

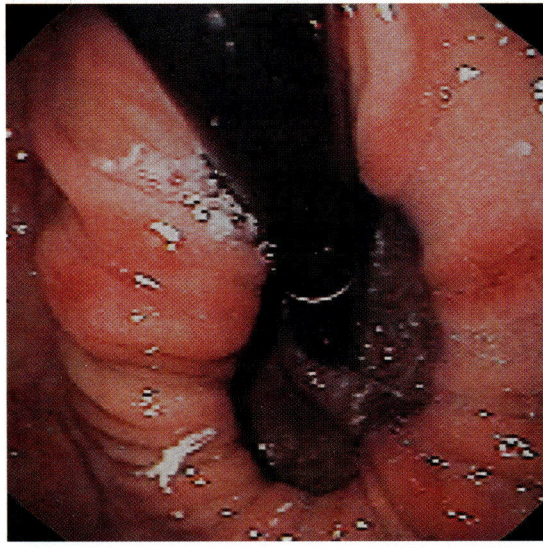

Figure 2-131: **Stomach. Cameron Erosion.** Multiple linear ulcers located at the distal end of the hiatal hernia, seen on retroflexed view.

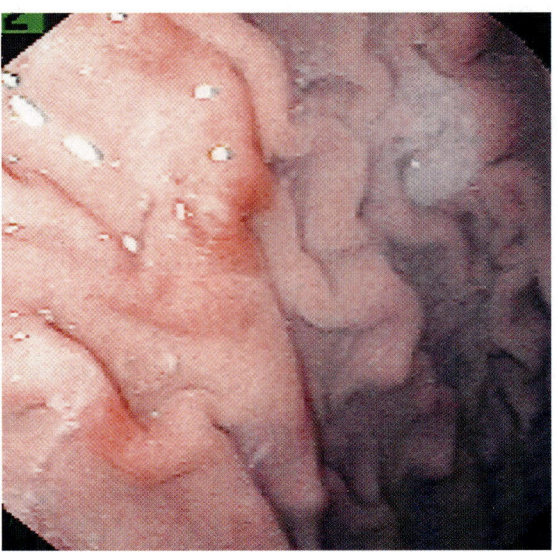

Figure 2-132: **Stomach. Cameron Erosion.** Surface erosion on gastric fold.

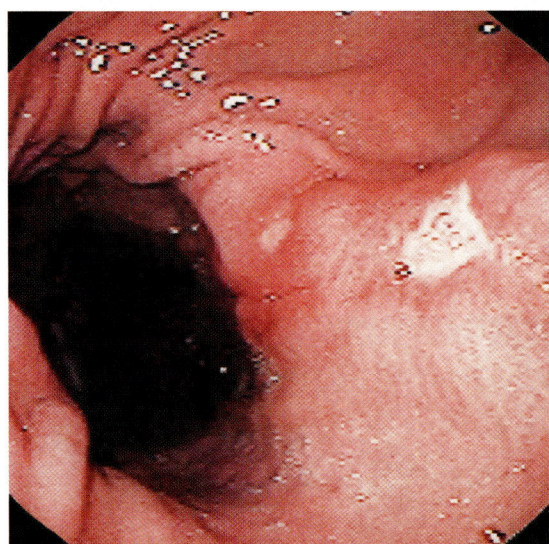

Figure 2-133: **Stomach. Cameron Erosion.** A discrete, shallow, clean-based ulcer with prominence of the surrounding mucosa. To the left of this ulcer is a smaller erosion with more erythema surrounding the margins. Both are located at the distal end of a large hiatal hernia.

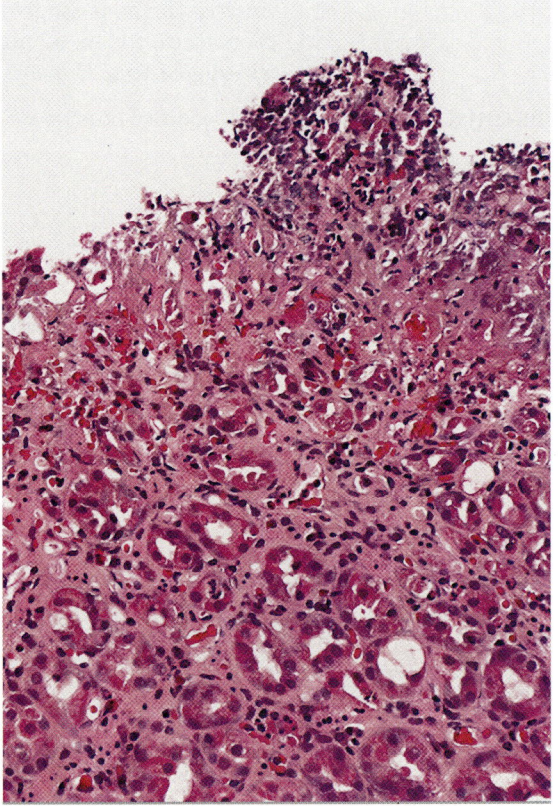

Figure 2-134: **Stomach. Cameron Erosion.** Superficial erosion in fundic mucosa.

DIEULAFOY LESION

- Morphology .... Vascular abnormality in which a muscular artery maintains a persistent large diameter as it penetrates the mucosa, where it may be traumatized and eroded.

- Endoscopic features .... The Dieulafoy lesion presents with active arterial bleeding from a pinpoint location. Nonbleeding lesions have a protruding artery or pigmented protuberance surrounded by normal mucosa or an attached fresh clot. These lesions are most commonly located within 6 cm of the esophagogastric junction. The surrounding mucosa typically appears normal, but there may be a visible mucosal defect no more than a few millimeters surrounding the lesion.

- Clinical features .... Acute, recurrent, upper gastrointestinal bleeding. Episodes are typically serious, with hematemesis, hematochezia, and significant drops in hemoglobin.

- Differential diagnosis ...... Clinical: Peptic ulcer and bleeding varices. Due to the nature and severity of bleeding and the difficulty of identifying these lesions, the diagnosis is best established by an endoscopy close to or during active bleeding. Multiple endoscopies are often needed for diagnosis.

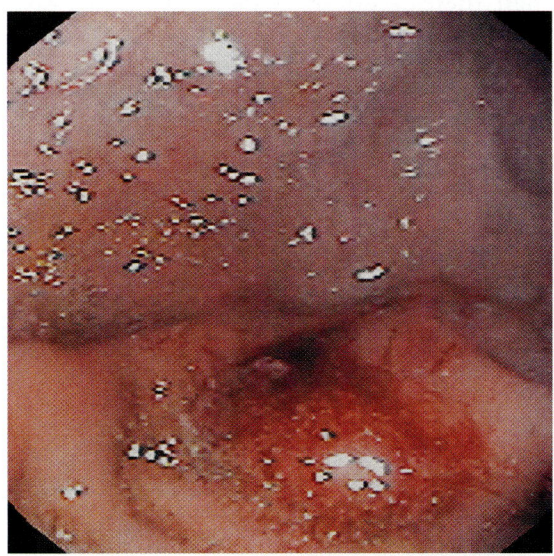

Figure 2-135: **Stomach. Dieulafoy Lesion.** A visible vessel presenting as a pale protuberance surrounded by a clot. The adjacent mucosa appears normal.

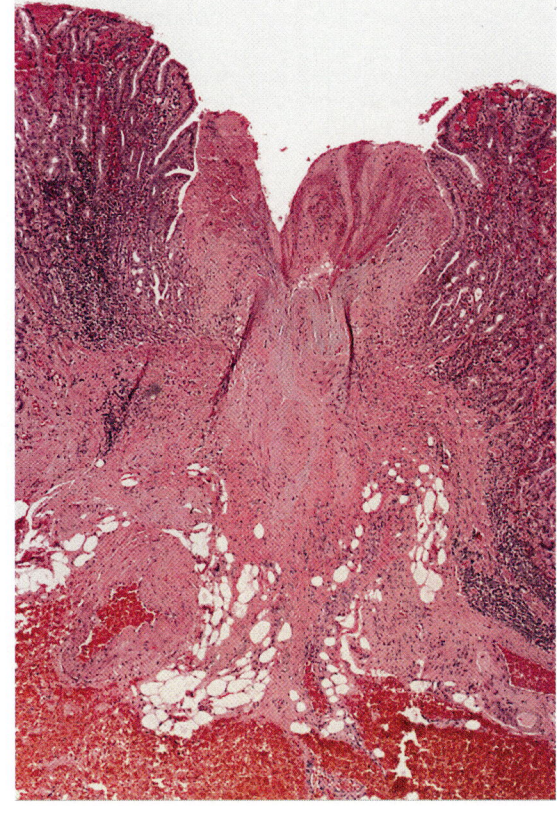

Figure 2-136: **Stomach. Dieulafoy Lesion.** Muscular artery penetrates mucosa. Wall of artery is eroded. No associated mucosal ulcer.

VARICES AND VASCULAR MALFORMATIONS

- Endoscopic features .... Gastric varices may be large bulging nodules or serpigenous venous trunks. Red color signs such as erythematous spots and wales suggest a high risk for bleeding. Mucosal vascular lesions are brightly erythematous and, when inspected closely, the vascular elements can be seen. The lesions may be single or multiple, as in hereditary syndromes such as Osler-Weber-Rendu (hereditary hemorrhagic telangiectasia). Larger vascular lesions, typically hereditary, are more easily identified because of their nodular or polypoid appearance and blue to purplish color due to their greater amount of venous elements.

- Clinical features .... Small mucosal vascular malformations or angiectasias, encountered with angiodysplasia, watermelon stomach, radiation, and Osler-Weber-Rendu syndrome, present with chronic iron deficiency anemia or melena, due to the chronic low volume of bleeding. Patients with larger macroscopic arteriovenous malformations, hemangiomas, and the blue-rubber bleb nevus syndrome also experience chronic iron deficiency anemia and chronic intermittent melena, but have a greater tendency for isolated episodes of overt bleeding.

- Differential diagnosis ...... Endoscopic: Small mucosal angiectasias must be differentiated from mucosal trauma and focally adherent clots. Suction and mucosal endoscope tip trauma, especially if very small (< 2 mm), can be difficult to distinguish from minute angiectasias. When there is doubt, a directed biopsy should be obtained.

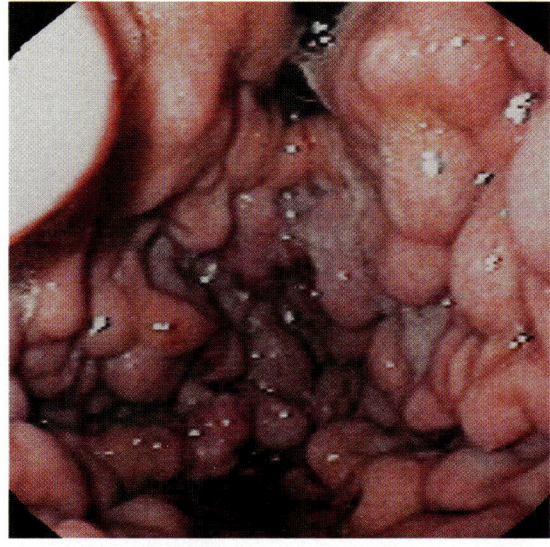

Figure 2-137: **Stomach. Varices.** Fundus and cardia packed with large nodular varices. Some contain red color signs such as red wales and hemocystic spots, which denote a high risk for bleeding.

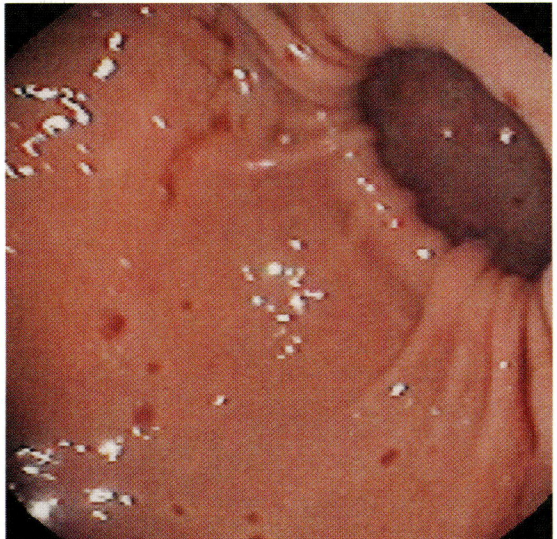

Figure 2-138: **Stomach. Osler-Weber-Rendu Syndrome.** Multiple telangiectasias with thin rims of pale mucosa. The multiplicity, presence throughout the stomach, and individual appearance are typical for Osler-Weber-Rendu syndrome. Upon closer inspection, the larger lesions appear as ectatic, tightly clustered blood vessels.

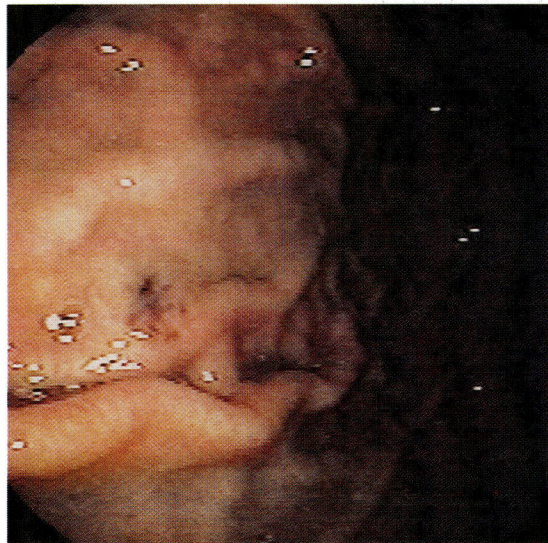

Figure 2-139: **Stomach. Blue-Rubber Bleb Nevus.** Bluish submucosal nodule with a central defect from which there had been bleeding.

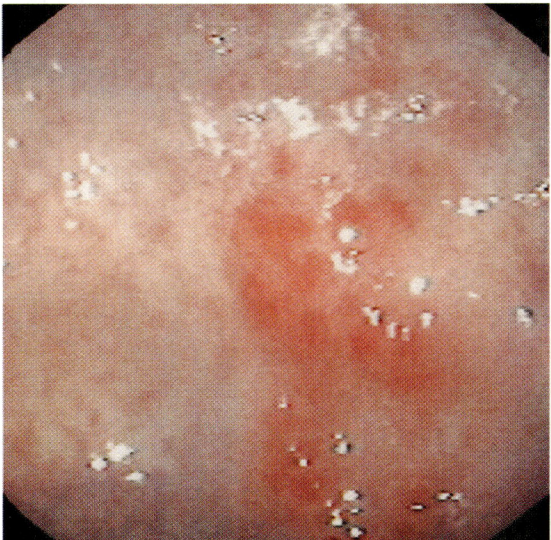

Figure 2-140: **Stomach. Angiectasia.** Unusual pattern of mucosal vascular malformations in the gastric body of a patient with portal hypertension, varices, and portal hypertensive gastropathy.

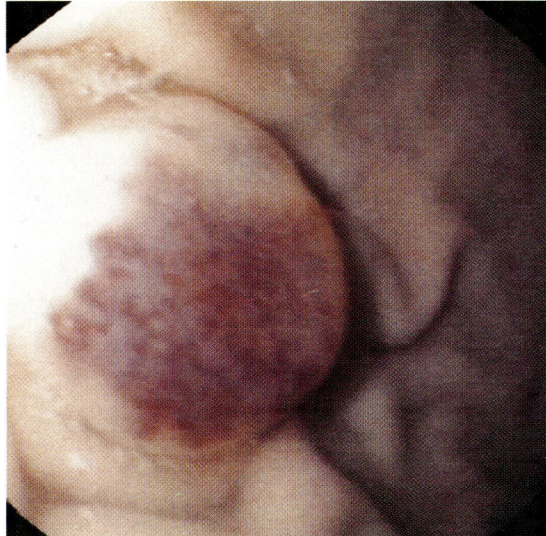

Figure 2-141: **Stomach. Hemangioma.** A vascular-appearing nodule along the greater curvature of the stomach in a patient with diffuse hemangiomatosis.

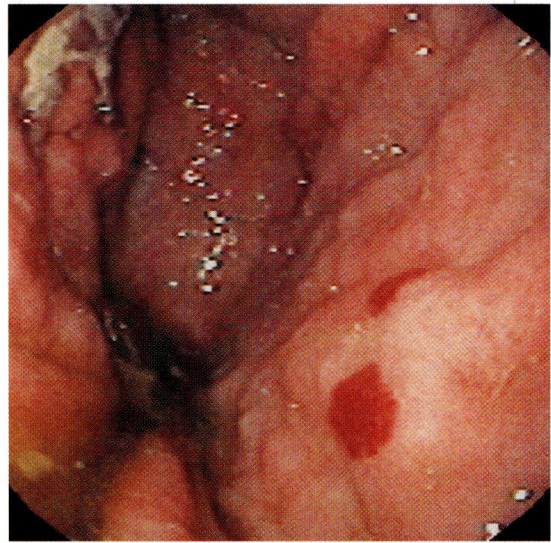

Figure 2-142: **Stomach. Angiectasia.** Two discrete angiectasias (angiodysplasia) are in the proximal body of the stomach.

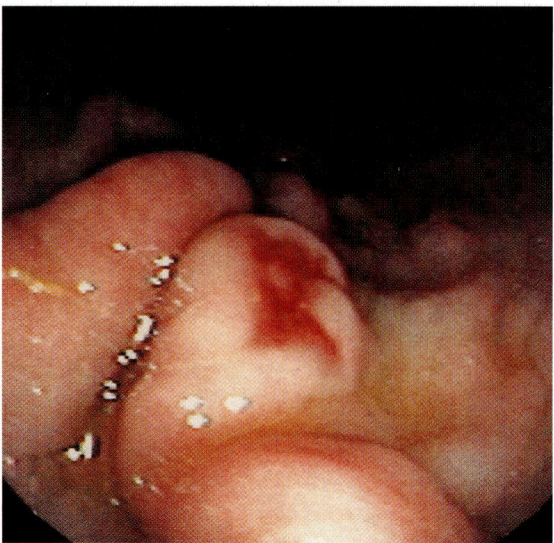

Figure 2-143: **Stomach. Angiectasia. Osler-Weber-Rendu Syndrome.** Discrete angiectasia with distinctive surrounding zone of pale mucosa. This "halo sign" is typical for these mucosal vascular malformations.

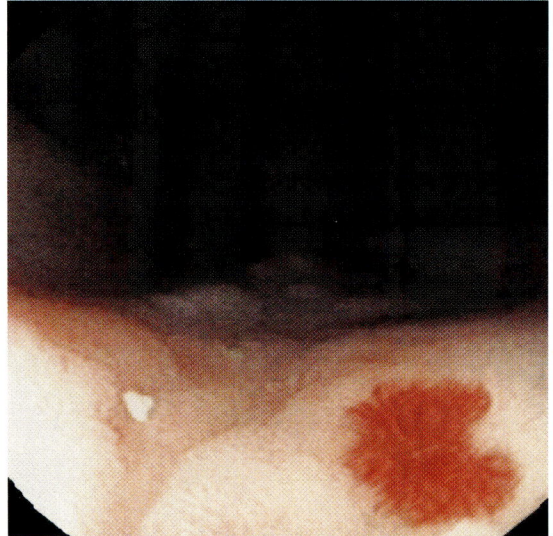

Figure 2-144: **Stomach. Angiectasia. Osler-Weber-Rendu Syndrome.** Close-up demonstrates the prominent ectatic, irregularly shaped mucosal vascular components, somewhat like miniature port-wine stains.

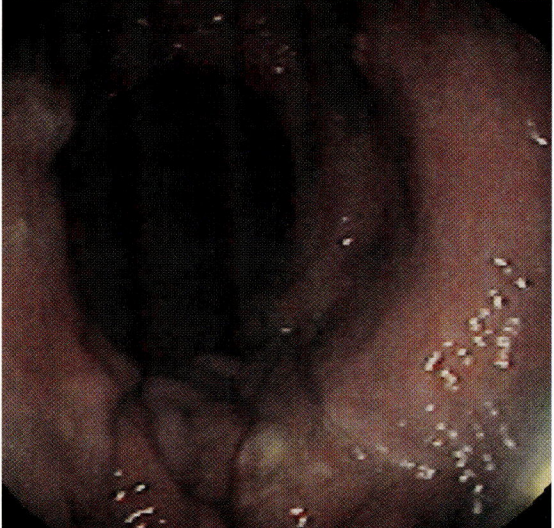

Figure 2-145: **Stomach. Angiectasia, Post-Treatment.** The lesions have been coagulated by a Nd:YAG laser and appear as a white, elevated coagulum. The elevation is due to edema caused by the thermal effect.

ATROPHIC GASTRITIS WITH CARCINOID TUMORS
Endocrine cell hyperplasia/micronests in atrophic gastritis

- Morphology .... Increased numbers of endocrine cells in glandular epithelium of the body of the stomach characterize enterochromaffinlike cell (ECL cell) hyperplasia—the response to continuous stimulation by gastrin in atrophic gastritis. Endocrine micronests/microcarcinoids, usually multiple in patients with atrophic gastritis/pernicious anemia, are clusters of cells in the lamina propria not forming a distinct tumor.

- Endoscopic features .... Thinned mucosa with loss of rugae, prominence of submucosal vascular pattern, and discrete erythematous nodules.

- Clinical features .... Endocrine hyperplasia/micronests/carcinoids are the result of prolonged hypergastrinemia, and are seen not only in atrophic gastritis/pernicious anemia, but also in Zollinger-Ellison syndrome. Endocrine proliferations in these settings behave in an indolent manner. Because of this, surveillance endoscopies are not warranted. High-risk groups include multiple endocrine neoplasia (MEN) syndromes and juvenile pernicious anemia.

- Differential diagnosis ...... Endoscopic: Hyperplastic polyps, fundic gland polyps, nodular intestinal metaplasia, and adenomas including small nodular adenocarcinomas. The coexistence of gastric atrophy with prominence of the submucosal vasculature can strengthen the possibility of a carcinoid.

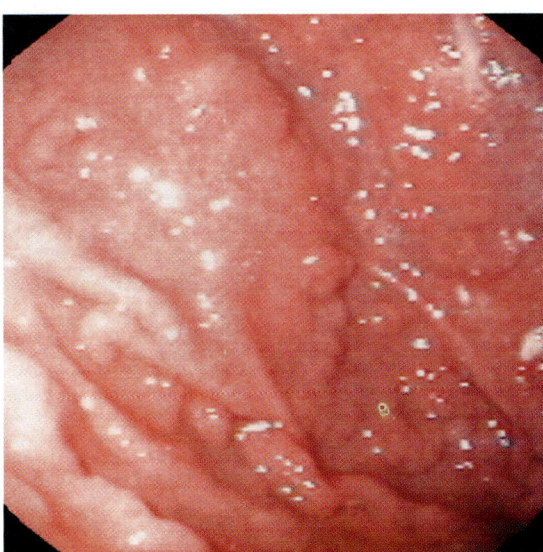

Figure 2-146: **Stomach. Atrophic Gastritis and Microcarcinoids.** Multiple polypoid nodules, mottled surrounding mucosa, and a prominent vasculature suggestive of atrophy.

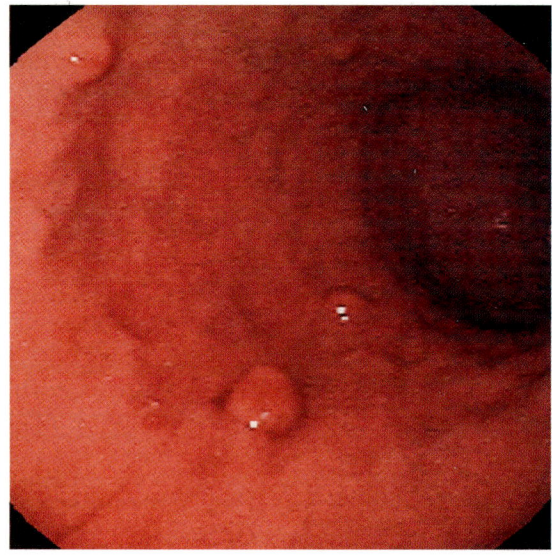

Figure 2-147: **Stomach. Atrophic Gastritis with Carcinoids.** Numerous semipedunculated polyps, 5 to 8 mm.

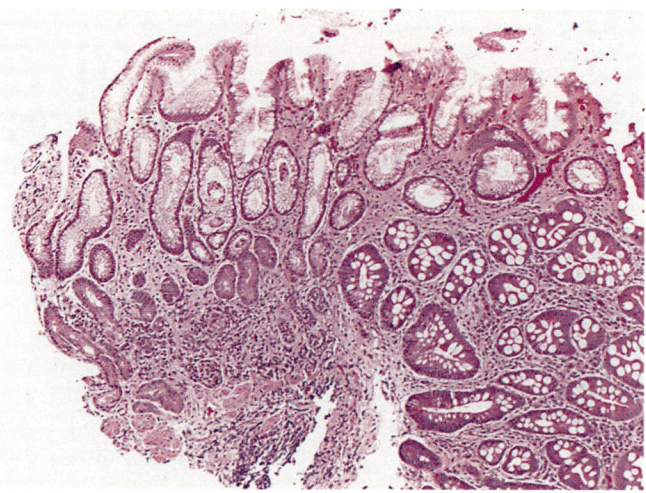

Figure 2-148: **Stomach. Carcinoid in Chronic Atrophic Gastritis.** Microcarcinoid in deep mucosa adjacent to large focus of intestinal metaplasia.

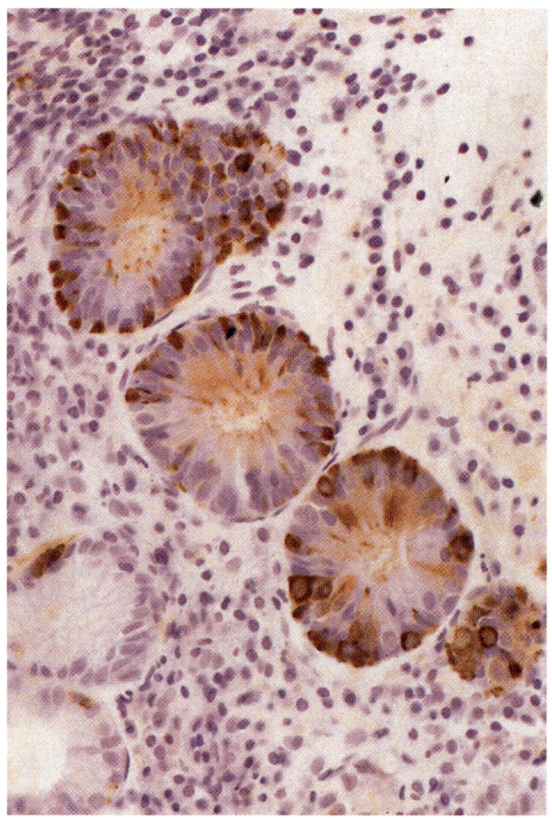

Figure 2-149: **Stomach. Endocrine Cell Hyperplasia, Atrophic Gastritis.** Increased numbers of chromogranin-positive cells in gastric glands (immunostain); background chronic inflammation.

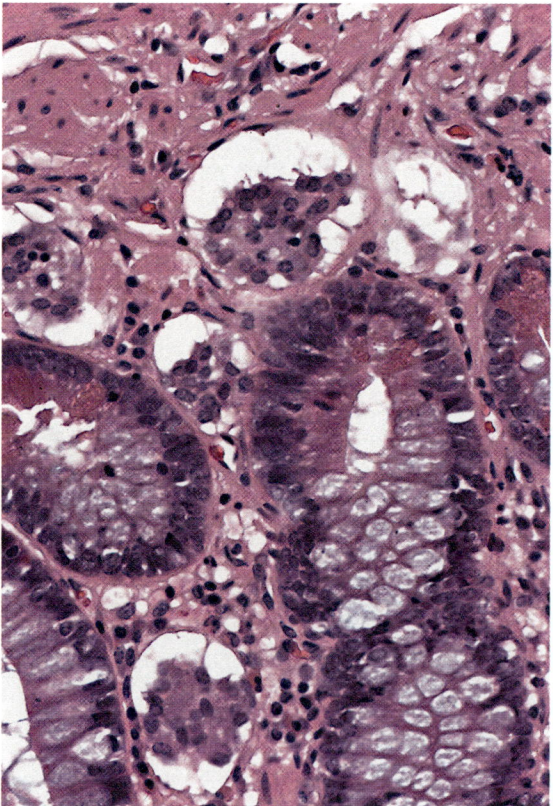

Figure 2-150: **Stomach. Endocrine Micronests, Atrophic Gastritis.** Clusters of endocrine cells surrounded by clear artifactual spaces in deep lamina propria. Small cells with amphophilic cytoplasm and round, uniform nuclei without nucleoli. Intestinalized glands with goblet and Paneth cells replace fundic epithelium.

CARCINOID TUMOR

- Morphology .... Gastric antral carcinoids are solid lesions that extend from the mucosa into the submucosa and rarely ulcerate. Growth patterns are more irregular with diffuse, trabecular, and glandular structures, compared to the typical midgut carcinoids which are insular (nests). Cytologically, the nuclei are bland with diffuse chromatin, inconspicuous nucleoli, and rare mitoses. Confirmatory histochemical or immunohistochemical reactions are only needed in the minority of cases where the histologic appearance is unusual. Chromogranin is the most reliable marker to identify gastric carcinoids. Association with syndromes such as Zollinger-Ellison require clinical correlation (e.g., serum gastrin levels and immunohistochemistry) to identify secretory products.

- Endoscopic features .... Sporadic carcinoid tumors tend to be solitary and are larger than carcinoids arising from prolonged hypergastrinemia. Endoscopic ultrasound can be helpful in the assessment of the carcinoid tumor. Lesions over 2 cm in size have a greater malignant potential.

- Clinical features .... Sporadic carcinoid tumors tend to be aggressive compared to carcinoids in chronic atrophic gastritis. Unless the carcinoid tumor has grown sufficiently to metastasize to the liver, the lesion is asymptomatic and incidentally encountered.

- Differential diagnosis...... Endoscopic: Hyperplastic or adenomatous polyp, leiomyoma.

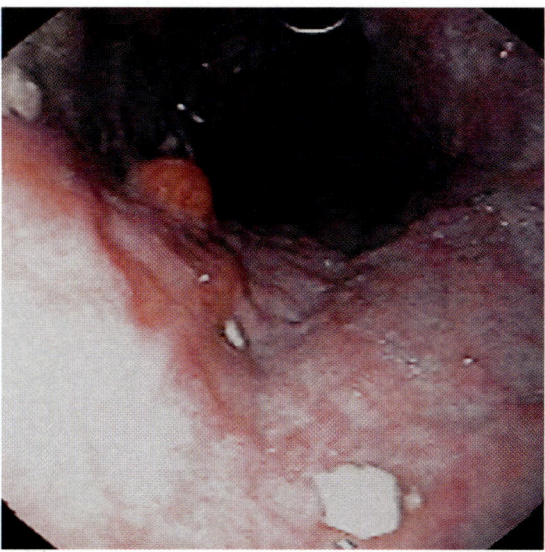

Figure 2-151: **Stomach, Antrum. Carcinoid in Chronic Atrophic Gastritis.** Discrete mucosal nodule in a background suggestive of gastric atrophy, with diffusely prominent submucosal vascular pattern.

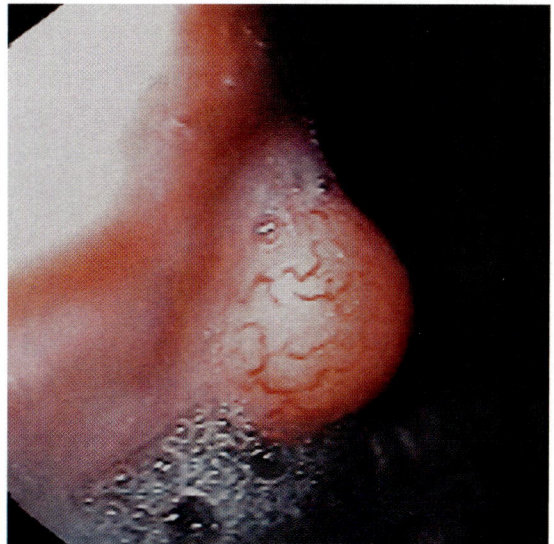

Figure 2-152: **Stomach, Antrum. Carcinoid in Chronic Atrophic Gastritis.** Smooth surface of nodule with multiple small mucosal microvessels.

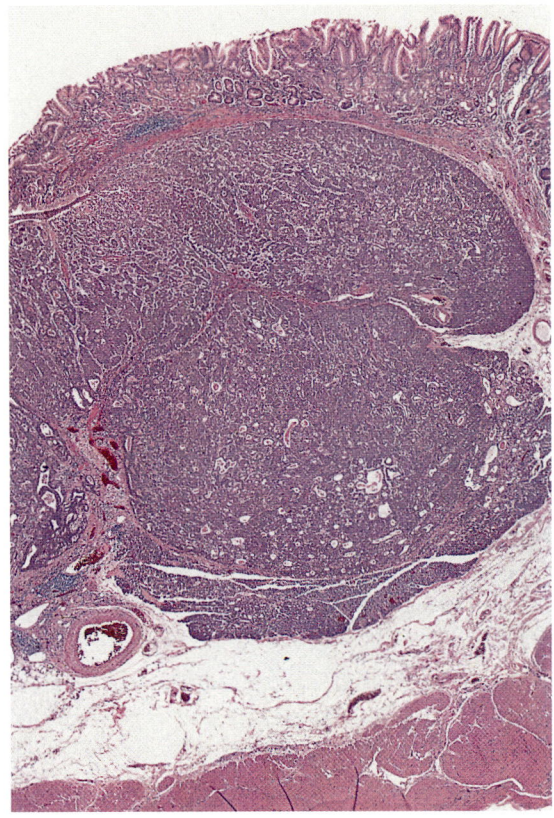

Figure 2-153: **Stomach, Antrum. Carcinoid Tumor.** Partially lobulated, solid, glandular, basophilic submucosal mass. Overlying mucosa inflamed and atrophic, but not ulcerated or eroded.

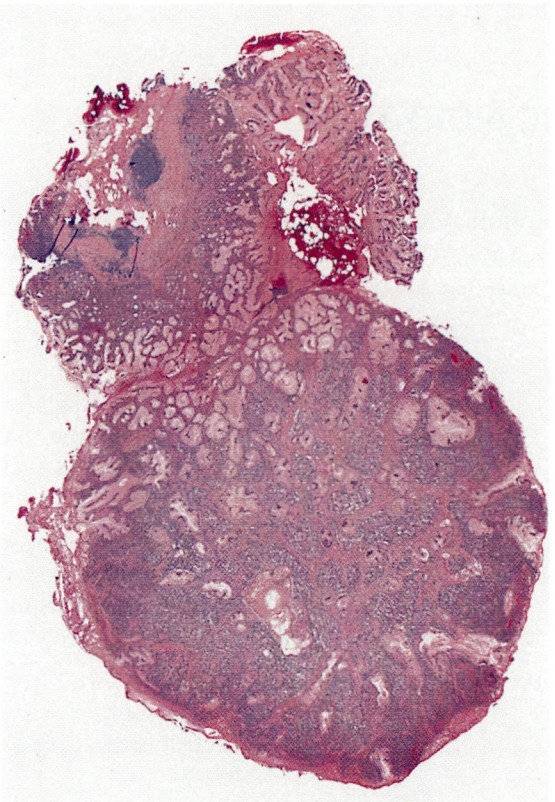

Figure 2-154: **Stomach. Carcinoid Tumor.** Polypoid growth with entrapment of foveolar glands.

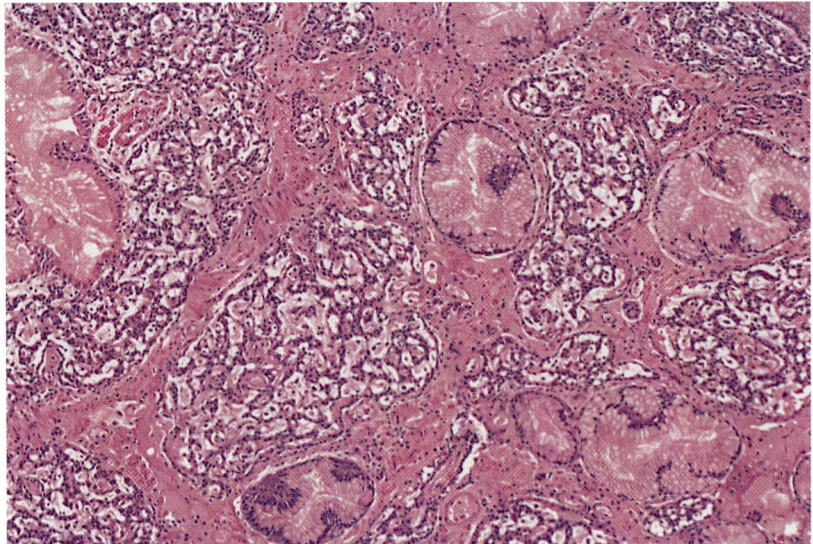

Figure 2-155: **Stomach. Carcinoid Tumor.** Complex growth pattern of carcinoid and entrapped foveolar glands.

PANCREATIC HETEROTOPIA AND METAPLASIA

- Morphology .... Heterotopic pancreatic tissue forms a tumorlike nodule, usually a nonencapsulated intramural nodule, that can reach several centimeters in size. Larger lesions often have central umbilication. The submucosa is the most frequent location, but some involve the muscularis propria. Both exocrine and endocrine pancreatic tissue may comprise the lesion, although ducts, often cystically dilated, usually dominate, with endocrine tissue being least common. Lobular structures are characteristic, often surrounded by or embedded in smooth muscle. The terms *myoepithelial hamartoma* and *adenomyoma* have been used as synonyms for lesions composed of only ducts and muscle. Pancreatic metaplasia differs from pancreatic heterotopia by its location in the mucosa, adjacent to or admixed with the gastric glands, and by the absence of prominent ducts and muscle bundles.

- Endoscopic features .... Pancreatic heterotopia presents as a submucosal nodule with a distinctive central depression corresponding to a duct. Pancreatic metaplasia is not evident endoscopically and is an incidental histologic finding.

- Clinical features .... The most distinctive heterotopic lesions occur in the antrum and are encountered in all age groups.

- Differential diagnosis...... Endoscopic: Other submucosal nodules, e.g., a carcinoid or a leiomyoma.

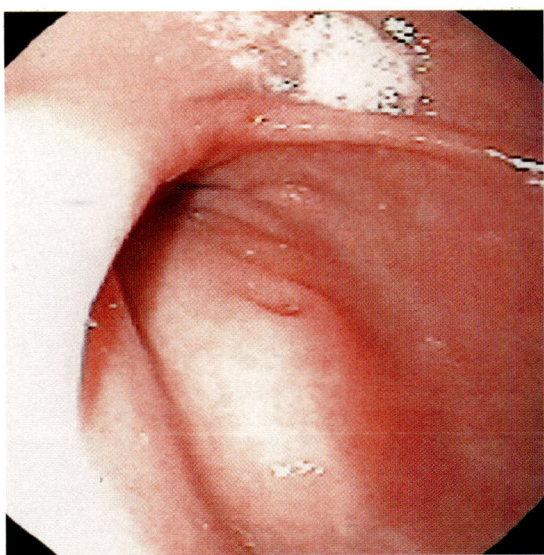

Figure 2-156: **Stomach. Pancreatic Heterotopia.** A 1-cm antral nodule with central depression and intact, overlying antral mucosa.

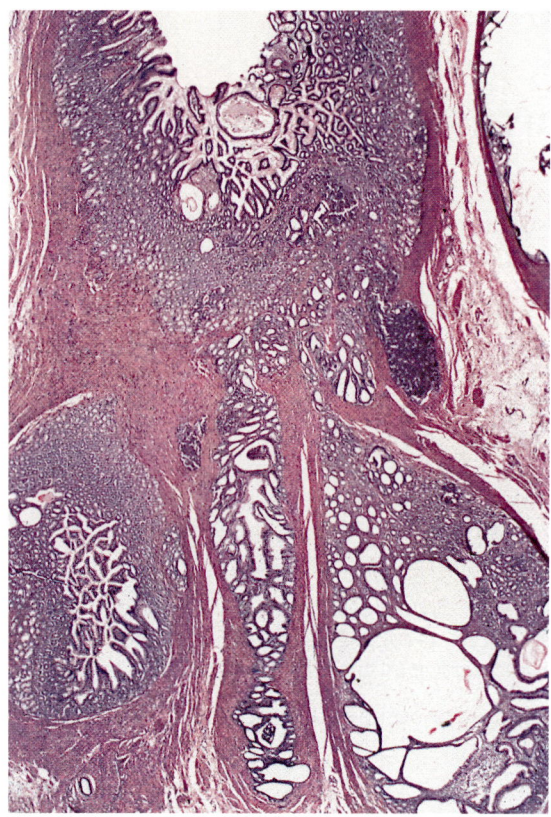

Figure 2-157: **Stomach. Pancreatic Heterotopia.** Mucosa has an indentation (dimpling) and overlies lobules of pancreatic acinar and ductal tissue.

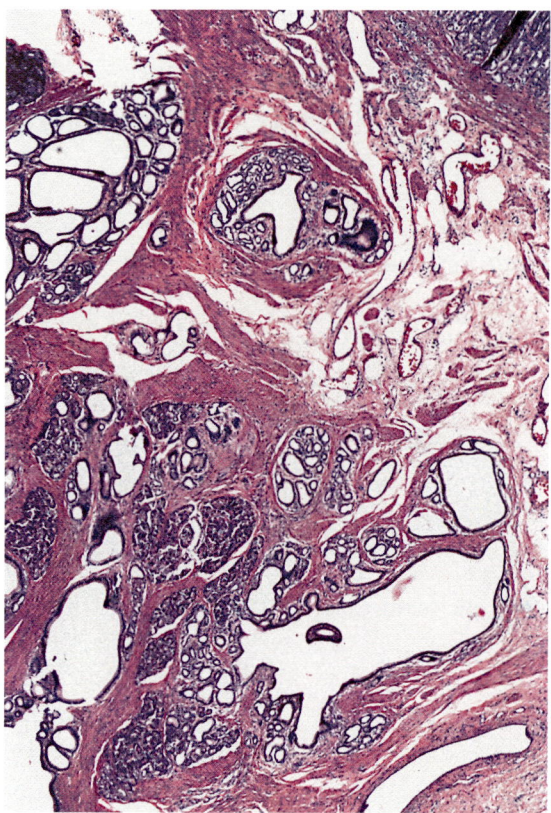

Figure 2-158: **Stomach. Pancreatic Heterotopia.** Lobules of ductal and acinar structures surrounded by smooth muscle form a mass in the submucosa. The lobular arrangement of the glandular tissue distinguishes this from carcinoma, even at low magnification.

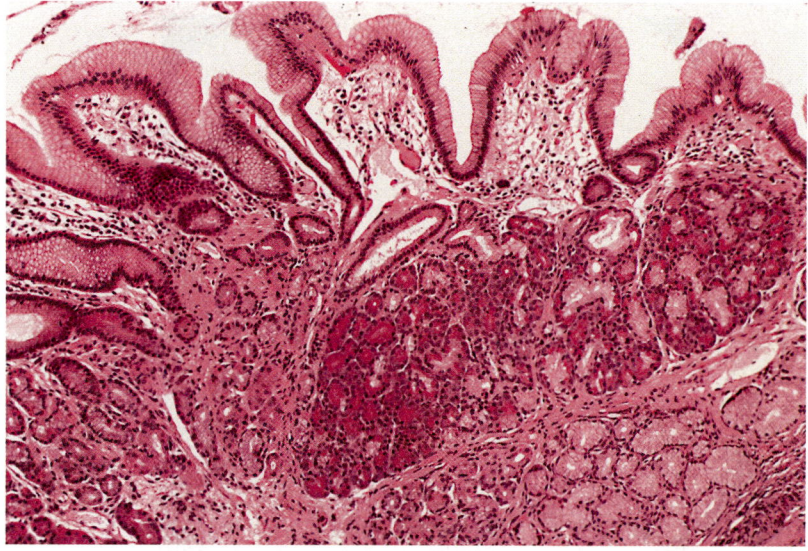

Figure 2-159: **Stomach. Pancreatic Metaplasia.** A lobule of pancreatic acini admixed with cardiac glands is in the lamina propria.

FUNDIC GLAND POLYP

- Morphology .... Fundic gland polyps are typically small, round, sessile lesions composed of mature surface and fundic glands that are often cystically dilated. They do not ulcerate, bleed, or become inflamed.

- Endoscopic features .... Although these polyps are associated with familial adenomatous polyposis, they occur sporadically as single or multiple lesions in nonpolyposis situations. Fundic gland polyps associated with familial adenomatous polyposis may carpet the proximal stomach. They are nonneoplastic, and, unlike the duodenum and periampullary area of these patients, do not require routine gastric endoscopic surveillance and histologic sampling.

- Clinical features .... When associated with familial adenomatous polyposis, they are multiple, often in great numbers, and show no gender predilection. In sporadic cases, they are about 5 times more common in females and are found in middle-aged persons.

- Differential diagnosis ...... Endoscopic: Hyperplastic polyp, adenoma, nodular adenocarcinoma, carcinoid, and intestinal metaplasia. Adjacent gastric atrophy with a striking submucosal vascular pattern beneath a thinned mucosa favors a hyperplastic polyp or carcinoid.

    In a patient with familial adenomatous polyposis, numerous gastric polyps may be misinterpreted endoscopically as adenomas. Biopsy invariably distinguishes between them because fundic gland polyps are devoid of dysplasia and adenomas are, by definition, dysplastic. Fundic gland polyps are distinguished from hyperplastic polyps by the presence of cystic fundic glands and little, if any, foveolar hyperplasia.

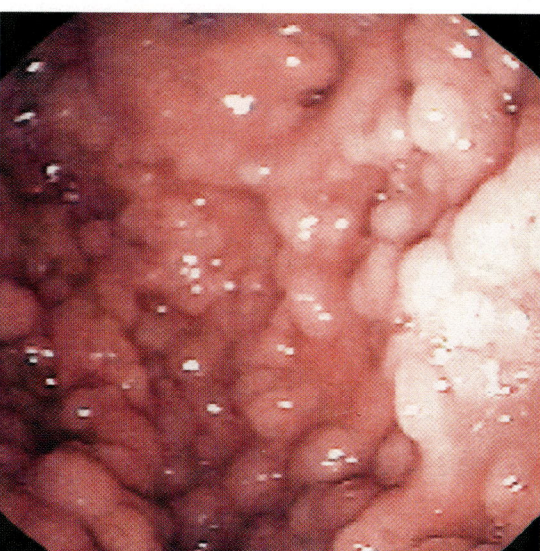

Figure 2-160: **Stomach. Fundic Gland Polyps.** Retroflexed view of the proximal stomach in a patient with familial adenomatous polyposis. Innumerable fundic gland polyps.

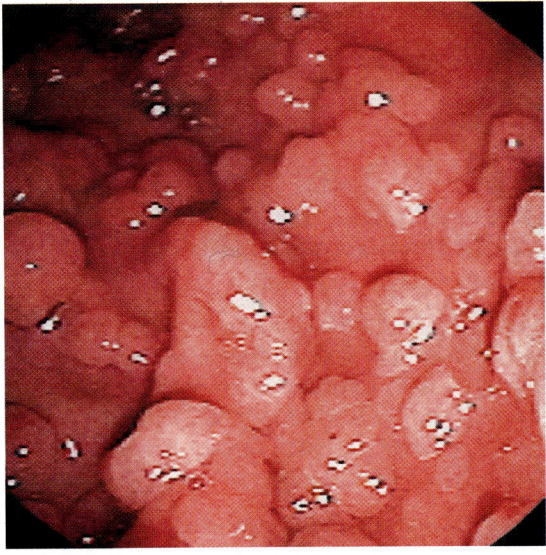

Figure 2-161: **Stomach. Fundic Gland Polyps.** Retroflexed view. Fundus carpeted with numerous diminutive polyps, some superimposed on others, classic for fundic gland polyps encountered in the setting of familial adenomatous polyposis syndrome.

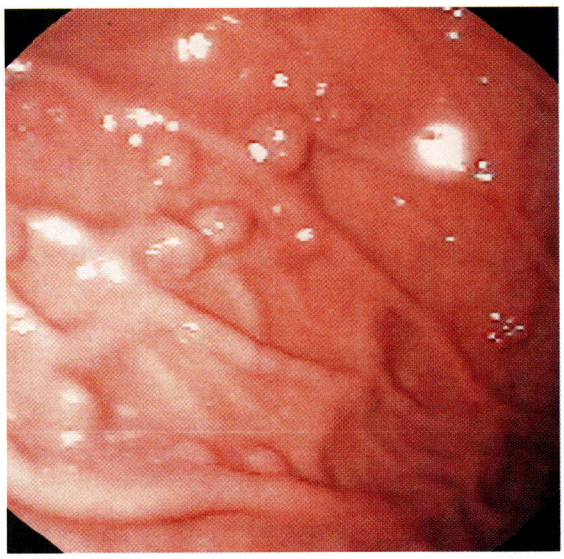

Figure 2-162: **Stomach. Fundic Gland Polyps.** Diminutive sessile polyps along the greater curvature within the proximal body. The size, location, and number of these polyps are suggestive of fundic gland polyps.

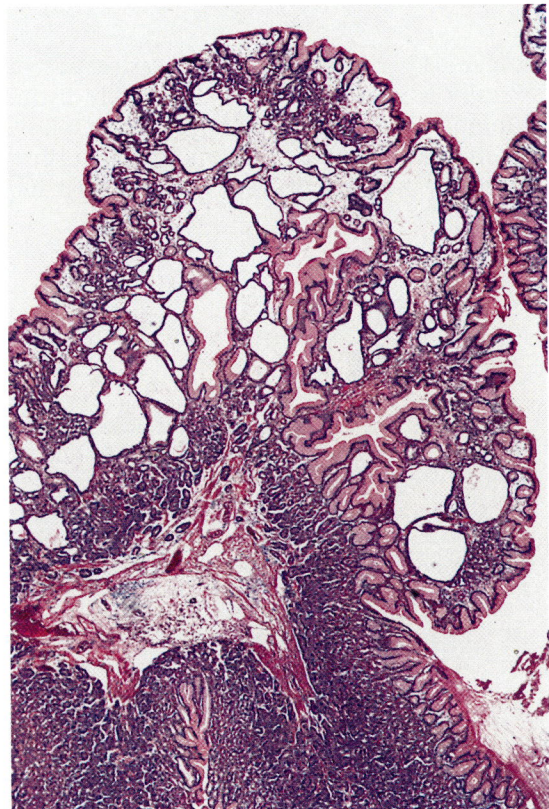

Figure 2-163: **Stomach. Fundic Gland Polyp.** A small, sessile, epithelial polyp with a mixture of fundic and foveolar glands, many of which are cystic.

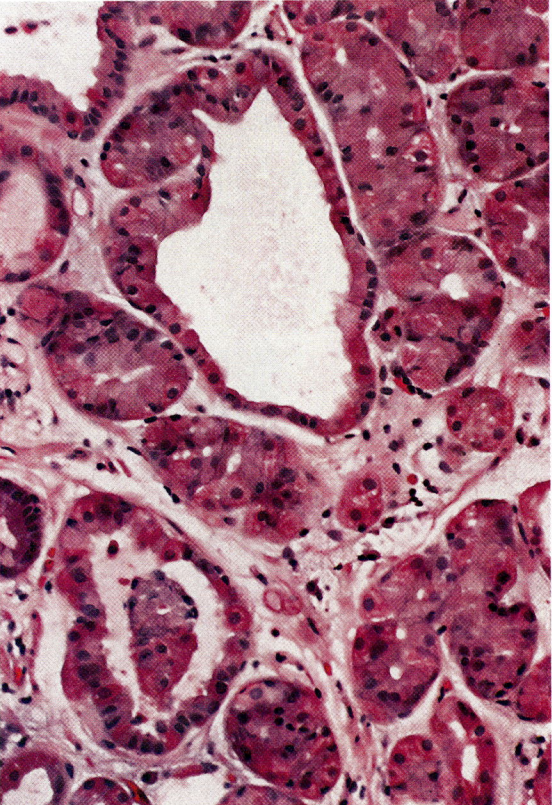

Figure 2-164: **Stomach. Fundic Gland Polyp.** Normal and dilated oxyntic (fundic/body) glands. No nuclear enlargement or other signs of cellular atypia.

HYPERPLASTIC POLYP

- Morphology .... Hyperplastic foveolar glands and inflamed, edematous lamina propria are the hallmarks of this lesion. Surface erosion is common and reactive inflammatory and regenerative epithelial changes are frequent. Single or multiple, they are most common in the antrum and may be associated with chronic gastritis. They may be found near carcinomas.

- Endoscopic features .... The polyps can become quite large and eroded. Current endoscopic management guidelines do not recommend mandatory removal or surveillance for these lesions. They may grow in any location but tend to be found most often in the antrum and cardia.

- Clinical features .... Large hyperplastic polyps are friable and can give rise to GI blood loss with anemia. These polyps may develop at sites of repeated thermal injury, for example, in patients with watermelon stomach who undergo endoscopic laser ablation for bleeding antral vasculopathy. Giant hyperplastic polyps located in either the proximal stomach or distal antrum may cause obstructive symptoms.

- Differential diagnosis ...... Histologic: Mucosal lesions producing foveolar hyperplasia, edematous lamina propria, and inflammation, e.g., Cronkhite-Canada polyps, juvenile polyps, Menetrier disease, and stomal polypoid hyperplasia at gastroenteric anastomotic sites, and hypertrophic gastritis. Regenerative atypia following erosion may simulate dysplasia. Fundic gland polyps may have foveolar hyperplasia, but the predominant component is oxyntic glands. Furthermore, fundic gland polyps lack inflammation and surface erosions.

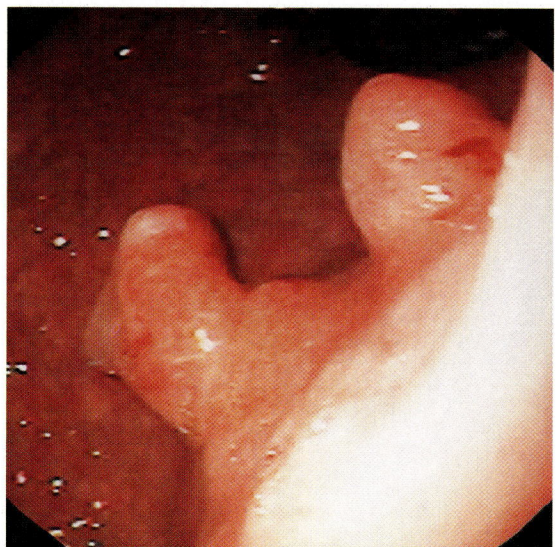

Figure 2-165: **Stomach. Hyperplastic Polyp.** Irregular shape and surface erosion, typical of hyperplastic polyps.

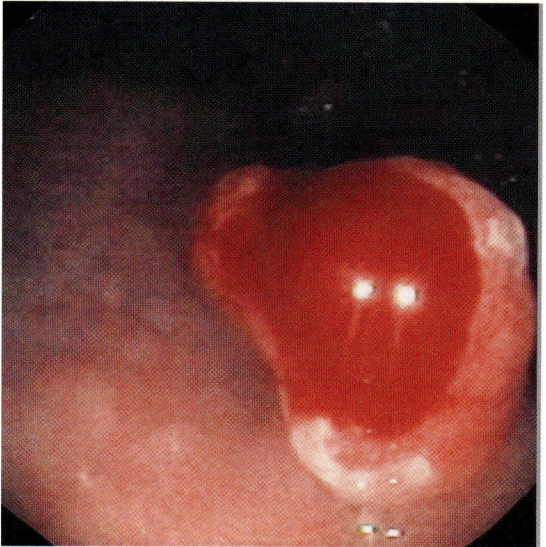

Figure 2-166: **Stomach, Proximal Body. Hyperplastic Polyp.** Friable, erythematous, sessile polyp oozing blood.

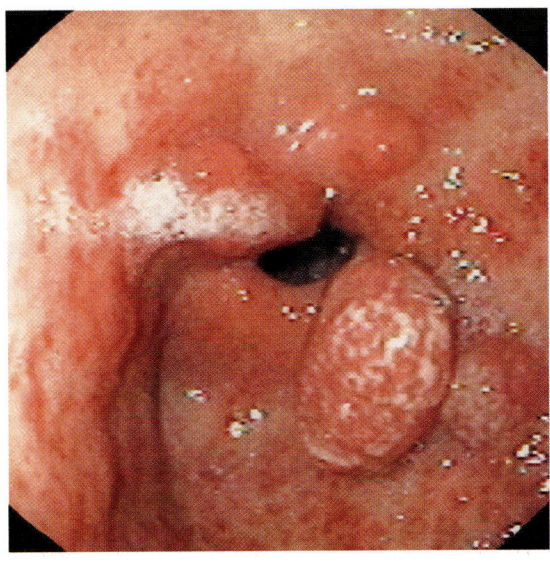

Figure 2-167: **Stomach. Hyperplastic Polyps.** Eroded surface on larger of multiple polyps in patient with watermelon stomach.

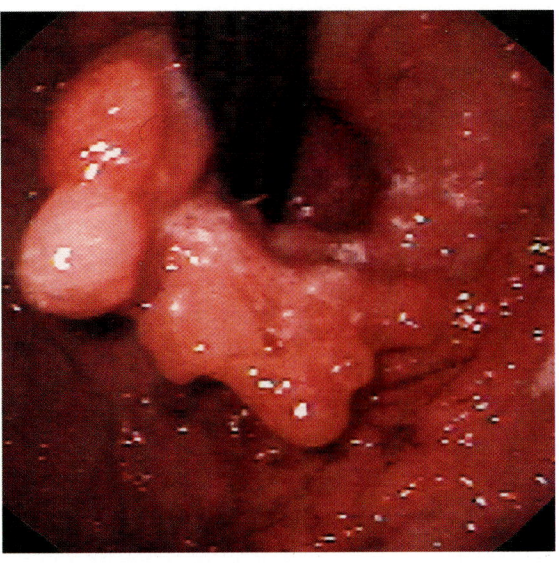

Figure 2-168: **Stomach, Proximal. Hyperplastic Polyps.** Several sessile polyps with irregular surfaces.

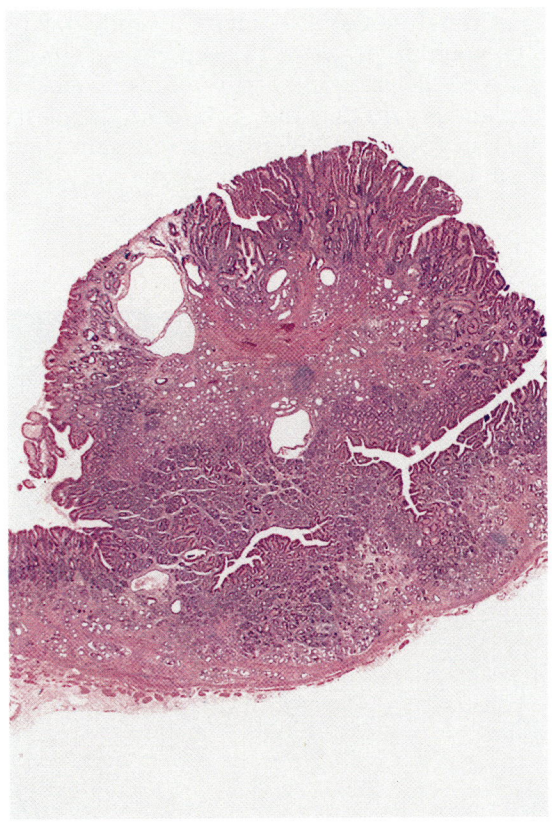

Figure 2-169: **Stomach. Hyperplastic Polyp.** Polypoid lesion without a well-defined stalk, with elongated foveolar glands and focal cystic dilatation.

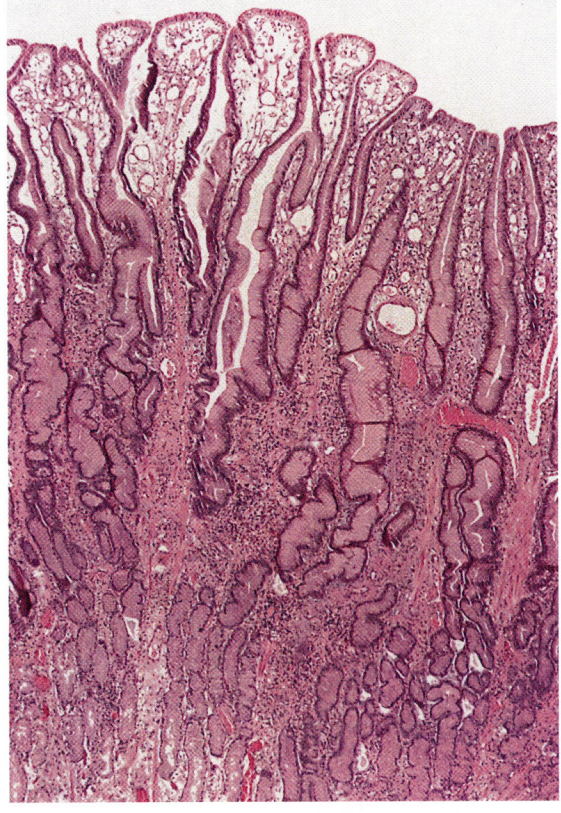

Figure 2-170: **Stomach. Hyperplastic Polyp.** Greatly elongated foveolar glands, edematous, vascularized, and chronically inflamed lamina propria. Splays of muscle extend perpendicularly between the glands.

JUVENILE POLYP AND PEUTZ-JEGHERS POLYP

- Morphology .... Juvenile polyp—Gastric juvenile polyps are indistinguishable histologically from the more common gastric hyperplastic polyp and the uncommon Cronkite-Canada polyp. All 3 contain hyperplastic foveolar epithelium and edematous lamina propria. The glands of a juvenile polyp are more disorganized than the elongated foveolar glands typical of Menetrier disease. The irregular contour of the gastric juvenile polyp differs from the typical sporadic colonic juvenile polyp, which has a smooth, often eroded surface.

   Peutz-Jeghers polyp—Throughout the gastrointestinal tract, Peutz-Jeghers polyps are hamartomatous lesions composed of a smooth muscle infrastructure covered by indigenous glands. Juvenile polyps are also considered hamartomas but do not have a significant smooth muscle component.

- Endoscopic features .... Juvenile polyps are clustered, extremely soft, and markedly irregular in size and shape. A prominent frondlike surface pattern is characteristic but not distinctive.

   The Peutz-Jeghers polyp is typically pedunculated and has a surface appearance similar to adenomatous polyps. The polyps tend to be of appreciable size (greater than 1 cm) and are friable. They are sessile in the stomach.

- Clinical features .... Both juvenile and Peutz-Jeghers polyps are encountered in pediatric patients. Gastric Peutz-Jeghers polyps, unlike those of the small intestine, are not associated with intussusception and intermittent obstructive symptoms. Occult chronic blood loss associated with Peutz-Jeghers polyps may cause iron deficiency anemia.

- Differential diagnosis ...... Endoscopic and histologic: Juvenile polyps are indistinguishable from the polyps of Cronkhite-Canada syndrome. However, Cronkhite-Canada syndrome is not seen below age 30, and juvenile polyposis is rare in older adults. The Peutz-Jeghers polyp is endoscopically indistinguishable from hyperplastic polyps and pedunculated adenomatous polyps.

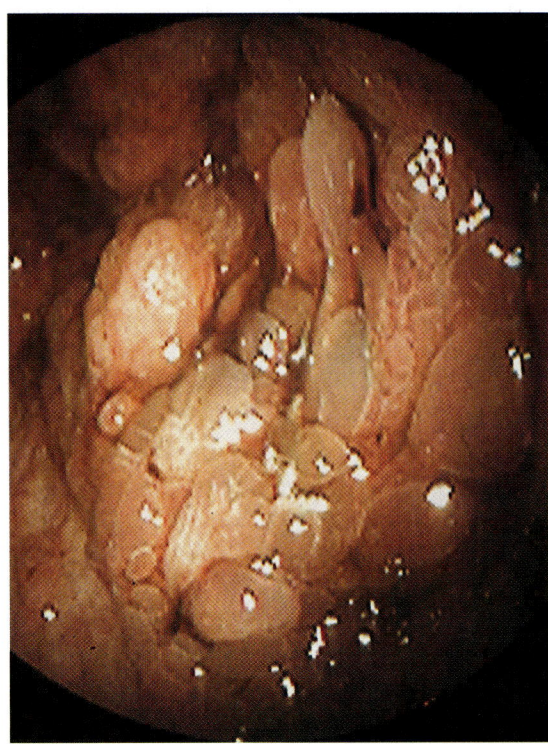

Figure 2-171: **Stomach. Juvenile Polyps.** The polyps are multiple, soft, and almost mucoid in appearance, with long, frondlike surface features varying in size, length, and configuration. These polyps tend to be clustered over large surface areas, and are distinctive from most other types of gastric polyps.

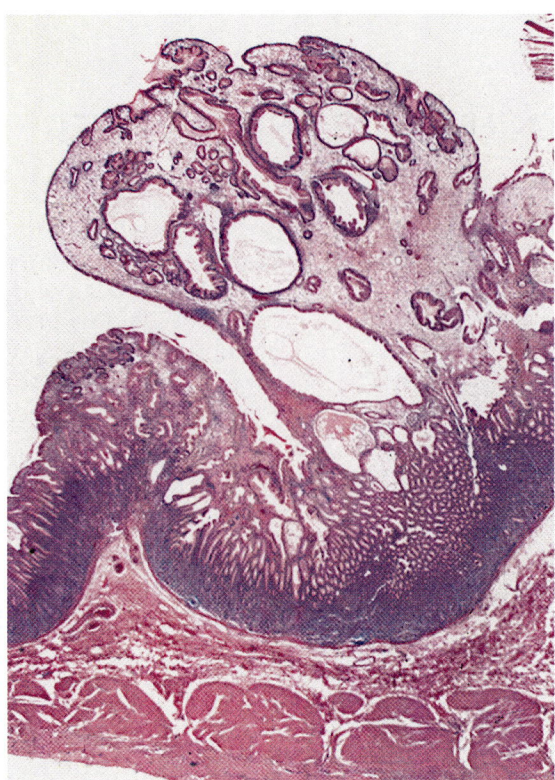

Figure 2-172: **Stomach. Juvenile Polyps.** Hyperplastic gastric foveolar epithelium and edematous lamina propria.

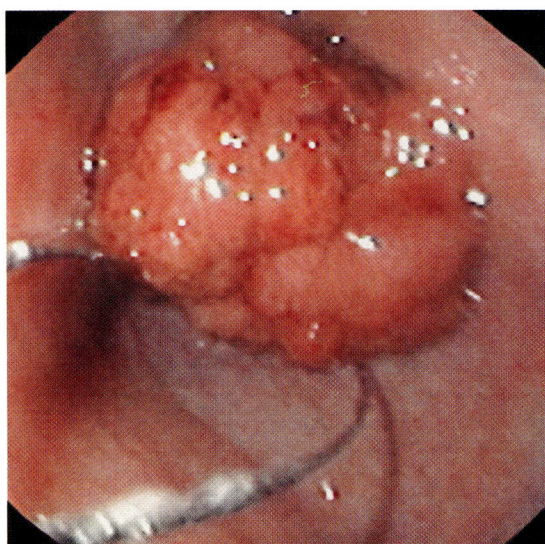

Figure 2-173: **Stomach. Peutz-Jeghers Polyp.** Polyp protrudes through the pylorus in a young patient.

Figure 2-174: **Stomach. Peutz-Jeghers Polyp.** A prominent smooth muscle infrastructure is covered by gastric mucosa. The latter contains hyperplastic foveolar epithelium overlying fundic glands.

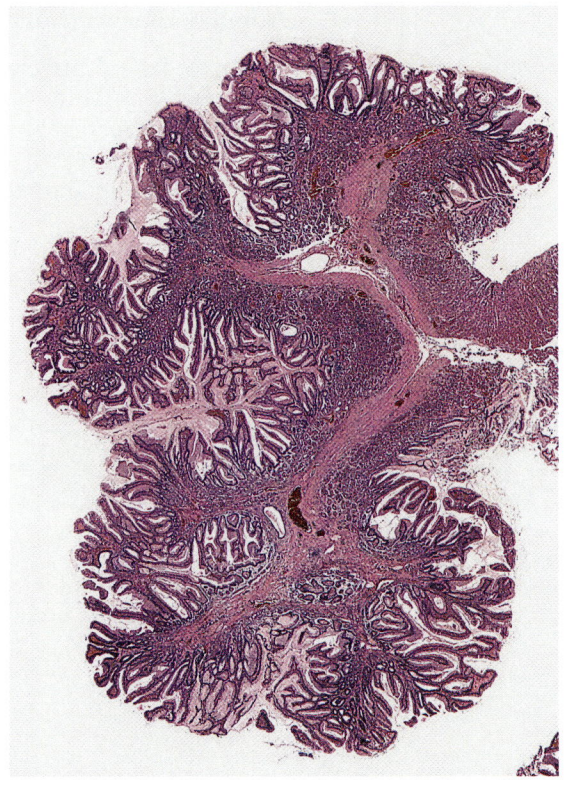

INFLAMMATORY FIBROID POLYP

- Morphology .... These sessile polyps arise in the submucosa, are composed of vascularized stroma, and are infiltrated by chronic inflammatory cells, particularly eosinophils. Surface erosion and glandular atrophy are frequent. Penetration into the underlying muscularis propria is minimal, in contrast to similar lesions in the small bowel. These benign, nonneoplastic lesions probably represent an unresolved reaction to injury.

- Endoscopic features .... The polyps are usually solitary, sessile, and without distinctive size or surface features.

- Clinical features .... The lesions occur in all age groups. The stomach is the main site, followed by the small bowel. The surface of the polyp may become eroded and give rise to occult GI blood loss. Peripheral eosinophilia is not a feature, despite the high concentration of tissue eosinophils in the lesion.

- Differential diagnosis ...... Endoscopic: Hyperplastic polyps, adenomas, adenocarcinomas, and lymphoma.

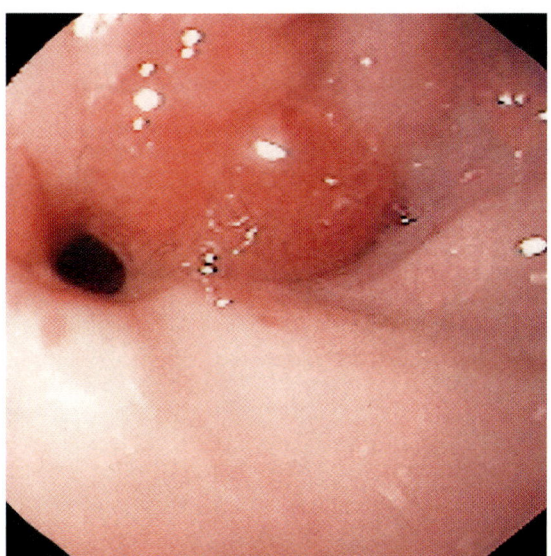

Figure 2-175: **Stomach. Inflammatory Fibroid Polyp.** A diminutive polyp located on the gastric side of the esophagogastric junction.

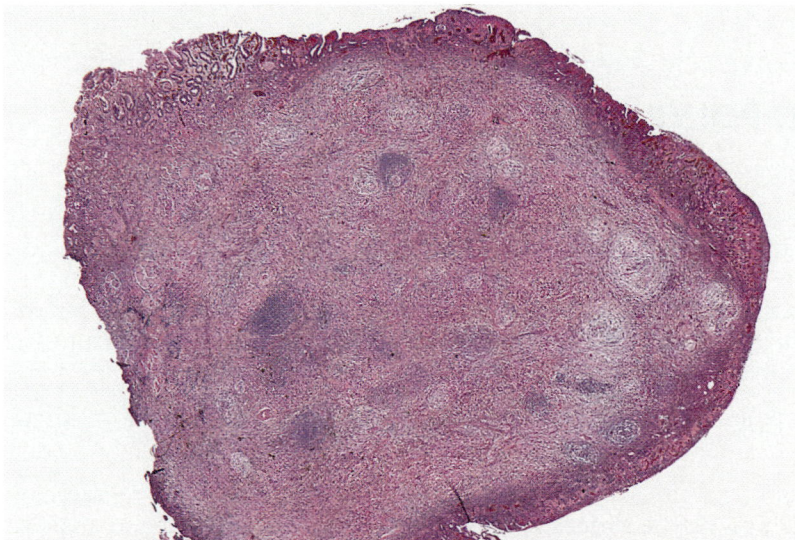

Figure 2-176: **Stomach. Inflammatory Fibroid Polyp.** Inflamed stroma expands the submucosa, causing a sessile polyp. Nodular collections of lymphoid tissue alternate with perivascular, pale, edematous stroma. The overlying mucosa is partially eroded and focally atrophic with considerable capillary congestion.

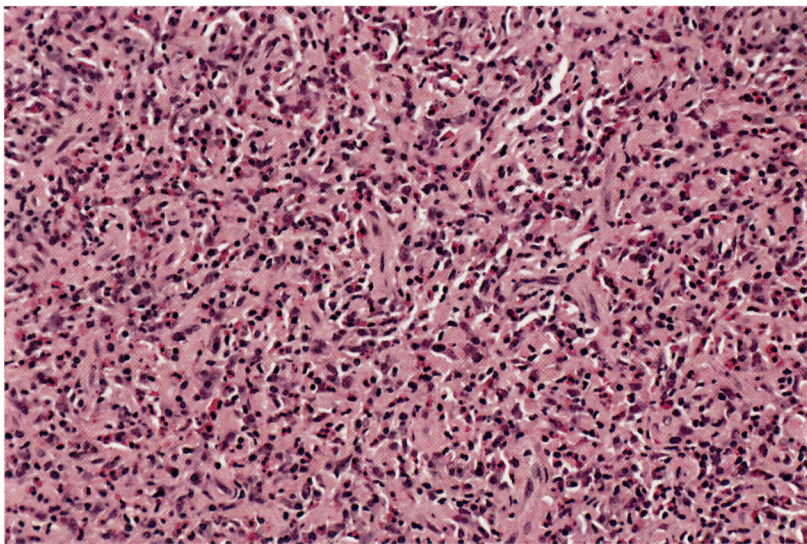

Figure 2-177: **Stomach. Inflammatory Fibroid Polyp.** Vascularized stroma heavily infiltrated by eosinophils.

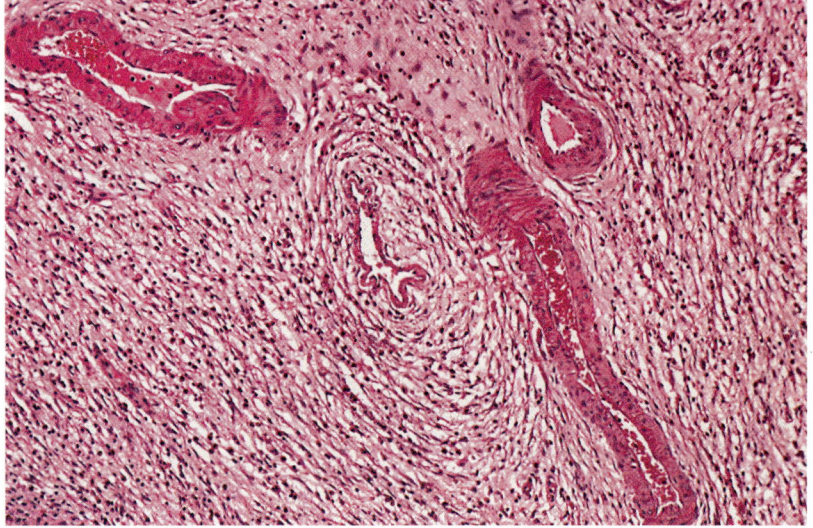

Figure 2-178: **Stomach. Inflammatory Fibroid Polyp.** Typical perivascular, concentric, fibrous whorls produce an "onion-skin" lesion. Eosinophils are the main inflammatory component.

DYSPLASIA

- Morphology .... Dysplastic cells have large, irregular, hyperchromatic nuclei, nuclear membrane irregularities, and often large, irregular nucleoli. Regenerating cells are basophilic and have smooth nuclear membranes. Regenerative atypia is generally limited to the deep basal zone; reactive atypia is accompanied by acute inflammation. Cellular and architectural uniformity favor regenerative/reactive atypia. Nuclear stratification and extension of the atypia to the gastric lumen favor dysplasia. Dysplasia commonly replaces intestinalized epithelium. Dysplasia in the flat mucosa is often multifocal and associated with atrophic gastritis. Focal, macroscopically visible dysplasia is an adenoma.

- Endoscopic features .... Dysplasia cannot be identified grossly during routine endoscopy. Dysplasia may be suspected in areas where there are focal plaques or nodular changes. Suspicion would be greatest when there are also findings of gastric atrophy within the body of the stomach. Intestinal metaplasia most often appears as small islands of nodular or polypoid tissue, or as bland plaques (Fig. 2-179). High-resolution endoscopy with vital dye staining (chromoscopy) and magnification endoscopy (10-X to 100-X) may help to differentiate dysplastic from normal tissue. These endoscopic techniques are currently under investigation.

- Clinical features .... Chronic atrophic gastritis with intestinal metaplasia is the usual precursor of dysplasia in the flat mucosa.

- Differential diagnosis .... Endoscopic: Intestinal metaplasia.

    Histologic: Reactive/regenerative atypia.

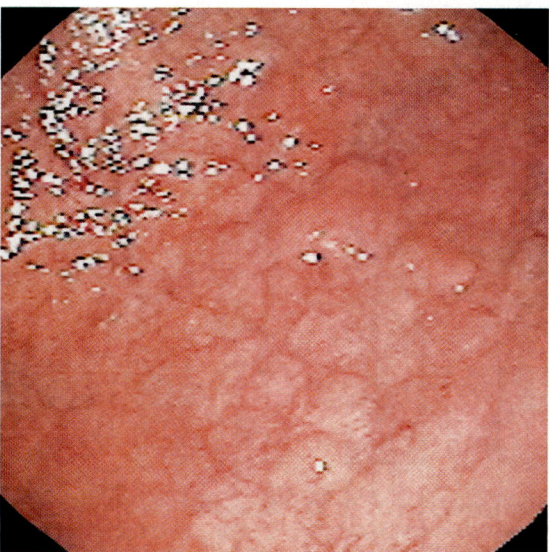

Figure 2-179: **Stomach, Fundus. Chronic Atrophic Gastritis with Dysplasia.** Prominent submucosal vascular network, loss of rugal folds, and multiple polypoid nodules consistent with atrophic gastritis. Biopsy showed dysplasia.

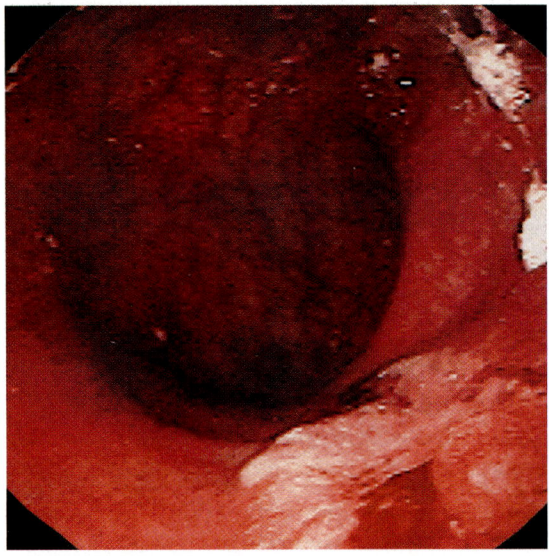

Figure 2-180: **Stomach, Fundus. Ulcer with Dysplasia.** A 2-cm shallow ulcer along the greater curvature of the stomach. Distal to the ulcer, a prominent vascular pattern is highly suggestive of atrophic gastritis. Dysplasia was present in the pale adjacent mucosa.

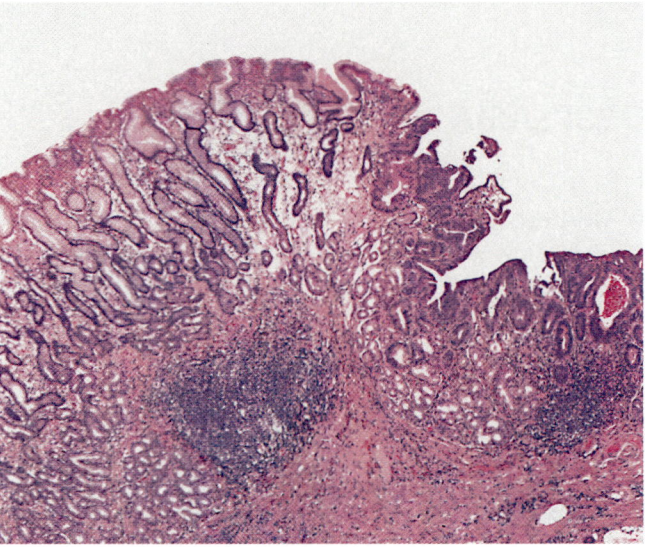

Figure 2-181: **Stomach. Dysplasia.** Basophilic dysplastic glands in the depressed right field contrast with the pale, elongated, hyperplastic foveolar glands in the edematous mucosa to the left.

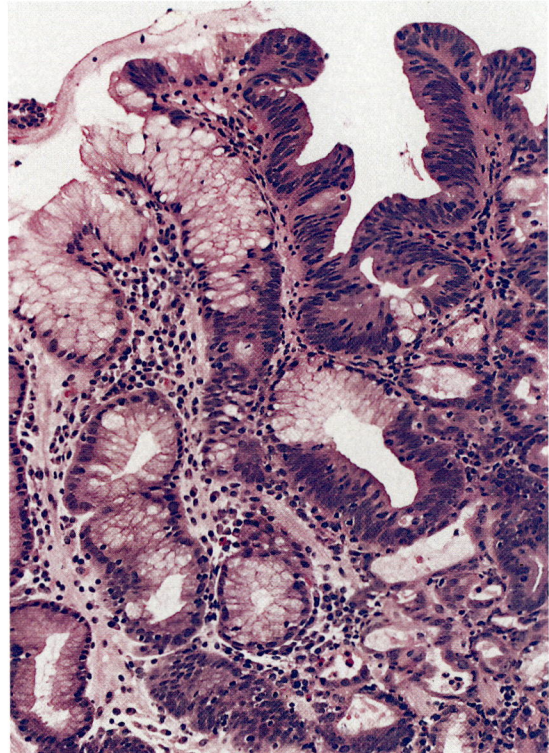

Figure 2-182: **Stomach. Low-Grade Dysplasia.** Abrupt transition between pale, mucus-filled foveolar cells and basophilic dysplastic epithelium with elongated hyperchromatic nuclei. Overall retention of nuclear polarity and apical cytoplasm are features of low-grade dysplasia.

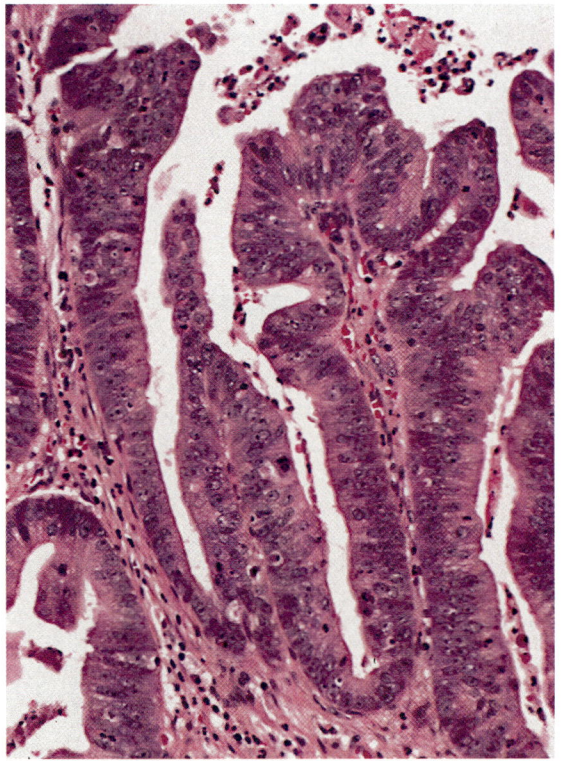

Figure 2-183: **Stomach. High-Grade Dysplasia.** Dysplastic glands with vesicular nuclei, prominent nucleoli, and mitotic activity. Loss of polarity, with nuclei extending to the surface, is a sign of high-grade dysplasia.

ADENOMA

- Morphology .... The dysplastic cells of adenomas usually arise near the surface of the mucosa and spread superficially as well as deeply. In the stomach, the superficial spread leads to flat or plateaulike sessile adenomas. Pedunculation is less common than in the colon. Distinguishing between dysplasia in the flat mucosa and a sessile adenoma in biopsy samples may be impossible because of the relatively flat nature and the lack of pedunculation. The distinction may be important because dysplasia in the flat mucosa is more likely multifocal. Carcinomas that develop in gastric adenomas and invade the lamina propria have a metastatic potential.

- Endoscopic features .... Adenomatous polyps are indistinguishable from hyperplastic polyps. Generally, adenomas are small and sessile, while large pedunculated polyps (> 2 cm) tend to be hyperplastic.

- Clinical features .... Adenomatous polyps are usually incidental. Gastric adenomas, while less common than in the colon, are more likely to become malignant.

- Differential diagnosis...... Endoscopic: Hyperplastic polyp.

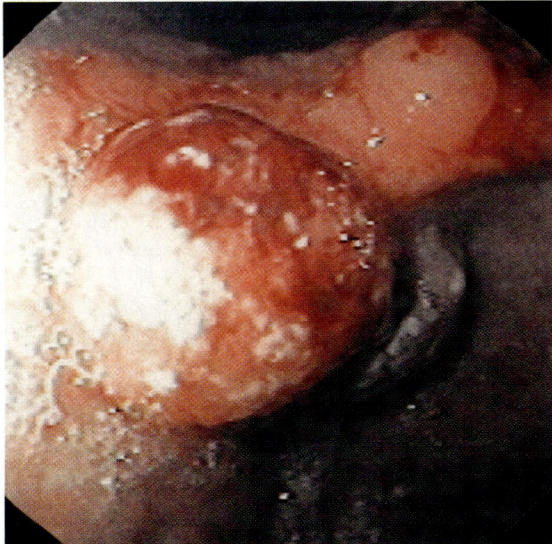

Figure 2-184: **Stomach, Antrum. Tubular Adenoma.** Sessile multilobed polyp on the incisura. Surface hemorrhage with a white exudate. Since this polyp is an isolated finding within the stomach, it requires removal.

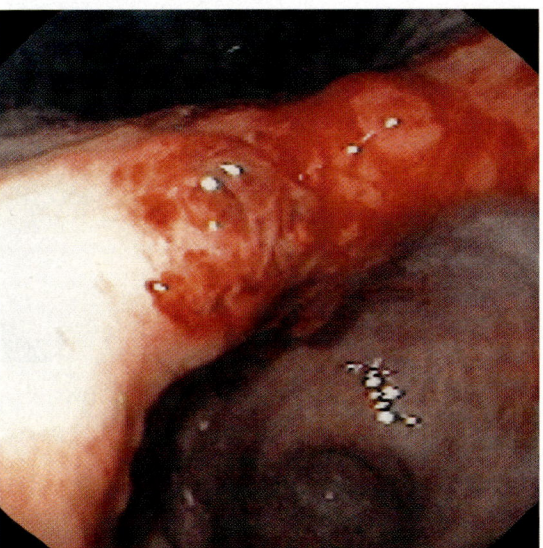

Figure 2-185: **Stomach, Antrum. Post-Polypectomy.** Same polyp as Fig. 2-184. The polyp was removed by snare excision after the base was injected with saline solution to enhance accessibility and minimize the depth of tissue injury. The remaining sessile polyp was coagulated.

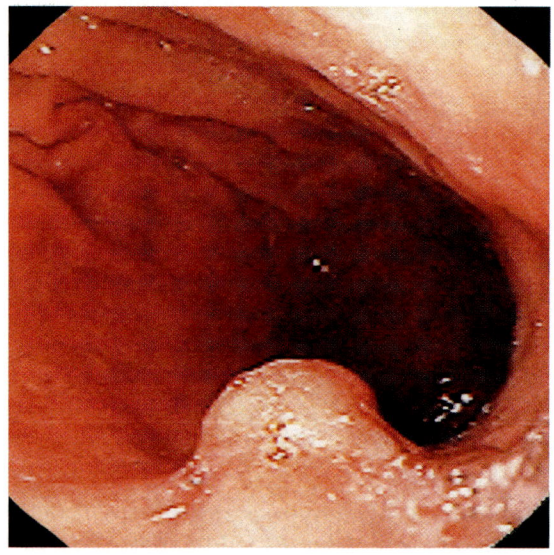

Figure 2-186: **Stomach, Body. Tubular Adenoma.** Posterior midbody, broad-based sessile, 2-cm polyp.

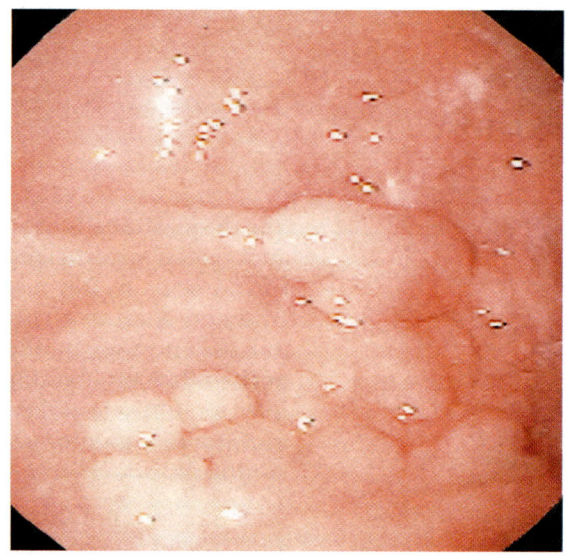

Figure 2-187: **Stomach, Body. Adenomas.** Multiple sessile polyps ranging from 3 mm to 1 cm.

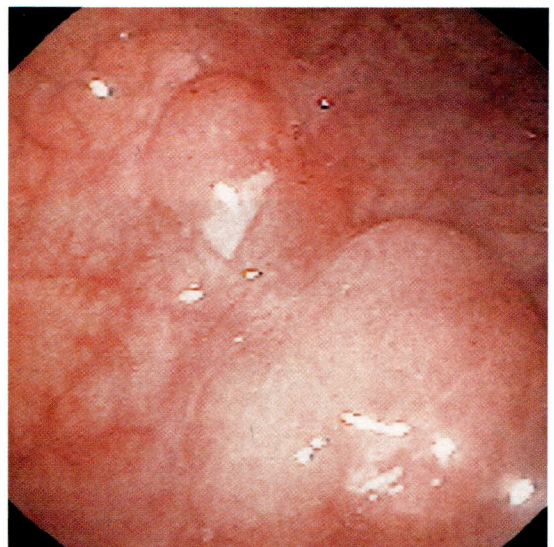

Figure 2-188: **Stomach, Body. Adenomas.** Two sessile polyps. The mucosa shows evidence of atrophy, i.e., prominent submucosal vasculature.

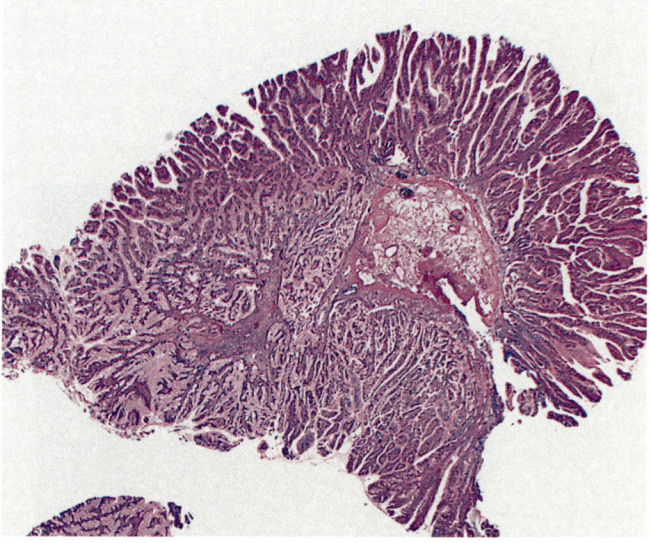

Figure 2-189: **Stomach. Tubulovillous Adenoma.** Basophilic papillary and glandular structures surround polyp's submucosal core. No evidence of invasion.

MALIGNANT ULCER

- Morphology .... Ulcerating carcinomas (malignant ulcers) have thick, irregular craters with heaped-up edges compared to benign peptic ulcers. A biopsy specimen taken from the periphery of the crater is more likely to contain identifiable tumor cells than one from the center, where exudate may predominate. A specimen from the edge of the ulcer showing only reactive mucosa in a clinically suspicious lesion does not exclude an underlying malignancy. Cells with foamy cytoplasm in a gastric ulcer simulating muciphages should be investigated further because muciphages are not present in the stomach (unlike the colon). A cytokeratin study is useful for this distinction. Xanthelasma cells have only fine PAS-positive granules in contrast to carcinoma. PAS with diastase is helpful because some carcinoma cells contain neutral mucin and will not react with mucicarmine or alcian blue.

- Endoscopic features .... The malignant ulcer is classically raised above the mucosa due to a mass effect of the neoplasm. The margins of the ulcer are typically firm and friable. Small malignant ulcers of early cancers are difficult to distinguish from benign gastric erosions and ulcers. Thickened or nodular surrounding tissue raises suspicion of malignancy, particularly in high-risk patients.

- Clinical features .... Malignant ulcers cause recalcitrant epigastric pain and chronic occult and overt GI blood loss. The bleeding is from the friable ulcer margins, not from discrete or visible vessels, as occurs in peptic ulcers.

- Differential diagnosis ...... Endoscopic: Adenocarcinoma, lymphoma, and intramural tumor.

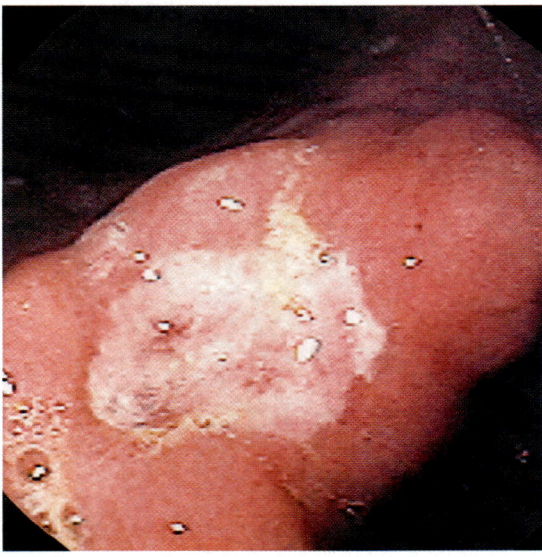

Figure 2-190: **Stomach. Ulcerating Adenocarcinoma.** Raised midbody gastric ulcer with irregular nodular margins suggestive of a neoplasm. Shallow ulcer with clean base.

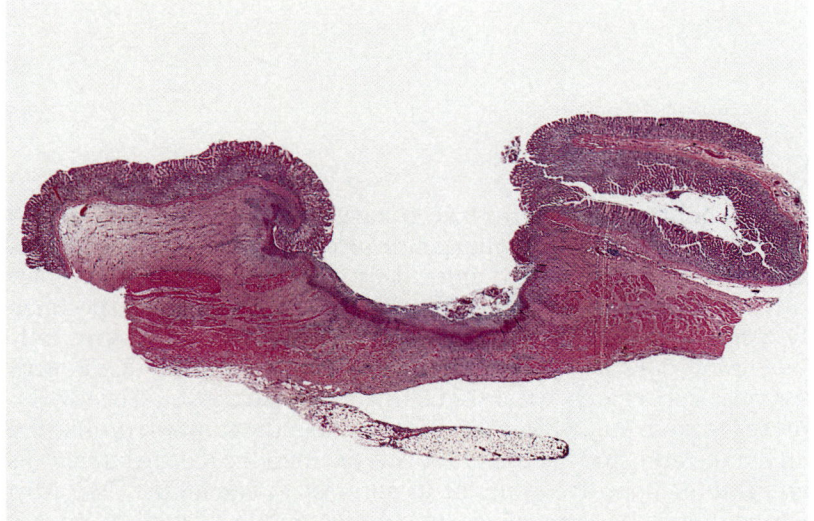

Figure 2-191: **Stomach. Chronic Peptic Ulcer, Benign.** Deep, sharp crater penetrates into muscularis propria. Normal mucosa overhangs edge. Marked edema of submucosa. Little muscle remains under crater.

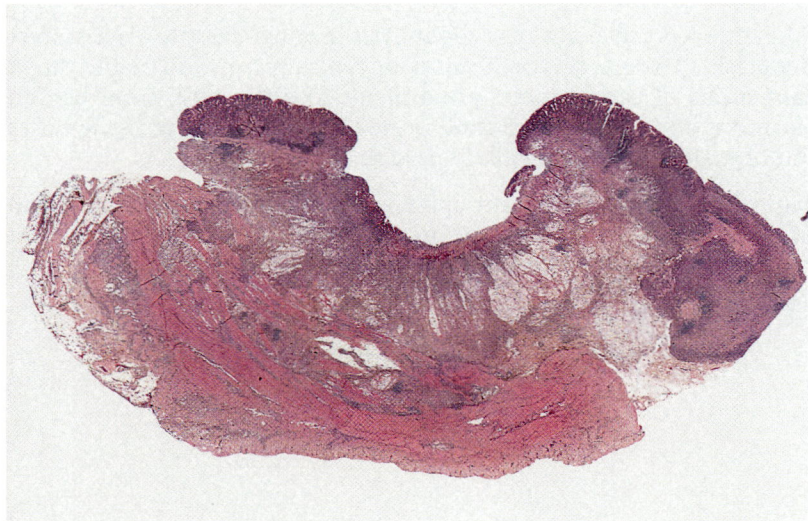

Figure 2-192: **Stomach. Ulcerating Adenocarcinoma.** Crater with partially nodular surface and raised, heaped-up edge penetrates into greatly thickened, cancer-filled submucosa. Muscularis propria partially separated by tumor.

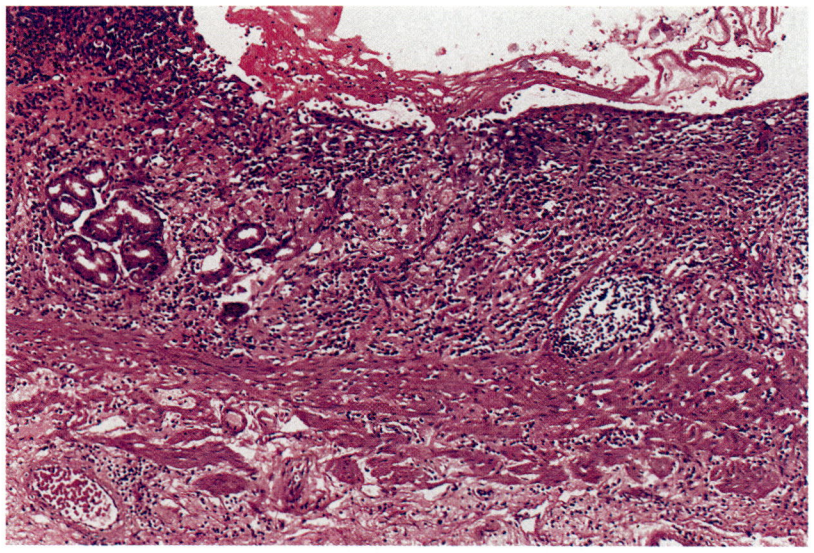

Figure 2-193: **Stomach. Adenocarcinoma, Poorly Differentiated.** Eroded mucosa contains pale, mucin-filled tumor cells with residual glands and lymphoid tissue. Muscularis mucosae intact; therefore, tumor is intramucosal carcinoma.

ADENOCARCINOMA

- Morphology .... Adenocarcinomas form glands, grow in solid sheets, or infiltrate as single cells. Stage is a more important prognosticator than grade. Intramucosal adenocarcinoma and adenocarcinoma limited to the submucosa (T1) are associated with a relatively good prognosis compared to more deeply invasive lesions, irrespective of histologic pattern. Interpretation of endoscopic biopsies may be difficult because of the scant and sometimes superficial material, e.g. adenomatous tissue may lie above an invasive carcinoma; papillary adenocarcinoma may be difficult to distinguish from a villous adenoma. It may be impossible on histology alone to distinguish a primary, poorly differentiated adenocarcinoma (Fig. 2-200) from a metastasis, particularly from the breast, or even metastatic melanoma. Diffusely infiltrative tumor cells that can expand the lamina propria between nondysplastic glands can simulate inflammatory cells. The size of the cells as well as an immunostain for cytokeratin can be helpful. Clinical information is often critical in biopsy interpretation.

- Endoscopic features .... Adenocarcinoma may be ulcerated, polypoid, fungating, flat, or infiltrative. Diffusely infiltrative carcinomas can produce large folds and/or a nondistensible stomach. While gross morphology does not always correspond to histologic appearance, polypoid lesions are generally of intestinal type, while a diffusely infiltrative pattern suggests signet-ring cell carcinoma.

    Linitis plastica usually presents as a poorly distensible, narrowed lumen occupying a portion or nearly all of the stomach. The mucosa may be intact and there may be no enlargement of the rugal folds. Advanced adenocarcinoma generally presents as a large (>2 cm), exophytic, ulcerated mass with evidence of bleeding from the irregular margins of the malignant ulcer. At times, a discrete neovessel in the ulcer can give rise to acute GI bleeding. The lesions are friable. Distal adenocarcinoma may obstruct the pylorus. Circumferential lesions reduce the gastric lumen and can create significant stenosis.

- Clinical features .... Pain, refractory dyspepsia, nausea, vomiting (outlet obstruction), early satiety, and occult and overt bleeding.

- Differential diagnosis .... Histologic: Metastatic carcinoma, carcinoid tumor, melanoma, lymphoma.

    Endoscopic: Multiple discrete, ulcerated nodules or markedly enlarged folds with an accentuated (areae gastricae) surface mosaic pattern favor lymphoma over adenocarcinoma.

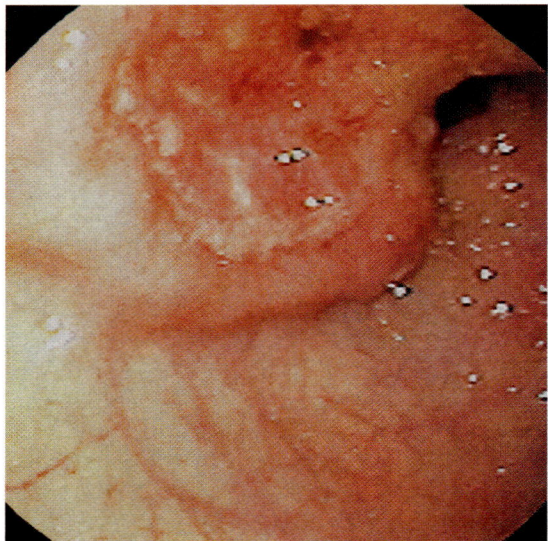

Figure 2-194: **Stomach, Antrum. Adenocarcinoma.** A large ulcer raised above surrounding mucosa suggests an ulcerated neoplasm.

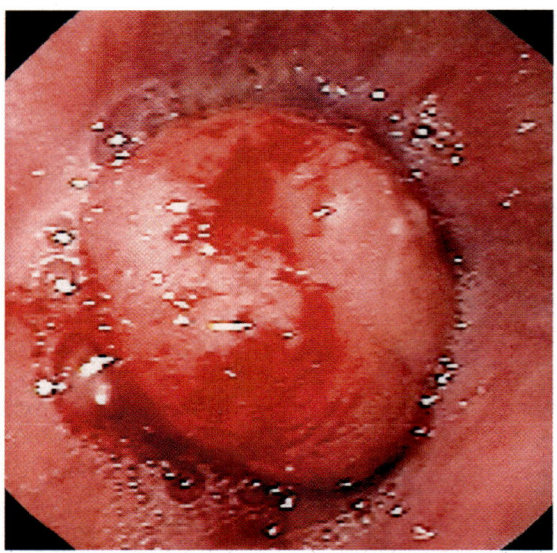

Figure 2-195: **Stomach, Cardia. Adenocarcinoma.** Nodular friable mass with superficial erosion seen during retroflexion.

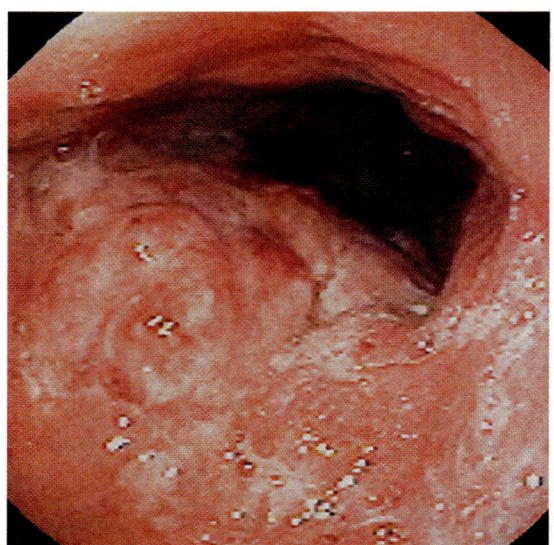

Figure 2-196: **Stomach. Signet-Ring Cell Carcinoma.** Lumen compromised by friable, infiltrating, and irregular neoplasm, which replaces the normal-appearing mucosa in the involved area.

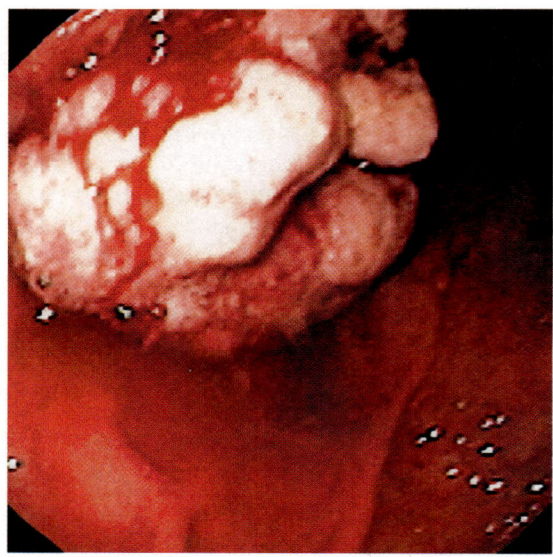

Figure 2-197: **Stomach, Cardia. Adenocarcinoma.** Friable, spontaneously bleeding, nodular polypoid mass.

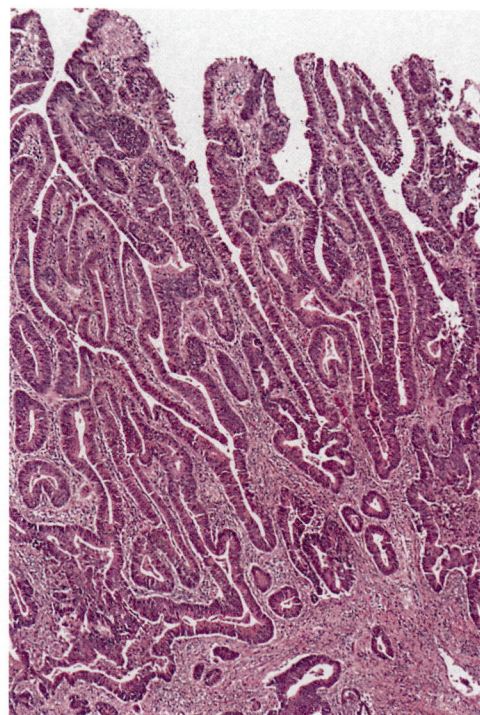

Figure 2-198: **Stomach. Adenocarcinoma.** Irregular glands invade stroma beneath highly dysplastic surface epithelium.

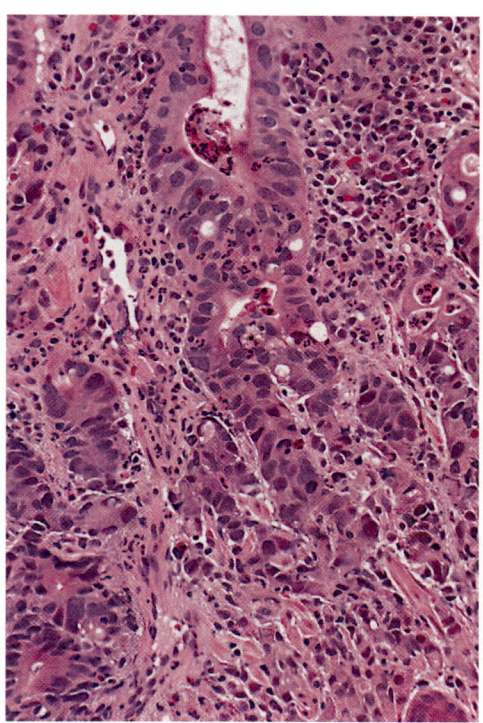

Figure 2-199: **Stomach. Adenocarcinoma.** Small irregular nests of malignant cells infiltrate inflamed stroma. Marked variation in nuclear size, shape, and polarity.

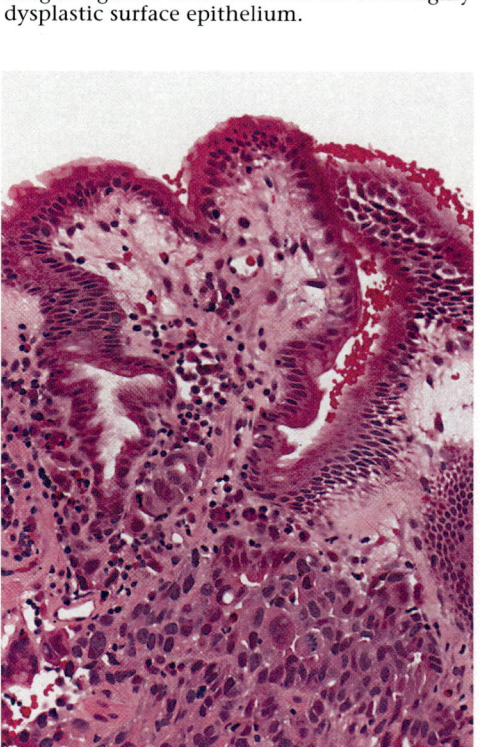

Figure 2-200: **Stomach. Adenocarcinoma.** Malignant cells beneath normal epithelium; no obvious gland formation. Pattern easily confused with carcinoid tumor, melanoma, or large cell lymphoma.

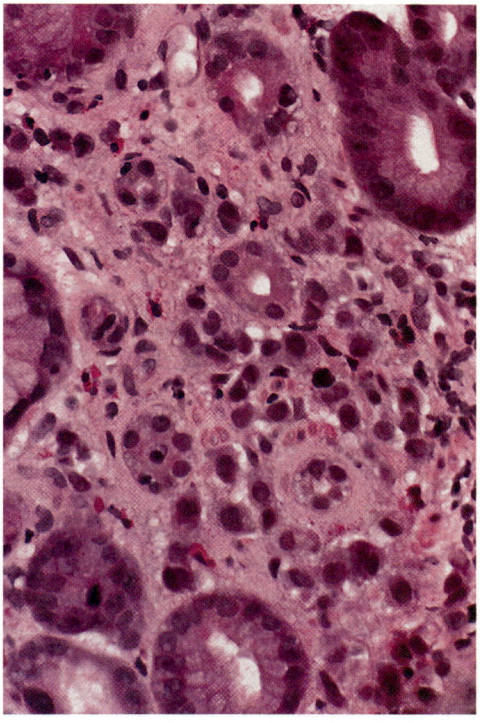

Figure 2-201: **Stomach. Adenocarcinoma.** Tumor cells infiltrate between nondysplastic glands. Large size of malignant cells distinguishes them from inflammatory cells.

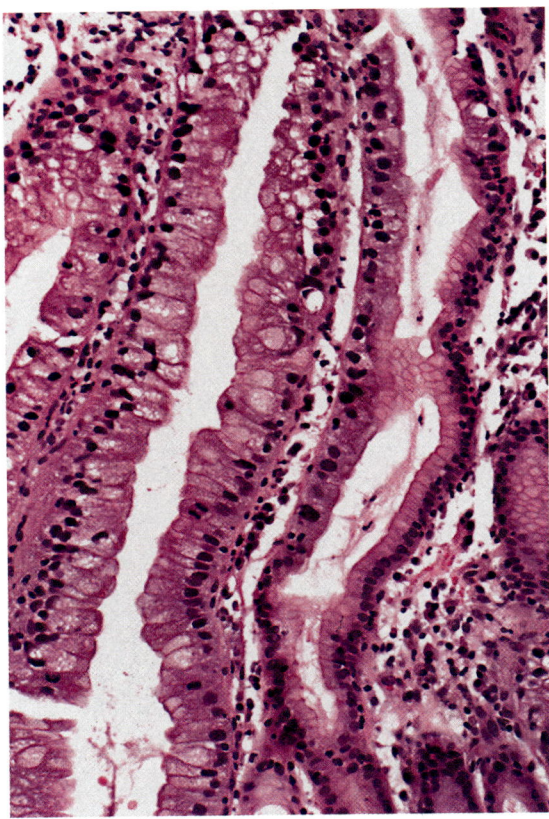

Figure 2-202: **Stomach. Adenocarcinoma.** Mild nuclear atypia in well-differentiated carcinoma cells. Contrast with remaining normal foveolar epithelium in gastric pit on left.

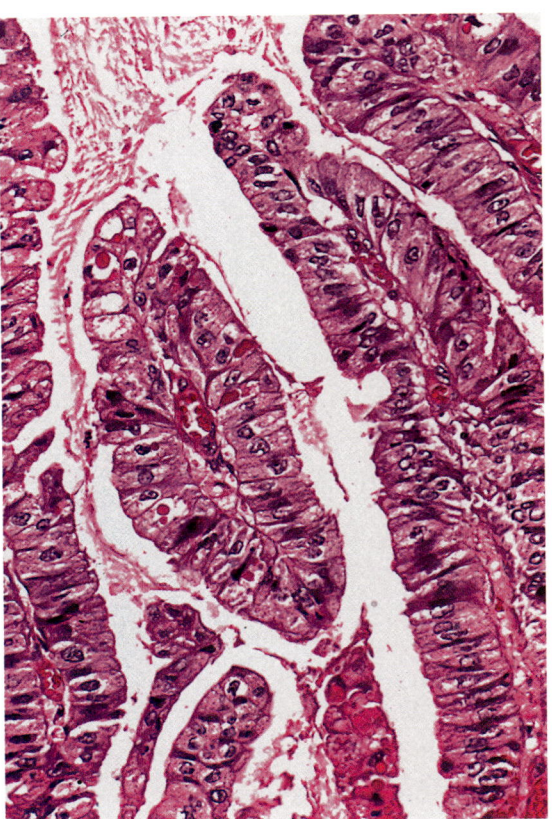

Figure 2-203: **Stomach. Adenocarcinoma.** Subtle dysplasia with papillary growth pattern could easily be confused with regenerative change. While this superficial sample could be from an adenoma, this is a well-differentiated papillary adenocarcinoma that invaded the muscular wall.

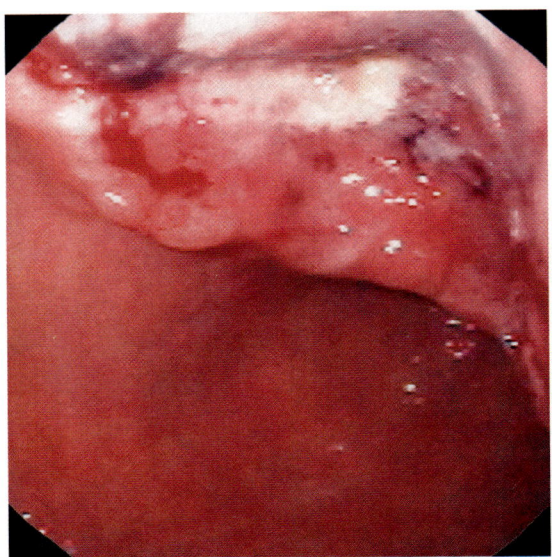

Figure 2-204: **Stomach. Adenocarcinoma.** Large, deeply ulcerated, friable and bleeding antral mass.

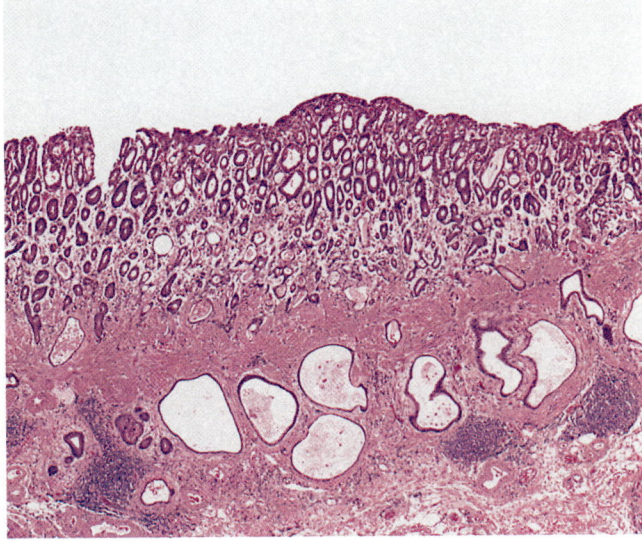

Figure 2-205: **Stomach. Adenocarcinoma.** Extremely well-differentiated invasive adenocarcinoma could not be diagnosed from superficial biopsy samples. Irregular, cystically dilated glands invade well into submucosa. This reinforces the need for clinicopathologic correlation in diagnosis.

SIGNET-RING CELL CARCINOMA

- Morphology .... Signet-ring cells may be widely dispersed and easily overlooked. At low power, their vesicular or compressed nuclei and pale cytoplasm provide easy camouflage. Multiple biopsy fragments from the edge of an ulcer may show only a few malignant cells in 1 or 2 fragments. Ulceration occurs as a secondary phenomenon. In this respect, it differs from ulcerating gland-forming adenocarcinoma, where the tumor itself becomes necrotic. These ulcers may appear endoscopically benign and even heal with therapy.

- Endoscopic features .... A poorly distensible stomach is the most obvious feature. The gastric folds may be enlarged, with scattered superficial ulceration and erosion. A prominent rugal mucosal mosaic pattern suggests an infiltrative process.

- Clinical features .... Diffuse adenocarcinoma or linitis plastica has a fairly typical presentation, with progressive weight loss, poorly defined upper abdominal discomfort, early satiety, nausea, and vomiting. The impairment of gastric motility due to the extensive infiltrating tumor may give rise to gastric outlet or retention symptoms, which include regurgitation, eructation, and emesis of retained food. Additionally, there is a sense of prolonged satiety. Symptoms or manifestations of overt gastrointestinal bleeding are not anticipated since the neoplastic process is largely submucosal.

- Differential diagnosis...... Histologic: Histiocytes (xanthelasma), metastatic lobular carcinoma of the breast.

    Endoscopic: Metastatic carcinoma, lymphoma, leukemia, Menetrier disease, and portal hypertensive gastropathy. Endoscopic ultrasound along with fine-needle aspiration can be useful in the diagnosis of enlarged rugal folds.

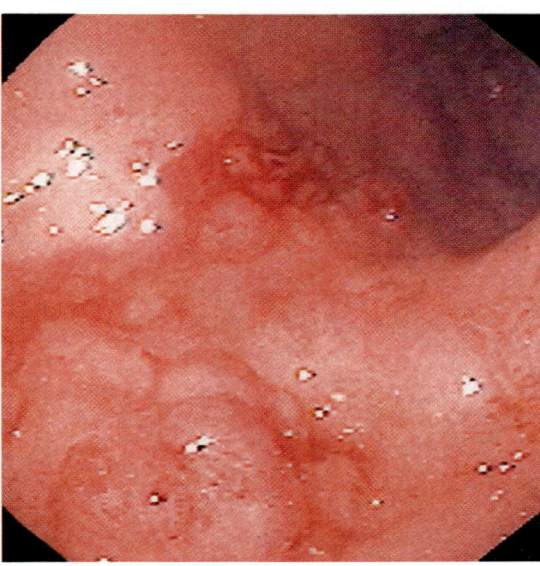

Figure 2-206: **Stomach, Body. Signet-Ring Cell Carcinoma.** Diffusely nodular tumor with a granular surface.

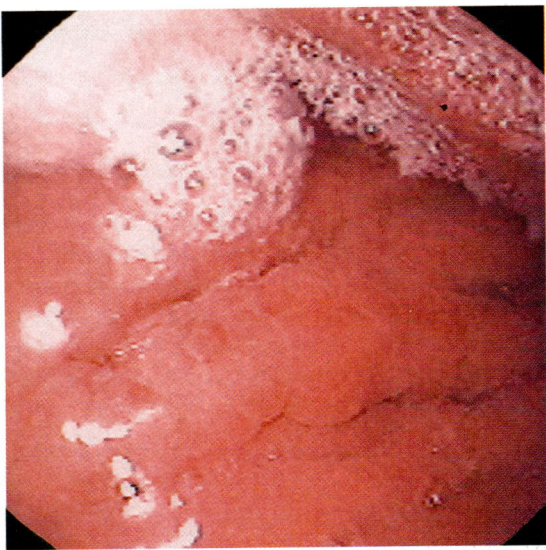

Figure 2-207: **Stomach. Signet-Ring Cell Carcinoma.** Enlarged nodular rugal folds and a prominent mosaic pattern due to an accentuation of the areae gastricae. The stomach did not distend well. These findings collectively suggest the possibility of a diffusely infiltrative disorder.

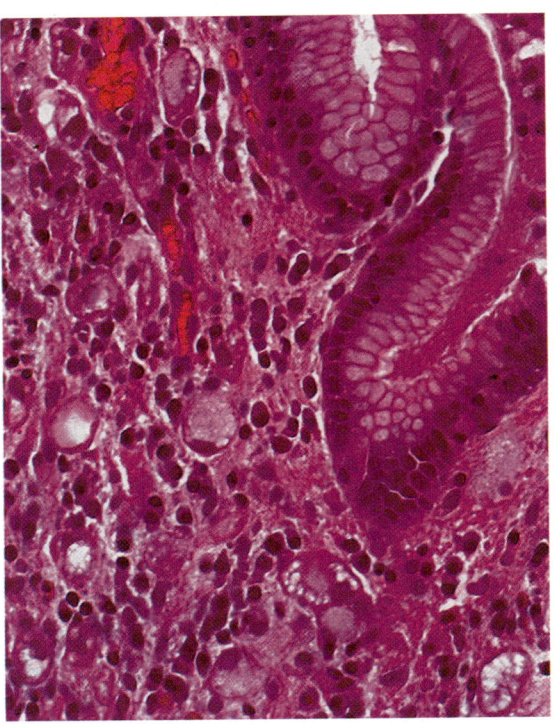

Figure 2-208: **Stomach. Signet-Ring Cell Carcinoma.** Tumor cells with voluminous cytoplasm are scattered in the lamina propria. Nuclei are large and eccentric.

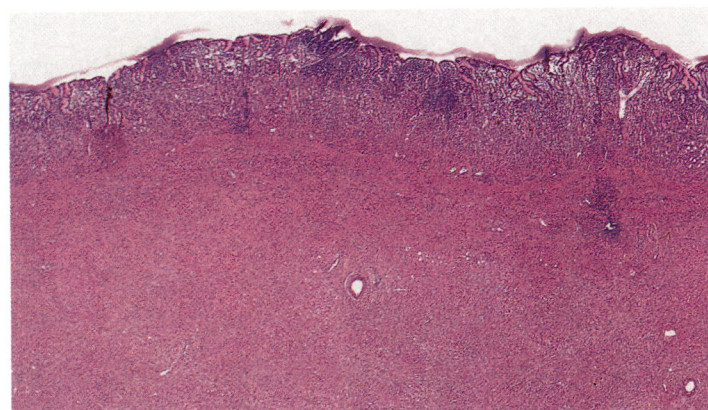

Figure 2-209: **Stomach. Linitis Plastica (Diffuse Adenocarcinoma).** Massive expansion of submucosa with loss of clearly defined separation of mucosa from submucosa. Surface epithelium is intact.

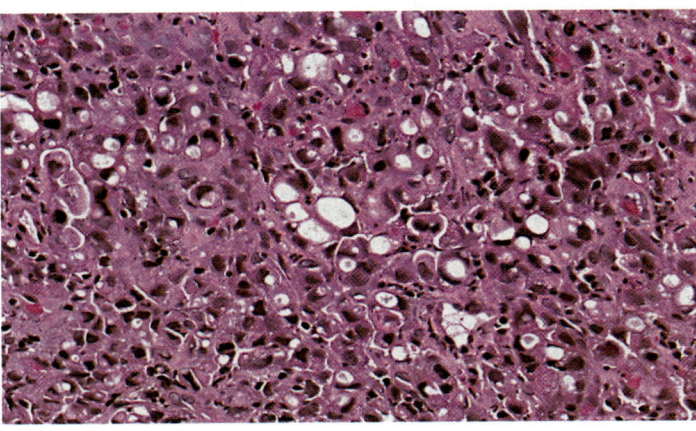

Figure 2-210: **Stomach. Signet-Ring Cell Carcinoma.** Tumor cells with varying degrees of cytoplasmic vacuolization fill lamina. Some have a central density giving a bull's-eye appearance.

MALIGNANT LYMPHOMA

- Morphology .... Small cell lymphomas may resemble reactive lymphoid hyperplasia. A monotonous lymphoid infiltrate, lymphoepithelial lesions (lymphoid clusters within the epithelium), degenerating eosinophilic glands, and destruction of reactive lymphoid follicles by the infiltrate characterize mucosa-associated lymphoid tissue (MALT) lymphoma. Large cell lymphoma can resemble undifferentiated carcinoma. Mucin stains or immunohistochemistry for cytokeratin and lymphoid markers usually resolve this distinction.

- Endoscopic features .... Lymphomatous involvement of the stomach may have a variety of manifestations, including large infiltrated rugae, eroded nodules, and exophytic and ulcerated masses. The infiltration of the rugal folds can be subtle or dramatic, with markedly enlarged folds containing a striking mucosal mosaic pattern. Enlarged rugal folds reflect the subepithelial infiltrative growth pattern of MALT lymphomas, particularly in early stages. Masses, erosions, and ulcers usually signify more extensive infiltration.

- Clinical features .... Gastric lymphoma may be associated with nonspecific dyspepsia, gastric outlet complaints due to obstruction or impairment of gastric motility, and anemia due to blood loss from ulceration.

- Differential diagnosis ...... Endoscopic: With solitary ulcers, benign peptic ulcer disease; with a large ulcerated mass, adenocarcinoma; with a single ulcerated nodule, an intramural soft tissue tumor; enlarged folds with a prominent mosaic pattern (areae gastricae), Menetrier disease, linitis plastica, leukemia, portal hypertensive gastropathy, and *H pylori* infection.

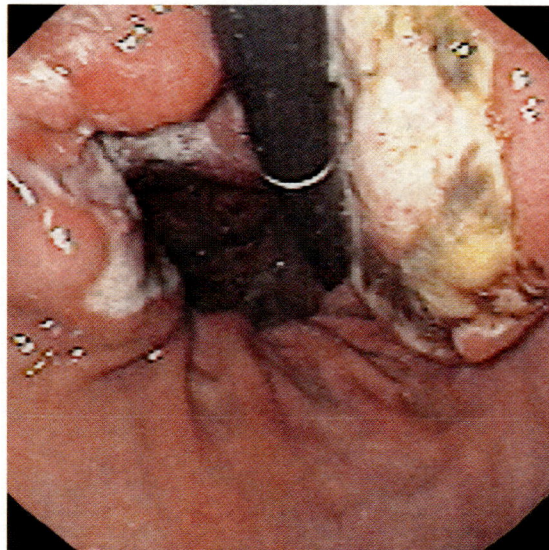

Figure 2-211: **Stomach, Proximal. Malignant Lymphoma, Large Cell.** Large mass encircling most of the lumen with surface ulcer.

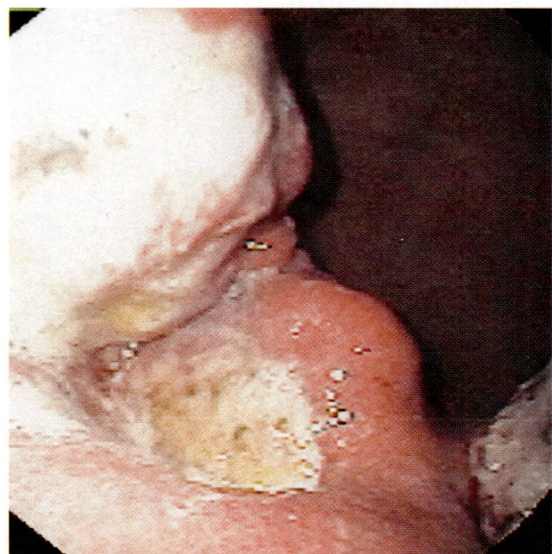

Figure 2-212: **Stomach, Proximal. Malignant Lymphoma, Large Cell.** Large submucosal mass with ulcer suggestive of an infiltrative process such as lymphoma.

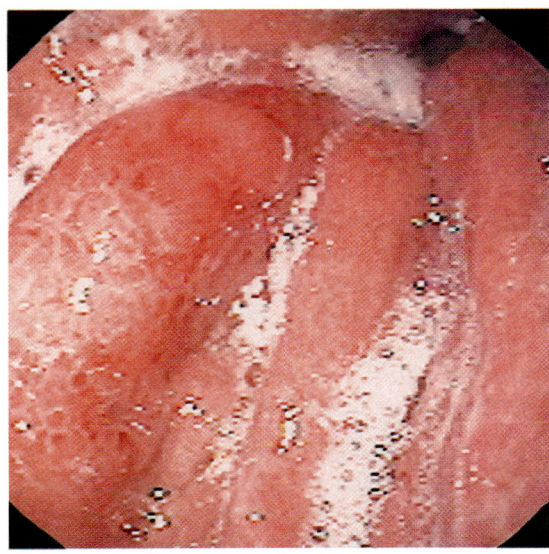

Figure 2-213: **Stomach. Malignant Lymphoma, Small Cell (MALT).** Enlarged rugal folds with a prominent mosaic pattern.

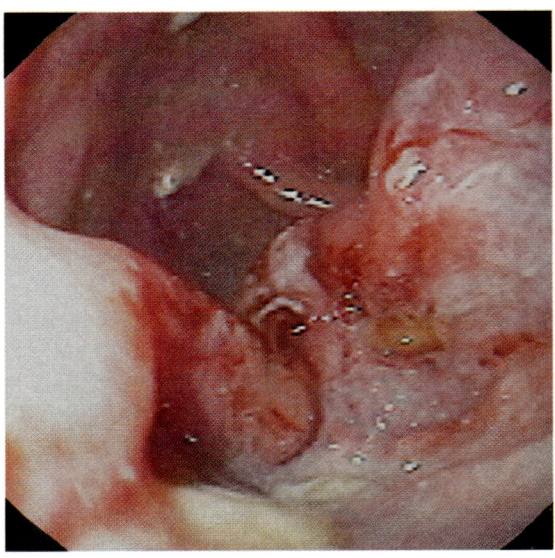

Figure 2-214: **Stomach. Malignant Lymphoma, Small Cell (MALT).** Large, irregular, ulcerating mass in the distal gastric body.

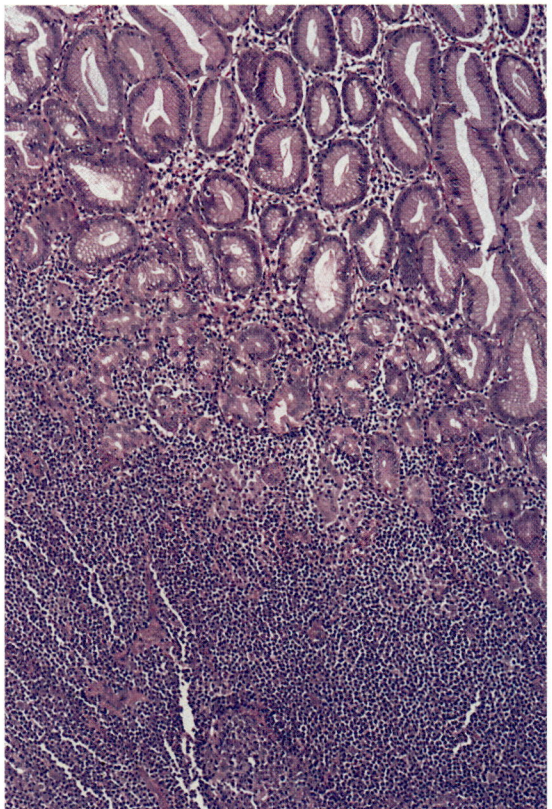

Figure 2-215: **Stomach. Malignant Lymphoma, Small Cell (MALT).** Dense basophilic infiltrate of small lymphoid cells obscures, disperses, and destroys deep gastric glands.

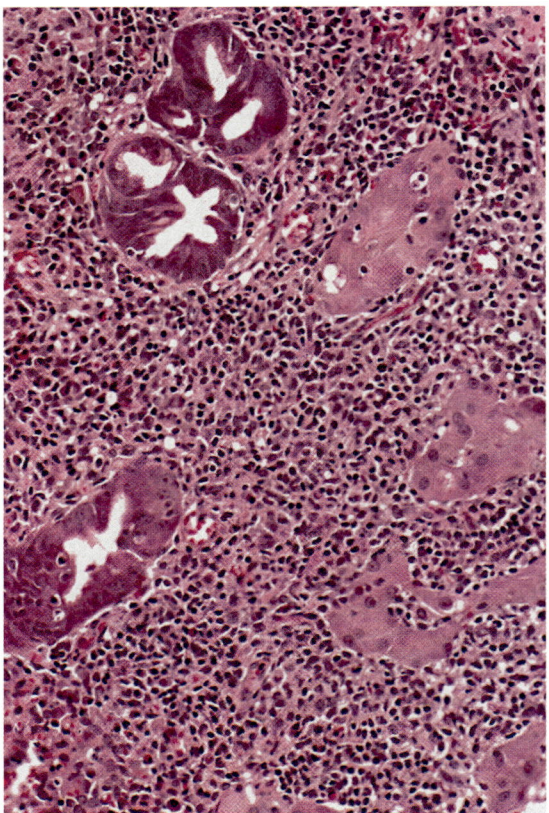

Figure 2-216: **Stomach. Malignant Lymphoma, Small Cell (MALT).** Small lymphoid cells surround and infiltrate gastric glands (lymphoepithelial lesions). Glandular eosinophilia, typical of destruction by MALT lymphoma.

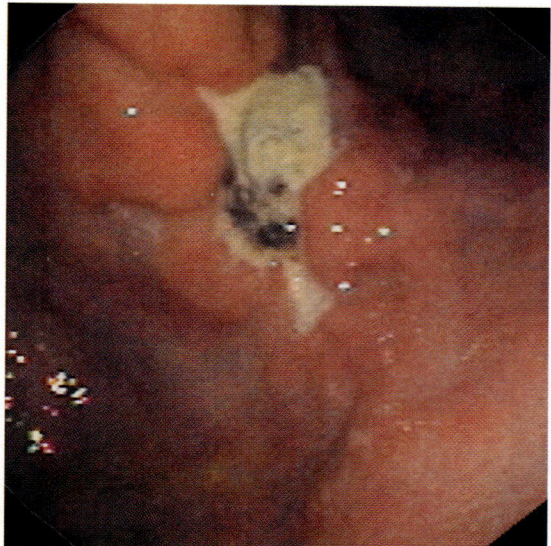 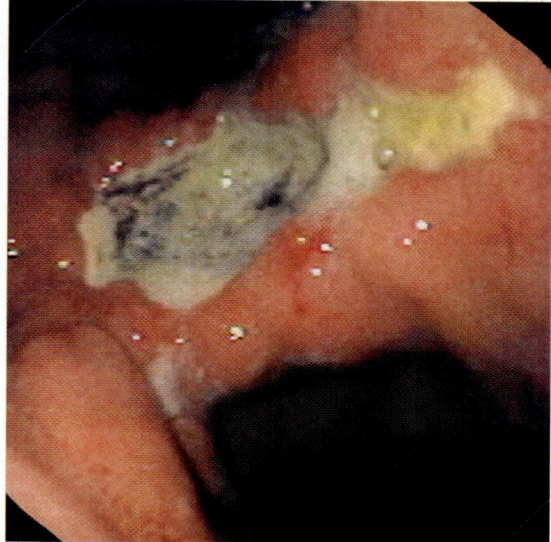

Figures 2-217 and 2-218: **Stomach. Malignant Lymphoma, Small Cell (MALT).** An irregular ulcer surrounded by heaped-up nodular folds. Close-up demonstrates ulcer depth. Lesion is situated along gastric folds and raised above surrounding mucosa. Appearance is suggestive of a neoplastic process.

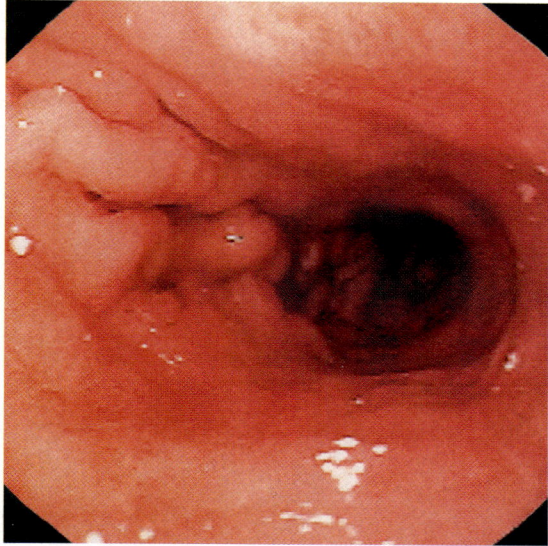

Figure 2-219: **Stomach. Malignant Lymphoma, Small Cell (MALT).** The folds along the greater curvature are slightly prominent but otherwise unremarkable.

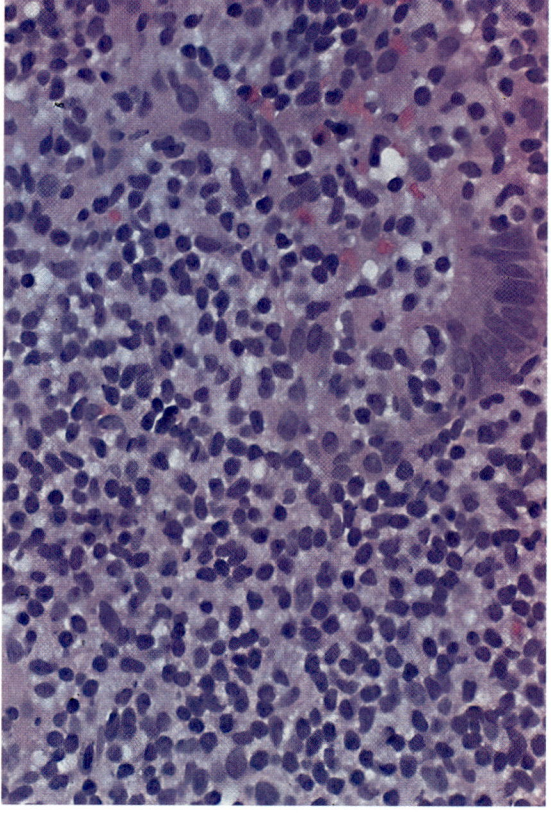

Figure 2-220: **Stomach. Malignant Lymphoma, Small Cell (MALT).** Clusters of small lymphoid cells infiltrate and destroy gastric glands, forming characteristic lymphoepithelial lesions.

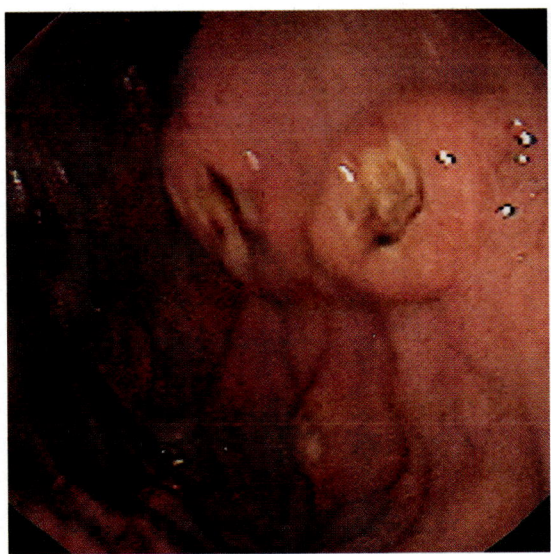 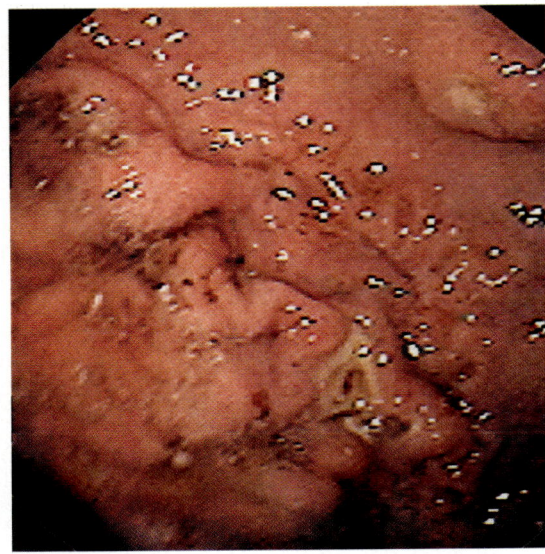

Figures 2-221 and 2-222: **Stomach. Malignant Lymphoma, Large Cell.** Ulcerated nodules and thickened folds with altered blood along greater curvature.

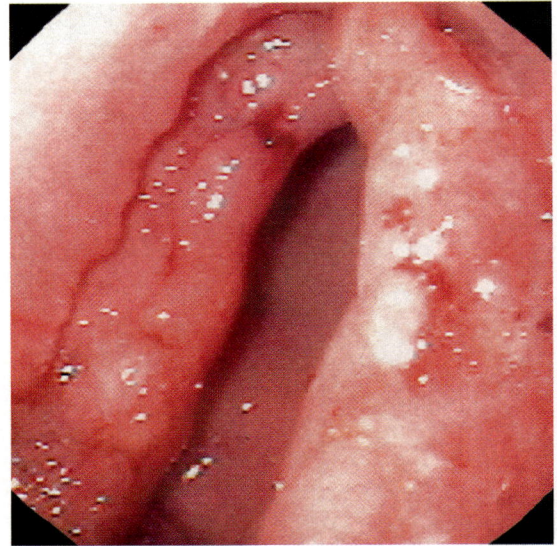 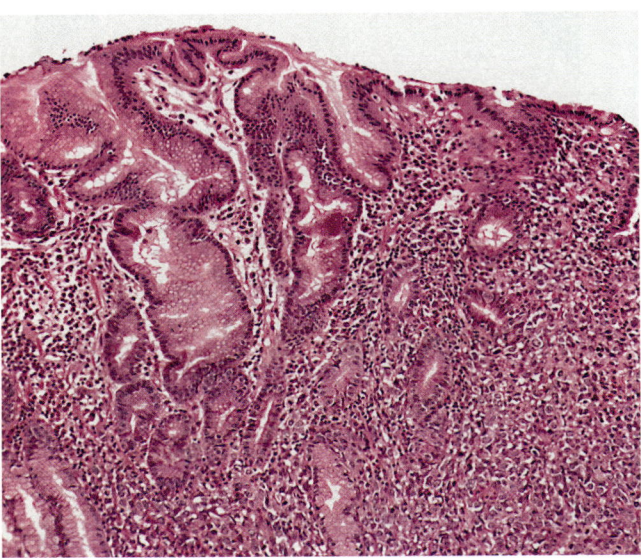

Figure 2-223: **Stomach. Malignant Lymphoma, Large Cell.** Coarse, superficial, ulcerated folds, with focal areas of hemorrhage and nodularity. The strikingly abnormal appearance is suggestive of a neoplastic process such as lymphoma.

Figure 2-224: **Stomach. Malignant Lymphoma, Large Cell.** Large lymphoid cells destroy and replace gastric mucosa.

STROMAL TUMORS (SMOOTH MUSCLE/STROMAL, NEUROGENIC, LIPOMATOUS)

- Morphology .... Stromal tumors, whether muscular, neurogenic, or lipomatous, generally are well-demarcated mural (as distinct from mucosal) nodules or masses. The overlying mucosa may be stretched and atrophic (Fig. 2-226), eroded or ulcerated (Fig. 2-232), or hyperplastic, as in a gastropathy (Fig. 2-233). Except for lipomas, the various stromal tumors cannot be distinguished endoscopically or grossly. The term *stromal tumor* is frequently used as a synonym for smooth muscle tumor in the gastrointestinal tract. Histologically, *smooth muscle/stromal tumors (GISTs)* are typically composed of spindle cells with blunt-ended nuclei and eosinophilic cytoplasm. They may have unipolar cytoplasmic vacuoles or be epithelioid (polygonal or round). The most important criterion for malignancy is the mitotic rate. Large size, infiltrative growth pattern, necrosis, and high cellularity are other important factors in evaluating smooth muscle tumors. In any case, it can be difficult to predict the behavior of smooth muscle/stromal tumors in the gastrointestinal tract. *Glomus tumors* appear to be related to smooth muscle tumors and may resemble the epithelioid variety. Their bland cytology, monotonous uniformity, and association with large, dilated blood spaces are typical features. They are virtually always benign. *Neurogenic tumors* are less common than smooth muscle tumors in the stomach. Schwannomas greatly outnumber neurofibromas. Schwannomas characteristically have spindle cells with elongated, angulated nuclei and are surrounded by or contain lymphoid aggregates and hyalinized blood vessels (features unusual in smooth muscle tumors). Nuclear palisading (Antoni type A pattern) is not a reliable feature of gastrointestinal schwannomas, as it is frequently absent and may be present in smooth muscle tumors. Immunohistochemical demonstration of S-100 protein is typical of schwannomas and is generally absent from smooth muscle tumors, where actin positivity is more characteristic. The distinction between schwannomas and smooth muscle tumors is important because the former rarely become malignant. *Lipomas* are less common in the stomach than in the intestines. Endoscopic biopsy may be unrewarding. Liposarcomas do not occur at this site.

- Endoscopic features .... Leiomyomas and leiomyosarcomas are the most commonly encountered stromal tumors and typically present within the proximal body or fundus as discretely demarcated submucosal nodules. These may be encountered incidentally during upper endoscopy for other indications, or, when ulcerated, present with acute GI bleeding. The ulceration in figure 2-228 is central, creating a dimpling or umbilication of the lesion very characteristic of ulcerated stromal tumors. Lesions less than 2 cm tend to be benign. Endoscopic ultrasound can be useful to assess size. Irregular margins, also seen by endoscopic ultrasound, suggest an aggressive lesion.

- Clinical features .... Can be an asymptomatic, incidental finding; acute episodic GI bleeding.

- Differential diagnosis ...... Endoscopic: Leiomyoma versus a leiomyosarcoma.

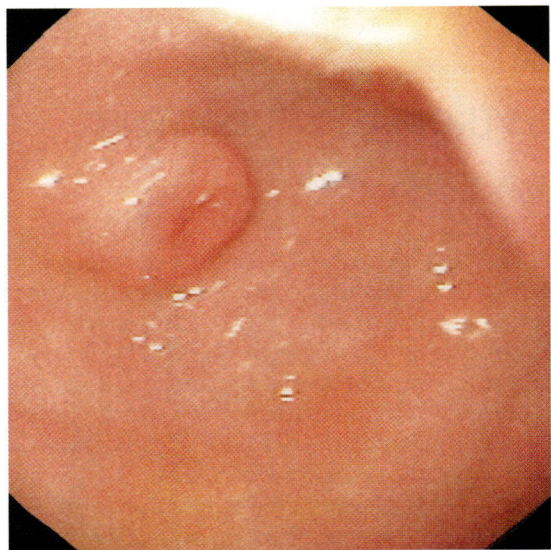

Figure 2-225: **Stomach. Smooth Muscle/Stromal Tumor.** A 1-cm nodule with central umbilication in antrum. Endoscopic differential is leiomyoma or pancreatic heterotopia.

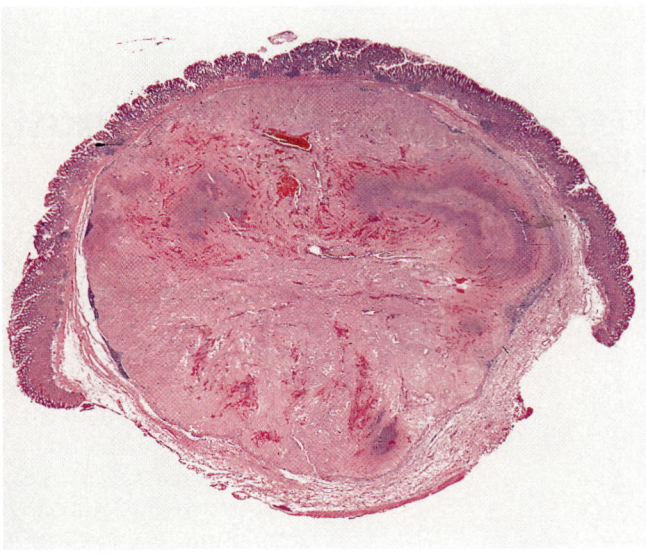

Figure 2-226: **Stomach. Smooth Muscle/Stromal Tumor.** Small, round, well-demarcated submucosal nodule with congestion, hemorrhage, and focal necrosis.

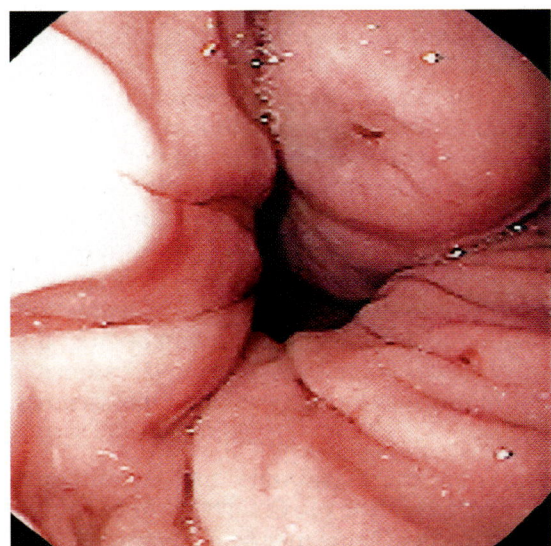

Figure 2-227: **Stomach. Smooth Muscle/Stromal Tumor.** Round submucosal mass with central dimple.

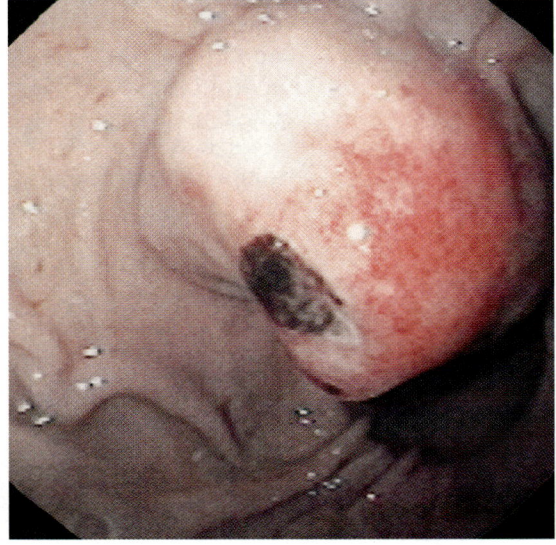

Figure 2-228: **Stomach. Smooth Muscle/Stromal Tumor.** A large submucosal nodule in proximal body with central ulceration. Patient presented with acute GI bleeding.

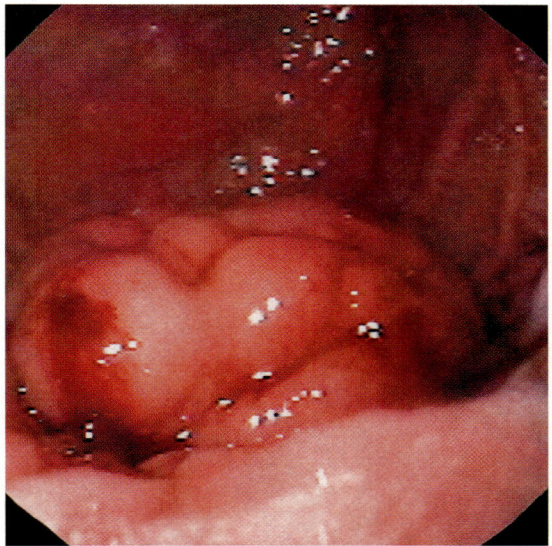

Figure 2-229: **Stomach. Smooth Muscle/Stromal Tumor.** Lobulated tumor covered by relatively normal-appearing mucosa without ulceration. Lobulation is uncommon in these tumors.

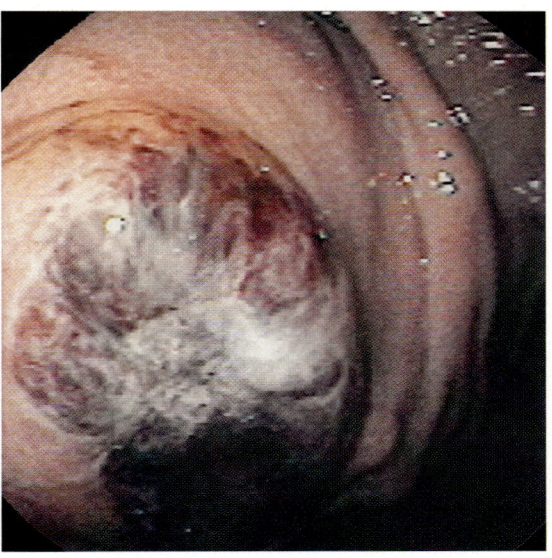

Figure 2-230: **Stomach. Leiomyosarcoma/Stromal Sarcoma.** Hemorrhagic ulcer over mural mass.

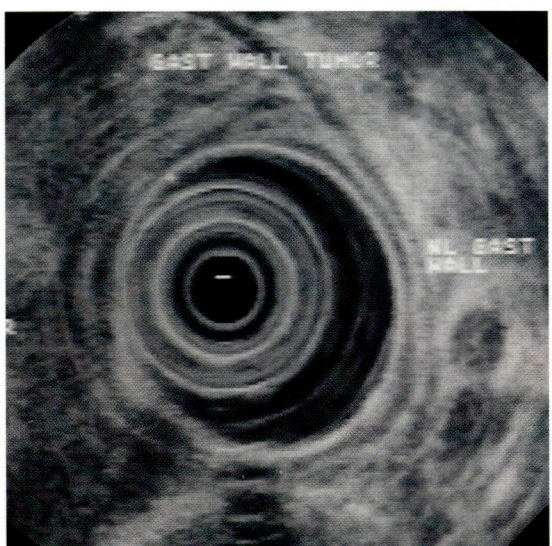

Figure 2-231: **Stomach. Leiomyosarcoma/Stromal Sarcoma.** Endoscopic ultrasound demonstrates lesion in Fig. 2-230. The lesion appears to arise from the muscularis propria echolayer, which expands as the mass increases in size, viewed from right to left across the upper portion of the photograph. Size exceeding 2 cm raises suspicion of a malignant intramural neoplasm. Tumor has inhomogeneous echo texture, consistent with a neoplasm. Outermost radiolucent endosonographic layer of gastric wall borders lesion, characteristic of an intramural tumor. If leiomyosarcoma is part of differential diagnosis, it is important to image entire tumor to determine whether margins are irregular and indistinct, especially the outermost sonolucent layer of gastric wall, which supports a malignant tumor.

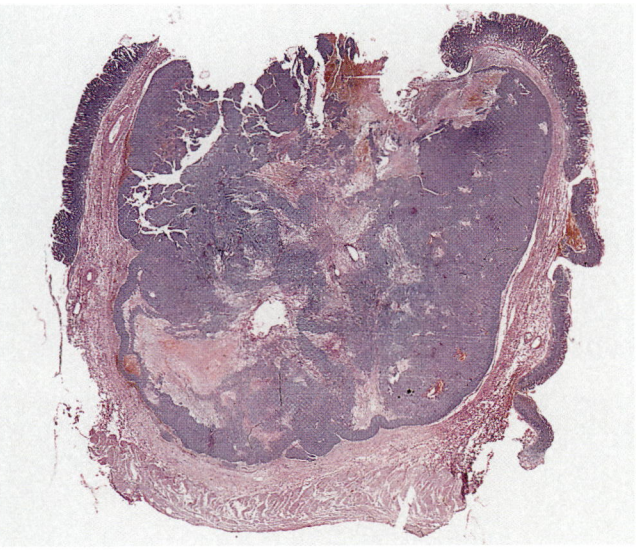

Figure 2-232: **Stomach. Smooth Muscle Tumor.** Well-demarcated submucosal nodule with ulceration and hemorrhage.

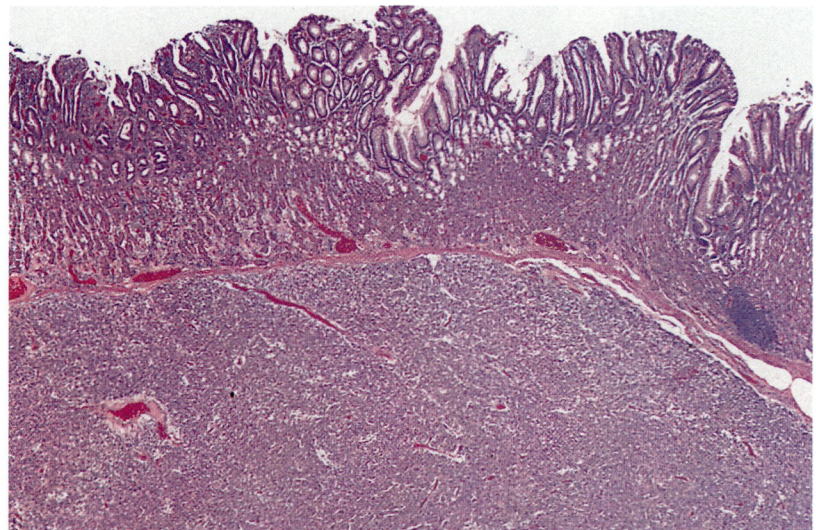

Figure 2-233: **Stomach. Leiomyosarcoma/Stromal Sarcoma, Low-Grade.** Cellular submucosal gastric tumor with intact muscularis mucosae and hyperplastic foveolae. Elevated mitotic rate justified diagnosis of sarcoma.

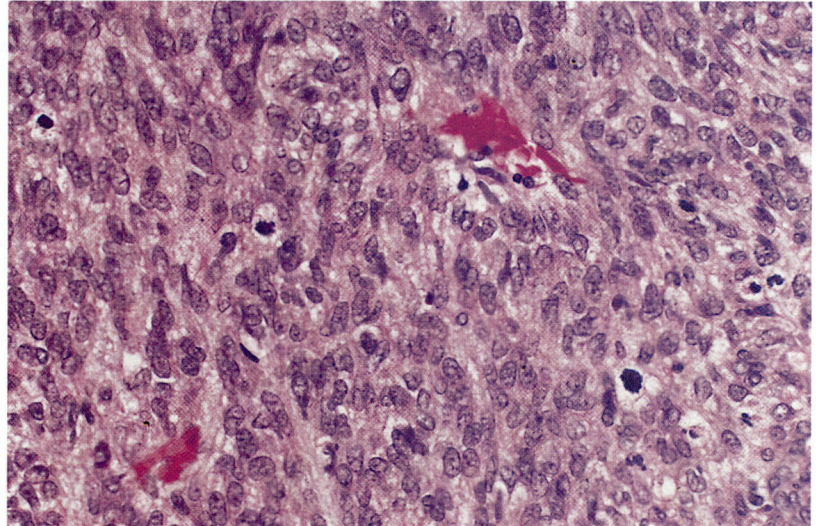

Figure 2-234: **Stomach. Leiomyosarcoma/Stromal Sarcoma, High-Grade.** Numerous mitoses indicate high-grade lesion.

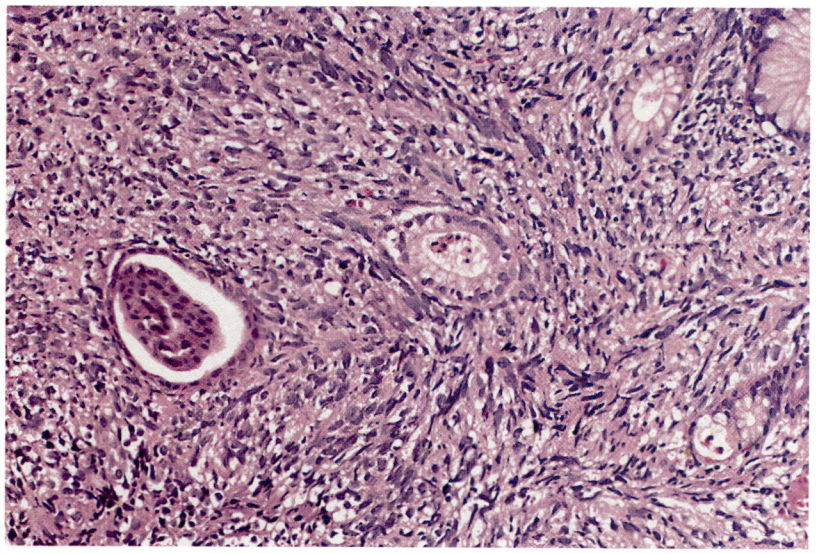

Figure 2-235: **Stomach. Leiomyosarcoma/Stromal Sarcoma.** Pleomorphic stromal cells infiltrate lamina propria separating gastric glands, a feature of malignancy.

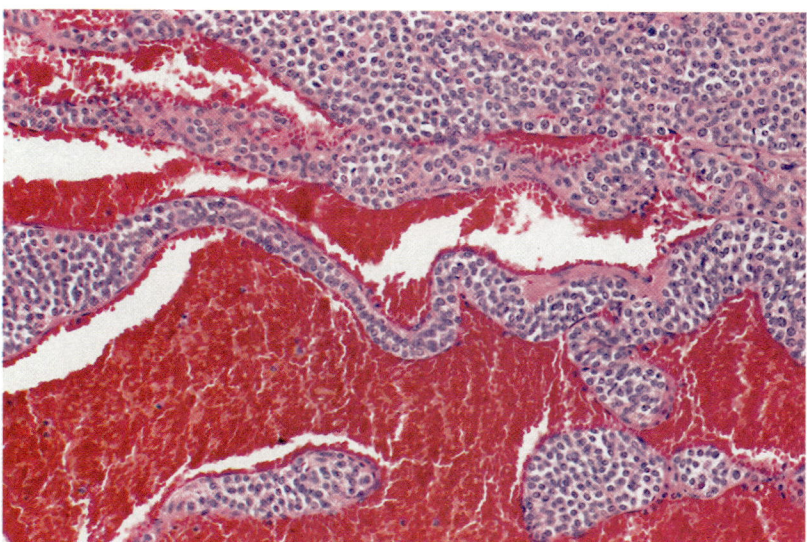

Figure 2-236: **Stomach. Glomus Tumor.** Large vascular spaces surrounded by uniform stromal cells with round, regular nuclei and clear cytoplasm.

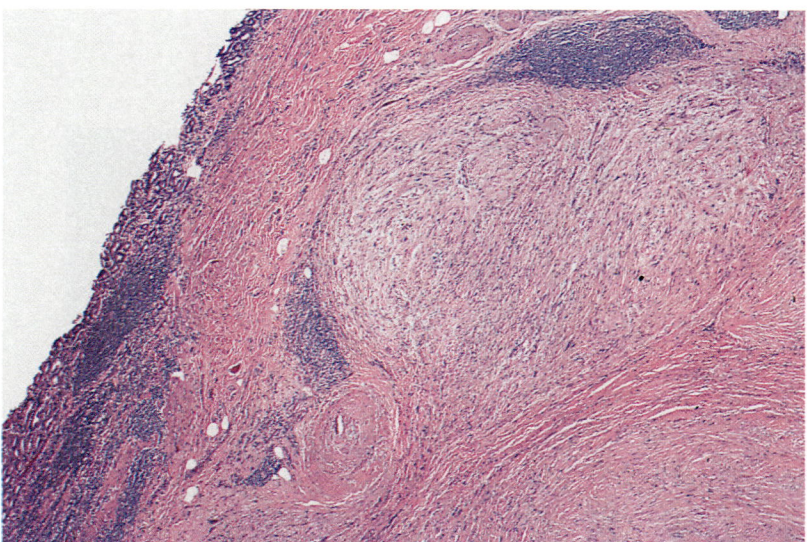

Figure 2-237: **Stomach. Schwannoma.** Submucosal stromal nodules with lymphoid aggregates and thickened, hyalinized arteries. Mucosa atrophic and chronically inflamed.

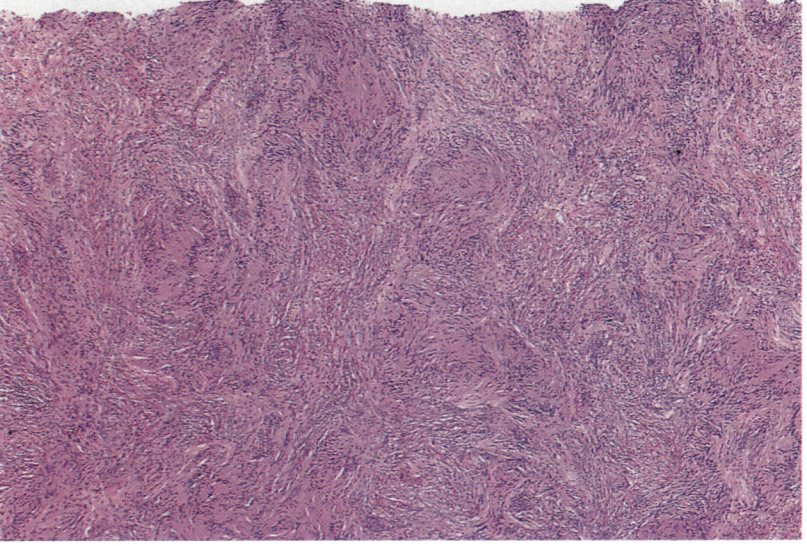

Figure 2-238: **Stomach. Schwannoma.** Antoni type A palisading.

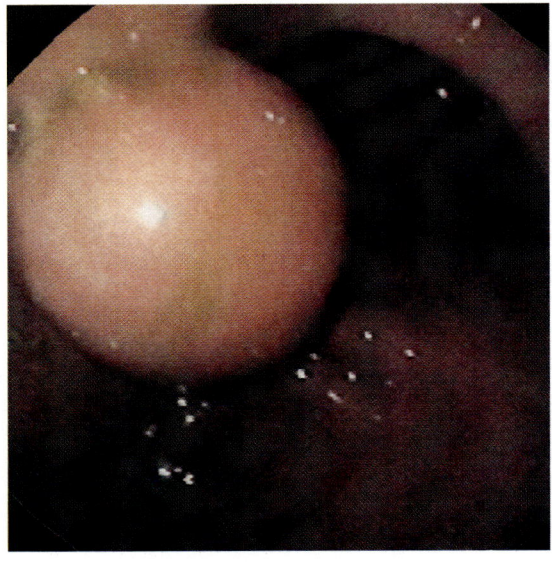

Figure 2-239: **Stomach. Submucosal Mass.** Large, round, submucosal mass with intact overlying mucosa.

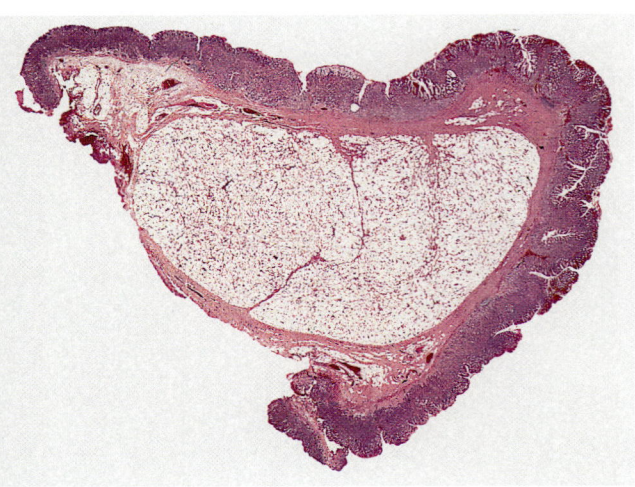

Figure 2-240: **Stomach. Lipoma.** Well-demarcated, ovoid, submucosal mass of mature adipose tissue.

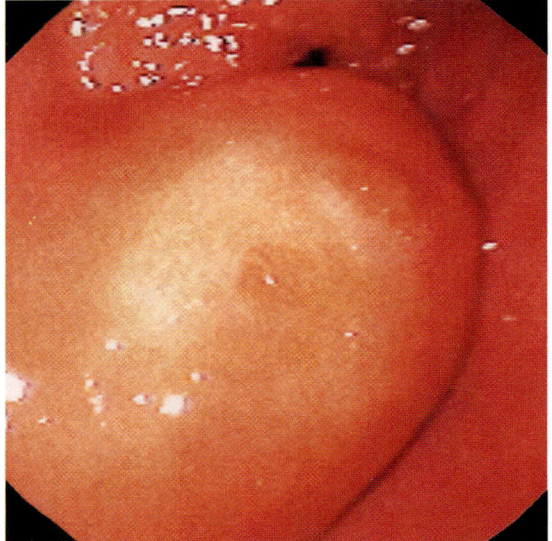

Figure 2-241: **Stomach. Submucosal Mass.** Large submucosal mass in antrum.

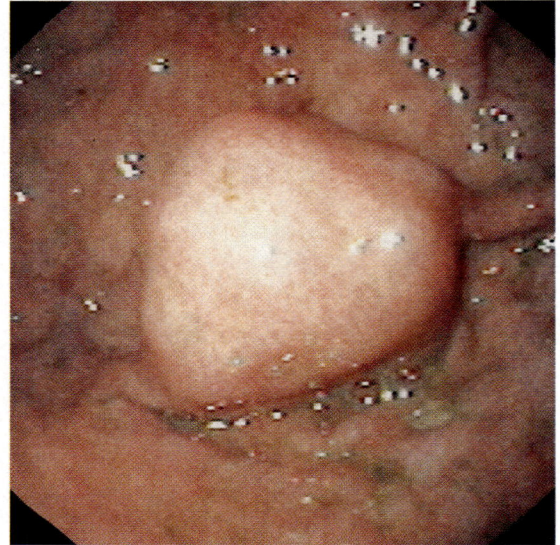

Figure 2-242: **Stomach. Submucosal Mass.** Slightly irregular submucosal nodule with intact overlying mucosa.

METASTATIC TUMORS

- Endoscopic features .... Localized metastatic neoplasms produce nodules that ulcerate centrally and cleave, dimple, or umbilicate. Diffuse infiltrative metastases enlarge folds and exaggerate the areae gastricae.
- Clinical features .... Metastatic disease to the stomach may be asymptomatic. Clinical presentation is often due to GI blood loss with anemia or overt bleeding. Outlet obstruction also occurs.
- Differential diagnosis ...... Histologic and endoscopic: Primary carcinoma.

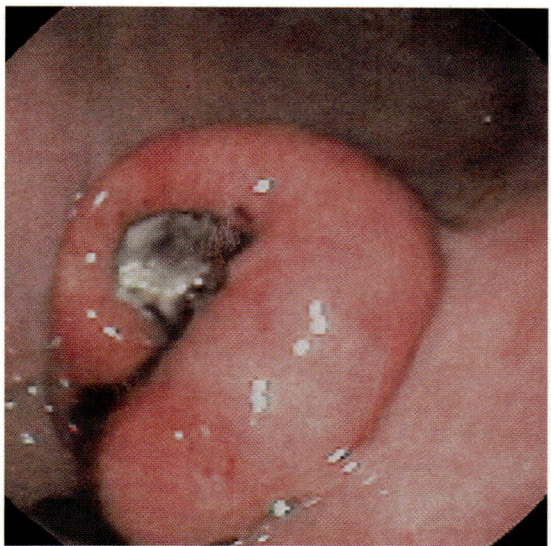

Figure 2-243: **Stomach. Metastatic Melanoma.** A centrally ulcerated, erythematous nodule in the distal body of the stomach. Both nodule and ulcer are raised above the surrounding mucosal surface. There is a scant amount of altered blood located along the margins of the ulcer.

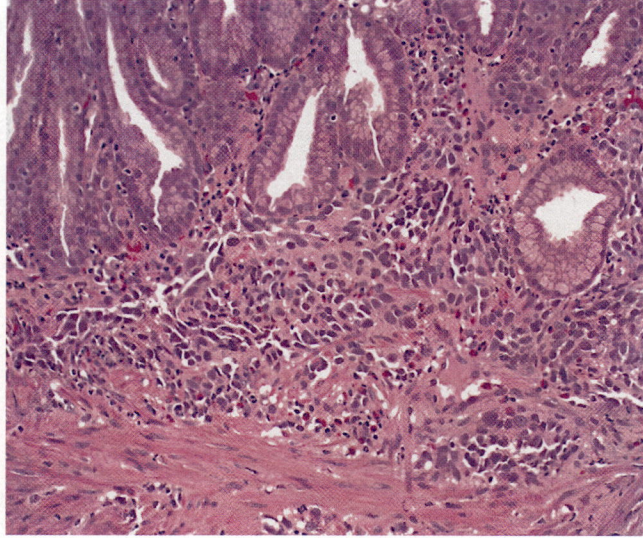

Figure 2-244: **Stomach. Metastatic Melanoma.** Cells with plasmacytoid appearance and large nuclei infiltrate beneath and between gastric glands.

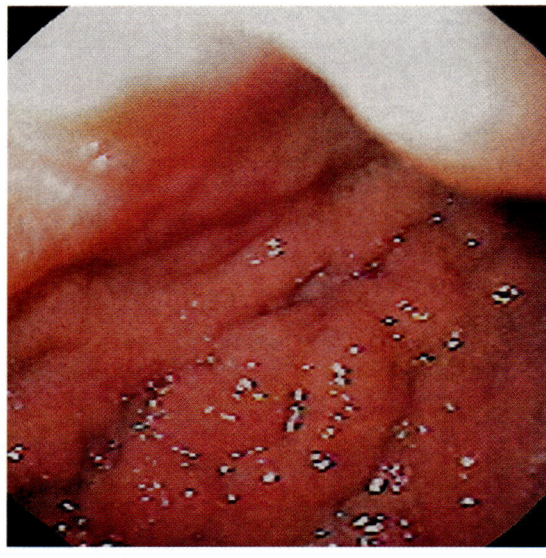

Figure 2-245: **Stomach. Metastatic Breast Carcinoma.** The gastric folds are enlarged and irregular and have a nodular surface.

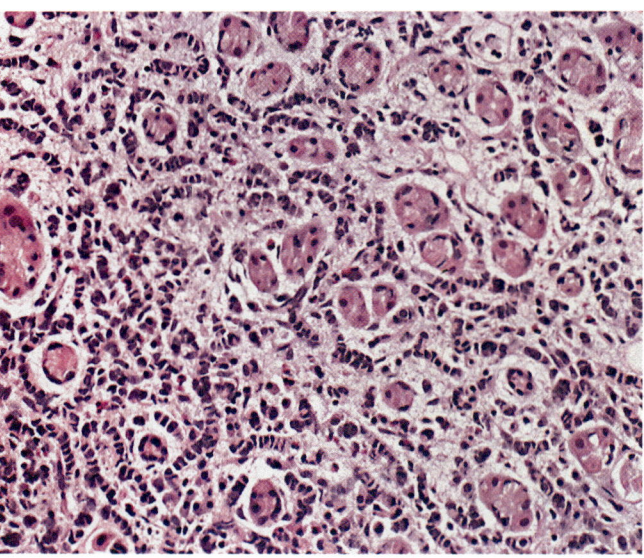

Figure 2-246: **Stomach. Metastatic Breast Carcinoma.** Small cells in single file infiltrate between glands, typical of lobular carcinoma of the breast.

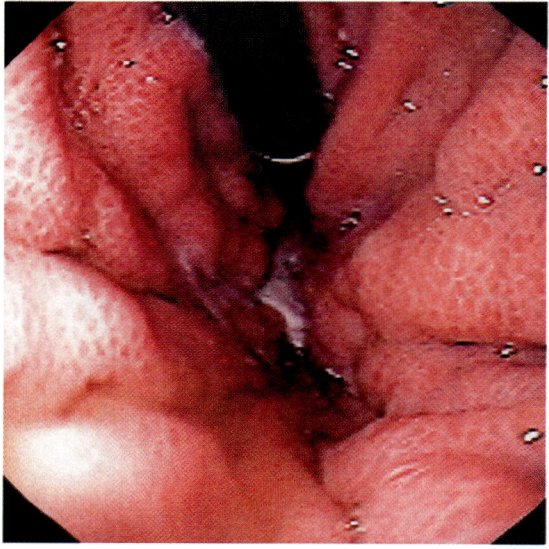

Figure 2-247: **Stomach. Leukemia.** Enlarged gastric folds with a striking mosaic pattern.

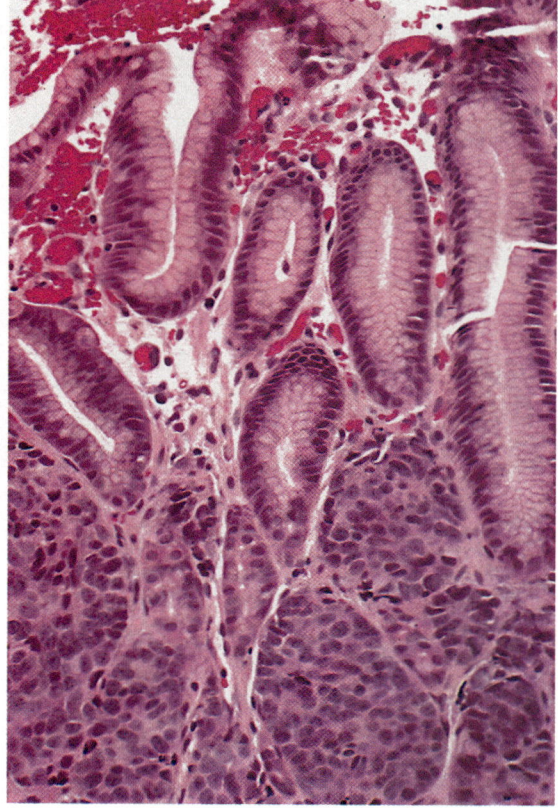

Figure 2-248: **Stomach. Metastatic Prostatic Adenocarcinoma.** Nests of tumor cells fill lower lamina propria, resembling carcinoid tumor. Prostate Specific Antigen (PSA)-positive, chromogranin-negative.

CHAPTER 3

SMALL INTESTINE

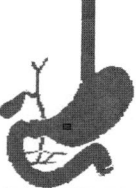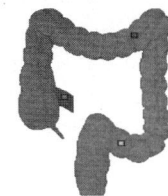

Endoscopic examination	174
Histology	175
Normal small intestine	176
Normal ileum	179
Patterns of injury	181
Duodenitis	182
Ulcers and erosions	184
Ileal ulcers and erosions	186
Eosinophilic enteritis	188
Granulomatous enteritis/Crohn's disease	190
Infections with normal mucosal pattern	193
Giardiasis	194
Cryptosporidia	196
Microsporidia	197
Isospora belli	198
Viral infections	199
Infections within histiocytes: *Mycobacterium avium-intracellulare*, Whipple disease	201
Infections within histiocytes: leishmania, histoplasma, typhoid	204
Candida infection	206
Parasites, worms	207
Common variable immunodeficiency/ hypogammaglobulinemia	208
Lymphoid hyperplasia	210
Malabsorption	212
Cronkhite-Canada syndrome: protein-losing enteropathy	216
Lymphatic dilatation	218
Congenital lymphatic dilatation	218
Vascular lesions	221
Vasculitis	224
Hemorrhagic enteropathy	226
Ischemia	227
Collagen vascular disease	230
Amyloid	231
Intussusception	232
Ostomy, diverticula	234
Anastomotic ulcers	236
Pouchitis	237
Pigments	239
Submucosal inflammatory mass	241
Heterotopic gastric mucosa	242
Brunner gland lesions	244
Lipoma	246
Hyperplastic polyp	247
Inflammatory fibroid polyp	248
Peutz-Jeghers polyp	250
Pancreatic heterotopia	252
Gangliocytic paraganglioma	254
Schwannoma	256
Neurofibroma	257
Carcinoid tumor	258
Adenoma	260
Ampullary adenoma	263
Adenocarcinoma	265
Malignant lymphoma	267
Smooth muscle/stromal tumors	271
Benign vascular neoplasms	272
Vascular malignancies	272
Lymphangioma	275
Metastatic tumors	276

ENDOSCOPIC EXAMINATION

Endoscopic examination of the small intestine beyond the duodenum is a challenge. Enteroscopy is performed using several techniques: push enteroscopy, sonde enteroscopy, and surgically assisted enteroscopy.

Push enteroscopy is performed with a specially designed jejunoscope, commonly used in conjunction with an overtube to prevent looping of the enteroscope in the stomach. Push enteroscope working lengths range from 230 to 260 cm. In experienced hands, the push enteroscope can easily be passed through the jejunum. A colonoscope may also be used in push enteroscopy. Successfully examining the jejunum depends on minimizing gastric loop formation.

The sonde enteroscope is approximately 300 cm in working length and travels passively through the small bowel. In 75% of examinations, the sonde enteroscope tip enters the ileum. A complete examination of the small intestine is possible in only 10% to 15% of patients; the remainder are unable to tolerate the procedure. Unlike push enteroscopy, sonde enteroscopy allows diagnosis only, not therapy. Inability to control tip movement and to readvance when desired greatly limits the ability to maintain an adequate view.

Surgical enteroscopy utilizes colonoscopes or push jejunoscopes passed orally or via a midbowel enterotomy. The surgeon passes the endoscope throughout the length of the small intestine by threading the bowel on to the endoscope as the endoscope is passed. Inspection during passage assures that iatrogenic mucosal injury due to intraoperative manipulations will not be mistaken for pathologic lesions.

The endoscopist must be able to recognize the anatomic features of the duodenum, jejunum, and ileum. The duodenal lumen is larger than the jejunum, and the circular folds (valvulae conniventes) are spaced farther apart. The villous structure of the jejunal mucosa creates a speckled or glittering appearance quite distinctive from that of the duodenum. The ileal mucosa appears smoother than the jejunum; the circular folds are shorter and spaced farther apart. The ileal lumen may be slightly smaller but not consistently so.

The villous pattern should always be assessed during enteroscopic examination. Villi may be easily seen when viewing the mucosa below any fluid accumulation or simply by instilling water. Fluids magnify the mucosal view, producing a striking villous pattern. This simple technique can readily identify spruelike conditions and help direct biopsy.

Commonly encountered abnormalities include diverticula and alterations in blood vascular and lymphatic systems. Duodenal diverticula are encountered typically in the postbulbar duodenum, and most commonly involve the papilla of Vater. Diverticula may be quite large and have very large openings. Vascular changes include phlebectasias and prominent submucosal venous structures. Focal collections of dilated lymphatics and xanthelasmas are also common.

The terminal ileum is assessed during colonoscopy. Intubation of the ileocecal valve permits, on average, an examination of up to 10 cm of terminal ileum. Lymphoid nodules are common, especially in young patients. Mucosal vessels may be prominent and can be mistaken for vascular abnormalities. Retrograde ileoscopy rarely, if ever, reaches a Meckel diverticulum. Examination of the terminal ileum is part of the evaluation of diarrhea, inflammatory bowel disease, and obscure GI bleeding.

Biopsy of the small intestine is accomplished with standard pinch avulsion-type biopsy forceps. Mucosectomy is infrequently performed and is limited to the duodenal bulb.

HISTOLOGY

Small bowel mucosa consists of crypts and villi. Secretion occurs in the crypts and absorption in the villi. Villi vary in size and shape depending on location, but are generally finger- or leaf-shaped and longer in the distal than in the proximal small bowel. They are short and flat over Brunner glands or lymphoid follicles. Superficial mucosal biopsies may appear flat when stretched.

Epithelial cells proliferate in the base of the crypt, migrate to the surface, and undergo apoptosis at the tip of the villus. Three crypts contribute to each villus. Goblet cells are regularly interspersed with surface absorptive cells. The microvillus border embedded in the glycocalyx appears as a refractile band on H&E sections and is best seen with PAS diastase. Paneth cells, endocrine cells, and undifferentiated crypt cells are located in the crypts.

Lymphocytes are either clustered in follicles (B and helper T cells) or dispersed in the epithelium (suppressor/cytotoxic T cells) in a ratio of 1 per 5 epithelial cells. Lymphoid follicles are commonly seen on endoscopic examination in the terminal ileum (and rectum), especially in young persons. Plasma cells dominate the physiologic inflammatory cell population in the lamina propria. Macrophages are clustered beneath the tips of the villi. Eosinophils are sprinkled throughout. Mast cells are sparsely but uniformly dispersed, and require special stains (e.g. tryptase) to be visualized. Neutrophils are abnormal outside of the vascular space. The density of the physiologic inflammatory infiltrate varies in individuals.

Smooth muscle cells from the muscularis mucosae are attached to the crypts and surface epithelium. They order the mucosa and express secretions.

Submucosal arteries follow the circular folds. An arteriole, accompanied by a venule and lymphatic course perpendicularly through the center of each villus. A cascade of capillaries arises from arterioles. It is separated by basement membrane from the surface epithelium and collects in a venule. The lymphatics extend close to the mucosal surface and transport absorbed fat and proteins. Lacteals are normally collapsed, but dilate when there is edema or lymphatic obstruction.

NORMAL SMALL INTESTINE

- Morphology .... Ideally, biopsy specimens are oriented on a filter or mesh prior to fixation. Proper histologic orientation is characterized by longitudinally oriented crypts. Minor variations in villus shape and size are caused by normal anatomic variations, stretching artifact, or tangential sectioning. Poorly oriented specimens may appear flat, but pathologic villus atrophy is almost always associated with epithelial damage and inflammation. Plasma cells are normal and should always be present. Neutrophils are never normal outside the vascular space. A few histiocytes in the villus tips are normal. Lacteals are not normally visible and when dilated indicate an abnormality. Submucosal vessels should be assessed for lymphangiectasia or amyloid. *Giardia, Cryptosporidium, Isospora,* Microsporidia, and adenovirus may cause no villus abnormality or mucosal response and can be difficult to detect.

    Biliary or pancreatic duct epithelial cells contain diffuse neutral mucin and are indistinguishable on light microscopy from gastric foveolar cell metaplasia. Biopsy specimens are usually too small to distinguish normal from hyperplastic Brunner glands. Dislodged Brunner gland epithelium in the ducts can simulate neoplasia, especially when crushed.

- Endoscopic features .... Normal endoscopic features include easily identified circular folds, villi, and the absence of a submucosal vascular pattern. Villi are best identified using water submersion magnification of the mucosal surface. A submucosal vascular network, if present, suggests a spruelike state.

    The papilla of Vater is rounded, fleshy, and averages 5 to 8 mm in diameter. It can be extremely small and minimally elevated from the surrounding duodenal surface, or large, polypoid, and irregular. The papilla may be located along the margin of a duodenal diverticulum or nestled deep within the duodenal hood. The duodenal hood is typically the size of the papilla but may be prominent and bulging or absent.

- Differential diagnosis ...... Histologic: Infections that do not cause inflammation, subtle immunodeficiency disorders such as IgA or common variable immunodeficiency, very mild inflammatory conditions, eosinophilic enteritis due to its patchy distribution.

    Histologic and endoscopic: Normal Brunner gland versus Brunner gland hyperplasia, cyst, or hamartoma.

    Papilla of Vater. Histologic: Biliary or pancreatic ductal epithelium versus gastric foveolar epithelium.

    Endoscopic: Normal ampulla versus adenoma.

SMALL INTESTINE

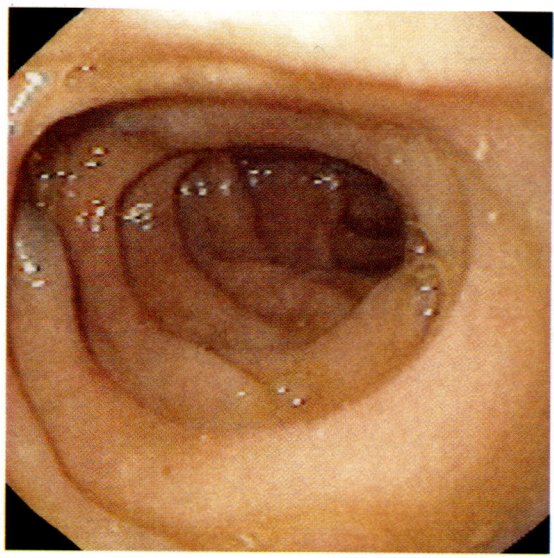

Figure 3-1: **Duodenum. Normal.** Distal duodenum with deep circular folds. In the extreme left portion of the photograph, there is a prominent submucosal venous structure.

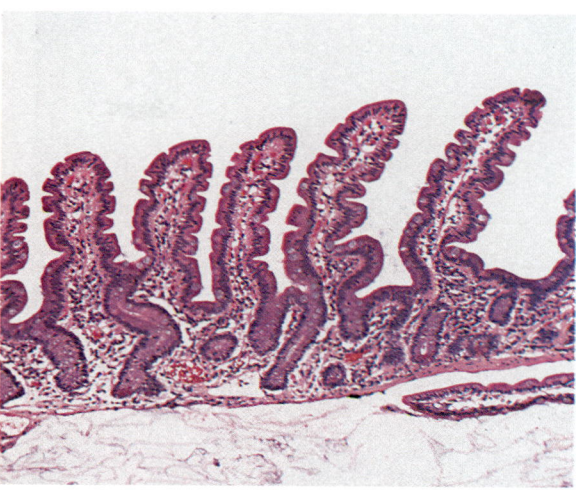

Figure 3-2: **Duodenum. Normal.** Well-oriented specimen with longitudinally sectioned crypts and more than 4 villi in a row. Villus-to-crypt ratio 3:1.

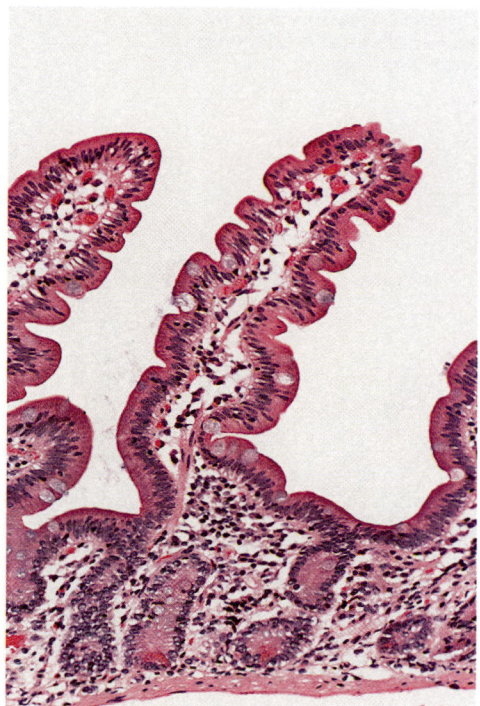

Figure 3-3: **Duodenum. Normal.** Tall columnar absorptive and goblet cells with basal nuclei. Crypt mitoses present; crypt nuclei uniform. Intraepithelial lymphocytes regularly dispersed, approximately 1 per 5 epithelial cells. Plasma cells in lamina propria. No neutrophils or macrophages. Smooth muscle strands extend into villus.

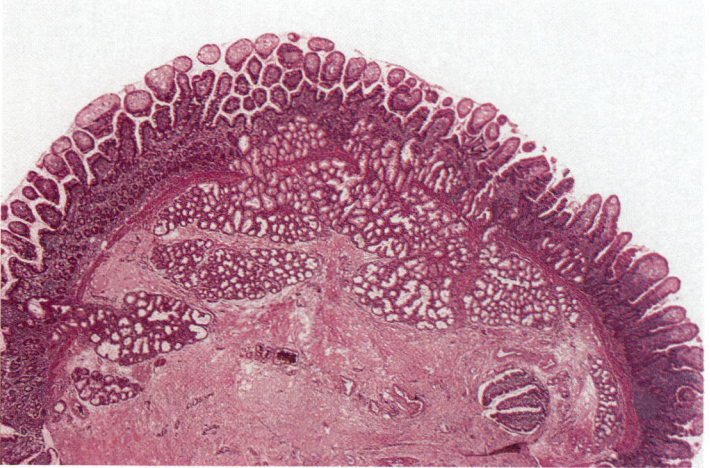

Figure 3-4: **Duodenum. Normal.** Brunner glands empty into crypt bases. Specimen is not well-oriented centrally, as evidenced by tangentially sectioned villi and crypts.

177

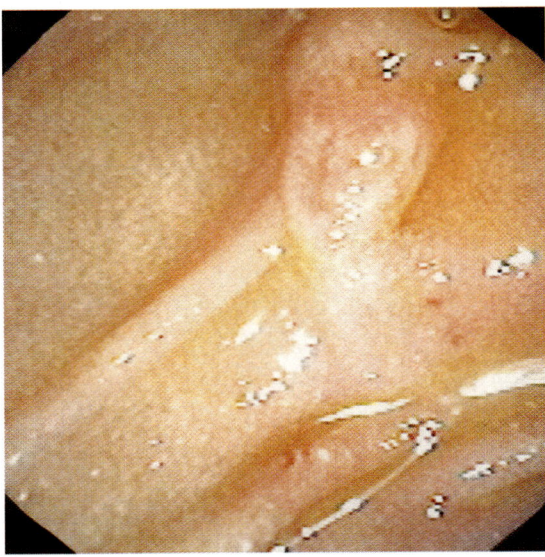

Figure 3-5: **Papilla of Vater. Normal.** The papilla is small, round, and fleshy. The duodenal hood, cephalad to the papilla, is small and conforms well to the papilla.

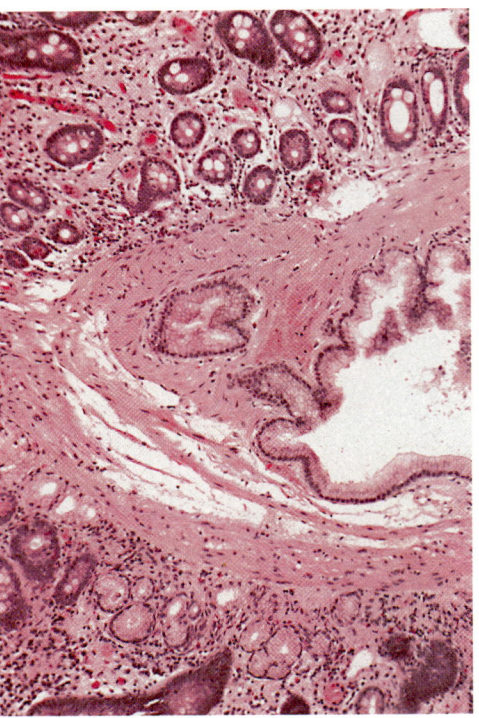

Figure 3-6: **Duodenum. Normal Accessory Duct.** Cross section of accessory duct in submucosa. Duct epithelium is tall columnar with diffuse cytoplasmic mucin.

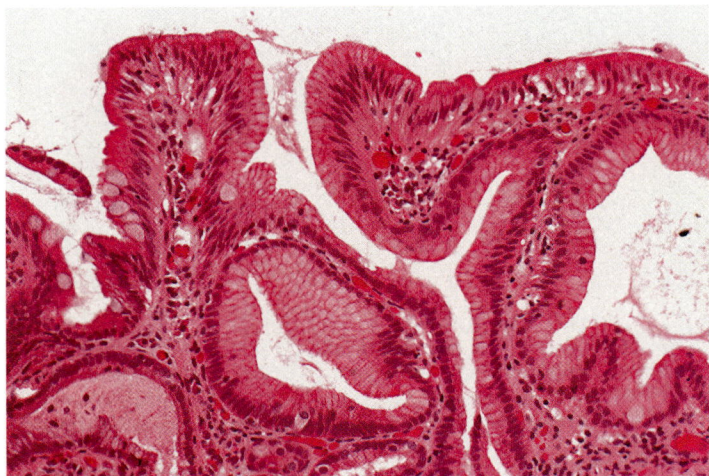

Figure 3-7: **Duodenum. Normal Accessory Duct.** Opening of accessory duct at the mucosal surface.

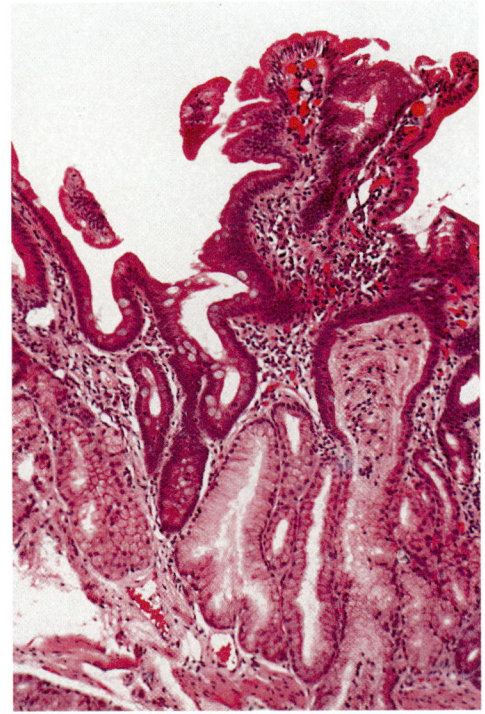

Figure 3-8: **Duodenum. Mechanical Artifact, Brunner Gland.** Dislodged Brunner gland epithelium plugs duct.

NORMAL ILEUM

- Morphology .... Villi appear short and blunt over Peyer patches. Peyer patches can be confused with chronic inflammation or lymphoma, particularly if the specimen does not include a germinal center. In chronic inflammatory conditions, other types of inflammatory cells, including neutrophils, are present. The lack of cytologic atypia together with typical endoscopic findings should prevent misinterpretation.

- Endoscopic features .... The terminal ileum is notable for the speckled light pattern due to the presence of villi and lymphoid nodules. This is less striking in the ileum than in the jejunum. Circular folds vary from widely spaced to frequent and complete.

- Differential diagnosis ...... Histologic: Peyer patches versus chronic ileitis, lymphoma.

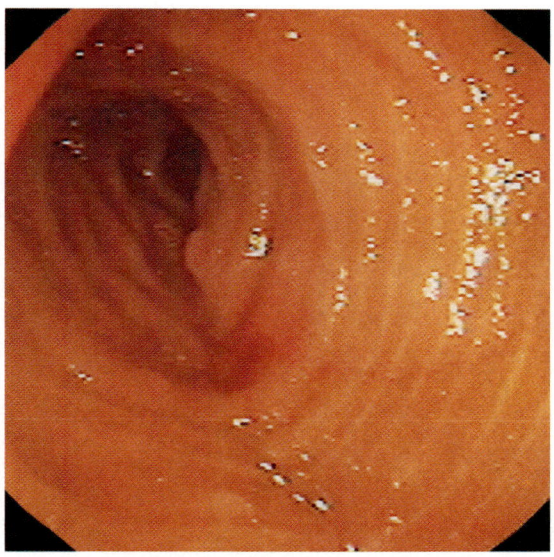

Figure 3-9: **Ileum. Normal.** Distal ileum with speckled light reflection off villi. Scattered subtle lymphoid nodules. Well-spaced and complete circular folds.

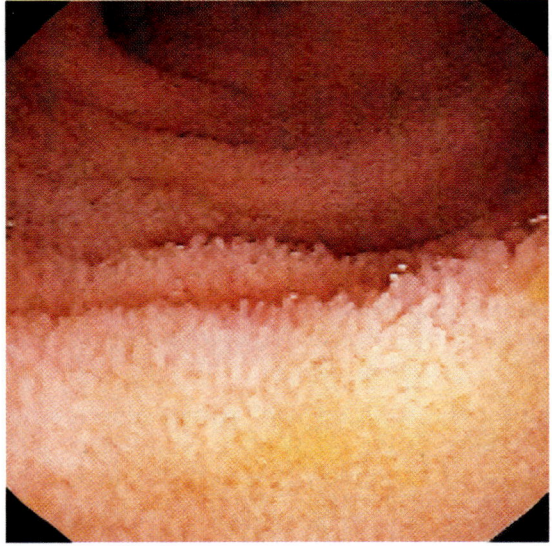

Figure 3-10: **Ileum. Normal.** Water-submerged mucosal magnification illustrates normal villi.

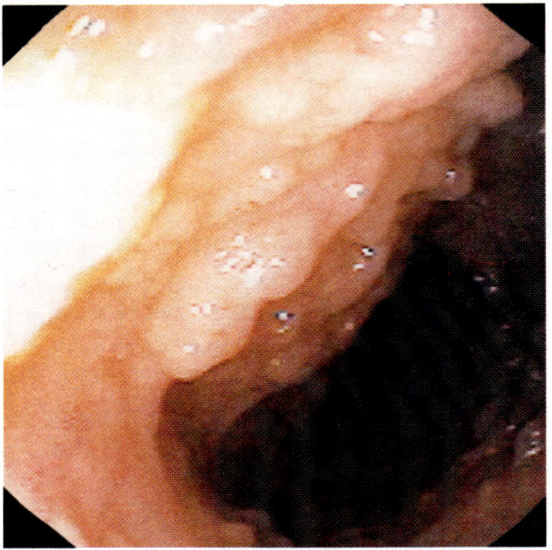

Figure 3-11: **Ileum. Normal Peyer Patch.** Multiple crowded and heaped-up lymphoid nodules.

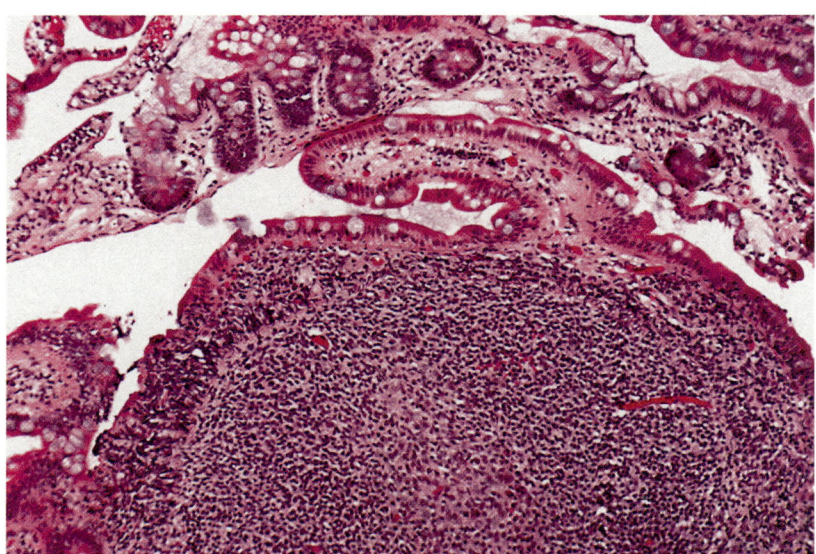

Figure 3-12: **Ileum. Normal Peyer Patch.** Villi are sparse and distorted over a lymphoid nodule.

PATTERNS OF INJURY

The presence of neutrophils in the lamina propria and/or epithelium serves to distinguish pathologic from physiologic inflammation. Chronic processes are generally associated with an increase of plasma cells, other mononuclear cells, and eosinophils, as well as epithelial regeneration. Specific criteria for separating acute from chronic inflammation have not been clearly defined for small intestine.

Inflammation in the upper small intestine is commonly due to peptic disease, NSAID injury, or malabsorption syndrome. Histologic features are overlapping, as all are associated with surface epithelial damage, chronic inflammation, crypt hyperplasia, and villous atrophy. The only additional feature characteristic of malabsorption inflammatory pattern is intraepithelial lymphocytosis. Clinical information, endoscopic appearance, and biopsy location (e.g. duodenal bulb versus distal duodenum or jejunum) are important in suggesting a cause of the mucosal injury and crypt hyperplasia/regeneration. The malabsorption pattern consisting of chronic inflammation, surface epithelial damage with intraepithelial lymphocytosis, villous atrophy, and crypt hyperplasia is characteristic, but not specific, for celiac sprue. It may be caused by hypersensitivity to other proteins, bacterial overgrowth, tropical sprue, severe protein calorie malnutrition, and autoimmunity. The proximal small bowel is typically affected, but in severe cases, the ileum may be involved.

Lesions of eosinophilic enteritis are most often in the upper tract and are generally associated with peripheral eosinophilia. The submucosa is usually heavily infiltrated by eosinophils, with minor multifocal penetration of the mucosa which, on endoscopic examination, appears as multifocal papules and erosions. Since eosinophils are increased as a component of nonspecific chronic inflammation, histologic diagnosis requires an exclusive increase in eosinophils. Pure collections of eosinophils, particularly in the deep lamina propria, suggest eosinophilic enteritis. The key to diagnosis is numerous biopsies.

Crohn's disease affects both upper and lower small bowel, but more commonly the ileum. Crohn's disease often lacks characteristic granulomas. If granulomas are present, tuberculosis, yersiniosis, histoplasmosis, and other systemic fungi should be considered. In the absence of granulomas, these, as well as infections with enterococcus, salmonella, and cytomegalovirus, are still considerations. Histochemical studies, cultures, and serology are important. Inflammation without granulomas may also be caused by NSAIDs and backwash ileitis, in the setting of chronic ulcerative colitis. NSAIDs are commonly used, often forgotten, and a frequent cause of terminal ileitis. In fact, terminal ileitis is probably a more common consequence of NSAIDs than are ulcers of the stomach and duodenum.

Erosions and ulcers are typically associated with mucosal inflammation, and are the result of diverse inflammatory conditions affecting the intestine. Multiple shallow linear or sharp punched-out ulcers suggest NSAIDs. Crohn ulcers may also be sharply punched-out or irregular, linear, or fissuring. In the ileum, shallow transverse and circumferential ulcers, with or without narrow diaphragm strictures, are caused by NSAIDs and tuberculosis. Large uniform and regularly spaced, oval, longitudinally oriented ulcers (ulcerated Peyer patches) are typical of typhoid; single or multiple ulcers without inflammation in surrounding mucosa are characteristic of cytomegalovirus infection.

DUODENITIS

- Morphology — The presence of neutrophils indicates an active inflammatory process, distinguishing pathologic from physiologic inflammation. Erosions are shallow mucosal defects, while ulcers involve the submucosa. Acute erosions are characterized by epithelial damage, hemorrhage, fibrin, and an influx of neutrophils. They are usually the result of peptic disease, NSAIDs, ischemic states, and infections. Microvascular ischemia probably plays an important role in some of these acute erosions.

- Endoscopic features — Duodenitis is characterized by patchy, punctate erythema located within the duodenal bulb and postbulbar duodenum. The erythema may be prominent on top of the circular folds and is often accompanied by erosions. Duodenal erosions vary in size up to 5 mm. They are shallow, multiple, and randomly distributed within the bulb. There is a tendency for erosions to occur on top of the circular folds in the postbulbar duodenum. Erosions may contain altered blood and have central areas of nonspecific pigmentation.

- Clinical features — Dyspepsia.

- Differential diagnosis — Histologic: Crohn's disease and, when there is villous damage, malabsorption.

  Etiologic: NSAIDs, peptic disease, ischemic erosions.

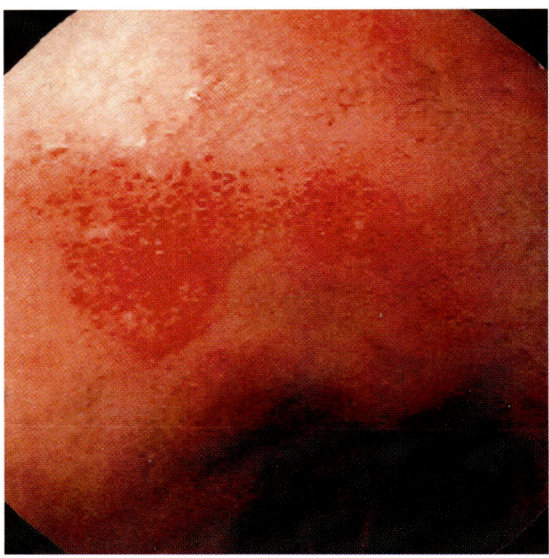

Figure 3-13: **Duodenum. Duodenitis.** Patchy erythema in duodenal bulb composed of a tight collection of pinpoint red spots. Minute erosion at periphery of the erythematous patch (left).

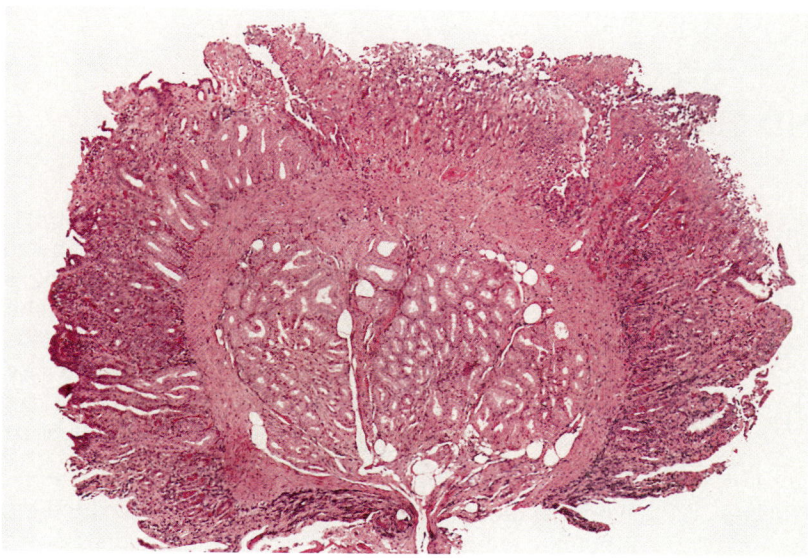

Figure 3-14: **Duodenum. Erosive Duodenitis.** Surface erosion, epithelial degeneration, and inflammation. Prominent Brunner gland.

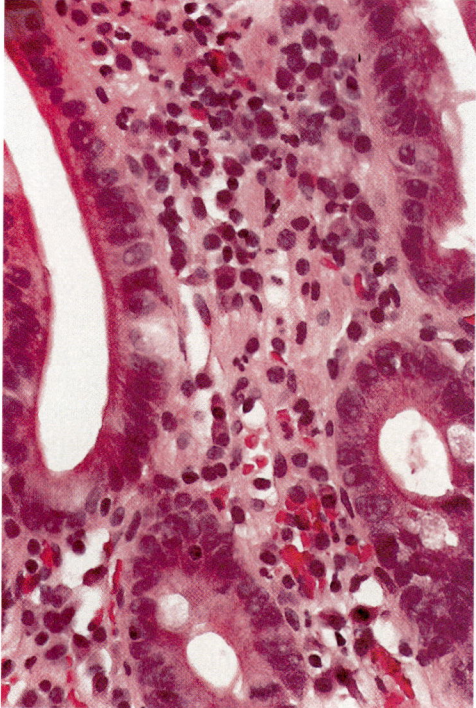

Figure 3-15: **Duodenum. Duodenitis.** A few scattered neutrophils indicate a mild active inflammatory process.

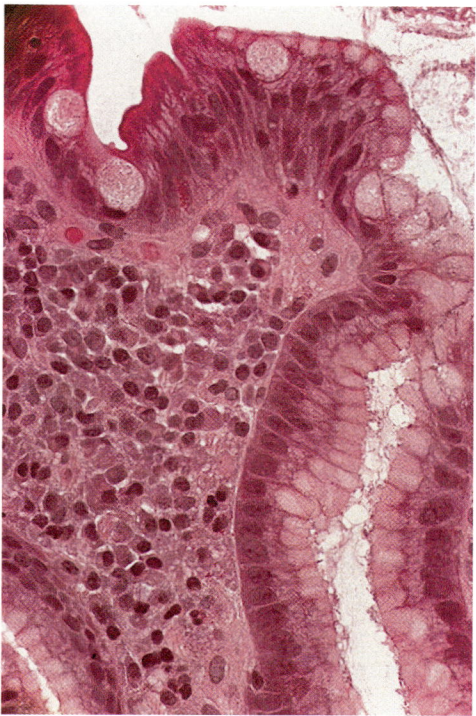

Figure 3-16: **Duodenum. Foveolar Metaplasia and *Helicobacter pylori*.** *Helicobacter pylori* cling to gastric foveolar cells.

ULCERS AND EROSIONS

- Morphology .... Erosions interrupt the mucosa; ulcers extend completely through the mucosa. Acute ulcers have submucosal hemorrhage and edema. Chronic ulcers typically show chronic inflammation on the edge of the ulcer and granulation tissue and fibrosis in the base. Etiologies include *Helicobacter pylori* infection, NSAIDs, ischemia, infections (mainly CMV), and lymphoma (enteropathy-associated T-cell lymphomas). Multiple discrete ulcers are often due to drugs, particularly NSAIDs. Single ulcers are typical of *H pylori* infection. Clinical history together with endoscopic appearance and gastric biopsy may suggest the etiology.

- Endoscopic features .... Duodenal ulcers are most common within the duodenal bulb. They may be difficult to identify when located in the immediate postbulbar area, especially posteriorly, where the angulation of the duodenal bulb and descending duodenum together with inflammatory edema reduce the ability to see this anatomic area. Ulcers are discrete, measuring greater than 5 mm in diameter. They have well-defined margins and a necrotic yellow to white base. In the base, there may be altered blood which appears dark. Discrete, punctate, flat, pigmented spots may represent exposed or visible vessels. A visible vessel is suspected when there is a protruding tubular structure, usually 1 to 2 mm in diameter, a pigmented, dark red or purple protuberance up to 4 mm in diameter, or a dense adherent clot with a focal point of attachment. These stigmata, in the setting of acute upper gastrointestinal bleeding, connote a high likelihood of rebleeding. Increasing ulcer size ($\geq$ 2 cm) and ulcer depth also carry an increased risk of rebleeding. Acute ulcers are shallow, with sharp margins and little or no edema in the surrounding mucosa (flat margins). Chronic ulcers have raised, erythematous margins and surrounding mucosa and are firm when probed or sampled.

    Distinguishing an acute from a chronic ulcer is important when endoscopic therapy is needed to stop bleeding. The risk of perforation with endoscopic therapy is greatest with an acute ulcer. A chronic, large, or penetrating ulcer that has previously perforated can be reopened. Endoscopic treatment of an exposed or visible vessel in a large, deeply penetrating, posterior duodenal bulb ulcer may cause significant bleeding if a large serosal artery, such as the gastroduodenal artery, is involved. It is therefore critical that the endoscopist determine whether an ulcer is in the anterior or posterior wall.

    Submucosal nodules such as leiomyomas and carcinoid tumors may ulcerate centrally. The ulcers are discrete and penetrate into the submucosal mass, causing umbilication.

- Clinical features .... Dyspepsia, acute gastrointestinal bleeding, which usually presents as melena and/or hematochezia. Hematemesis is uncommon. Patients presenting with hematochezia may initially be thought to have acute lower gastrointestinal bleeding. A history of duodenal ulcer, the use of NSAIDs, or a clinical presentation of orthostasis or significant anemia, consistent with a major bleeding event, raise suspicion of an acutely bleeding duodenal ulcer.

- Differential diagnosis...... Etiologic: *H pylori* gastritis, NSAIDs, ischemia, ulcerating neoplasms.

SMALL INTESTINE

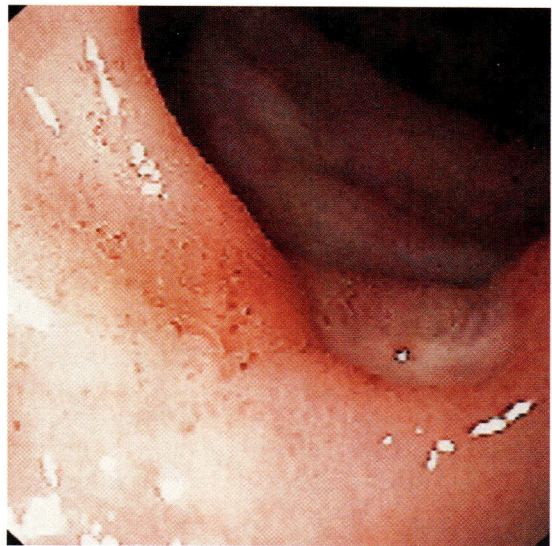

Figure 3-17: **Duodenum, Postbulbar. Ulcer**. A deep, 1-cm ulcer with thick margins and a small, flat, pigmented spot in the center of the ulcer base (pinpoint light reflexion).

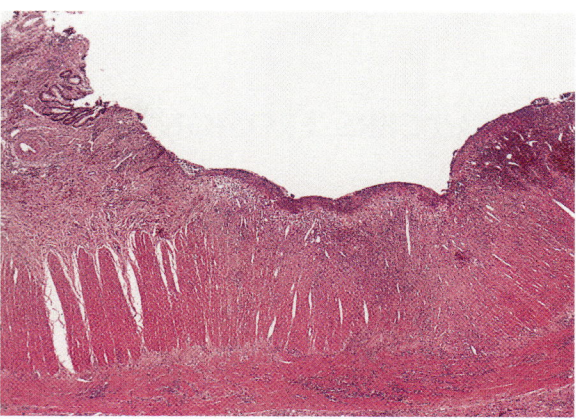

Figure 3-18: **Small Intestine. Chronic Ulcer**. Ulcer extends into muscularis propria. Submucosal fibrosis and chronic inflammation.

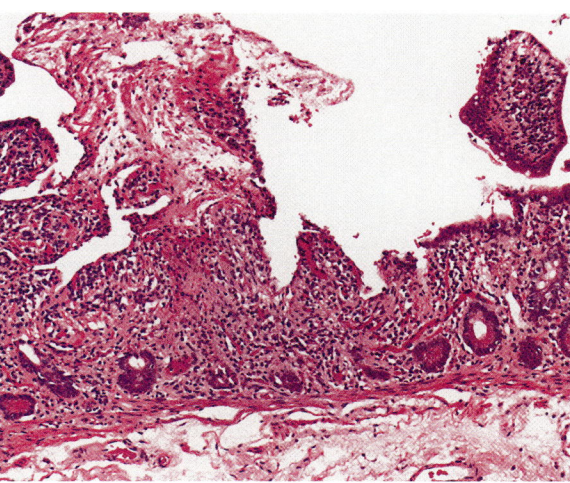

Figure 3-20: **Duodenum. Erosion**. Surface erosion and fibrinous exudate.

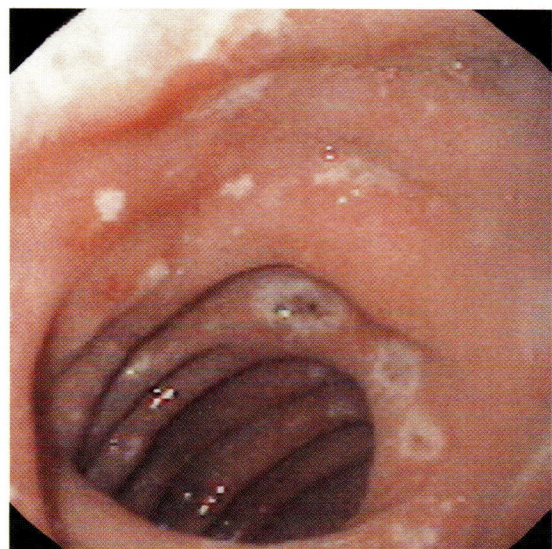

Figure 3-19: **Duodenum, Postbulbar. Multiple Erosions**. Multiple, variably sized, shallow erosions, some with white necrotic bases, others with dark altered blood. Erosions range from 1 to 5 mm. There is thickening of the circular folds in the foreground.

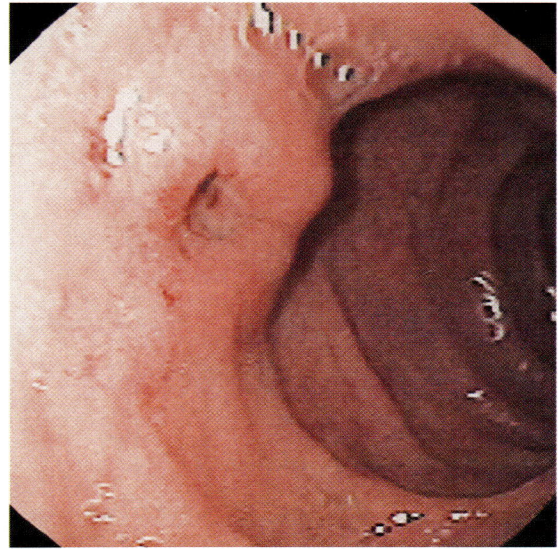

Figure 3-21: **Duodenum. Ulcer.** Nodule with a small, discrete, and penetrating central ulcer or umbilication.

185

ILEAL ULCERS/EROSIONS

- Morphology .... Ileal erosions and ulcers commonly occur in the setting of mucosal inflammation due to infection, NSAIDs, or Crohn's disease. Histologic features are usually not specific. Pyloric metaplasia, when present, is an indication of a long-standing chronic inflammatory process.

- Endoscopic features .... Ileal ulcers and erosions are most often encountered in the setting of Crohn's disease. They are discrete, generally not exceeding 2 cm. The base is yellow-white and the surrounding mucosa is often erythematous. The margins of the ulcer may or may not be raised. In patients with Crohn's disease who have had resections, recurrent erosions and ulcers occur predictably at and proximal to an anastomosis.

    NSAID erosions tend to be linear, discrete, and sharply punched-out, much like those of Crohn's disease. Sometimes NSAIDs produce multiple shallow circumferential ulcers that heal to narrow diaphragms, which may be circumferential and weblike, are morphologically striking, and similar to those of tuberculosis. In contrast, Crohn's ulcers tend to be oriented longitudinally along the mesenteric attachment, and the strictures are long. Both patterns likely reflect the anatomy of the underlying vascular injury. Irregular, atypical ulceration occurs in infections, e.g., *Yersinia, Campylobacter jejuni*, tuberculosis, systemic fungal infections, and CMV.

    Ileal ulceration associated with superior mesenteric artery ischemia is accompanied by edema, friability, spontaneous bleeding, and similar findings within the proximal colon.

    Highly irregular and atypical-appearing ulcers are encountered in neoplastic processes such as lymphoma. Submucosal tumors, such as carcinoids and leiomyomas, may ulcerate. Erosions vary in size, shape, and distribution.

- Clinical features .... Diarrhea, crampy abdominal pain, obstructive symptoms, hematochezia.

- Differential diagnosis ...... Etiologic: Crohn's, NSAIDs, infections, neoplasms.

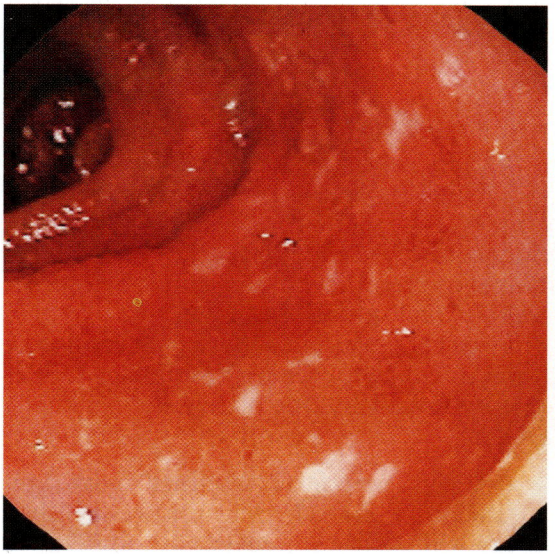

Figure 3-22: **Ileum. Multiple Erosions.** Multiple minute, shallow, white-based, irregular erosions in the terminal ileum.

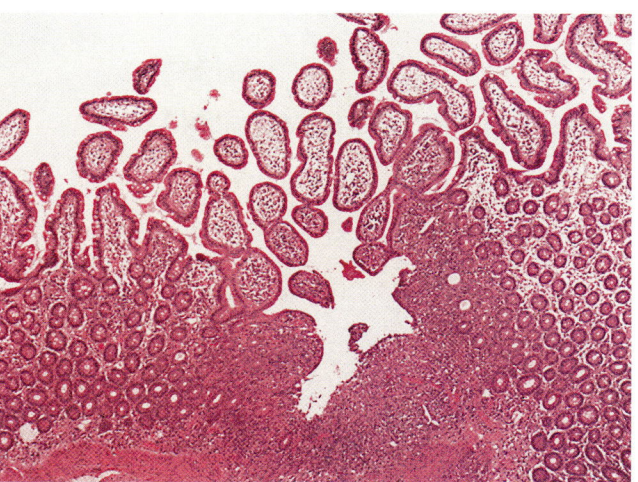

Figure 3-23: **Ileum. Ileal Erosion.** Discrete area of inflammation and erosion.

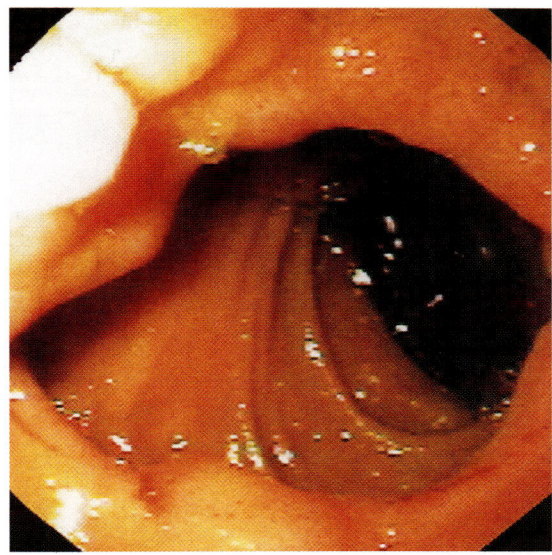

Figure 3-24: **Ileum. Stricture.** Circumferential nodular stricture in the distal ileum during ileoscopy (Brooke). Small ulcers within prominent nodular folds (left).

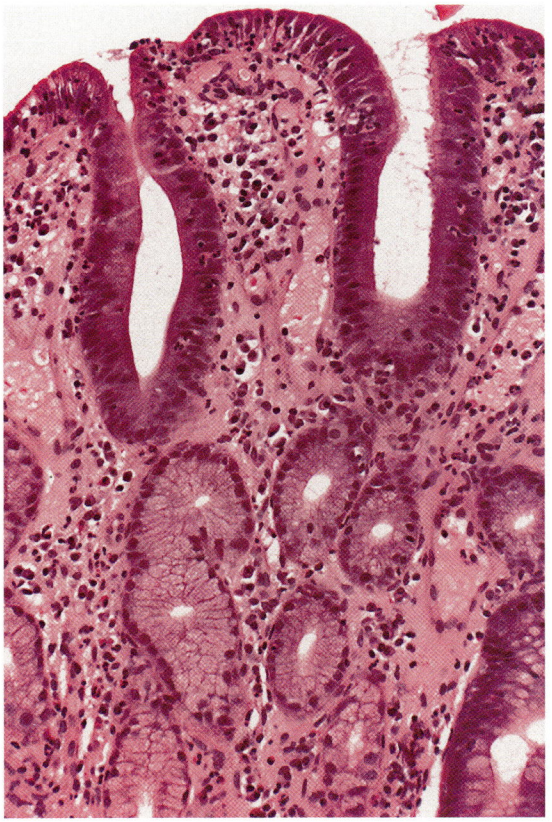

Figure 3-25: **Ileum. Ileitis.** Active inflammation and pyloric metaplasia.

EOSINOPHILIC ENTERITIS

- Morphology — Eosinophilic enteritis usually involves the submucosa, with multifocal mucosal infiltration that may be widely scattered and subtle. Clusters of eosinophils in the deep lamina propria and crypt epithelium are significant features. Multiple biopsies are often necessary for diagnosis. Eosinophils are a component of any chronic inflammatory cell population, so that a pure eosinophil infiltrate is necessary for diagnosis. Submucosal edema is a prominent feature but is not usually evident in biopsy specimens. The presence of peripheral eosinophilia supports the diagnosis.

- Endoscopic features — Eosinophilic enteritis is associated with nonspecific findings, most commonly erythema. The mucosa is usually normal. The diagnosis is established with random biopsies in patients with refractory upper GI symptoms of unknown cause. Abnormal findings can include thickening or blunting of the circular folds due to edema or infiltration and ulceration/erosions.

- Clinical features — Dyspepsia, periumbilical cramping, diarrhea.

- Differential diagnosis — Histologic: Inflammatory fibroid polyp, other chronic inflammatory conditions with increased eosinophils.

  Endoscopic: Erosions/ulcers of any cause.

  Clinical: Idiopathic, parasites, drugs, food allergies, vasculitis, hypereosinophilic syndromes.

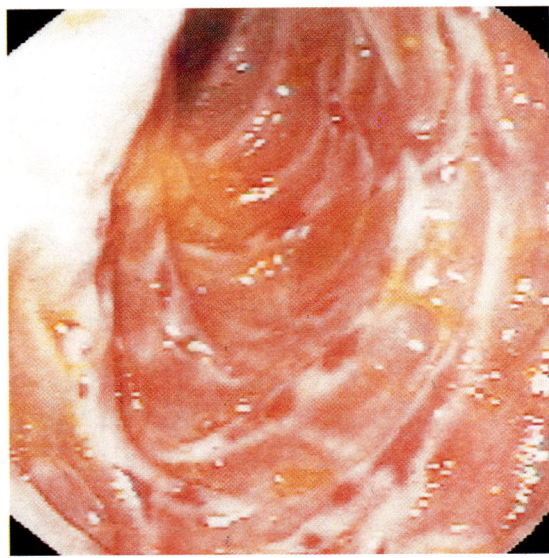

Figure 3-26: **Duodenum. Eosinophilic Enteritis.**
Nonspecific patchy erythema within the duodenum.

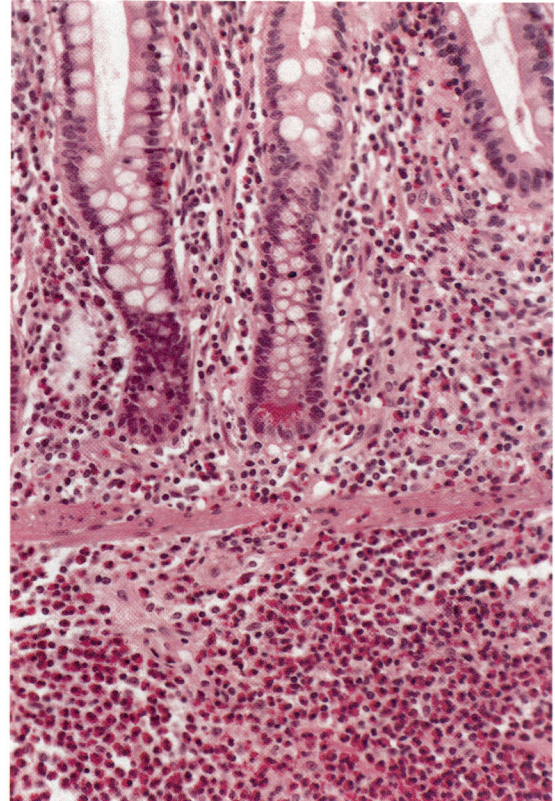

Figure 3-27: **Small Intestine. Eosinophilic Enteritis.** Eosinophilic infiltrate in submucosa and lower lamina propria.

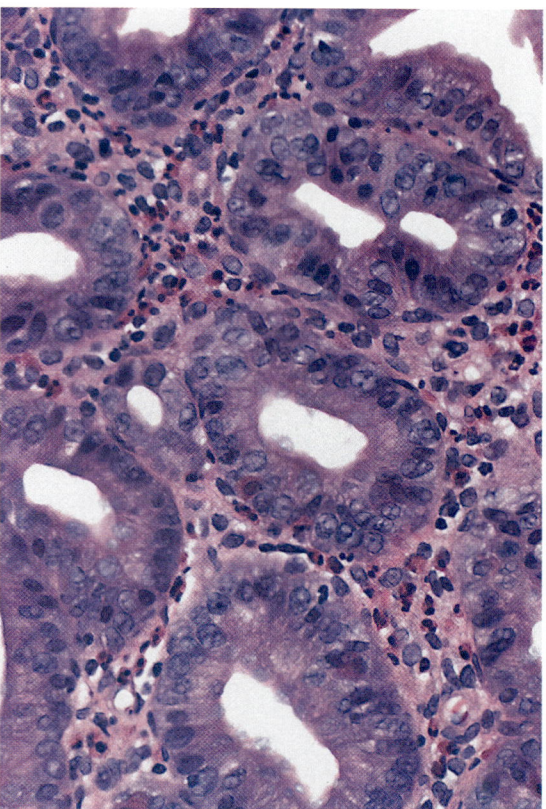

Figure 3-28: **Small Intestine. Eosinophilic Enteritis.** Clusters of eosinophils in mucosa.

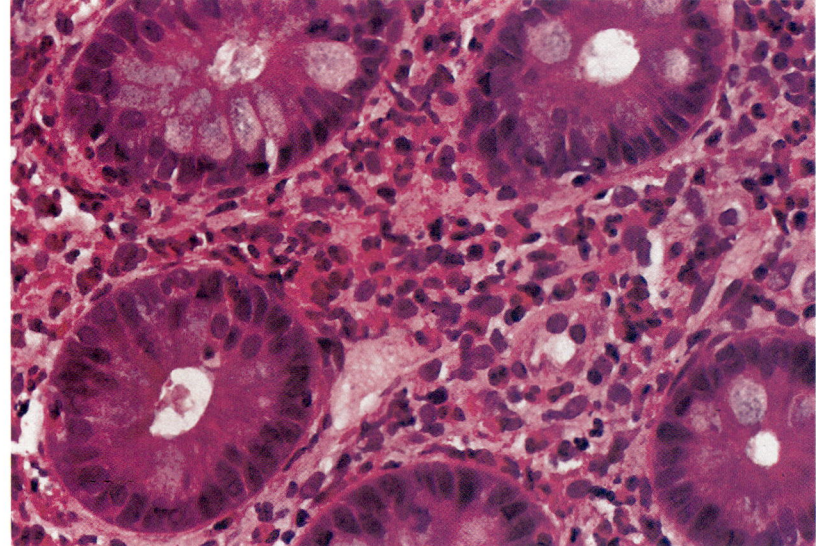

Figure 3-29: **Small Intestine. Eosinophilic Enteritis.** Eosinophilic infiltrate fills lamina propria between crypts.

GRANULOMATOUS ENTERITIS/CROHN'S DISEASE

- Morphology .... Granulomas occur in Crohn's disease, sarcoid, and infections. Typically, Crohn is characterized by areas of focal active, chronic, destructive epithelial injury with inflammation and occasionally loose, poorly formed epithelioid granulomas. When granulomas are numerous, an infectious etiology is more likely. The lack of granulomas does not exclude Crohn or any infection characteristically associated with granulomas. Noncaseating epithelioid granulomas with little inflammation are characteristic of sarcoid. While sarcoidosis commonly involves the gastrointestinal tract, it seldom causes clinical symptoms. Epithelioid granulomas occur in infections such as tuberculosis, histoplasmosis, and yersiniosis, where they may be suppurative and caseating. Organisms are most often demonstrated by special stains in areas of necrosis. Negative stains do not exclude infection. Cultures and serologic tests are important for diagnosis.

- Endoscopic features .... There is a spectrum of abnormalities ranging from multiple erosions to stenosis, with or without ulceration. Crohn's ulcers are discrete and may be friable and actively bleeding, and not associated with surrounding inflammatory changes such as erythema and edema. Cobblestoning or nodularity of the mucosa is common. The distinctive Crohn ulcer is the linear or "rake-type". The long segmental stenoses characteristic of healing Crohn's disease contrasts with the short diaphragn strictures caused by NSAIDs. Focal stenosis is also encountered at the sites of anastomoses and with long-standing disease with minimal activity.

- Clinical features .... Diarrhea, abdominal cramping, partial or complete small bowel obstruction, hematochezia. Deep fissuring ulcerations of the ileum can give rise to acute gastrointestinal bleeding, resulting in the need for surgical resection.

- Differential diagnosis ...... Endoscopic: Tuberculosis and other infections, lymphoma, NSAIDs.

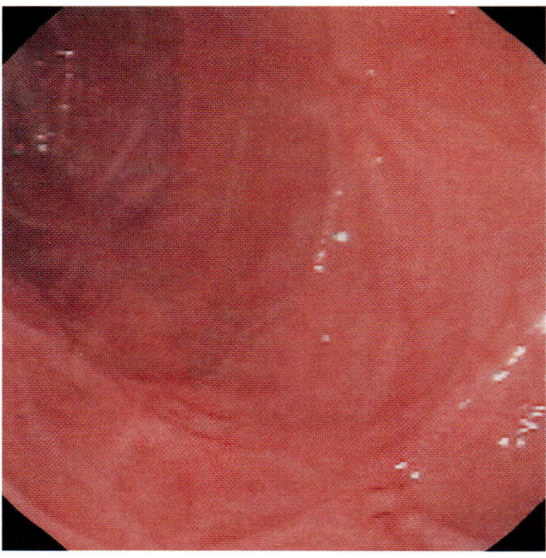

Figure 3-30: **Duodenum. Crohn's Disease**. Multiple small, shallow, and irregular ulcers within the postbulbar duodenum. The circular fold pattern of the duodenum is disrupted and replaced by folds radiating from these ulcers (cicatricial scarring).

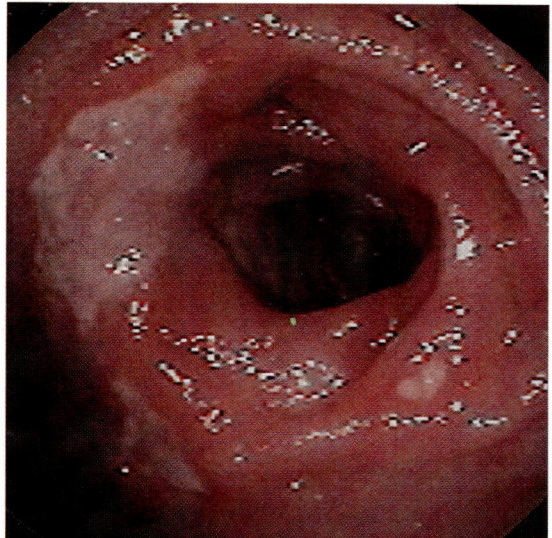

Figure 3-31: **Duodenum. Crohn's Disease.** Multiple, discrete, shallow and irregular ileal ulcers, minute to large. The surrounding mucosa appears normal.

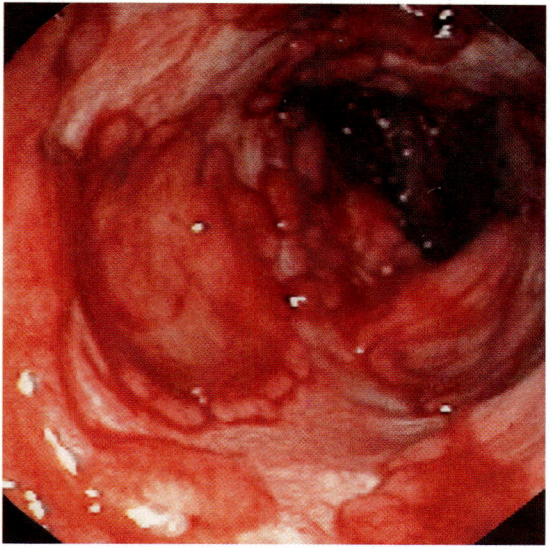

Figure 3-32: **Ileum. Crohn's Disease.** Extensive "rake-type" linear ulceration characteristic of Crohn's disease. Mucosa at margin is nodular or cobblestoned. There is spontaneous bleeding. The lumen is not compromised.

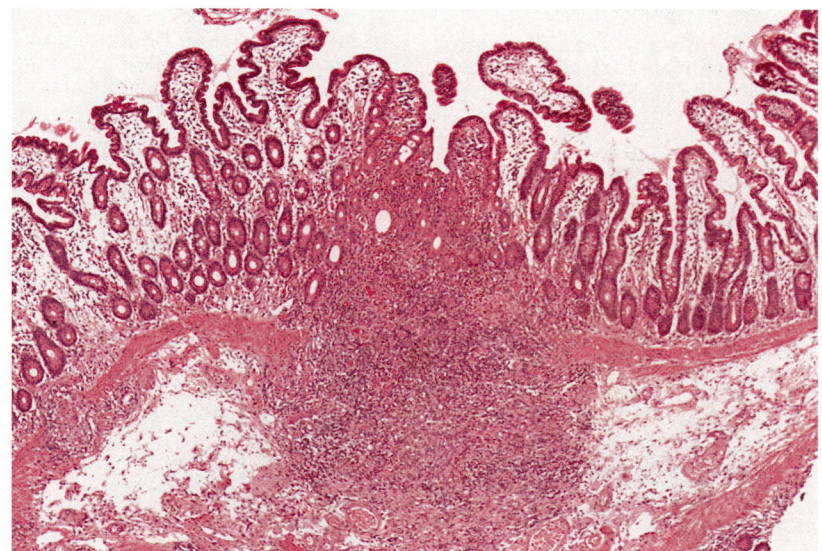

Figure 3-33: **Ileum. Active Chronic Ileitis with Aphthous Erosion.** Discrete mucosal and submucosal inflammation with uninvolved adjacent mucosa, consistent with Crohn's disease.

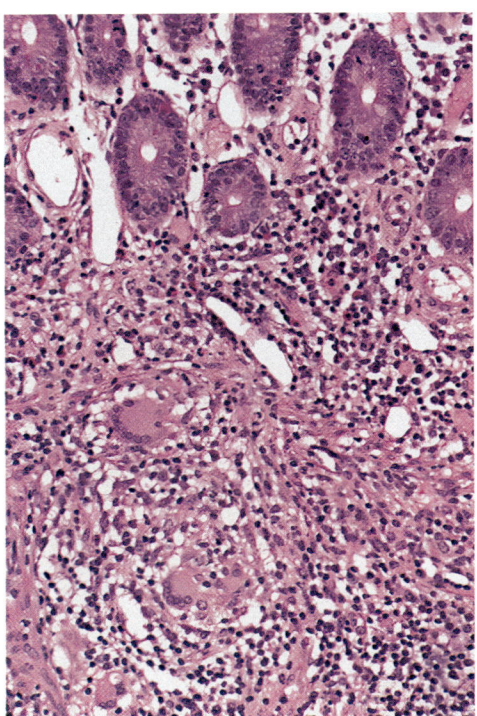

Figure 3-34: **Small Intestine. Granulomatous Inflammation.** Epithelioid granuloma deep in lamina propria.

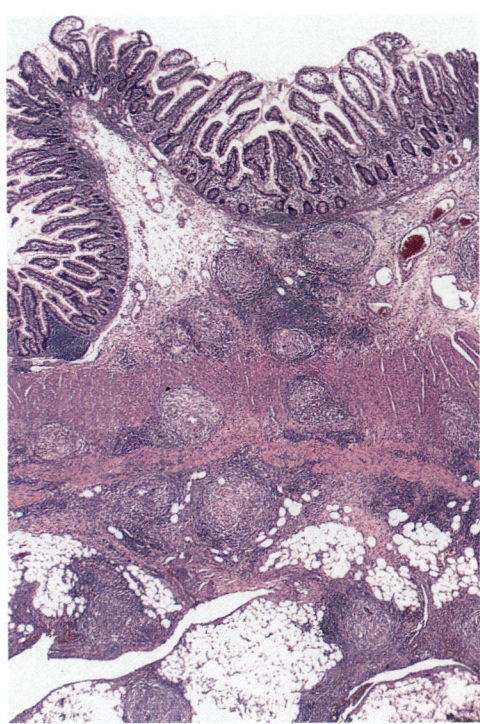

Figure 3-35: **Ileum. Granulomatous Inflammation.** Transmural granulomatous inflammation. Overlying mucosa uninvolved.

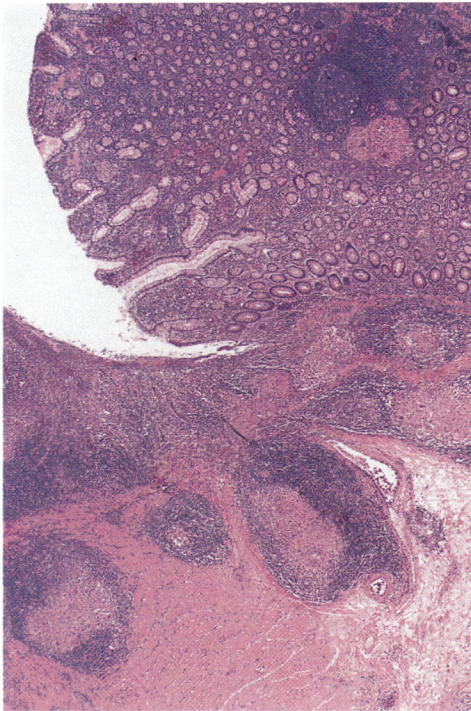

Figure 3-36: **Ileum. Granulomatous Inflammation.** Well-defined ulcer with granulomatous inflammation centered in lymphoid aggregates, probable yersiniosis.

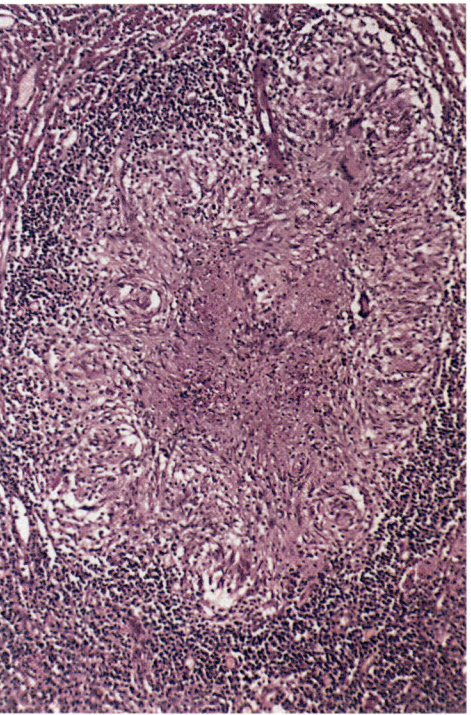

Figure 3-37: **Ileum. Granulomatous Inflammation.** Necrotizing granuloma.

INFECTIONS WITH NORMAL MUCOSAL PATTERN

- Morphology .... While most infections elicit an inflammatory response, some infectious agents cause no or minimal mucosal inflammation. The most common of these agents are *Giardia lamblia*, *Cryptosporidium*, Microsporidia, and *Isospora belli*. A careful search for these organisms is necessary for diagnosis.

- Endoscopic features .... Color of the mucosa is uniform. Circular folds are evident and well-demarcated. Light from the endoscope reflects from the villi in a speckled pattern. Viewing the duodenal mucosa under instilled water or pooled secretions magnifies surface features and demonstrates villi, allowing detection of abnormal villous patterns.

- Clinical features .... Diarrhea, weight loss, malabsorption.

- Differential diagnosis ...... Histologic: Normal versus infection.

    Clinical: Infection versus malabsorption syndrome versus pancreatic insufficiency.

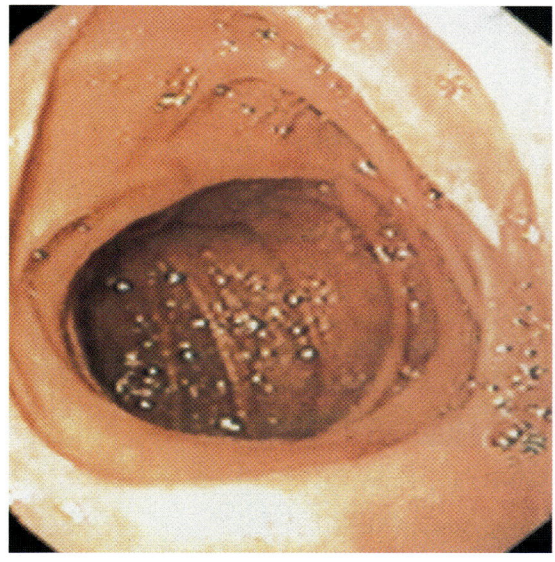

Figure 3-38: **Duodenum. Normal Duodenum.** Normal duodenum with uniform mucosal appearance. Circular folds are complete and of normal height. Secretions are present.

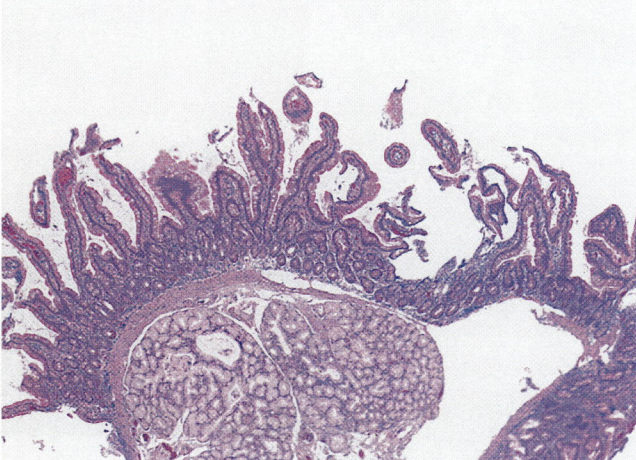

Figure 3-39: **Duodenum. *Giardia*.** Villi of normal height, normal surface epithelium, no inflammation. *Giardia* between villi, but not visualized at this magnification.

GIARDIASIS

- Morphology .... *Giardia* may be scarce and easily overlooked. They are commonly found over the sides of the villi. The mucosa is usually normal but may be inflamed or otherwise altered in immunosuppressed individuals. A search for *Giardia* should be part of every small bowel biopsy evaluation.

- Endoscopic features .... Normal-appearing small intestinal mucosa is a common finding. With severe infection or in immunocompromised patients, there may be inflammatory changes including erythema, ulceration, and coarsening of the mucosa with a granular or nodular appearance.

- Clinical features .... Diarrhea, bloating, nausea, weight loss, malabsorption.

- Differential diagnosis ...... Histologic: Normal.

  Endoscopic: Normal, Crohn's disease (with linear erosions), peptic duodenitis.

  Clinical: Peptic duodenitis, malabsorption syndromes.

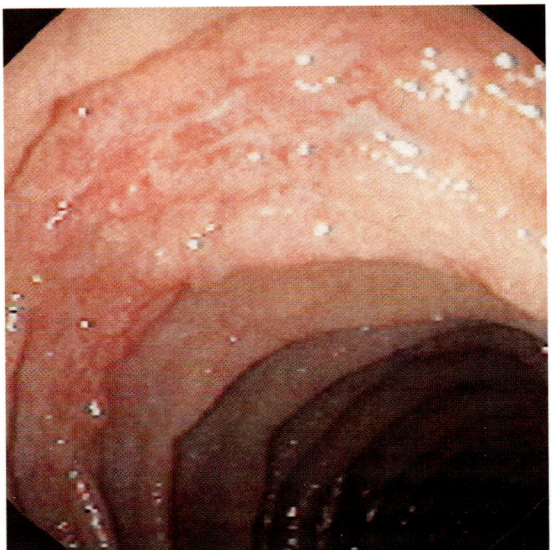

Figure 3-40: **Jejunum.** *Giardia*. Jejunal view during push enteroscopy. Focally nodular mucosa with patchy erythema and fine linear erosions disrupt the circular folds (upper).

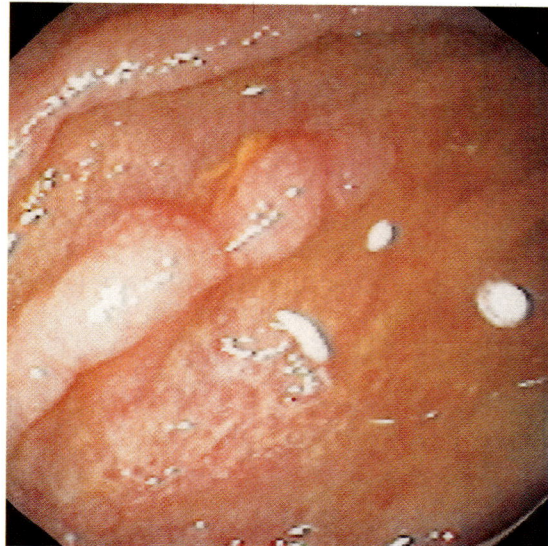

Figure 3-41: **Jejunum.** *Giardia.* Circular folds are interrupted and nodular due to fine interlacing linear ulceration (lower central). Other features are erythema and coarsening of the mucosa.

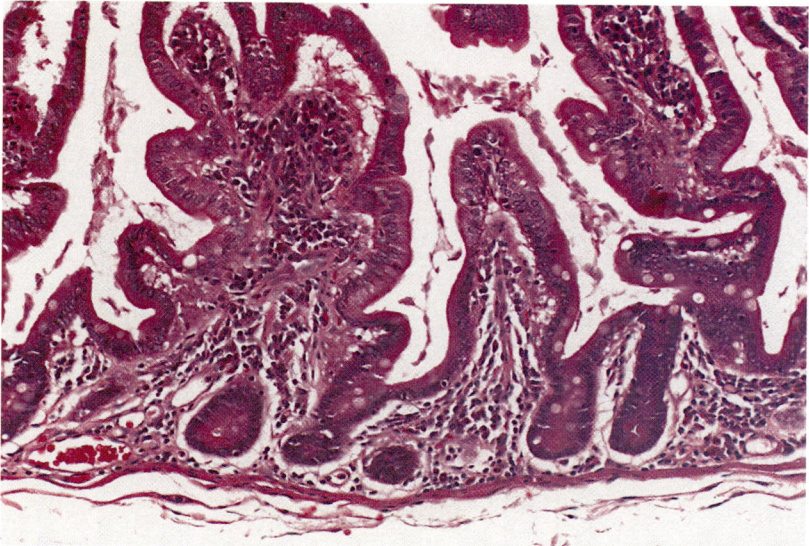

Figure 3-42: **Jejunum.** *Giardia.* Normal small bowel mucosa with numerous *Giardia* lying free over the villi.

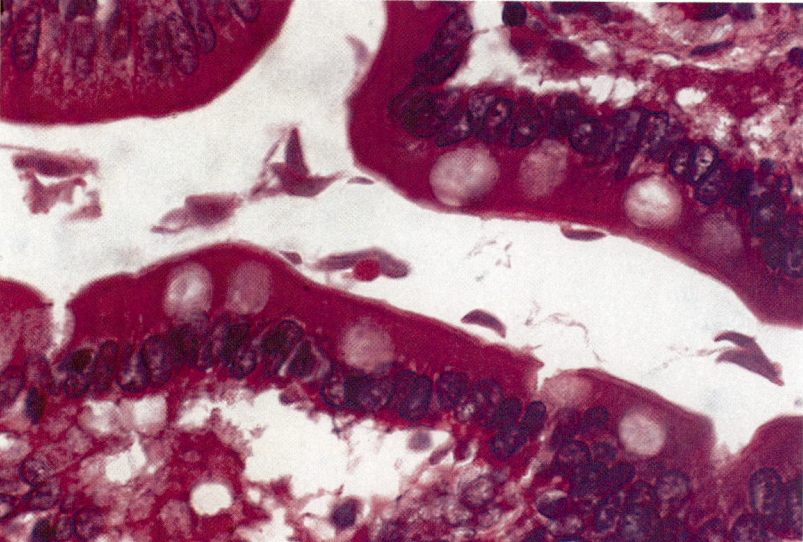

Figure 3-43: **Jejunum.** *Giardia.* Curved, flattened profile, suggestion of flagella, and small eyelike double nuclei are characteristic features. Surface epithelium is normal.

CRYPTOSPORIDIA

- Morphology .... Cryptosporidia are small, uniform, dotlike organisms that adhere to the surface epithelium. Small size and uniformity distinguish them from extruded mucin droplets. In the small bowel the organisms are found most frequently on the villi and may have a patchy distribution.
- Endoscopic features .... The small intestine typically appears normal.
- Clinical features .... Watery diarrhea, weight loss. Cryptosporidiosis is usually diagnosed in immunosuppressed patients with chronic watery diarrhea.
- Differential diagnosis ...... Histologic: Extruded mucin.

    Clinical: Other coccidian parasites (*Isospora*, Microsporidia).

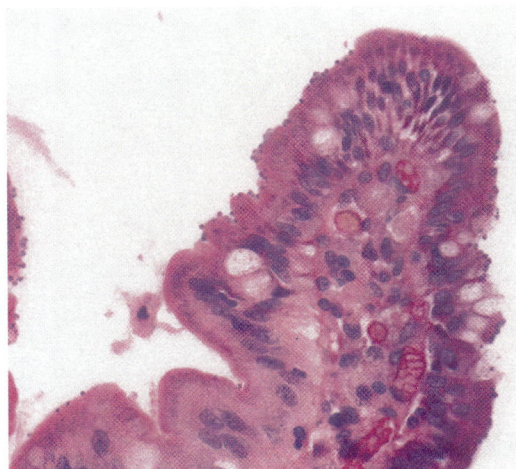

Figure 3-44: **Duodenum. Cryptosporidia.** Intact villus without inflammation. Cryptosporidia on epithelial surface.

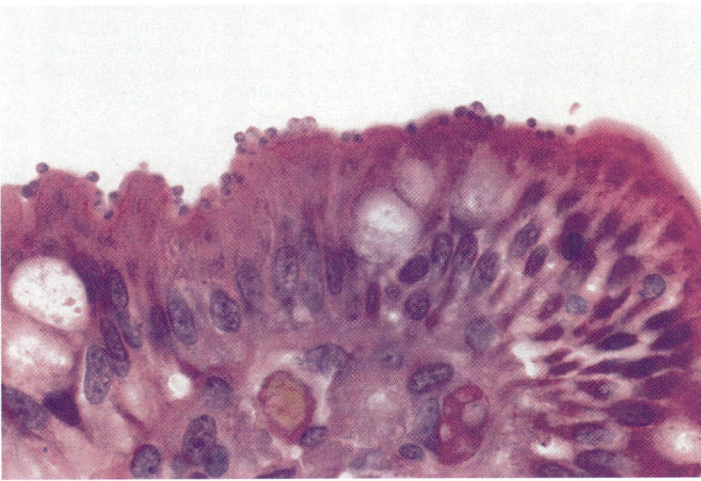

Figure 3-45: **Duodenum. Cryptosporidia.** High magnification illustrating amphophilic, uniform, round organisms on epithelial surface.

MICROSPORIDIA

- Morphology .... Microsporidial infection is most commonly caused by *Enterocytozoon bieneusi*. Most common in the distal duodenum and proximal jejunum, the organisms are difficult to identify on routine biopsies because they do not stain well with hematoxylin and eosin. There may be no mucosal injury or slight villous atrophy. The spores are located supranuclearly in the apical cytoplasm of the villous enterocytes. They stain with tissue Gram stain and Giemsa, and are birefringent under polarized light.

- Endoscopic features .... The small intestine usually appears normal.

- Clinical features .... Watery diarrhea, weight loss in immunocompromised hosts, for example HIV-infected individuals.

- Differential diagnosis ...... Histologic: Apoptotic fragments in the surface epithelium.

  Clinical: Other infections in immunosuppressed patients, e.g., giardiasis, cryptosporidiosis.

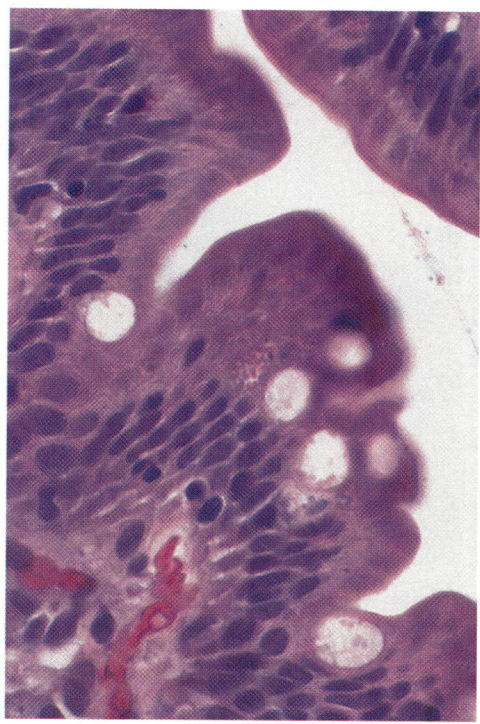

Figure 3-46: **Small Intestine. Microsporidia.** Numerous spores in the apical cytoplasm of villous enterocytes.

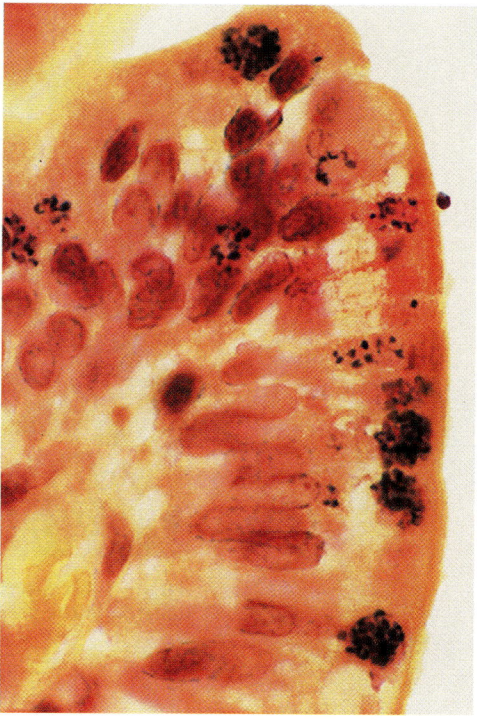

Figure 3-47: **Small Intestine. Microsporidia, Brown-Hopps Stain.** Spores in supranuclear location positive with tissue Gram stain.

ISOSPORA BELLI

- Morphology .... Spores are located in the subnuclear basal cytoplasm of surface enterocytes.
- Endoscopic features .... The small intestine usually appears normal.
- Clinical features .... Watery diarrhea, colicky abdominal pain, nausea, and weight loss. Most common in immunodeficient patients.
- Differential diagnosis ...... Clinical: Other infections in the immunosuppressed, e.g., giardiasis, cryptosporidiosis, microsporidiosis.

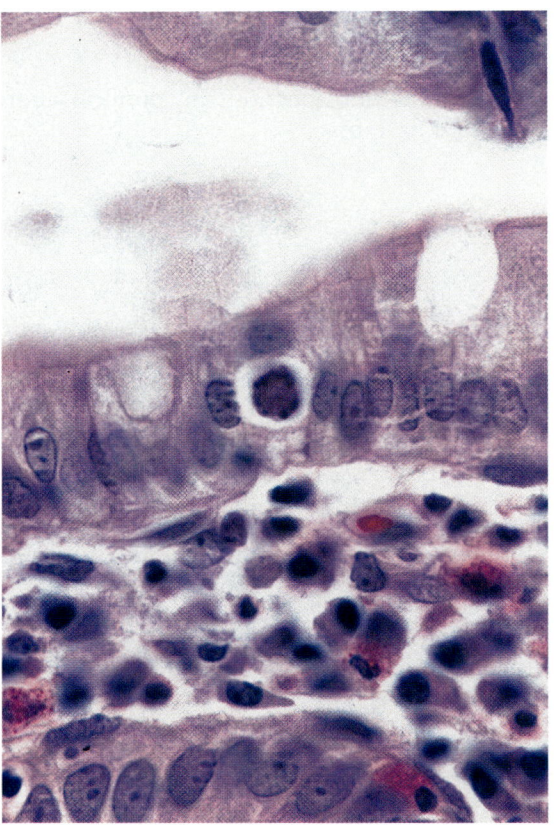

Figure 3-48: **Small Intestine. *Isospora belli*.** Large spore located in the subnuclear cytoplasm.

VIRAL INFECTIONS

- Morphology .... Most viruses lack specific cytopathic features that can be readily seen on light microscopic examination. Cytomegalovirus infection is the exception. Adenovirus and herpesviruses produce characteristic nuclear changes, but these are very difficult to see in endoscopic biopsy samples. They may be revealed by electron microscopy, immunostains, or in situ hybridization when there is a high index of suspicion.
- Endoscopic features .... Erosions, inflammation or normal-appearing small intestine.
- Clinical features .... Crampy abdominal pain, diarrhea, preceding fever and myalgias.
- Differential diagnosis ...... Histologic: Multifocal ischemic lesions, ulcers, atypical reactive epithelial and stromal cells.

    Endoscopic: In the presence of erosions and inflammatory changes, vasculitis or ischemic injury are considerations.

    Clinical: Other enteric infections.

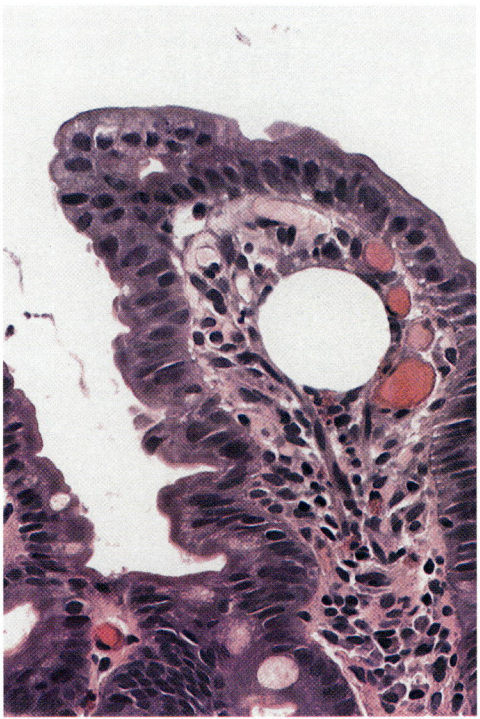

Figure 3-49: **Small Intestine. Adenovirus.** Epithelial cells appear slightly reactive. Viral epithelial cell nuclear inclusions are present but not evident. There is no inflammation.

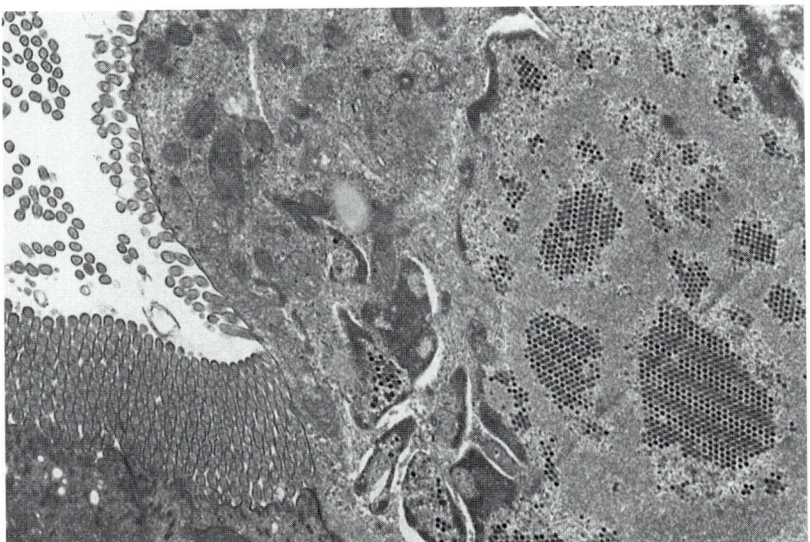

Figure 3-50: **Small Intestine. Adenovirus.** Electron photomicrograph of previous biopsy specimen shows geometric nuclear inclusions typical of adenovirus.

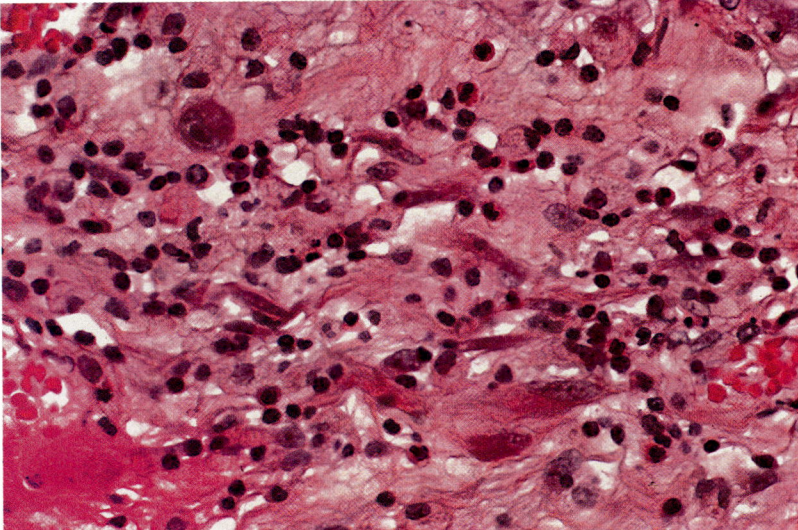

Figure 3-51: **Ileum. Cytomegalovirus.** Stromal cells with characteristic nuclear and cytoplasmic inclusions.

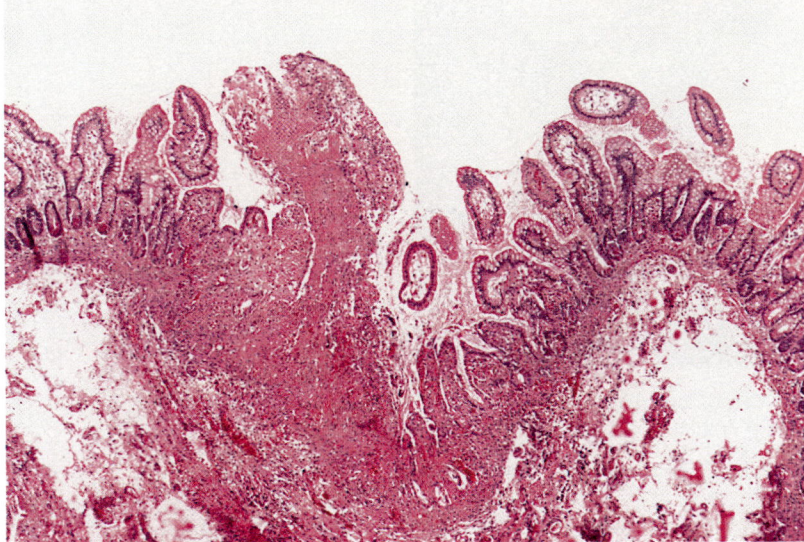

Figure 3-52: **Small Intestine. Varicella.** Focal ischemic erosion clinically due to varicella.

INFECTIONS WITHIN HISTIOCYTES: *Mycobacterium avium-intracellulare*, Whipple Disease

- Morphology .... Histologic features of *Tropheryma whippelii* and MAI infections are similar. Whipple bacillus is a short, curved rod; MAI is a long, straight, beaded, more delicate rod. Both are intracytoplasmic and stain with PAS after diastase, but only MAI is acid-fast. The histiocytes in Whipple infection are typically foamy on H&E. Often, neutral fat is present in the lamina propria and lacteals are dilated. The histiocytes of MAI are described as striated blue histiocytes on H&E.

- Endoscopic features .... The appearance of MAI infection varies from normal-appearing mucosa to the nodular mucosal changes seen in figure 3-53. Dilated lacteals may cause a blunting of villi which can sometimes be identified during endoscopy. The blunted villi are prominent and whitish, creating a nonreflective speckled pattern on the duodenal mucosa.

- Clinical features .... Whipple disease is most commonly seen in middle-aged men. MAI infections are common in AIDS.

- Differential diagnosis ...... Histologic: Whipple, MAI, histoplasmosis, macroglobulinemia.

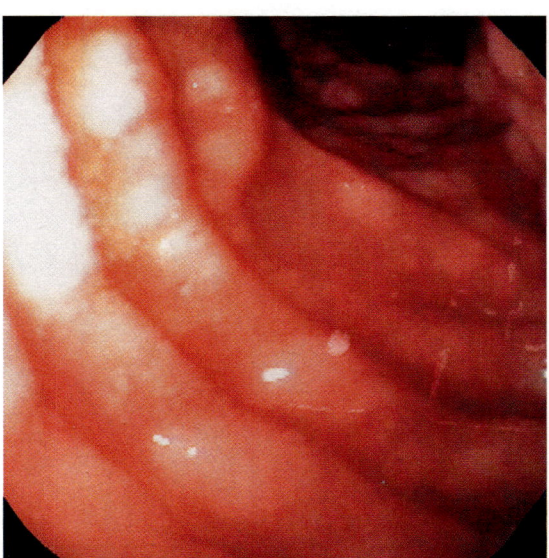

Figure 3-53: **Duodenum. *Mycobacterium avium-intracellulare*.** Circular folds of the postbulbar duodenum are thickened and contain yellowish nodules.

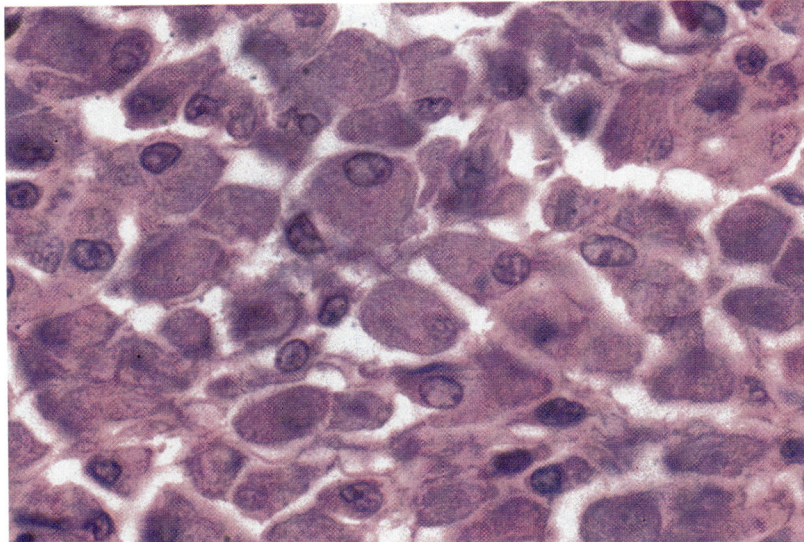

Figure 3-54: **Small Intestine. *Mycobacterium avium-intracellulare*.** Histiocytes with abundant pale, foamy cytoplasm.

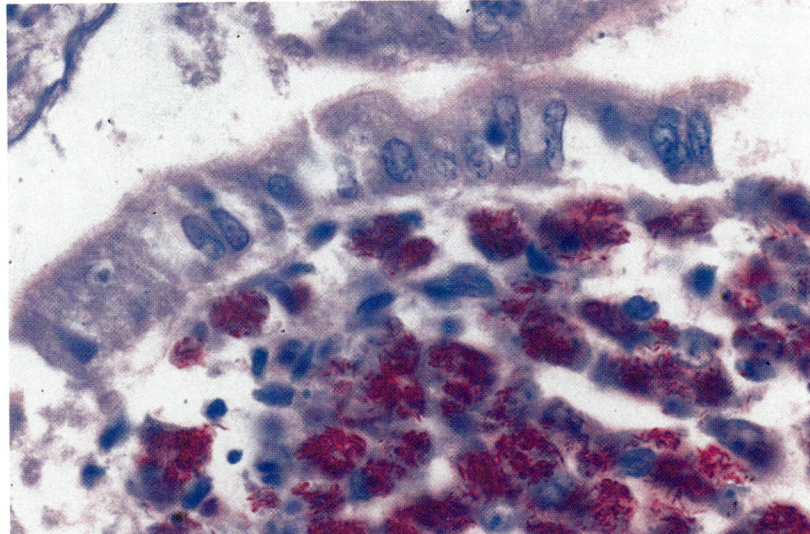

Figure 3-55: **Small Intestine. *Mycobacterium avium-intracellulare*.** Histiocytes filled with acid-fast bacterial rods.

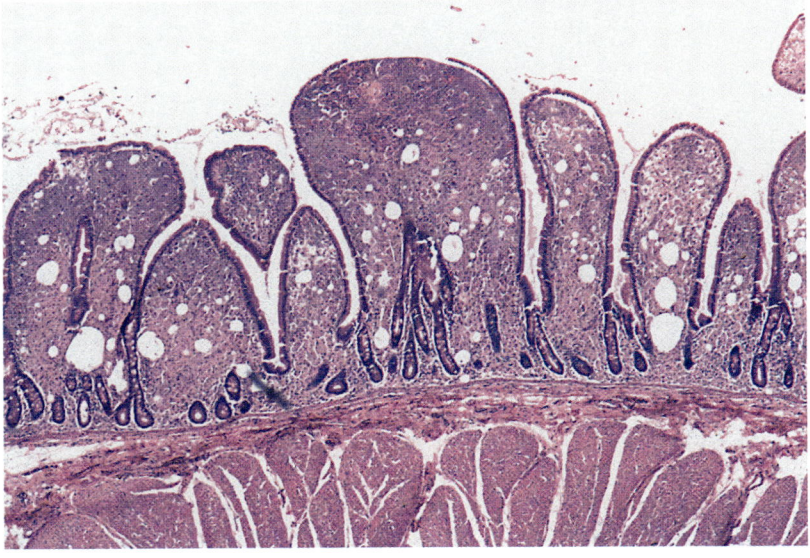

Figure 3-56: **Duodenum. Whipple Disease.** Lamina propria is distended with histiocytes. Swollen villi are compressed so the surface appears flat. Clear globules in dilated lacteals and lamina propria.

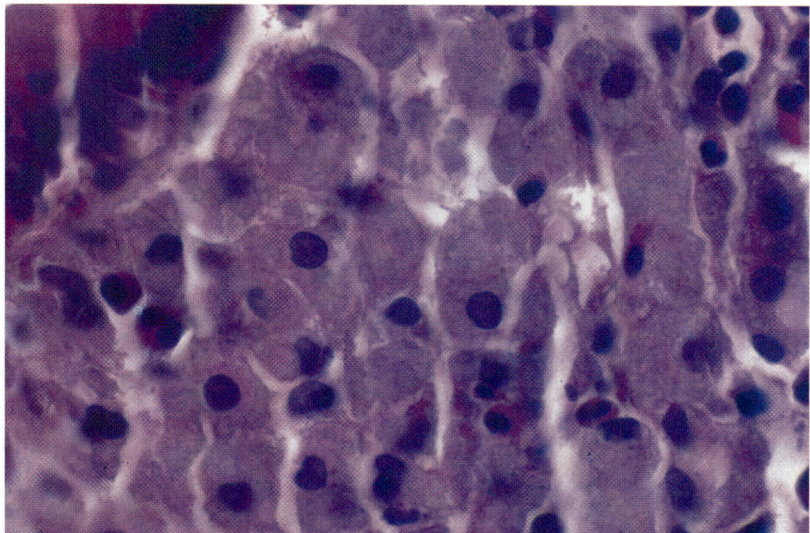

Figure 3-57: **Duodenum. Whipple Disease.** Numerous histiocytes with foamy cytoplasm.

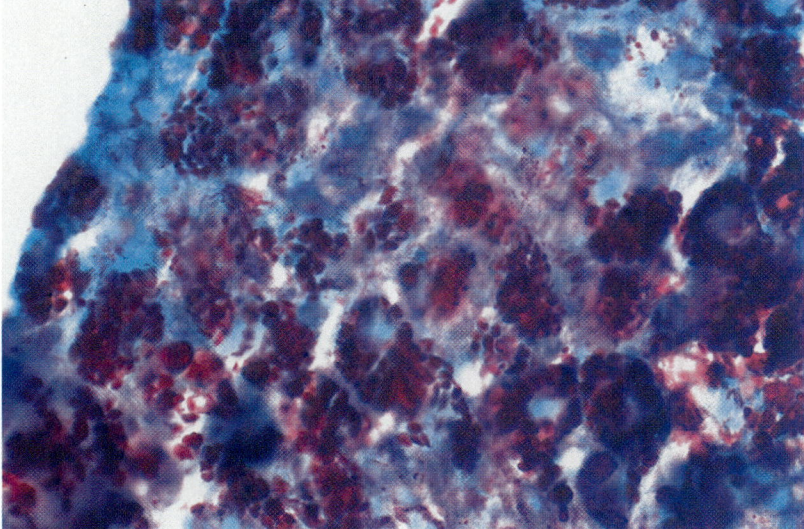

Figure 3-58: **Duodenum. Whipple Disease.** Characteristic PAS-positive Whipple bacilli in cytoplasm.

INFECTIONS WITHIN HISTIOCYTES: Leishmania, Histoplasma, Typhoid

- Morphology .... In endemic areas, visceral leishmaniasis occurs in immunocompetent individuals; in North America, cases occur in the immunosuppressed. The appearance of leishmania and disseminated *Histoplasma capsulatum* is similar. Histoplasma are slightly larger, less basophilic, and surrounded by a clear capsule that stains with PAS diastase. Patients with disseminated histoplasmosis may be normal or immunosuppressed. *Salmonella typhi* invade Peyer patches. Organisms are in sheets of histiocytes. The Peyer patches ultimately ulcerate and bleed.

- Endoscopic features .... Endoscopic findings range from normal (leishmaniasis, histoplasmosis) to nonspecific inflammatory changes (typhoid-salmonella) which include erythema, coarsening of mucosal folds, and aphthous ulcerations.

- Clinical features .... Fever (salmonella), abdominal pain, weight loss, diarrhea.

- Differential diagnosis ...... Endoscopic: Enteric infection versus systemic infection and idiopathic disease including Crohn's.

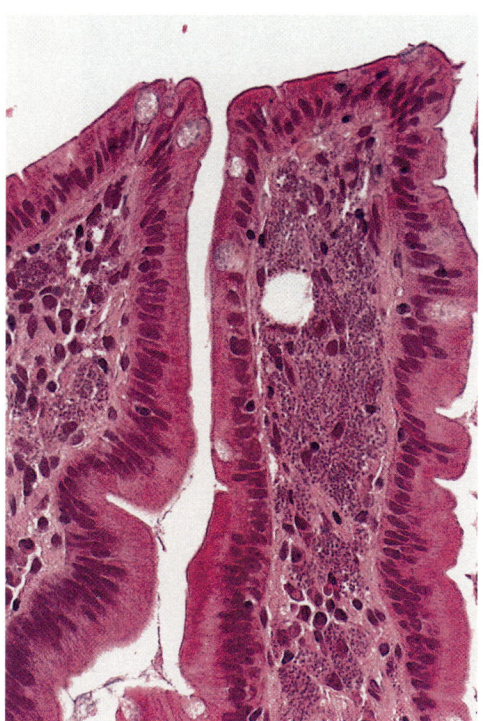

Figure 3-59: **Duodenum. Leishmania.**
Discrete, uniform, round, blue leishmania fill histiocytes.

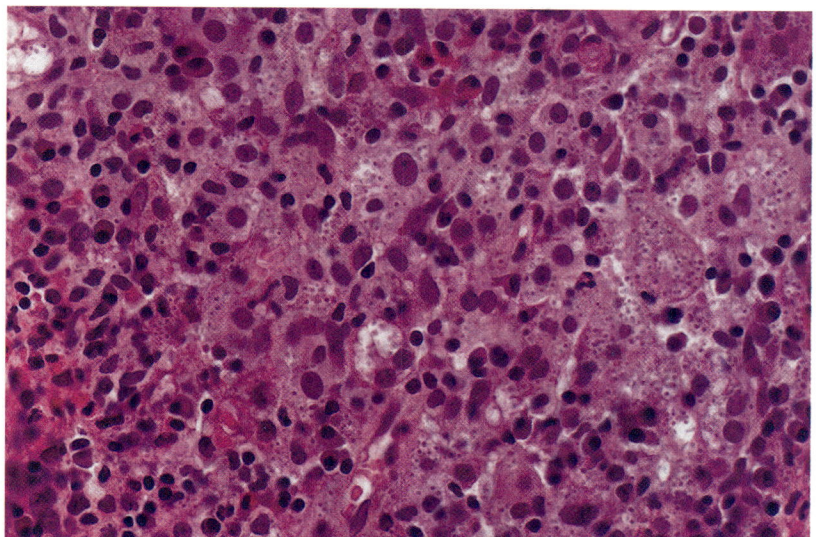

Figure 3-60: **Duodenum.** *Histoplasma*. *Histoplasma* appear as dots with halos filling histiocytes. They are slightly larger than leishmania.

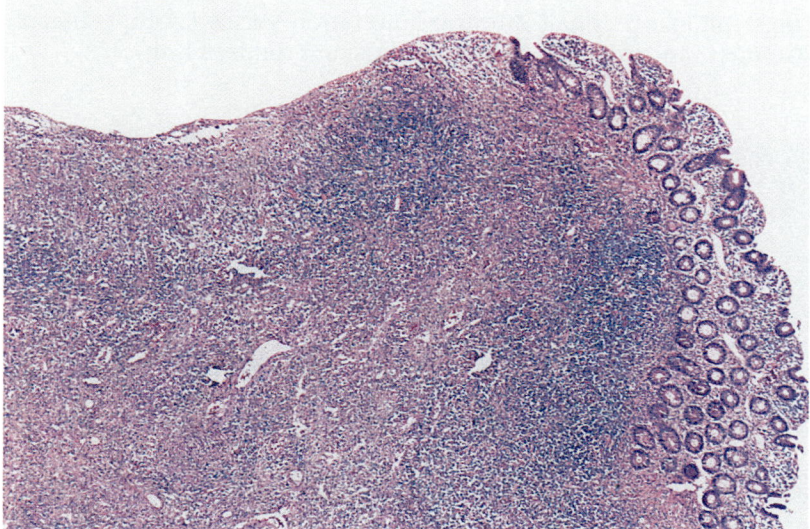

Figure 3-61: **Ileum. Typhoid.** Ulcerated Peyer patch.

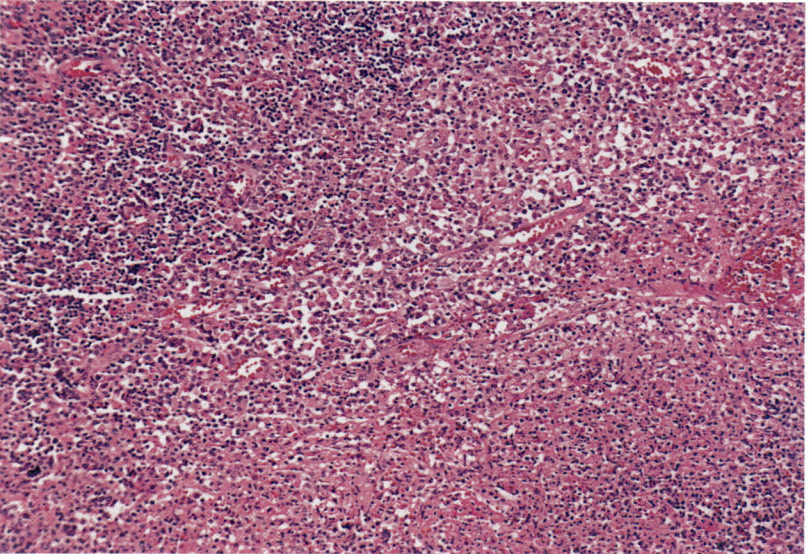

Figure 3-62: **Ileum. Typhoid.** Histiocytes infiltrate Peyer patch.

CANDIDA INFECTION

- Morphology .... *Candida* species often colonize ulcers in the small intestine without invading. Treatment involves anti-ulcer therapy without the need for anti-fungal agents. Rarely, *Candida* invades ulcers and causes mucosal microabscesses. In the neutropenic host, intestinal candidiasis may present with multiple ulcers and watery diarrhea. Invasion must be demonstrated to ascribe *Candida* as the cause of an ulcer.

- Endoscopic features .... Nonspecific ulceration.

- Clinical features .... None with colonization. Symptoms relate to the ulcer and ulcer site and include dyspepsia, abdominal pain, and acute and chronic gastrointestinal blood loss. In neutropenic immunocompromised individuals, watery diarrhea.

- Differential diagnosis ...... Endoscopic: Idiopathic small intestinal ulceration versus Crohn's disease, vasculitis, or enteric infection in an immunocompromised host.

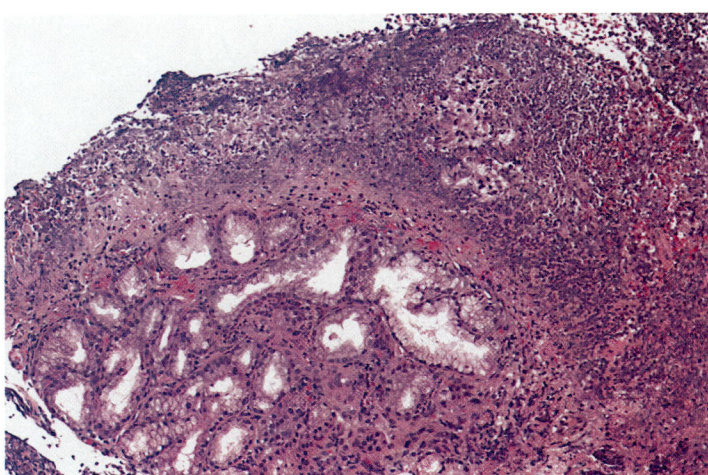

Figure 3-63: **Duodenum. Ulcer with *Candida*.** Inflammation and bluish debris in the ulcer base.

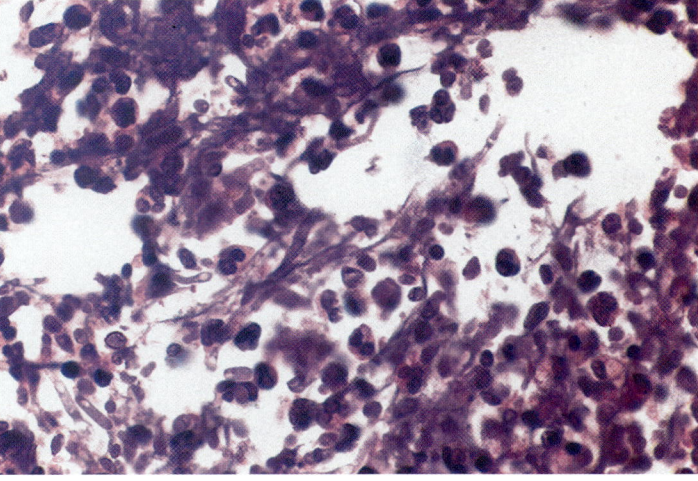

Figure 3-64: **Duodenum. Ulcer with *Candida*.** Acute inflammatory exudate and pseudohyphae of *Candida* species in base of ulcer.

PARASITES, WORMS

- Morphology .... A variety of parasitic worms/larvae (e.g. *Ancylostoma, Capillaria*, and *Strongyloides*) may be found in upper small bowel biopsy specimens.
- Endoscopic features .... None.
- Clinical features .... Nonspecific abdominal discomfort, iron deficiency anemia. In immunocompromised patient, unexplained diarrhea.
- Differential diagnosis...... Other parasitic worms and/or larvae.

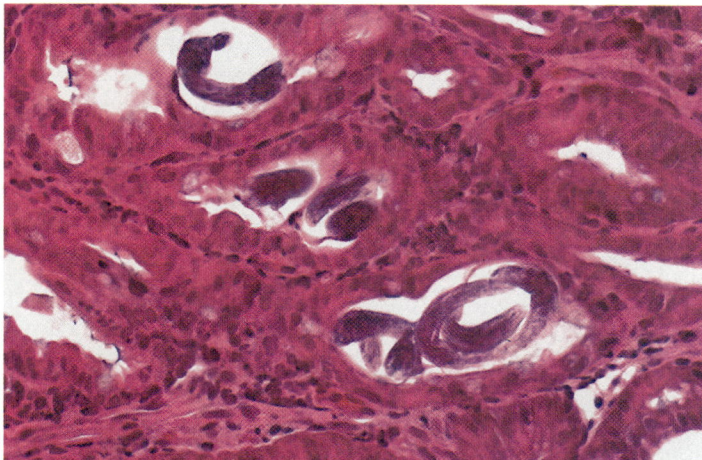

Figure 3-65: **Small Intestine. *Capillaria philippinensis*.** Parasitic worms in crypts.

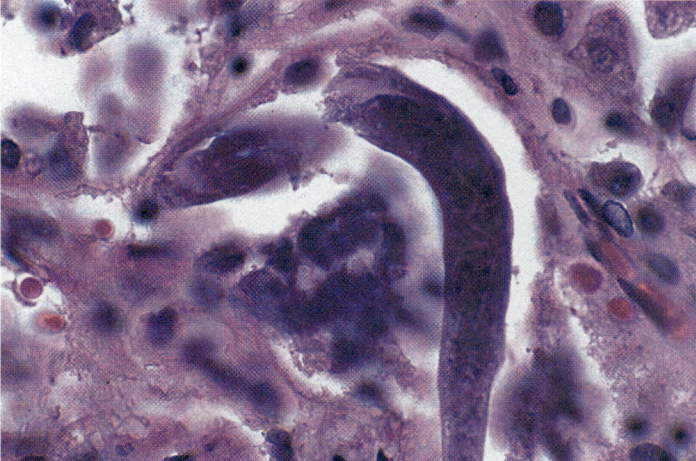

Figure 3-66: **Small Intestine. *Strongyloides stercoralis*.** Worm and cellular debris in mucosa.

COMMON VARIABLE IMMUNODEFICIENCY/ HYPOGAMMAGLOBULINEMIA

- **Morphology** — Small bowel histology is often normal except for the absence of plasma cells in the lamina propria. Instead of plasma cells, there are small lymphocytes with plasmacytoid nuclei. In selective IgA immunodeficiency, plasma cells may not be decreased due to a compensatory increase in IgM-secreting plasma cells. Lymphoid hyperplasia is a prominent finding. There may be villous flattening (atrophy) and inflammation, features resembling celiac sprue. Villi are usually flattened over lymphoid nodules. Associated *Giardia* infection is frequent.

- **Endoscopic features** — Large numbers of prominent lymphoid nodules, flattening of the circular folds and villi, best seen with mucosal magnification produced by the instillation of water. Endoscopic features are identical to those of sprue, partially or completely developed. In severe disease there is complete absence of villi, a mosaic mucosal pattern, and visible submucosal vasculature.

- **Clinical features** — Diarrhea, weight loss, malabsorption, hypogammaglobulinemia.

- **Differential diagnosis** — Histologic: Normal mucosa, malabsorption pattern.

    Endoscopic: Celiac sprue.

    Clinical: Malabsorption of other cause.

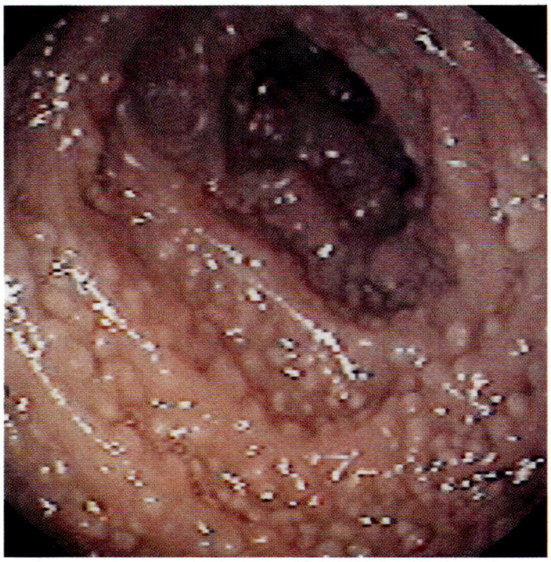

Figure 3-67: **Jejunum. Common Variable Immunodeficiency/Hypogammaglobulinemia.** Atypical jejunum with innumerable mucosal nodules.

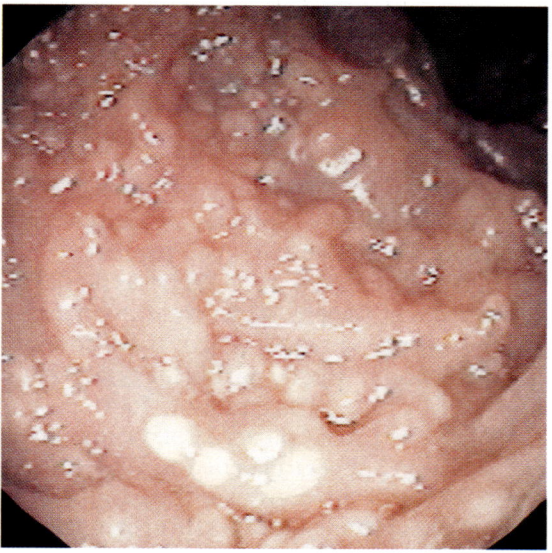

Figure 3-68: **Jejunum. Common Variable Immunodeficiency/Hypogammaglobulinemia.** Innumerable and prominent diffusely distributed lymphoid nodules.

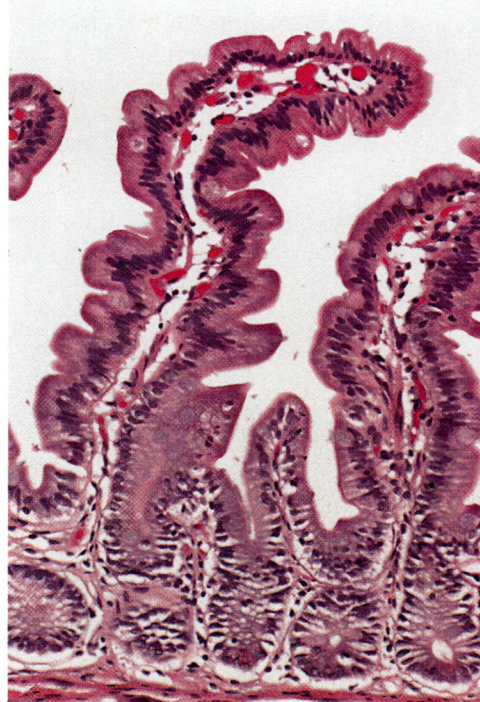

Figure 3-69: **Small Intestine. Common Variable Immunodeficiency/Hypogammaglobulinemia.** Normal small bowel mucosa, but no plasma cells.

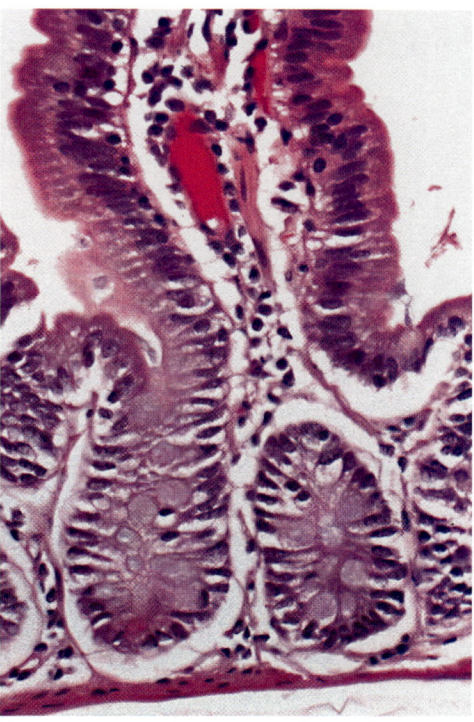

Figure 3-70: **Small Intestine. Common Variable Immunodeficiency/Hypogammaglobulinemia.** Lamina propria has small lymphoid cells but no plasma cells.

LYMPHOID HYPERPLASIA

- Morphology .... Lymphoid nodules/follicles are normal findings and are often prominent in the terminal ileum (Peyer patches). On mucosal biopsy they may be overinterpreted as lymphoid hyperplasia. The diagnosis requires endoscopic evidence of hyperplasia such as nodularity, thickening, or luminal narrowing. Lymphoid hyperplasia is more common in young patients than in the elderly and is usually of no clinical significance. Histologically, it is characterized by numerous lymphoid follicles often with large and irregular germinal centers. Lymphoid hyperplasia may be confused with Crohn's disease; the bowel may appear thickened and the lumen narrowed, the villi flattened, and there may be erosions over the lymphoid follicles. Lack of active inflammation and epithelial regeneration characterize lymphoid hyperplasia. Neutrophilic inflammation or crypt destruction suggest infection or inflammatory bowel disease (Crohn).

    Lymphoid hyperplasia in the proximal small bowel is rare. When present, it may cause luminal narrowing and thickening. Reactive germinal centers and mature bland lymphocytes distinguish hyperplasia from malignant lymphoma.

- Endoscopic features .... Lymphoid hyperplasia is common in the ileum. A rare lymphoid nodule may be seen in the jejunum during push enteroscopy in a young patient. Lymphoid hyperplasia appears as small mucosal nodules, scattered or innumerable. When numerous, they may be crowded and heaped up, creating a masslike appearance. Characteristically, there is no evidence of mucosal inflammation.

- Clinical features .... Lymphoid hyperplasia is usually an incidental finding. It is more prominent in the young and in patients with immunodeficiency-related malabsorption/diarrhea.

- Differential diagnosis ...... Histologic: Crohn's disease, malignant lymphoma, infectious ileitis.

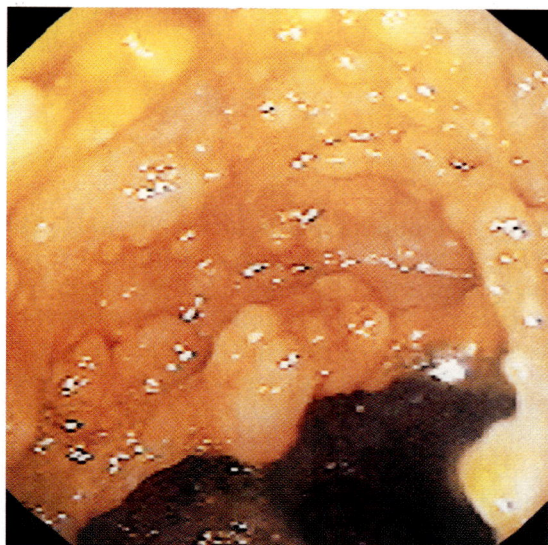

Figure 3-71: **Ileum. Lymphoid Hyperplasia.** Multiple variably sized nodules, some crowded and heaped up. The mucosa is normal without inflammatory changes. There are no findings suggestive of active inflammation.

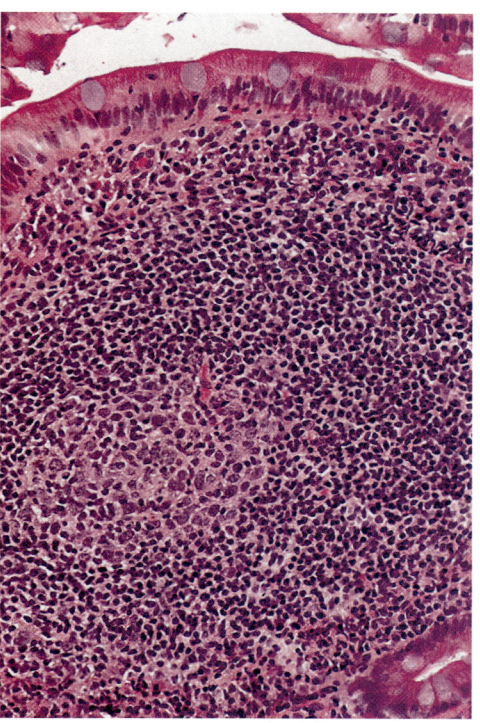

Figure 3-72: **Ileum. Lymphoid Hyperplasia.** Flattened epithelium over reactive lymphoid follicle with an active germinal center and small, mature lymphocytes.

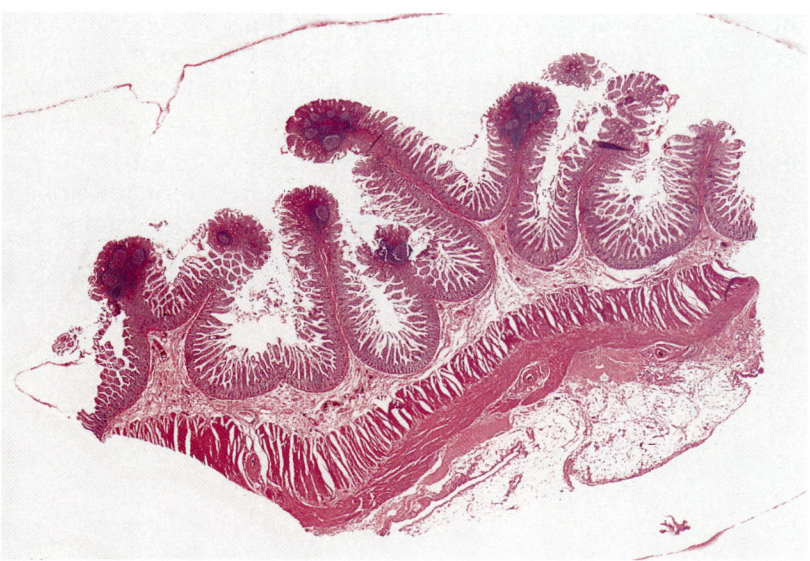

Figure 3-73: **Ileum. Lymphoid Hyperplasia.** Lymphoid nodules form bulbous structures at crests of circular folds resembling polyps.

MALABSORPTION

- Morphology .... Partial or total villous atrophy, crypt hyperplasia, active chronic inflammation and intraepithelial lymphocytosis are characteristic histologic features of the intestinal malabsorption pattern. Histologic changes may be patchy. This pattern, while characteristic of malabsorption, is nonspecific with regard to etiology and may be seen not only with celiac sprue but with hypersensitivity to other proteins such as soy or milk, bacterial overgrowth, tropical sprue, and severe protein calorie malnutrition. A thickened subepithelial collagen band characterizes collagenous sprue; whether this is a severe form of celiac sprue or a separate entity remains unclear. Submucosal edema is characteristic of sprue and may be seen radiographically. Complications of celiac sprue include ulcerative enteritis, T-cell lymphoma, and adenocarcinoma.

  Since peptic duodenitis and other inflammatory conditions may mimic a malabsorption pattern, specimens should be taken from the distal duodenum or jejunum. Multiple biopsy specimens may be necessary. Poorly oriented biopsy specimens may appear flat, but attention to other histologic features (e.g. orientation of crypts) will aid interpretation.

- Endoscopic features .... Characteristic of malabsorption are flattened circular folds, a mosaic or cobblestoned appearance of the mucosa, prominence of the submucosal vasculature, and loss of villi. Villi normally appear as discrete, fingerlike projections when magnified by secretions or instilled water (Fig. 3-77).

- Clinical features .... Weight loss, diarrhea, bloating, cramping, iron deficiency anemia, folate deficiency; with extensive malabsorption involving the terminal ileum, B_{12} deficiency. Associations include lymphocytic gastritis, lymphocytic colitis, and autoimmune disorders.

- Differential diagnosis ...... Clinical: Malabsorption due to hypersensitivity to gluten, soy, milk, other proteins; bacterial overgrowth, severe protein calorie malnutrition, immunodeficiency, autoimmune disease, tropical sprue.

SMALL INTESTINE

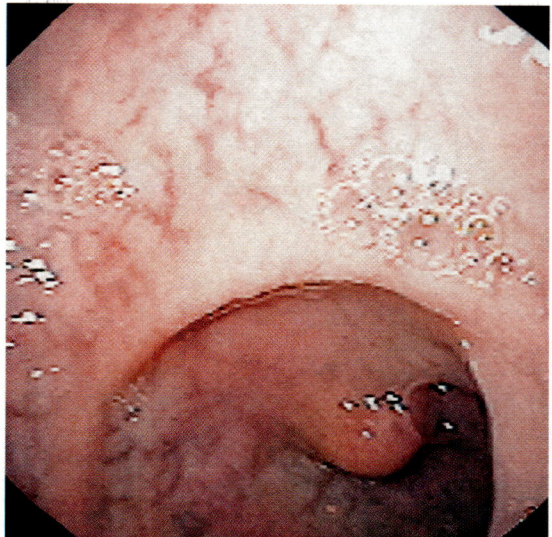

Figure 3-74: **Duodenum. Malabsorption.** Abnormal presence of the submucosal vascular pattern. The single circular fold in view is flattened. A nonspecific, discrete, diminutive sessile polyp is in the distance.

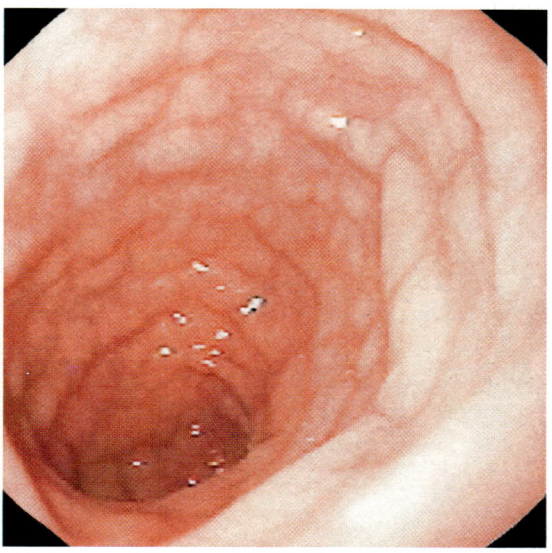

Figure 3-75: **Duodenum. Malabsorption.** Flattening of circular folds and disruption of the folds with a mosaic or cobblestone mucosal pattern.

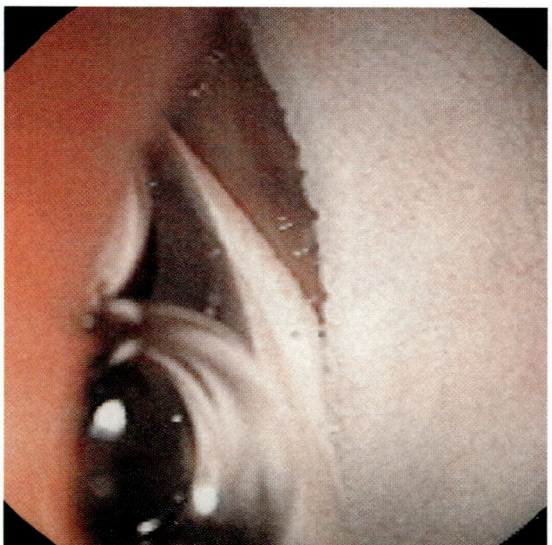

Figure 3-76: **Small Intestine. Malabsorption.** Water-submerged magnified view of the mucosa demonstrates the absence of villi which normally appear as discrete, fingerlike projections. Compare with Fig. 3-77.

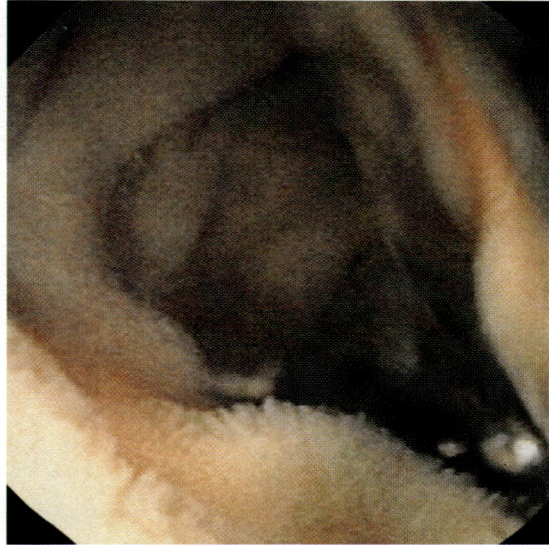

Figure 3-77: **Small Intestine. Normal.** Normal villi seen with water magnification.

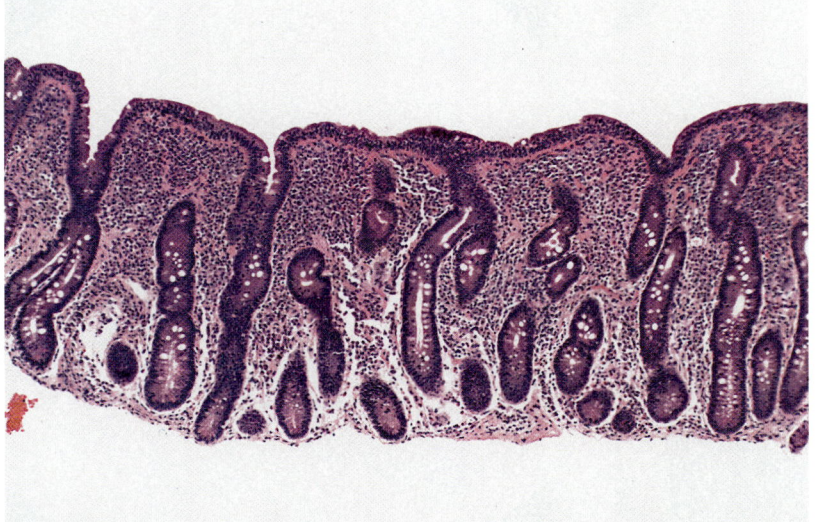

Figure 3-78: **Small Intestine. Malabsorption Pattern.** Total villous atrophy, crypt hyperplasia, active chronic inflammation, and intraepithelial lymphocytosis characterize the well-developed malabsorption pattern.

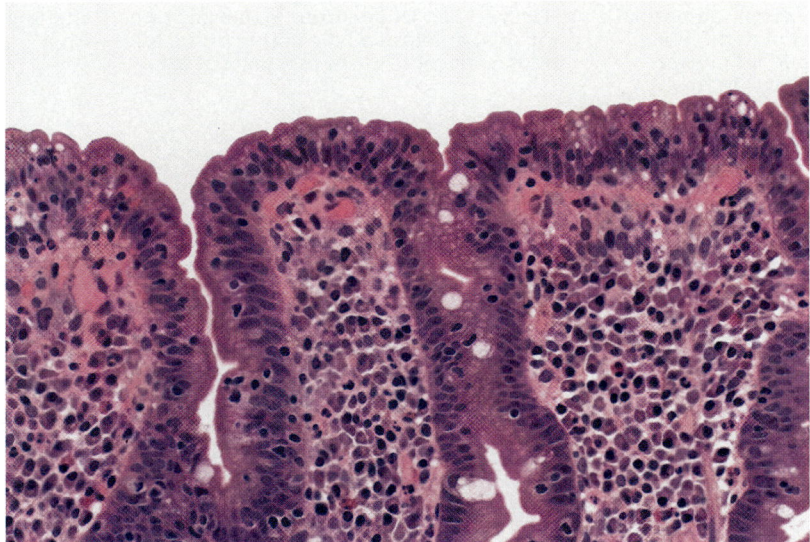

Figure 3-79: **Small Intestine. Malabsorption Pattern, Sprue.** Total villous atrophy, chronic inflammation, and intraepithelial lymphocytosis.

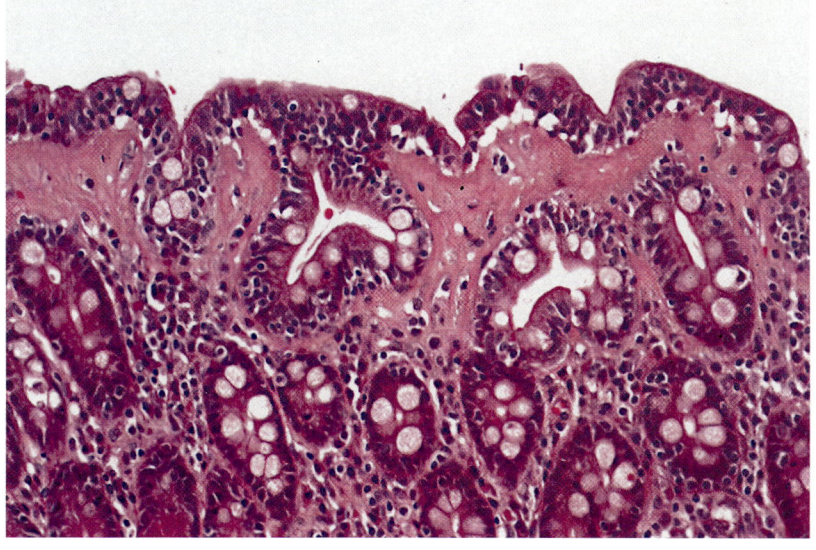

Figure 3-80: **Small Intestine. Collagenous Sprue.** Thick subepithelial collagen band, villous atrophy, and intraepithelial lymphocytes.

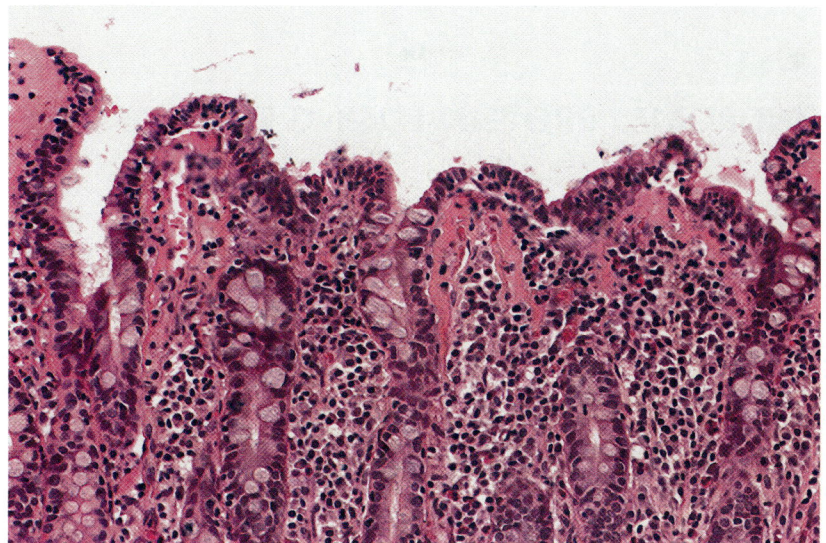

Figure 3-81: **Small Intestine. Collagenous Sprue.** Flat mucosa with crypt hyperplasia, chronic inflammation, intraepithelial lymphocytosis, and subepithelial collagenous band.

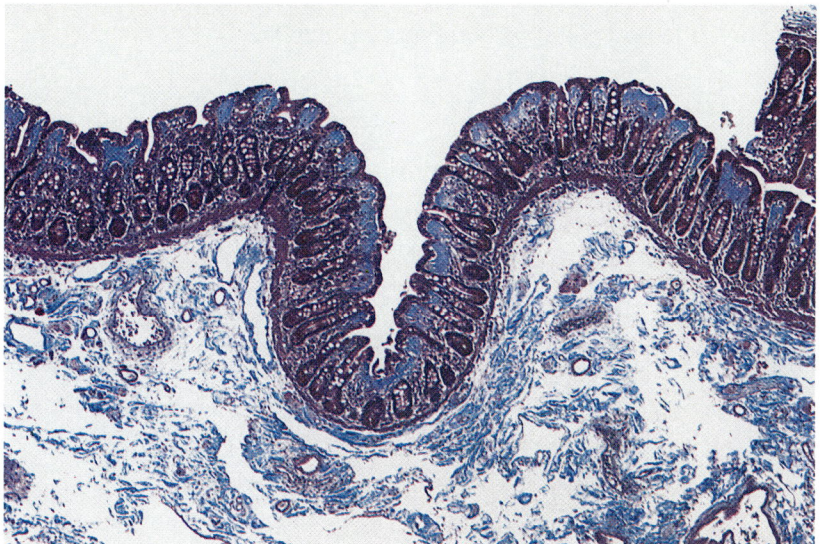

Figure 3-82: **Small Intestine. Collagenous Sprue, Trichrome.** Total villous atrophy, diffuse subepithelial collagen band, and submucosal edema.

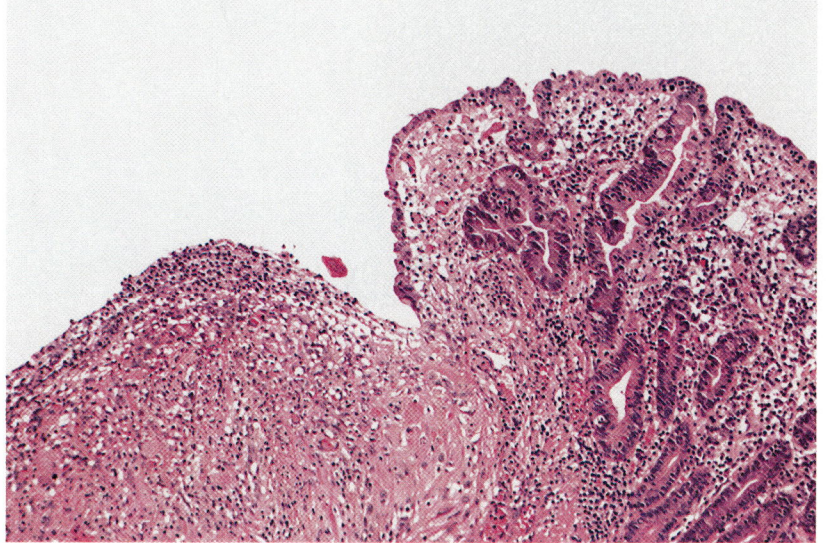

Figure 3-83: **Small Intestine. Malabsorption Pattern with Ulcer.** Ulcer arising in mucosa with a malabsorption pattern of injury.

CRONKHITE-CANADA SYNDROME: PROTEIN-LOSING ENTEROPATHY

- Morphology .... Protein-losing enteropathy with attendant nail and hair changes, when associated with diffusely edematous and distorted polypoid mucosa involving part or all of the gastrointestinal tract, constitute the Cronkhite-Canada syndrome. Cronkhite-Canada and juvenile polyposis may have overlapping endoscopic and histologic features.
- Endoscopic features .... The mucosa may be markedly edematous, polypoid, or even villous with patchy erythema and sometimes erosions. Dilated or engorged villi form long, enlarged, fingerlike projections. Dilated lacteals appear as punctate or miliary white nodules.
- Clinical features .... Diarrhea, weight loss, peripheral edema, hypoproteinemia, anemia, pigmentation of skin, nail and hair changes.
- Differential diagnosis ...... Histologic: Juvenile polyposis, inflammatory polyposis.

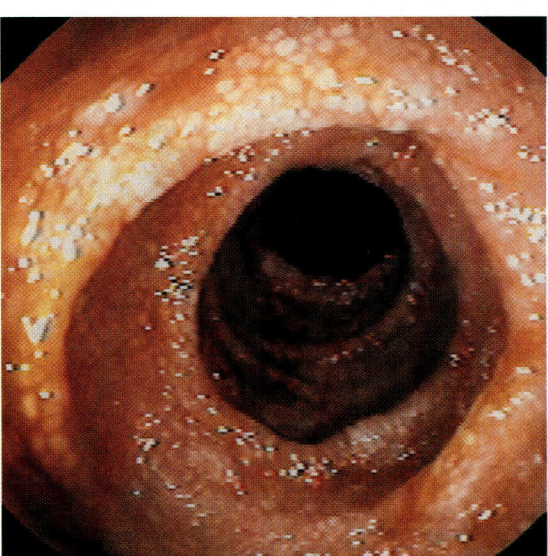

Figure 3-84: **Small Intestine. Cronkhite-Canada Protein-Losing Enteropathy.** There are innumerable enlarged lacteals appearing as multiple minute, elevated, punctate nodules.

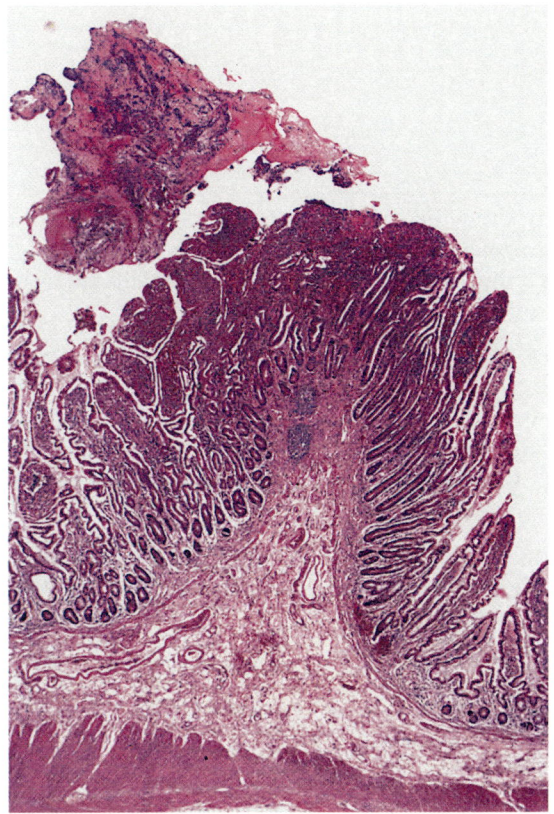

Figure 3-85: **Small Intestine. Cronkhite-Canada Protein-Losing Enteropathy.** Mucosal edema, inflammation, and ulceration over a circular fold. Villi are broad and distorted.

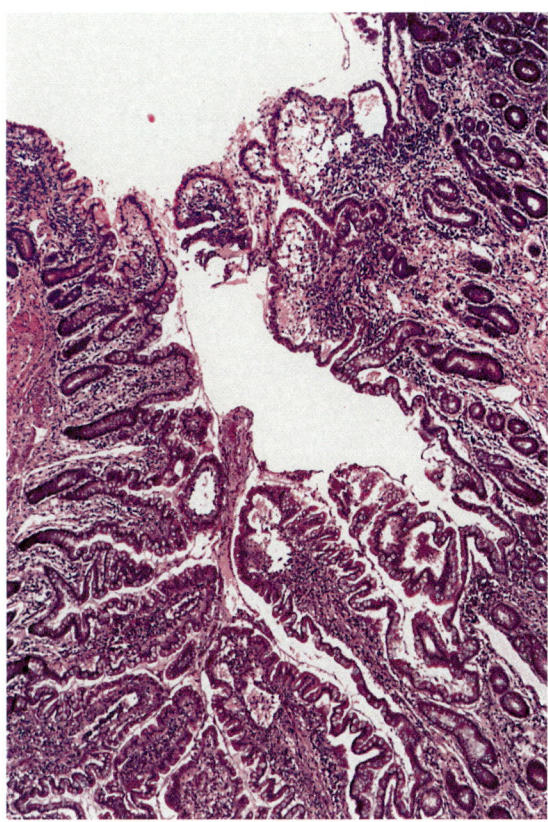

Figure 3-86: **Small Intestine. Cronkhite-Canada Protein-Losing Enteropathy.** Serrated villi enlarged by inflammation and edema. Lacteals are dilated.

LYMPHATIC DILATATION

- Morphology .... Dilated lacteals/lymphatics may be focal and of little consequence, a manifestation of localized lymphatic obstruction, or a generalized congenital process. The diagnosis of lymphangiectasia rests on finding dilated lacteals in several contiguous villi, or submucosal lymphatic dilatation.

- Endoscopic features .... Lymphangiectasia is fairly commonly encountered as a focal finding in the distal duodenum and beyond. It appears as a small mucosal nodule with multiple punctate white-to-yellow spots. At times, the spots are absent and the nodule is yellow. Biopsy in either circumstance will release milky lymphatic fluid (see Fig. 3-90). Sometimes nodules are absent and dilated lacteals appear as numerous white miliary dots.

- Clinical features .... None when an incidental finding; peripheral edema and chylous ascites when associated with significant lymphatic obstruction, e.g., due to extensive malignancy.

- Differential diagnosis ...... Histologic: Normal mucosa, lymphatic obstruction due to neoplasm, congenital lymphangiectasia.

CONGENITAL LYMPHATIC DILATATION

- Morphology .... Congenital lymphangiectasia is a rare cause of malabsorption. Biopsy specimens show nonspecific generalized but patchy lacteal dilation. Histologic examination cannot distinguish congenital lymphangiectasia from localized or secondary lymphangiectasia.

- Endoscopic features .... Enlarged (engorged), blunted, whitish villi encountered diffusely throughout or within segments of small intestine.

- Clinical features .... Malabsorption, protein-losing enteropathy, chylous ascites, chylous pleural effusions, and peripheral edema involving the lower extremities.

- Differential diagnosis ...... Histologic: Secondary lymphangiectasia.

SMALL INTESTINE

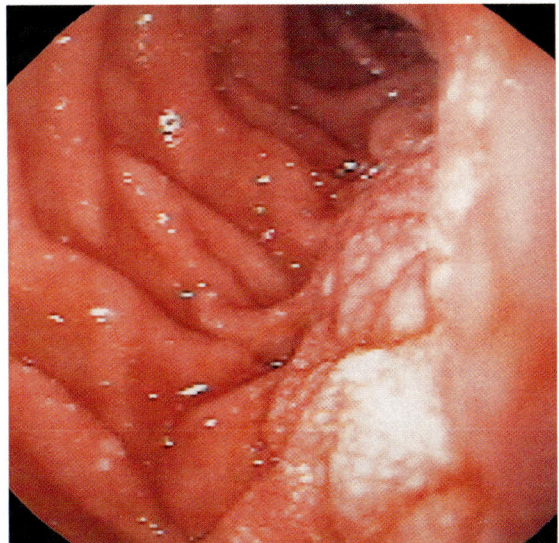

Figure 3-87: **Duodenum. Lymphangiectasia.** Disruption of distal duodenal mucosa, which appears thickened and nodular with numerous elevated, punctate, white spots.

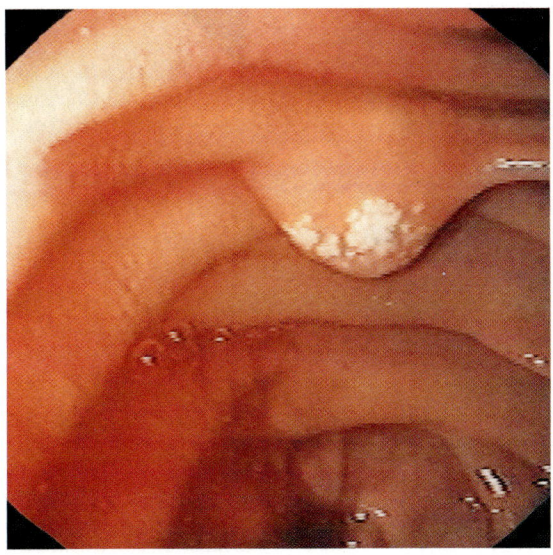

Figure 3-88: **Jejunum. Lymphangiectasia.** Diminutive nodule with distinctive collection of miliary, white, punctate spots.

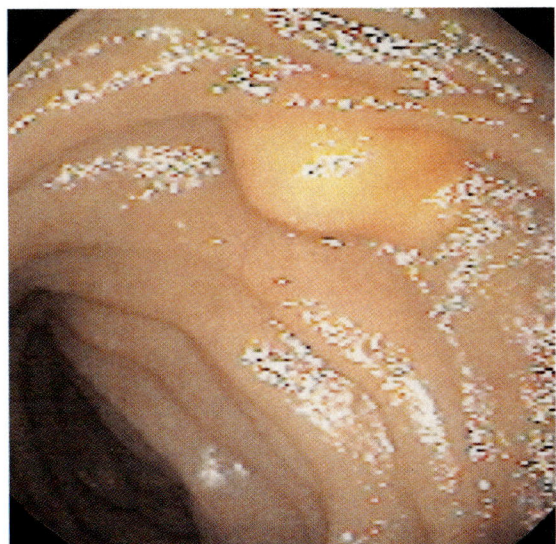

Figure 3-89: **Jejunum. Lymphangiectasia.** Discrete, diminutive, yellowish jejunal nodule, commonly encountered during push enteroscopy.

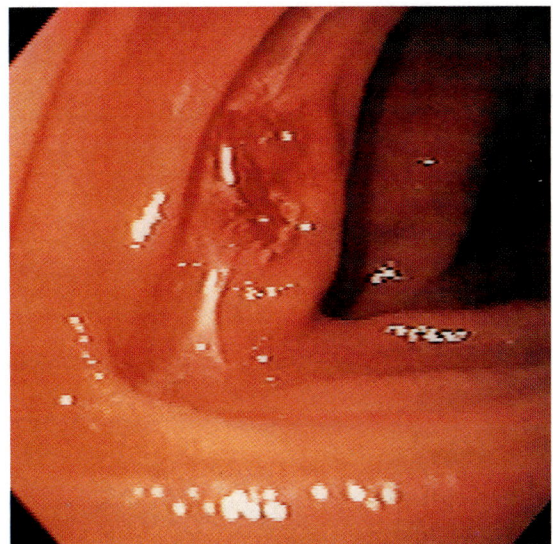

Figure 3-90: **Duodenum. Lymphangiectasia.** Focal collection of dilated lacteals/lymphatics sampled with release of milky lymphatic fluid.

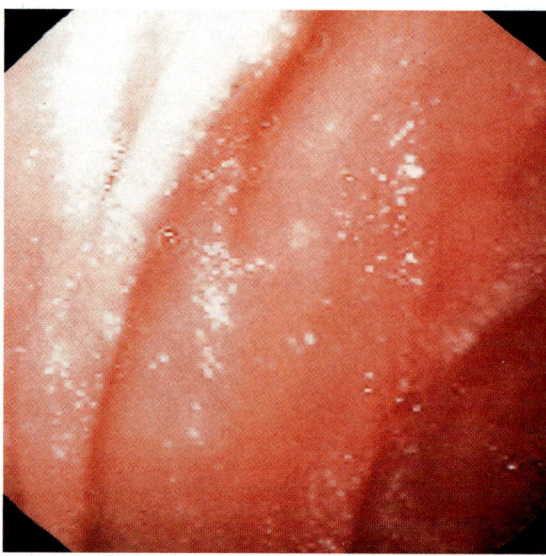

Figure 3-91: **Duodenum. Lymphangiectasia.** Multiple prominent villi with a white, punctate appearance consistent with dilated lacteals.

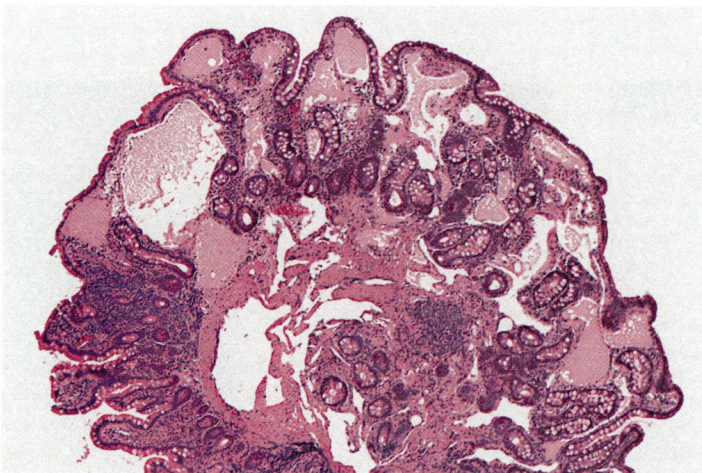

Figure 3-92: **Duodenum. Lymphangiectasia.** Cluster of markedly dilated lacteals expanding villi and forming a polypoid mass.

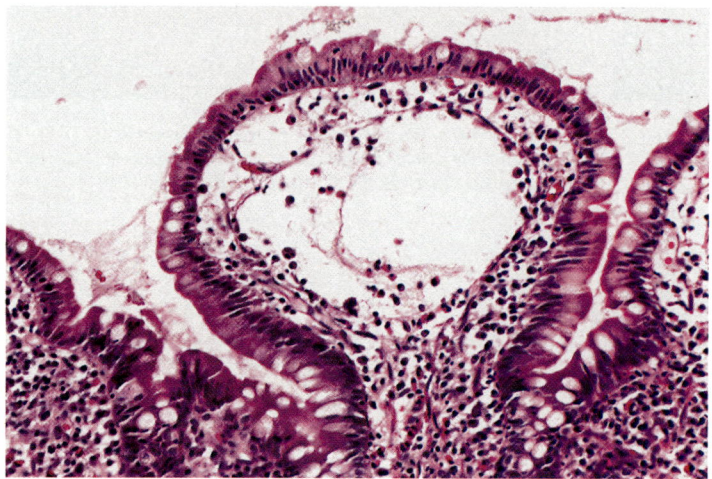

Figure 3-93: **Duodenum. Lymphangiectasia.** Dilated lacteal contains lymphoid cells.

VASCULAR LESIONS

- Morphology .... *Ectasia:* Superficial mucosal vascular ectasia is a consequence of chronic venous hypertension, local or remote. Ectatic vessels are dilated and sclerotic, distinguishing ectasia from transient vascular dilatation. Superficial vascular ectasias are found in a wide variety of conditions in which there is either chronic venous obstruction or increased blood flow, e.g., portal hypertension, angiodysplasia, telangiectasia, arteriovenous malformations, vascular tumors, or inflammatory or neoplastic masses. Histologic features of these various lesions are indistinguishable. Angiodysplasia in late stages affects the arteriole as well.

  Vascular malformation: Arteriovenous malformations are transmural knots of large, abnormally thick arteries and veins commonly present as a mucosal or submucosal mass. *Vascular neoplasms* are composed of proliferating vessels and form mucosal and submucosal masses, including hemangiomas, angiosarcomas, and Kaposi sarcoma. They may be misinterpreted as vascular malformations. See vascular neoplasms, page 272.

- Endoscopic features .... The vascular *ectasias* encountered in portal hypertensive enteropathy most often appear as multiple, very minute, petechial, discrete or coalescing erythematous spots. Occasionally, there may be a larger (e.g., 2 to 4 mm in diameter), isolated, focal, vascular ectatic lesion.

  Angiodysplasia, on the other hand, presents as discrete diminutive collections of ectatic mucosal microvessels. The lesions have a distinctive vascular pattern or a homogeneous, irregular shape, resembling a miniature cutaneous port-wine stain. Angiodysplastic lesions may have a characteristic thin, pale rim of mucosa surrounding the vascular lesion, referred to as the "halo sign."

  Arteriovenous malformations are discrete submucosal nodules, with a purple or bluish color due to a significant venous component. In some patients, these malformations may be located deep in the wall and present as submucosal nodules, sometimes with small ectasias involving the overlying mucosa.

- Clinical features .... *Portal hypertensive enteropathy* is a cause of refractory GI blood loss anemia and chronic melena. Small intestinal *angiodysplasia* is associated with iron deficiency anemia with or without overt bleeding (melena). Angiodysplasia of the small bowel tends to concentrate in the duodenum and proximal jejunum. They may be few and isolated or multiple, and in some cases, distributed throughout the small bowel. Active bleeding is rarely encountered. *Arteriovenous malformations,* when located in the small bowel, especially in children and young adults, are associated with iron deficiency anemia, and episodic overt bleeding with either melena or hematochezia. They are often multiple and diffusely scattered throughout the small intestine.

- Differential diagnosis ...... Histologic and endoscopic: *Angiodysplasia* versus focal mucosal trauma with adherent blood. *Arteriovenous malformations* versus ectopic varices and submucosal neoplasms.

  Clinical: Numerous angiodysplastic lesions raise the possibility of Osler-Weber-Rendu syndrome (hereditary hemorrhagic telangiectasia).

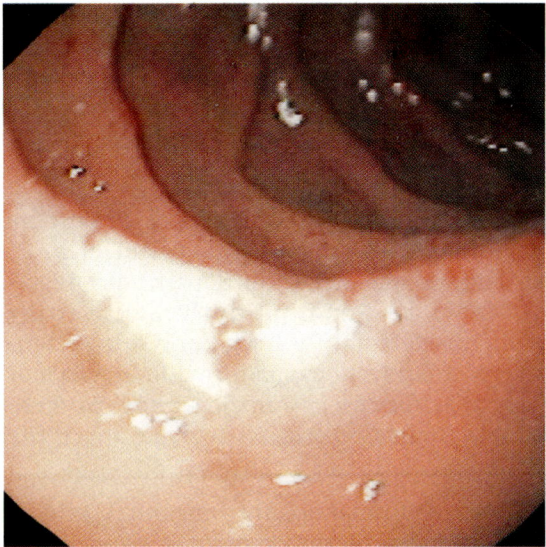

Figure 3-94: **Duodenum. Portal Hypertensive Ectasias.** Multiple punctate erythematous spots with some coalescence (center) in a patient with known portal hypertension and iron deficiency anemia.

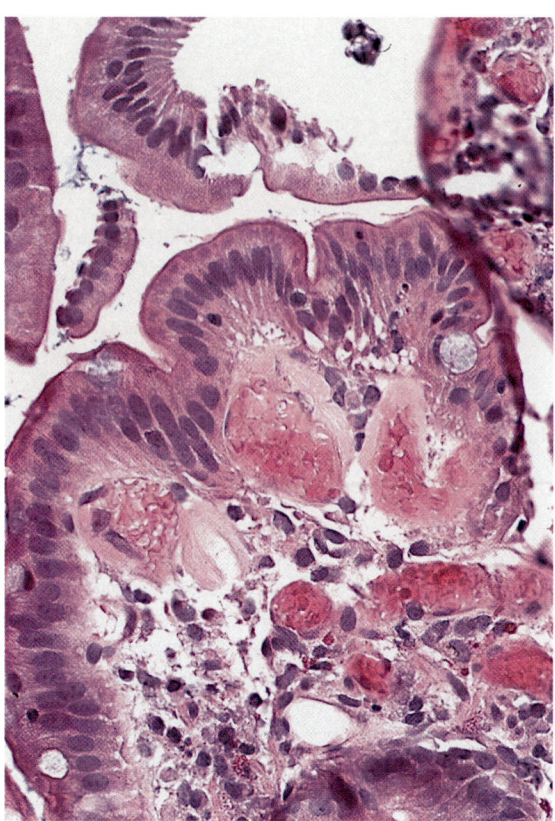

Figure 3-95: **Duodenum. Vascular Ectasias.** Ectatic capillaries with thickened sclerotic walls.

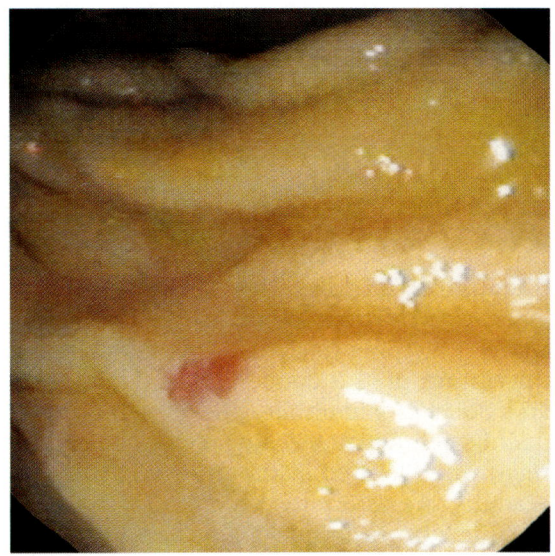

Figure 3-96: **Duodenum. Angiodysplasia.** Discrete, minute, mucosal angioectasia. The margins are irregular and the lesion resembles a miniature port-wine stain.

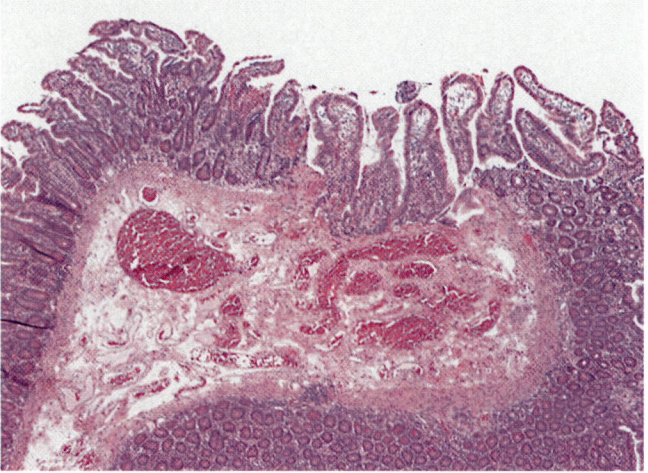

Figure 3-97: **Duodenum. Telangiectasia in Osler-Weber-Rendu Syndrome.** Submucosal vessels are greatly dilated.

SMALL INTESTINE

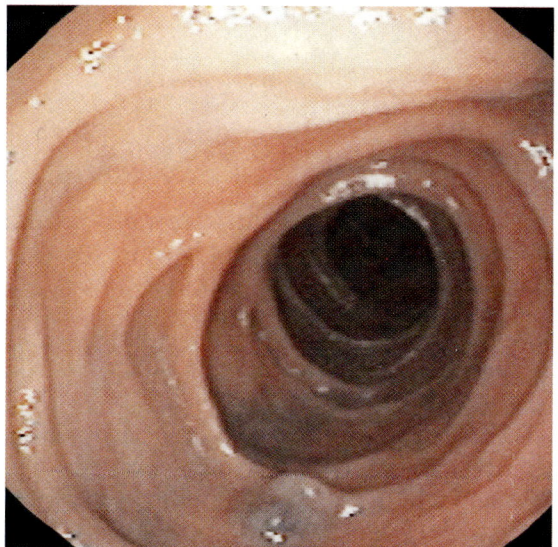

Figure 3-98: **Duodenum. Arteriovenous Malformation.** Irregular small nodule (lower center) with distinctive bluish coloration consistent with an arteriovenous malformation in a patient with chronic GI blood loss anemia.

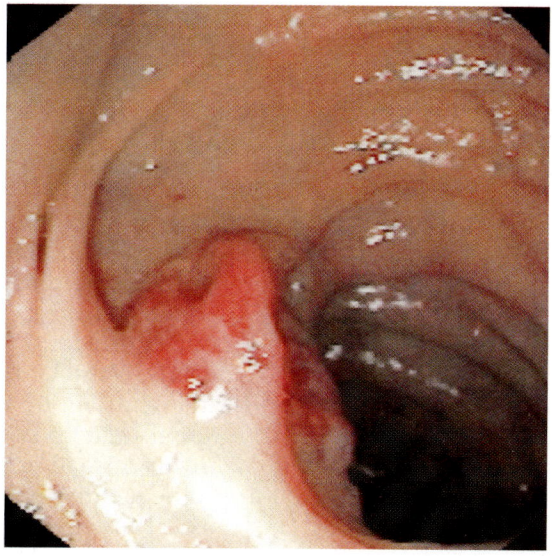

Figure 3-99: **Jejunum. Arteriovenous Malformation.** Arteriovenous malformation forming a submucosal polypoid mass with irregular patchy mucosal erythema. It is unclear whether the erythema represents ectatic mucosal microvascular extensions of the arteriovenous malformation. Push enteroscopy in a patient with obscure GI blood loss anemia.

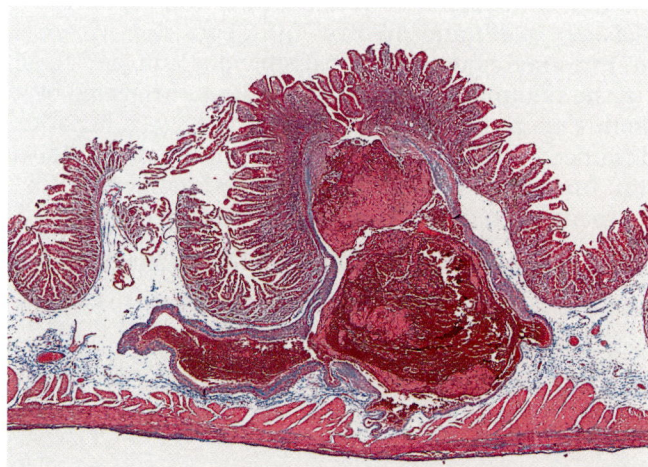

Figure 3-100: **Duodenum. Arteriovenous Malformation.** Large, dilated thrombosed vessels form a tumorlike mass in the submucosa.

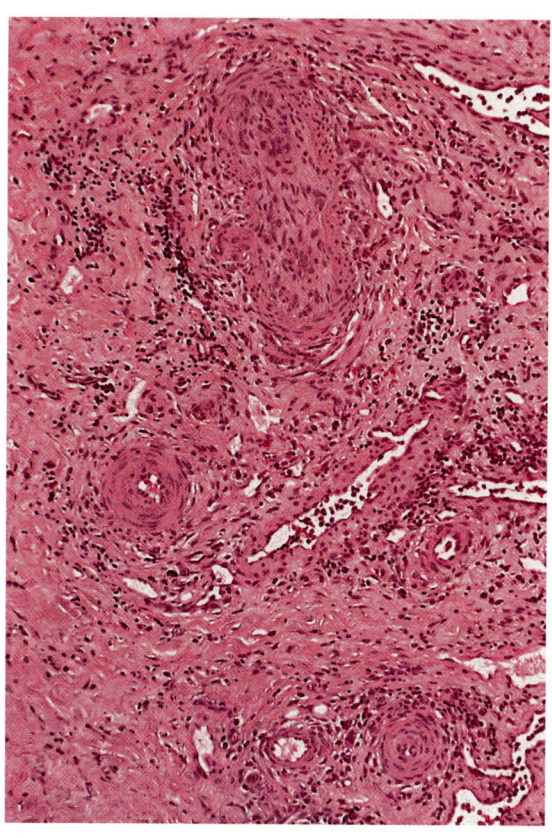

Figure 3-101: **Duodenum. Malignant Hypertension.** Submucosal arteries and arterioles with marked concentric intimal proliferation.

VASCULITIS

- **Morphology** — Biopsy specimens diagnostic of primary vasculitis are rare, because the diagnosis is usually established by other means, and because the vasculitis involves submucosal vessels missed in shallow mucosal biopsies. *Henoch-Schoenlein leukocytoclastic vasculitis* commonly involves the intestine and causes bleeding. The venules are infiltrated by neutrophils and nuclear debris. Vascular thrombosis and hemorrhagic mucosal necrosis accompany the neutrophilic inflammation. IgA deposition may be demonstrated in vessel walls of skin, renal glomeruli, and the intestine. *Polyarteritis nodosa* involves small or large arteries. The vessel walls undergo fibrinoid necrosis. Subsequently, lymphocytes and histiocytes surround and consume the affected vessel segment. The consequence is ischemic ulcers and bleeding. All layers of the wall are affected, so there may be perforation. Secondary vasculitis or nonspecific vascular inflammation in the base of ulcers of other cause is more common than primary vasculitis. To establish a diagnosis of primary rather than secondary vasculitis, a characteristic histologic pattern and involvement of vessels in otherwise normal intestine are useful features.

- **Endoscopic features** — Vasculitis has several endoscopic manifestations, including patchy erythema, petechial mucosal hemorrhage, and ulceration due to ischemia.

- **Clinical features** — Henoch-Schoenlein vasculitis is triggered by bacterial infection (e.g. streptococcus, *E coli*, *Campylobacter jejuni*) and involves IgA deposition in vessel walls. Abdominal pain, intestinal hemorrhage, palpable purpura, and renal insufficiency are part of the syndrome. Polyarteritis nodosa is triggered by a variety of insults, including streptococcal and viral infections (e.g. hepatitis B), drug reactions, and connective tissue diseases. Gastrointestinal symptoms include abdominal pain, intestinal hemorrhage, and intestinal perforation. Kidney or brain involvement often dominates the clinical picture.

- **Differential diagnosis** — Clinical: Primary versus secondary vasculitis, CMV enteritis, Crohn's disease.

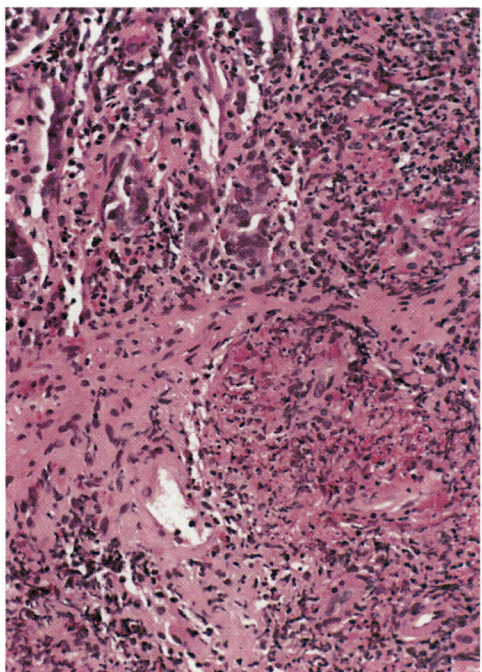

Figure 3-102: **Small Intestine. Henoch-Schoenlein Vasculitis.** Thrombosed submucosal venule with neutrophilic destruction of the vessel wall (leukocytoclastic vasculitis). Mucosa is acutely inflamed, making it difficult to see that a mucosal venule is also affected.

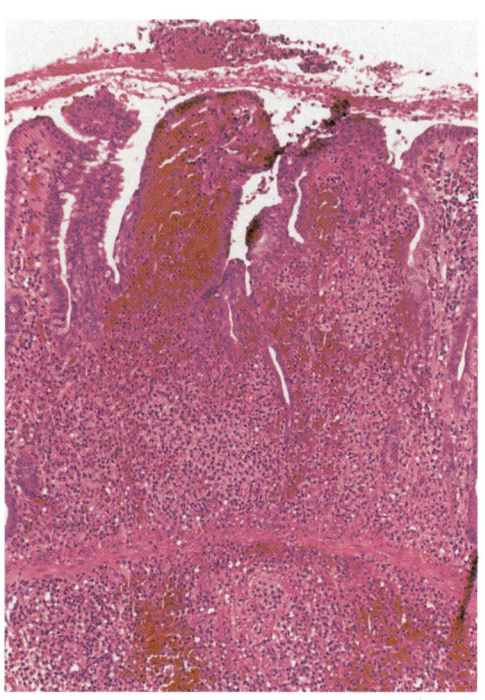

Figure 3-103: **Small Intestine. Henoch-Schoenlein Vasculitis.** Massive acute mucosal/submucosal inflammation with hemorrhagic mucosal necrosis. Vague round configuration of submucosal inflammation reflects the destroyed venule.

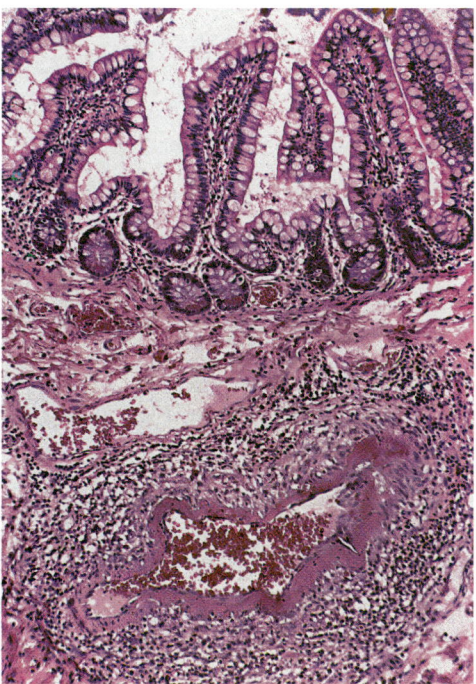

Figure 3-104: **Small Intestine. Polyarteritis Nodosa.** Fibrinoid necrosis of the submucosal arterial wall with surrounding lymphohistiocytic inflammation. Mucosa is normal.

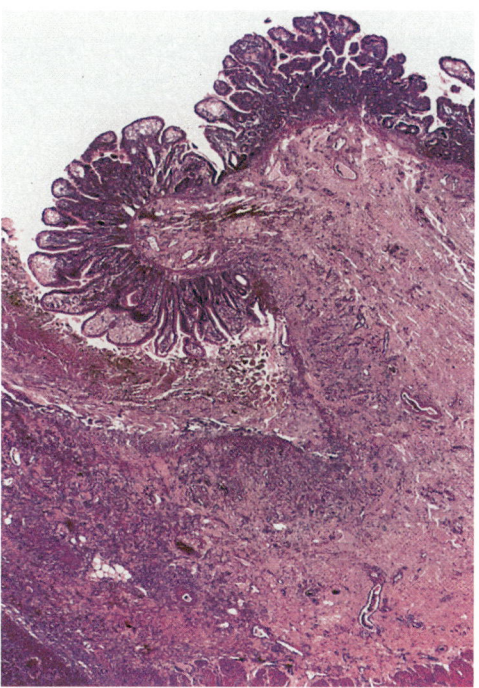

Figure 3-105: **Small Intestine. Polyarteritis Nodosa.** Discrete ulcer in edematous small bowel. Vasculitis is present in base but difficult to see and easily overlooked.

HEMORRHAGIC ENTEROPATHY

- Morphology .... Edema, congestion, and hemorrhage are manifestations of arterial or venous obstruction or occlusion, but may also be secondary to abnormalities in clotting.
- Endoscopic features .... Marked distortion of the small intestinal architecture, with thickening, edema and blunting of the circular folds, stenosis of the lumen, coarsening of the mucosal villous pattern, and discoloration ranging from maroon to cyanotic. The mucosa is friable and may bleed spontaneously or there may be intramucosal hemorrhage.
- Clinical features .... Abrupt onset of abdominal pain, nausea, vomiting, and diarrhea; eventually hematochezia.
- Differential diagnosis ...... Endoscopic and clinical: Overanticoagulation with intramural hemorrhage, mesenteric venous thrombosis, superior mesenteric artery occlusion, small vessel vasculitis with infarction, and ischemia secondary to mechanical obstruction (strangulation).

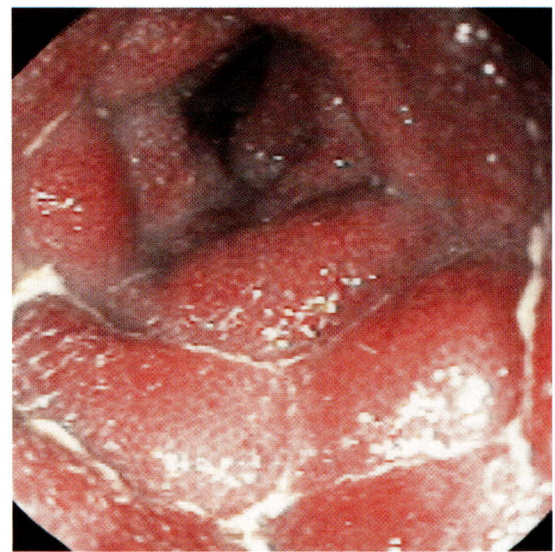

Figure 3-106: **Small Intestine. Hemorrhagic Enteropathy**. The small bowel is markedly abnormal, with mucosal thickening, enlargement and blunting of the circular folds, and narrowing of the lumen. The villous mucosal surface is coarse and diffusely erythematous, consistent with extensive intramural hemorrhage and congestion, features of ischemia.

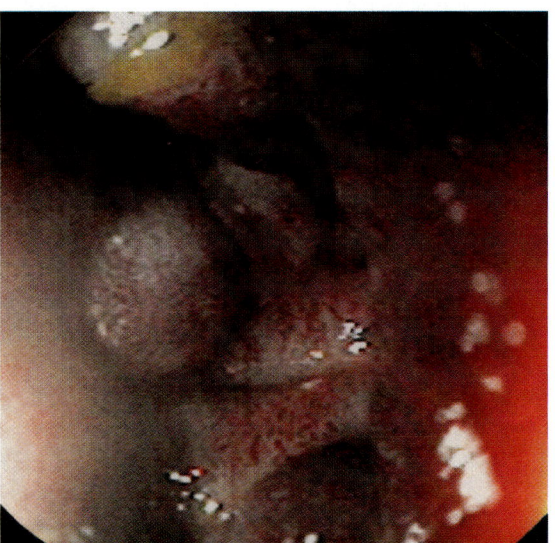

Figure 3-107: **Jejunum. Hemorrhagic Enteropathy.** Dusky congestion and hemorrhagic mucosa with distortion of circular folds and marked luminal stenosis. The patient was overanticoagulated and presented with abdominal pain and hematochezia.

ISCHEMIA

- Morphology — Ischemic enteritis has many causes: hypotension, peripheral vascular disease, thrombosis, or atheromatous emboli; drugs (e.g. NSAIDs, ergotamines, estrogen, and cocaine), viruses, (e.g. vaccinia, CMV), and toxin-producing bacteria. Radiation enteritis occurs with doses over 4500 RADs. The mucosal changes in acute radiation injury are similar to any other ischemic injury and include epithelial necrosis with preservation of the crypt outlines, mucosal hemorrhage, edema, and acute inflammation. Epithelial and stromal cell degenerative changes (cellular and nuclear enlargement, vacuolation, and macronucleoli), characteristic of radiation injury, are sometimes evident.

    In chronic ischemia, mucosal atrophy, architectural distortion, mucosal and submucosal fibrosis, and ulceration occur. Chronic radiation injury may be indistinguishable from ischemia of another cause. Atypical radiation fibroblasts with nuclear and cytoplasmic enlargement or submucosal arterial intimal proliferation with hyalinization of the media suggest radiation. Chronic radiation enteritis with stricture may be indistinguishable from Crohn's disease.

- Endoscopic features — Acute arterial ischemia (ischemic enteritis) causes focal or segmental infarction. In early ischemia, the mucosa is dark red with an irregular mottled appearance, often with superficial exudative ulcers. As the ischemic injury progresses, the mucosa becomes hemorrhagic and covered with a diffuse yellow exudate. Beneath, and in the intervening nonexudative areas, the mucosa is dusky, dark maroon to black, an appearance indicative of infarction. Chronic radiation changes consist of numerous mucosal angiectasias, which vary in size from punctate to discrete ectatic microvessels measuring 4 to 5 mm. The duodenal bulb and postbulbar duodenum are frequently affected following radiation for biliary tract malignancies. These vascular lesions may also be encountered within pelvic loops of ileum in patients who have undergone pelvic radiation. Chronic ulcers and enlarged, blunt villi with engorged lymphatics/lacteals may be present.

- Clinical features — Ischemia: Abdominal pain, nausea, cramping, diarrhea, hematochezia. Radiation: GI blood loss anemia, occult or overt bleeding, obstructive symptoms, diarrhea, bacterial overgrowth syndrome due to dysmotility and stasis.

- Differential diagnosis — Histologic: Crohn's disease, collagenous sprue.

    Endoscopic: Small bowel ischemic ulceration must be differentiated from neoplasm.

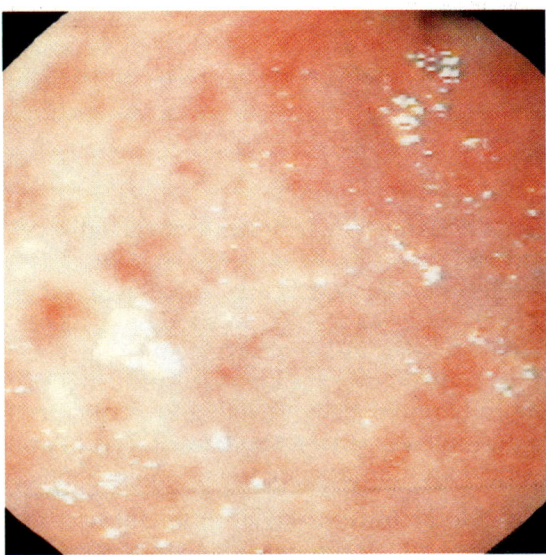

Figure 3-108: **Duodenum. Chronic Ischemia, Radiation.** Multiple, varying-sized angiectasias within the duodenal bulb in a patient irradiated for gallbladder cancer.

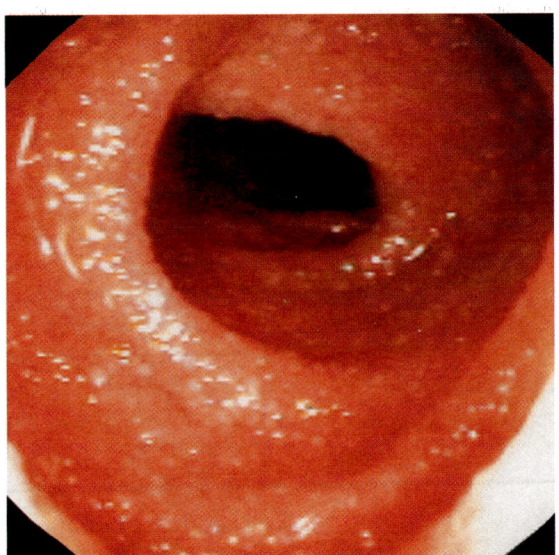

Figure 3-109: **Ileum. Chronic Ischemia, Radiation.** Coarsened, blunted, engorged villi. Blunt or granular appearance of villi can persist long after radiation injury.

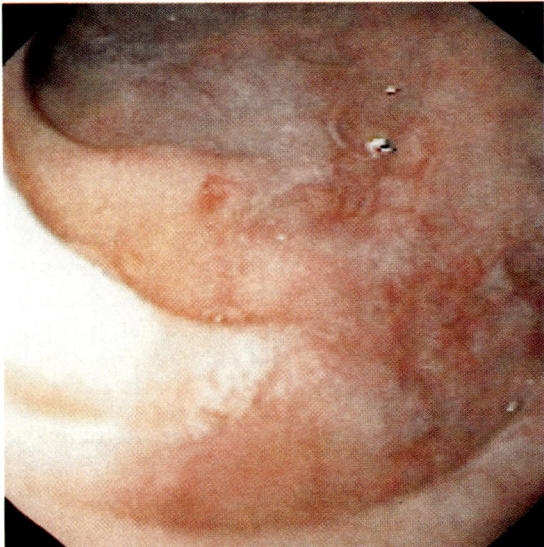

Figure 3-110: **Duodenum. Chronic Ischemia, Radiation.** Focal patch of early acute ischemia in the distal duodenum. Dark, mottled, and erythematous mucosa with superficial exudative ulceration. The margins of the involved area are irregular.

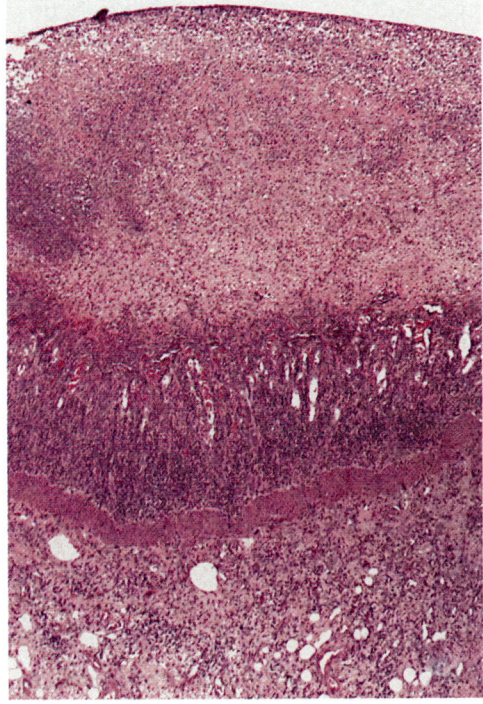

Figure 3-111: **Small Intestine. Chronic Ischemia.** Ulcer, necroinflammatory debris, submucosal fibrosis, and inflammation.

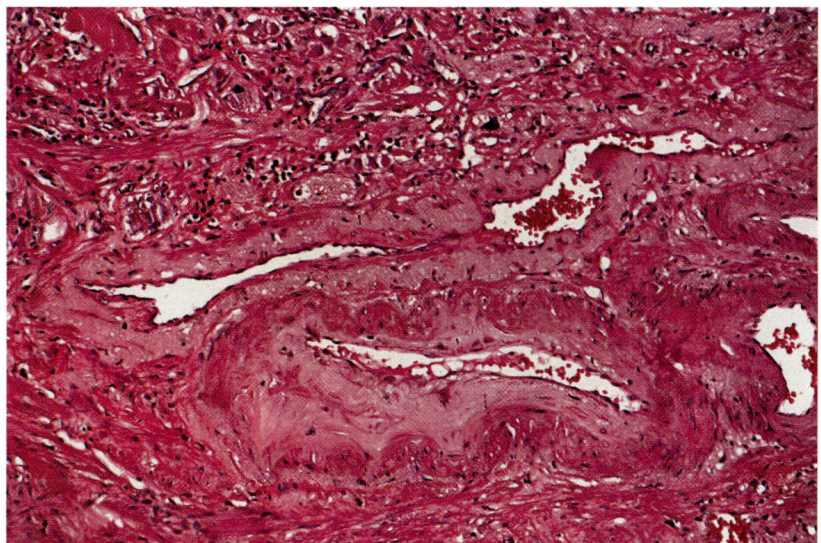

Figure 3-112: **Small Intestine. Chronic Ischemia, Radiation.** Submucosal arterioles with intimal thickening and hyalinized media.

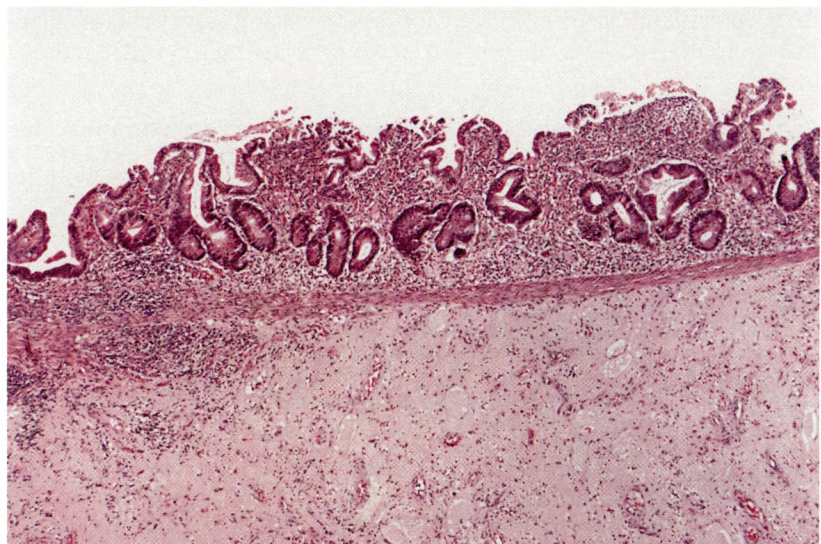

Figure 3-113: **Small Intestine. Chronic Ischemia.** Villous atrophy and crypt architectural distortion, inflamed lamina propria, and submucosal edema; changes of chronic ischemia.

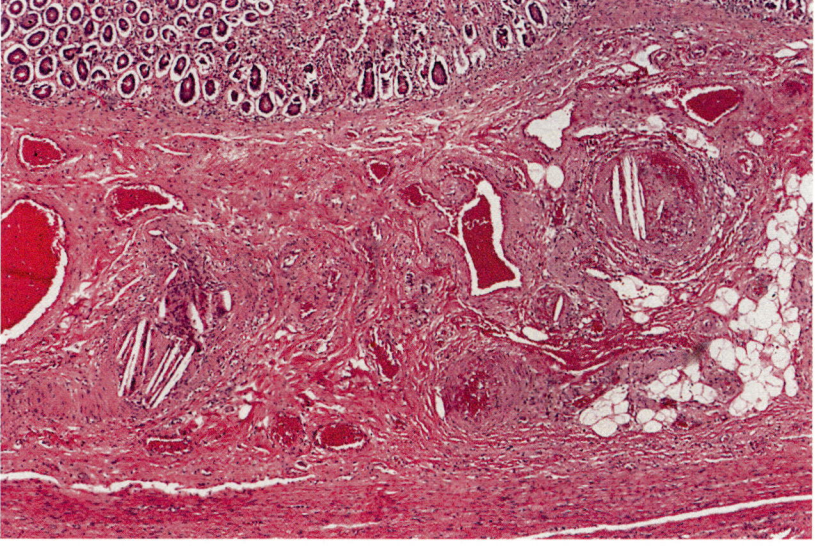

Figure 3-114: **Small Intestine. Chronic Ischemia with Cholesterol Emboli.** Clear, needlelike spaces, typical of cholesterol emboli in submucosal vessels.

COLLAGEN VASCULAR DISEASE

- Morphology .... In the small intestine, sclerodermal fibrosis of the muscularis propria leads to pseudo-obstruction, bacterial overgrowth, and malabsorption. Arterial concentric intimal hyperplasia results in ischemia. Dermatomyositis causes muscular damage. Hollow visceral myopathy, a familial myodegenerative disorder, affects the muscularis propria but causes vacuolar degeneration of the muscle cells rather than fibrosis, and involves the outer rather than the inner layer of the muscularis propria, unlike scleroderma. Skeletal muscular dystrophies may also affect the smooth muscle of the gut.

- Endoscopic features .... The distinctive endoscopic feature of scleroderma is a markedly dilated small intestinal lumen. Diverticula and accentuation of the circular folds are other findings. There are no distinctive mucosal changes.

- Clinical features .... Chronic or episodic abdominal distention and bloating with nausea, diarrhea, and weight loss. Malabsorption secondary to stasis and bacterial overgrowth.

- Differential diagnosis ...... Clinical: Malabsorption due to celiac sprue, bacterial overgrowth, muscular dystrophies, dermatomyositis, or hollow visceral myopathy.

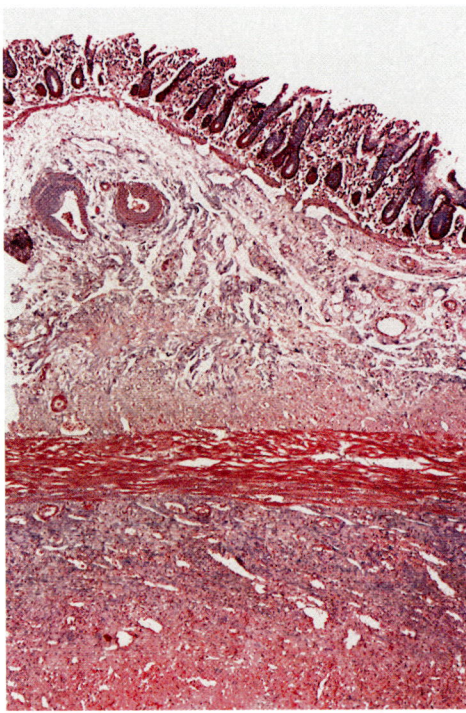

Figure 3-115: **Small Intestine. Scleroderma, Trichrome Stain**. Thick-walled submucosal vessels and loss of muscle cells in the inner circular layer of the muscularis propria. Mild mucosal inflammation.

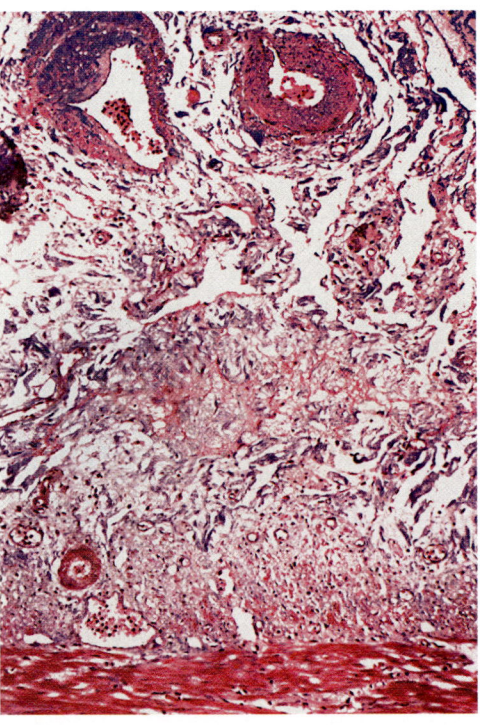

Figure 3-116: **Small Intestine. Scleroderma, Trichrome Stain**. Arterial concentric intimal hyperplasia and irregular venous intimal fibrosis. Atrophy and fibrosis of circular layer of muscularis propria.

AMYLOID

- Morphology .... Amyloid appears as an amorphous eosinophilic deposit in submucosal vessels, muscularis mucosae, and muscularis propria. AA (chronic disease) amyloid usually involves vessels and is more likely than AL (light chain) amyloid to deposit in lamina propria. AL amyloid has a propensity for muscularis mucosae and muscularis propria. Samples of submucosa are required to detect early arterial deposits. AL amyloid is PAS-diastase positive while AA amyloid is not. Congo red stain under polarized light demonstrates the characteristic apple-green birefringence. The sulfated alcian blue stain separates collagen from amyloid. Subclassification of amyloid with immunostains is definitive, but interpretation requires experience. Amyloid subtyping is important since AL amyloid may be associated with a systemic myeloproliferative disorder (light chain disease, multiple myeloma) requiring aggressive treatment. Amyloid of chronic disease (AA) is usually insidious, progressive, and unresponsive to therapy. Amyloid uncommonly narrows arterioles sufficiently to produce ischemic mucosal erosions and ulcers.

- Endoscopic features .... Usually no endoscopic abnormalities are encountered, even in symptomatic patients. In patients with gastrointestinal bleeding, the mucosa may be friable and bleed spontaneously in the absence of a discrete abnormality.

- Clinical features .... Asymptomatic, pseudo-obstruction with bacterial overgrowth, mucosal hemorrhage, and ulcers.

- Differential diagnosis...... Histologic: Ischemic fibrosis of lamina propria, arteriolosclerosis, degenerating fibrotic muscle.

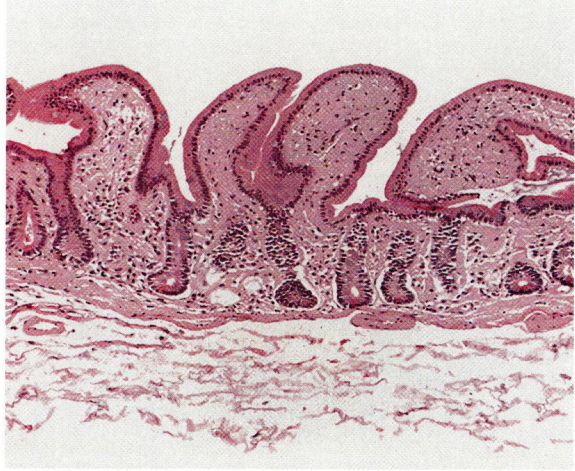

Figure 3-117: **Small Intestine. Amyloid.** Lamina propria expanded by pink amorphous material consistent with amyloid.

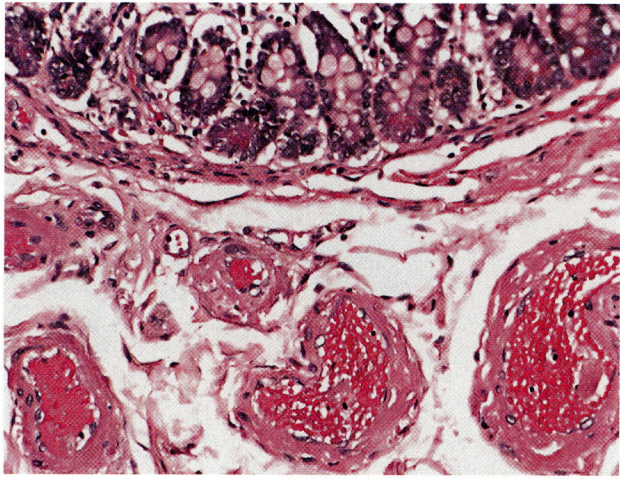

Figure 3-118: **Small Intestine. Amyloid.** Superficial submucosal arterioles with eosinophilic amyloid deposits.

INTUSSUSCEPTION

- Morphology .... Meckel diverticula and tumors may cause intussusception. Common tumors are adenomas, carcinomas, lipomas, stromal tumors, lymphomas, Peutz-Jeghers polyps, and inflammatory fibroid polyps. Ileal carcinoids do not commonly intussuscept due to dense fibrosis that anchors the tumor to the mesentery.
- Endoscopic features .... Chronic intussusception creates mucosal thickening and marked dark, beefy hyperemia, either patchy or diffuse. Mucosal friability, ulceration, and spontaneous bleeding due to mechanical ischemia are common features.
- Clinical features .... Recurrent obstructive symptoms with crampy abdominal pain, abdominal distention, nausea, and vomiting.
- Differential diagnosis ...... Endoscopic: Infiltrative disorder, ischemia (arterial or venous), intramural hemorrhage.

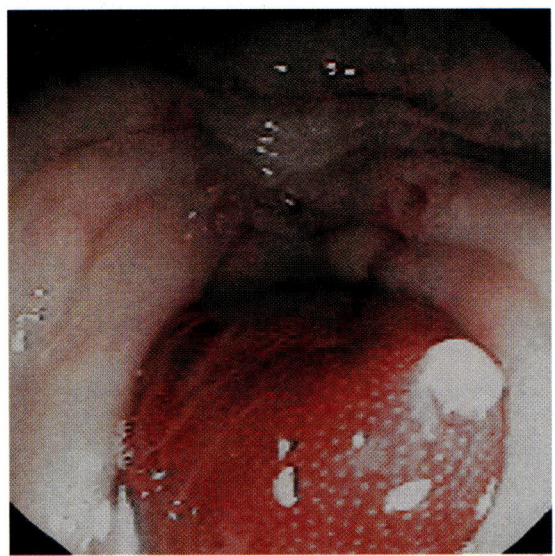

Figure 3-119: **Ileum. Intussusception.** Markedly congested and edematous cecum. The congestion and edema has accentuated the colonic crypt pattern to appear as a honeycomb arrangement of white dots.

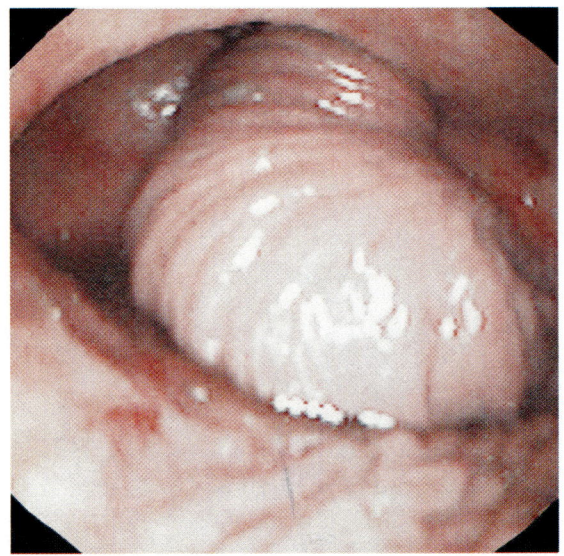

Figure 3-120: **Jejunum. Intussusception**. Afferent limb of a Billroth II anastomosis intussuscepted into the gastric remnant. Patient with postoperative nausea and vomiting.

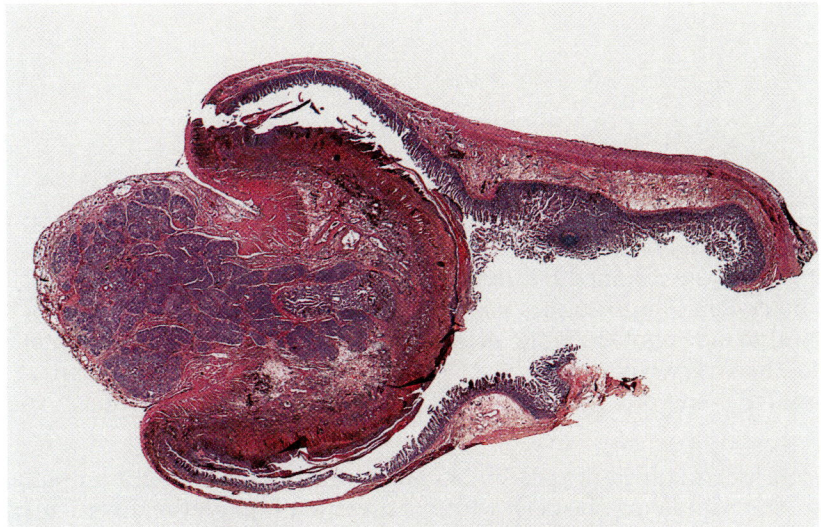

Figure 3-121: **Ileum. Intussusception, Meckel Diverticulum.** Leading edge is a Meckel diverticulum with ectopic pancreatic tissue.

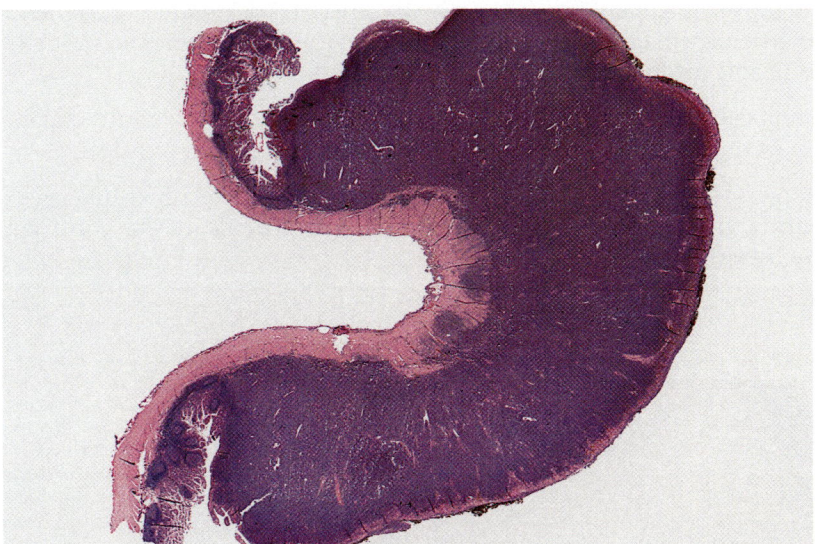

Figure 3-122: **Ileum. Intussusception, Lymphoma.** Lymphoma is the lead point.

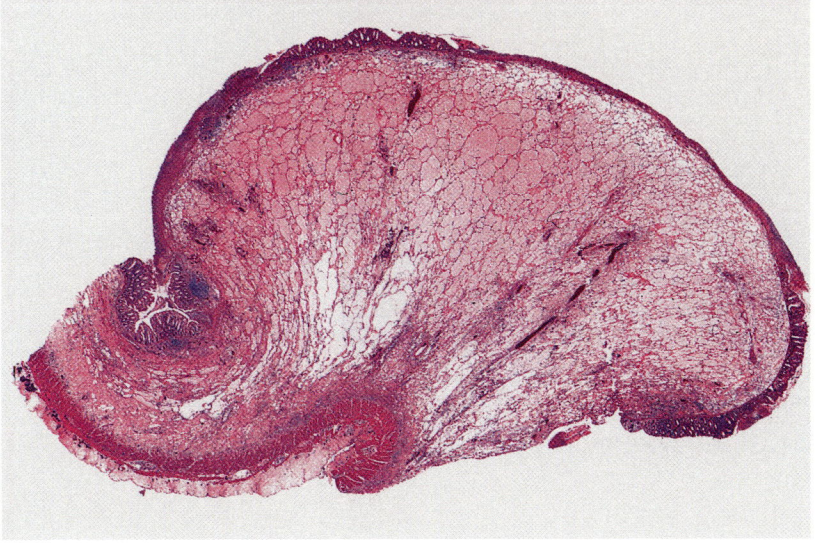

Figure 3-123: **Ileum. Intussusception, Lymphangioma.** Surface erosion and dilated vascular spaces in submucosa.

OSTOMY, DIVERTICULA

- Endoscopic features .... Biliary enteric anastomoses are discrete, round openings. Choledochoduodenostomies are usually in the apical portion of the duodenal bulb, where the common bile duct is in natural proximity to the duodenal wall. Choledochojejunostomies may be end-to-end or end-to-side constructions. End-to-side choledochojejunostomies are usually several centimeters distal to the oversewn stump of a Roux-en-Y limb. Anastomoses in all locations have smooth margins. Biliary epithelium is pale, smooth, or granular.

    Diverticula are usually in the postbulbar duodenum, adjacent to the ampulla of Vater. The papilla may be deep within a diverticulum, on the diverticular margin, or within the rim of the diverticulum. Small bowel diverticula typically have wide openings. They may be clustered or isolated. Extremely large diverticula will have mucosal ridges within the diverticular sac, and may contain sizable arteries that may erode and bleed.

- Clinical features .... Diverticula can be asymptomatic, produce acute bleeding, or cause malabsorption from bacterial overgrowth when they are large and multiple.

- Differential diagnosis ...... Endoscopic: A choledochoduodenostomy may resemble a small diverticulum. During the passage of the endoscope, large diverticula may be confused with the intestinal lumen.

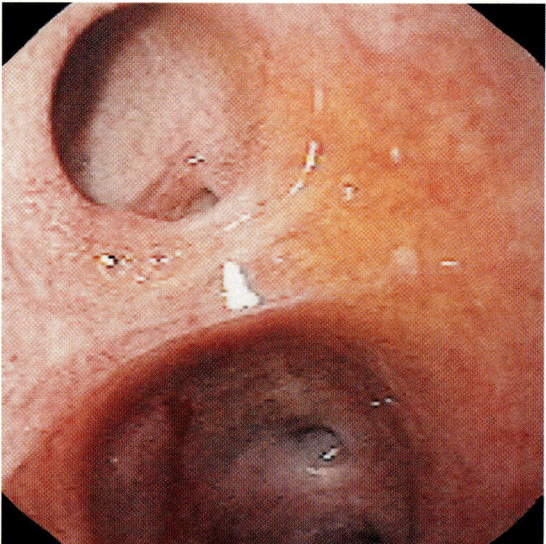

Figure 3-124: **Small Intestine. Choledochoduodenostomy**. The ostomy has a typical smooth, round margin. Biliary epithelium seen on the other side of the ostomy is paler than the bowel mucosa.

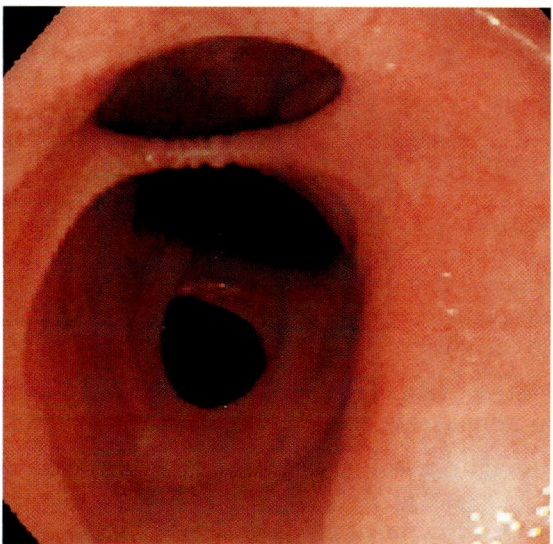

Figure 3-125: **Duodenum. Choledochoduodenostomy.** A view at and beyond the bifurcation from within a choledochoduodenostomy.

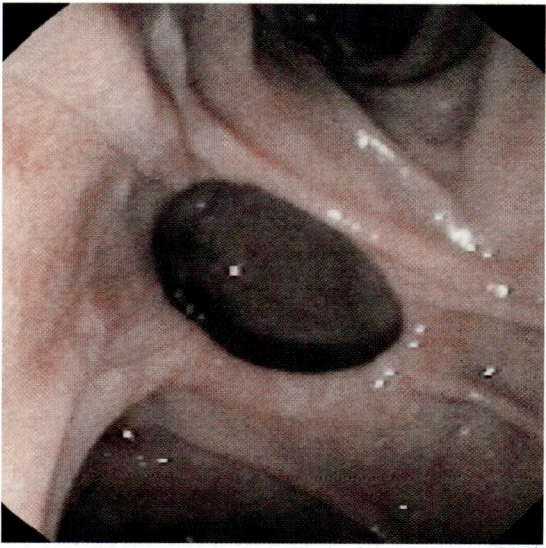

Figure 3-126: **Duodenum. Diverticulum.** Large postbulbar duodenal diverticulum with wide opening, free of retained debris.

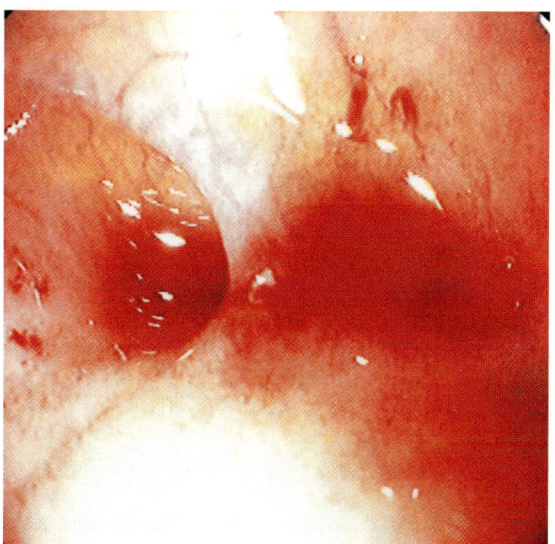

Figure 3-127: **Duodenum. Diverticulum.** View within a large duodenal diverticulum in a patient with acute GI bleeding. In the exact center of the photograph is a small mucosal defect from which arterial spurting has just ceased. A ridge sweeps up into the left of this bleeding point. The bleeding artery is presumed to be located within this mucosal ridge.

ANASTOMOTIC ULCERS

- Endoscopic features .... Gastrojejunal anastomotic ulcers are typically located on the margin or on the jejunal side of the anastomosis. In Billroth II anastomoses, ulcers commonly develop in the saddle area (jejunal wall opposing the anastomosis). Ulcers are solitary or multiple and are usually shallow. Deeper ulcers may contain an exposed or visible vessel.

- Clinical features .... Abdominal pain, acute gastrointestinal bleeding, iron deficiency anemia, or gastric outlet obstruction from edema and stenosis of the anastomosis.

- Differential diagnosis ...... Endoscopic: Idiopathic ulceration, incomplete vagotomy with retained antral tissue, NSAID use with ulceration on the gastric side of the anastomosis, ulcerated adenocarcinoma (stump cancer).

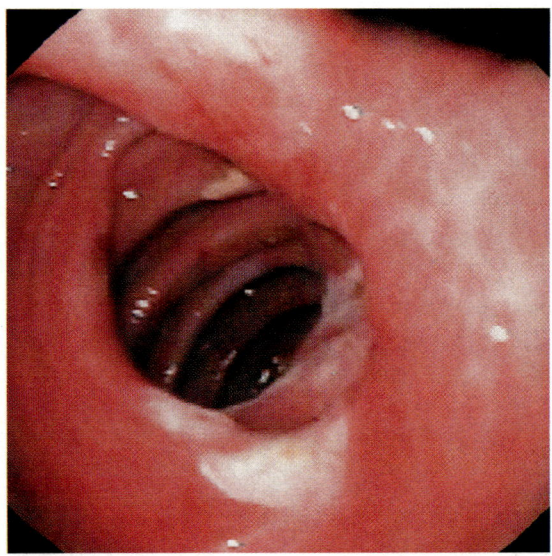

Figure 3-128: **Jejunum. Anastomotic Ulcer.** Gastrojejunal anastomosis with ulceration on the rim and on the jejunal ("saddle") side.

POUCHITIS

- Morphology .... The inflammation is nonspecific and varies in intensity. There may be chronic colitis or ileitis, with or without crypt destruction, with regeneration.
- Endoscopic features .... The mucosa is erythematous and friable but rarely bleeds spontaneously. There are usually shallow ulcers which vary in size and are irregularly shaped. The ulcers are often located at anastomotic suture lines, but may be on the free wall of the pouch or on the nipple of a Koch pouch. Severe pouchitis may have features indistinguishable from recurrent inflammatory bowel disease, including edema, granularity, ulcers, friability, and spontaneous bleeding.
- Clinical features .... Symptoms are similar to inflammatory bowel disease and include increased rate of stooling and incontinence, bleeding, cramping, and tenesmus.
- Differential diagnosis ...... Endoscopic: Recurrent inflammatory bowel disease, enteric infection.

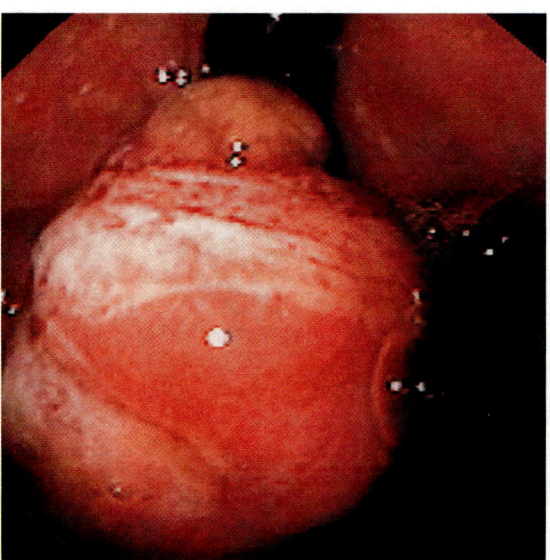

Figure 3-129: **Ileum. Pouchitis.** Retroflexed view within Koch pouch reveals shallow, friable ulceration of the nipple.

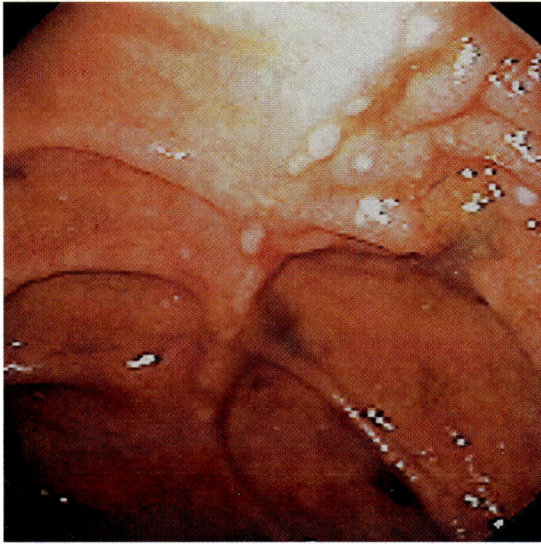

Figure 3-130: **Ileum. Pouchitis.** Shallow linear ulcerations along an anastomotic suture line within an ileoanal J-pouch.

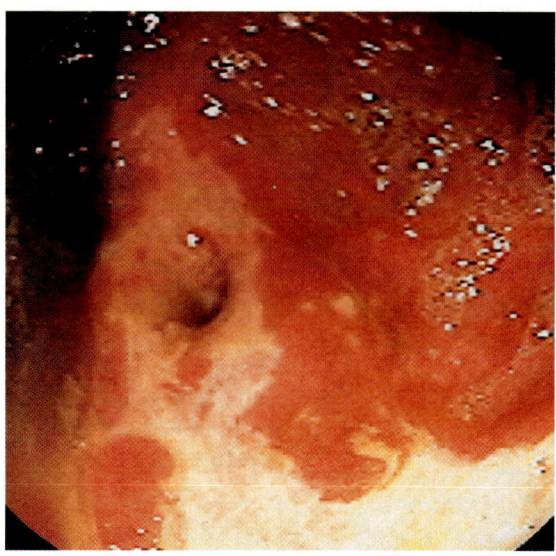

Figure 3-131: **Ileum. Pouchitis.** Large, flat, irregular ulceration in the ileoanal J-pouch. The ileum is ulcerated and stenotic as it enters the pouch.

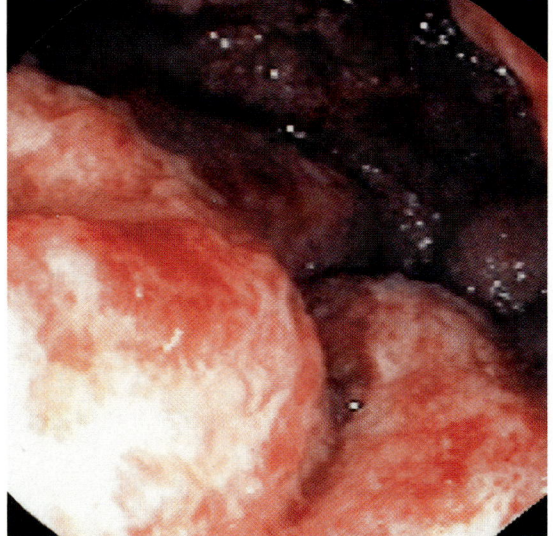

Figure 3-132: **Ileum. Pouchitis.** Severe diffuse pouchitis with edematous, granular, ulcerated mucosa that is friable and bleeds spontaneously. The appearance is identical to active inflammatory bowel disease.

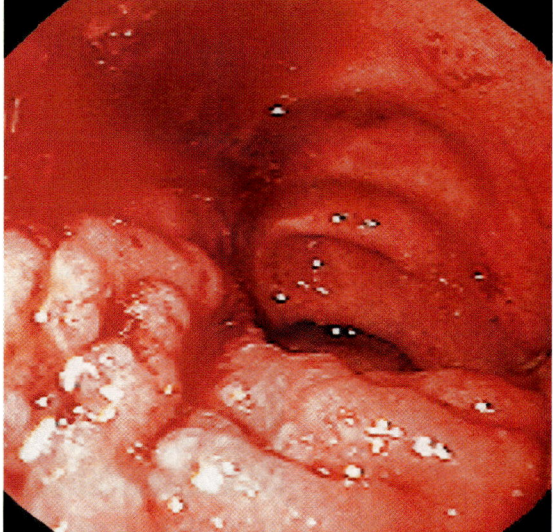

Figure 3-133: **Ileum. Pouchitis.** Thickened, nodular, ulcerated and friable patch of mucosa.

PIGMENTS

- Morphology .... Melanosis duodeni is rare. The cause is unknown but may be the result of several conditions with a similar histologic appearance. The pigment, a mixture of iron, ceroid, sulfur, and melanin, is contained in histiocytes. It is important to exclude melanin incontinence in a patient with metastatic melanoma to the small bowel. S-100 protein and HMB-45 immunostains are useful as they stain malignant melanoma cells which might otherwise be overlooked or mistaken for histiocytes.

  Iron deposition may be exogenous or the result of blood loss. Carbon pigment may be found in the mucosa and submucosa and is commonly associated with carbon (charcoal) ingestion for dyspepsia and from swallowed pulmonary secretions in smokers.

- Endoscopic features .... The "black duodenum" is distinctive, with varying shades of mucosal discoloration ranging from a subtle gray to a dark black. On close inspection, innumerable miliary pigment spots create this effect. The discoloration pattern caused by these miliary pigment spots is markedly different from the broad pigmentation of melanosis coli. Very mild cases can be overlooked.

- Clinical features .... Associated with renal dialysis, idiopathic.

- Differential diagnosis ...... Histologic and endoscopic: Malignant melanoma, hemosiderin, carbon pigment.

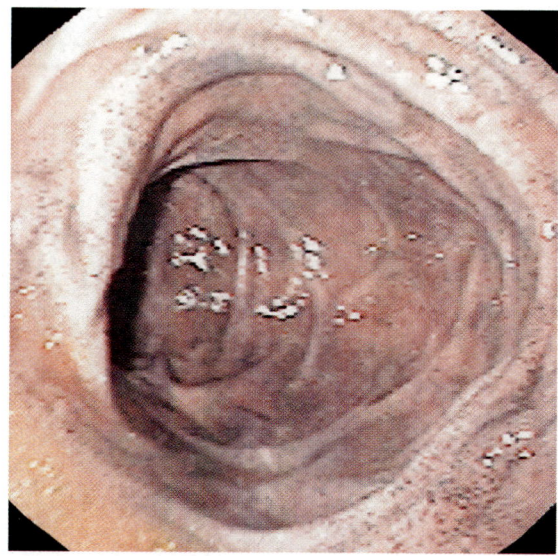

Figure 3-134: **Duodenum. Melanosis Duodeni.** The mucosa is discolored, darkened by a collection of miliary or pinpoint pigment spots. Duodenal architecture and mucosa are otherwise normal.

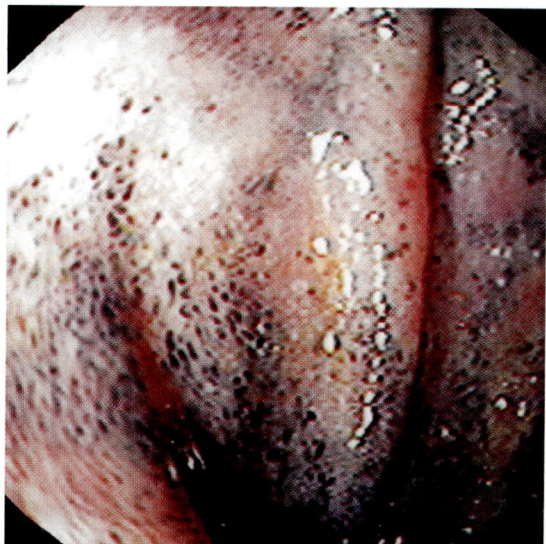

Figure 3-135: **Duodenum. Melanosis Duodeni.** Close-up of duodenal mucosa revealing numerous black miliary pigment spots. (Courtesy of Y. M. Tagouri, MD)

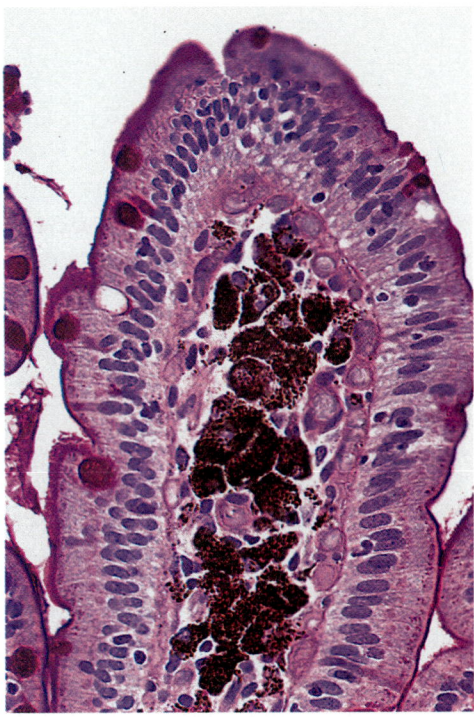

Figure 3-136: **Duodenum. Melanosis Duodeni.** Histiocytes with brown/black pigment.

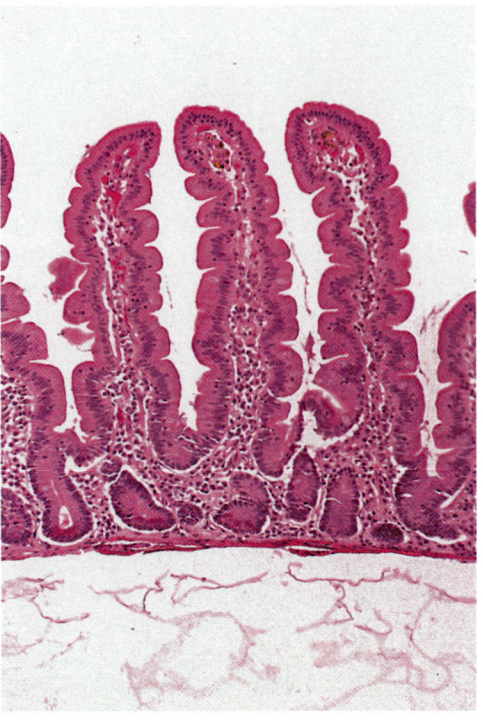

Figure 3-137: **Duodenum. Iron.** Brown pigment at tips of villi.

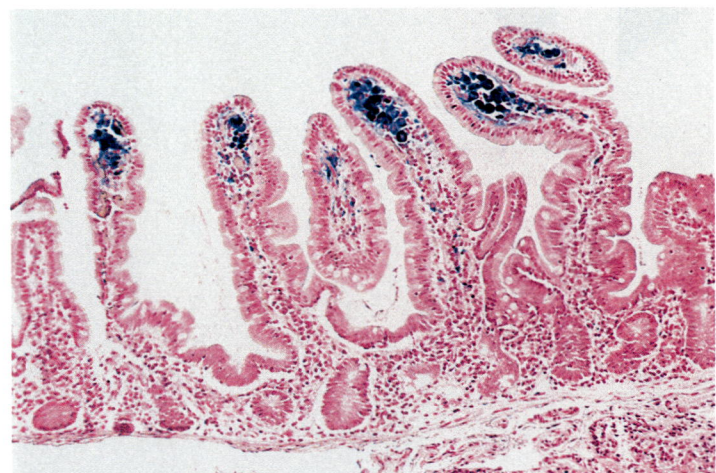

Figure 3-138: **Duodenum. Iron, Prussian Blue Stain.** Heavy staining indicating large quantity of iron at tips of villi.

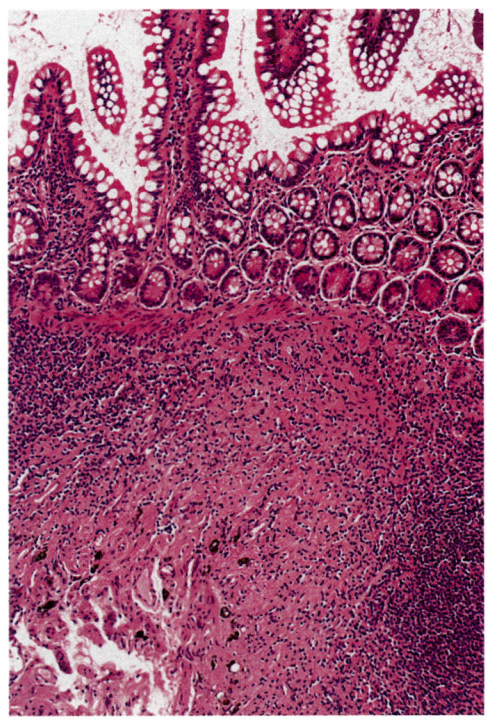

Figure 3-139: **Ileum. Carbon.** Carbon deposits in Peyer patches.

SUBMUCOSAL INFLAMMATORY MASS

- Endoscopic features .... Submucosal mass effect or marked thickening, with patchy or diffuse erythema with or without ulceration, and a purulent exudate.
- Clinical features .... Abdominal pain and sepsis.
- Differential diagnosis ...... Endoscopic: Malignant neoplasm, foreign body with intramural abscess.

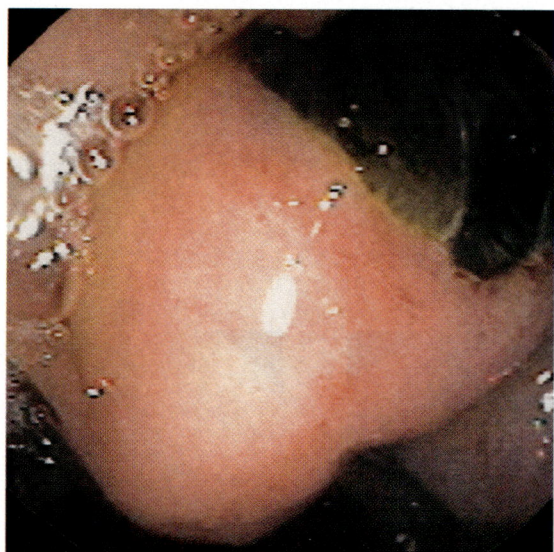

Figure 3-140: **Duodenum. Submucosal Inflammatory Mass.** Submucosal inflammatory mass in the postbulbar duodenum contiguous to the papilla of Vater. The overlying mucosa is erythematous. There is an ulcerated break in the mucosa with a bile-stained necrotic exudate. The location is suspicious for abscess and fistula related to choledocholithiasis with erosion into the intraduodenal segment of the common bile duct.

HETEROTOPIC GASTRIC MUCOSA

- Morphology .... Gastric mucosa found in the duodenum may be composed of foveolar, fundic, or antral glands. Foveolar metaplasia is common around peptic ulcers. Gastric fundic heterotopia is more common than antral heterotopia. Throughout the small bowel, antral (pyloric) metaplasia is a common consequence of chronic inflammation. Gastric antral and fundic metaplasia/heterotopia occur in Meckel diverticulum and occasionally elsewhere in the ileum or jejunum.

- Endoscopic features .... Gastric heterotopia appears as irregular sessile polypoid tissue, typically in the proximal duodenal bulb. Discrete localized nodules can resemble Brunner gland hyperplasia or various larger mucosal polyps.

- Clinical features .... None. The findings are incidental.

- Differential diagnosis ...... Histologic: Foveolar metaplasia versus pancreatic or biliary duct epithelium.

    Endoscopic: Brunner gland hyperplasia, adenomatous polyps, or other neoplastic or hamartomatous (mucosal or submucosal) lesions.

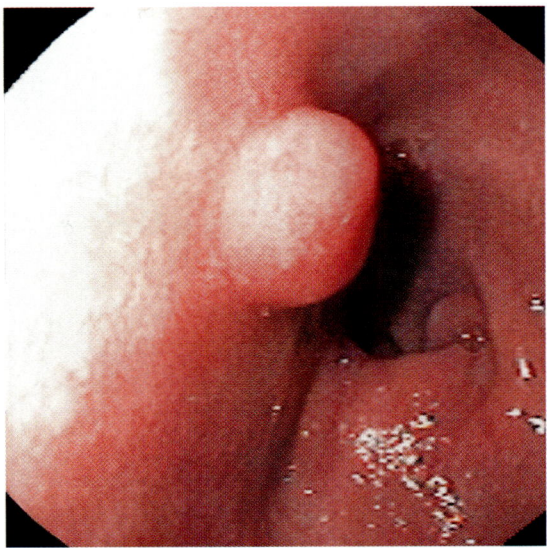

Figure 3-141: **Duodenum. Gastric Heterotopia.** Discrete, diminutive (≤ 5 mm diameter) sessile duodenal bulb polyp without hemorrhagic or ulcerative features.

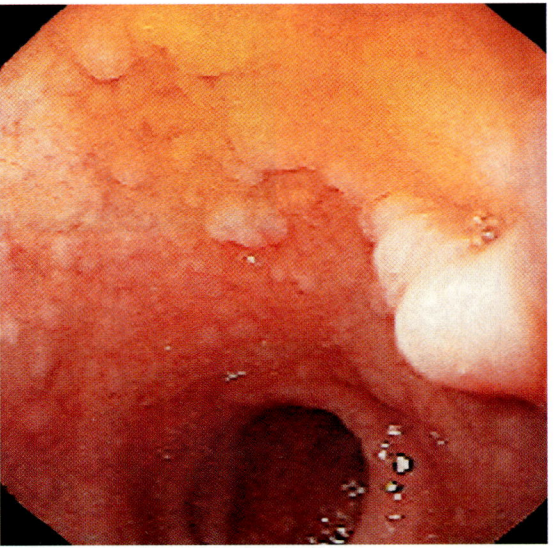

Figure 3-142: **Duodenum. Gastric Heterotopia.** A prominent ridge of polypoid tissue in the proximal duodenal bulb (right). Smaller sessile nodules in the proximal to midduodenal bulb (top).

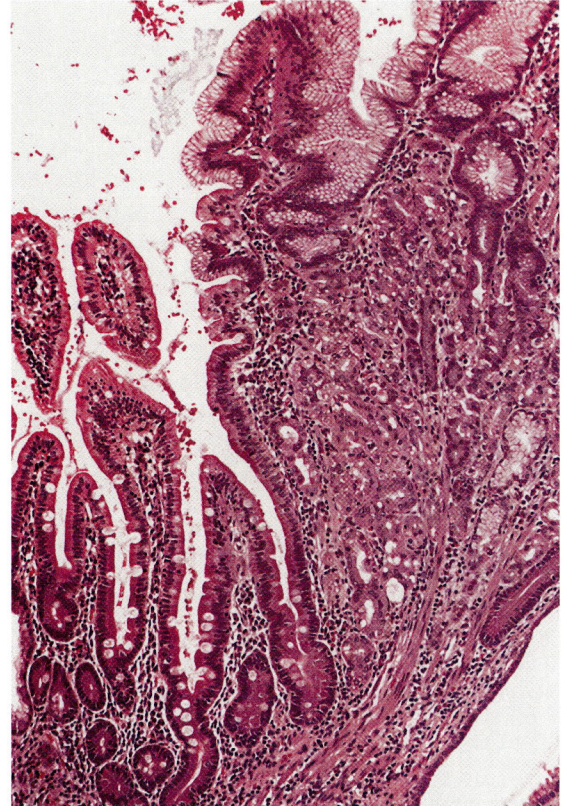

Figure 3-143: **Duodenum. Gastric Heterotopia.** Gastric foveolar epithelium and fundic glands form a nodule in small bowel mucosa.

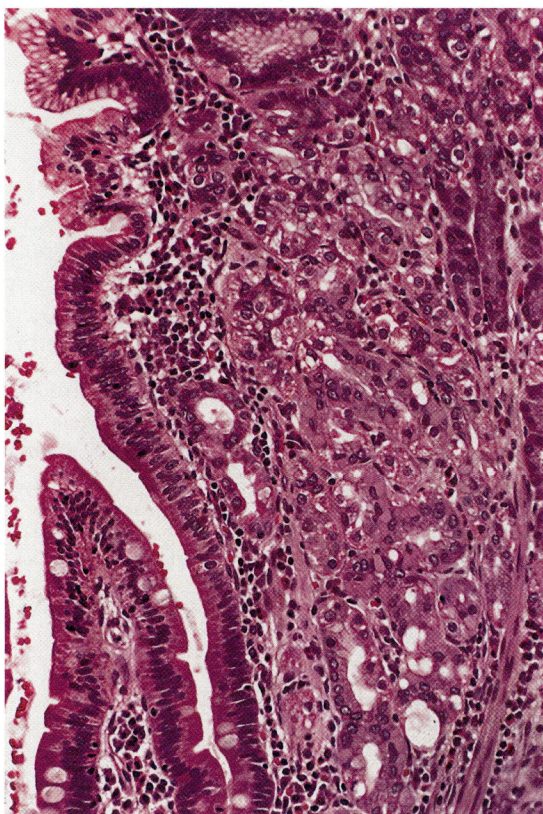

Figure 3-144: **Duodenum. Gastric Heterotopia.** Higher magnification showing gastric-type mucosa next to small bowel villus.

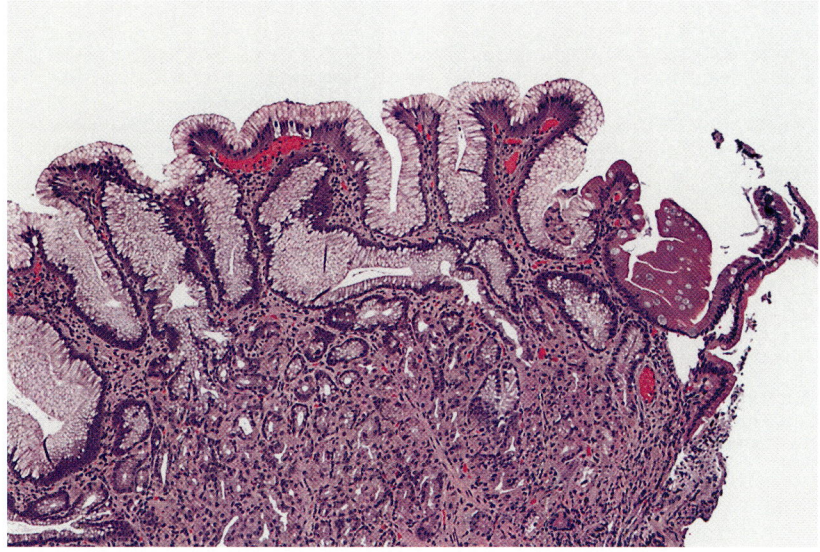

Figure 3-145: **Duodenum. Gastric Heterotopia.** Normal gastric fundic-type mucosa.

BRUNNER GLAND LESIONS

- Morphology .... Brunner gland hamartomas ("adenomas") are different from Brunner gland nodules or hyperplasia. Hamartomas are usually single, located in the bulb, and may be as large as 3 cm. They are present in mucosa and fill submucosa. Rarely, they form cystic masses that are identified by finding typical Brunner glands in the fibrous wall of the lesion.

- Endoscopic features .... Brunner gland hamartomas are discrete polypoid, sessile mucosal or submucosal nodules. They are usually in the distal duodenal bulb. When encountered in the immediate postbulbar duodenum, if they appear mucosal, they can be differentiated from a prominent minor papilla by using side-viewing duodenoscopy.

- Clinical features .... Incidental finding. Rarely, patients present with GI bleeding.

- Differential diagnosis ...... Endoscopic: Gastric heterotopia, submucosal tumors, prominent minor papilla.

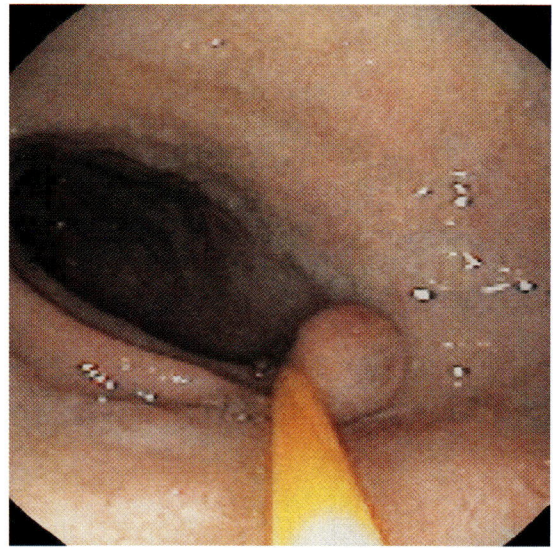

Figure 3-146: **Duodenum. Brunner Gland Hamartoma.** Discrete distal duodenal bulb submucosal nodule with intact overlying mucosa. The nodule is mobile when probed.

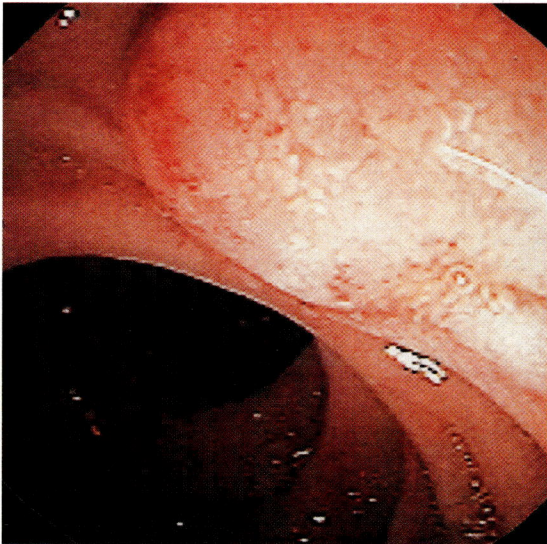

Figure 4-147: **Duodenum. Brunner Gland Hamartoma.** Small (< 1 cm in diameter) mucosal nodule in the postbulbar duodenum. The appearance is nonspecific.

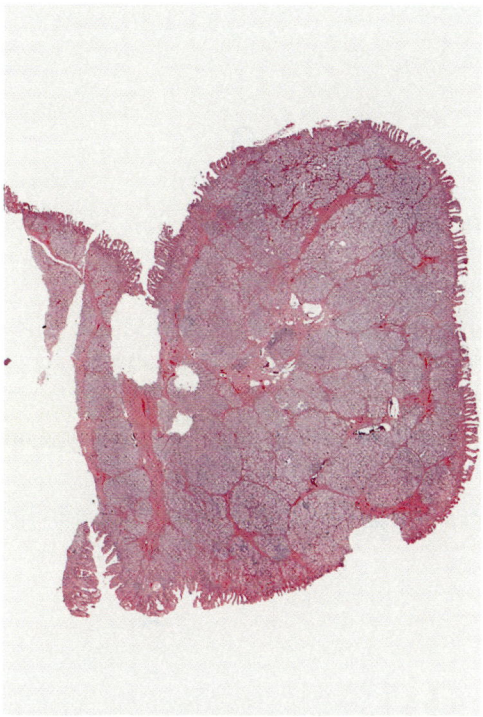

Figure 3-148: **Duodenum. Brunner Gland Hamartoma.** Large submucosal mass of Brunner gland tissue.

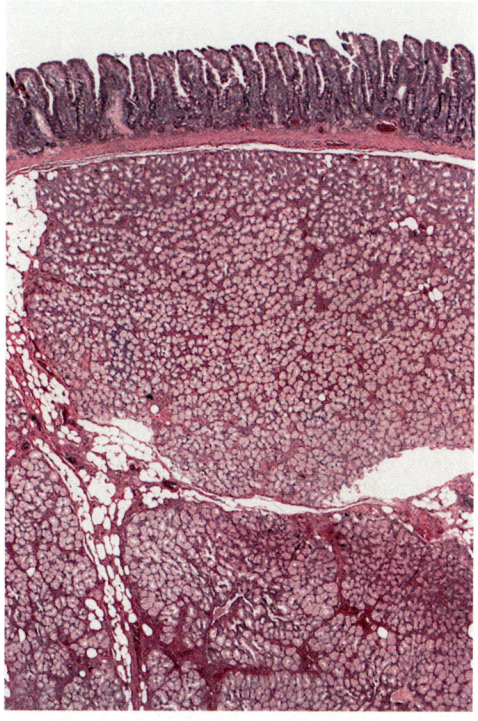

Figure 3-149: **Duodenum. Brunner Gland Hamartoma.** Typical mucous glands in lobules beneath the muscularis mucosae.

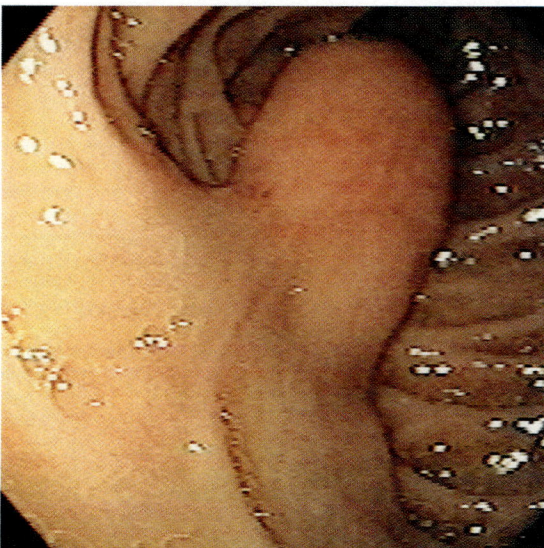

Figure 3-150: **Duodenum, Brunner Gland (Cystic) Hamartoma.** Submucosal cystic structure several centimeters in size.

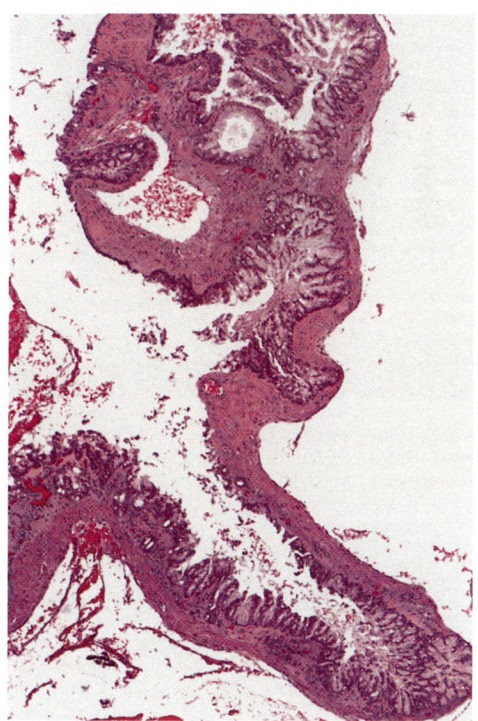

Figure 3-151: **Duodenum. Brunner Gland (Cystic) Hamartoma.** Cystically dilated Brunner glands. The cyst is lined by duct epithelium. Compressed, but otherwise typical, Brunner gland lobules were found elsewhere in the fibrous capsule.

LIPOMA

- Morphology .... Lipomas occur anywhere in the gastrointestinal tract. Biopsies of lipomas may show only normal mucosa or minimal fat. Biopsy from an ulcerated lipoma can resemble a spindle cell neoplasm.
- Endoscopic features .... Lipomas present as smooth, localized, submucosal nodules. They are mobile and the overlying mucosa is almost always intact. They may have a yellowish hue. Large lipomas tend to be pedunculated or ulcerated.
- Clinical features .... Lipomas are most often incidental findings. They may cause anemia when ulcerated, nausea and vomiting when obstructing.
- Differential diagnosis ...... Endoscopic: Leiomyoma, other submucosal tumors, e.g., carcinoid.

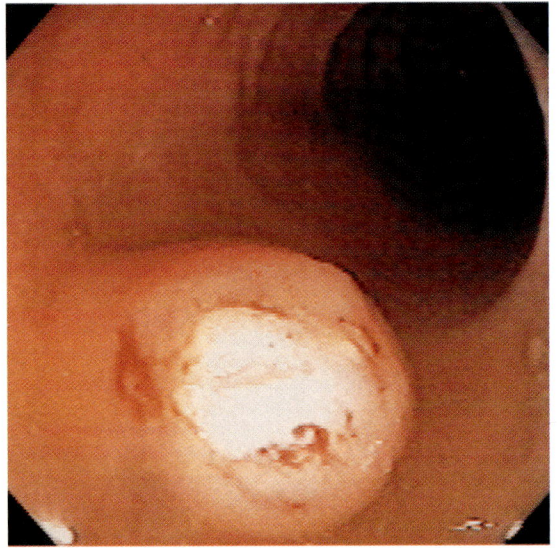

Figure 3-152: **Duodenum. Lipoma.** A 1-cm submucosal nodule in the distal duodenum encountered during push enteroscopy. Biopsy revealed fatty tissue.

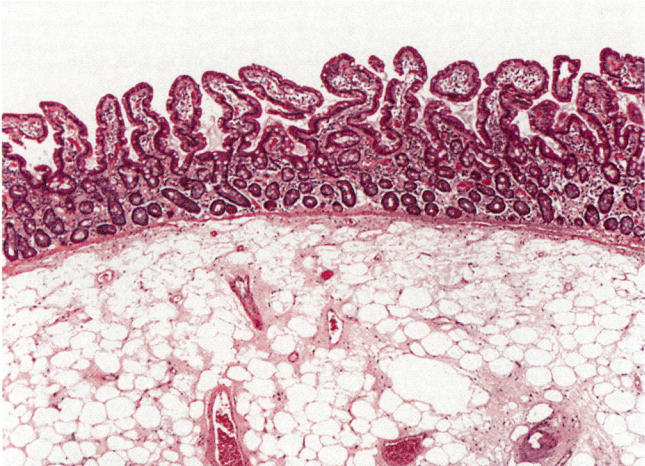

Figure 3-153: **Small Intestine. Lipoma.** Submucosal fat compresses the muscularis mucosae.

HYPERPLASTIC POLYP

- Morphology .... Hyperplastic polyps of the small intestine arise from gastric heterotopia in the duodenum. They are identical to hyperplastic polyps of the stomach and are characterized by marked foveolar hyperplasia with cystic dilatation and expanded, edematous, and inflamed lamina propria. They may be up to 6 cm in diameter.
- Endoscopic features .... Hyperplastic polyps vary in size and may be extremely large and friable. When located in the duodenal bulb, large polyps can prolapse into the stomach and cause obstruction.
- Clinical features .... Gastric outlet obstruction due to large polyps, occult GI blood loss.
- Differential diagnosis ...... Histologic and endoscopic: Other hamartomatous polyps and inflammatory polyps.

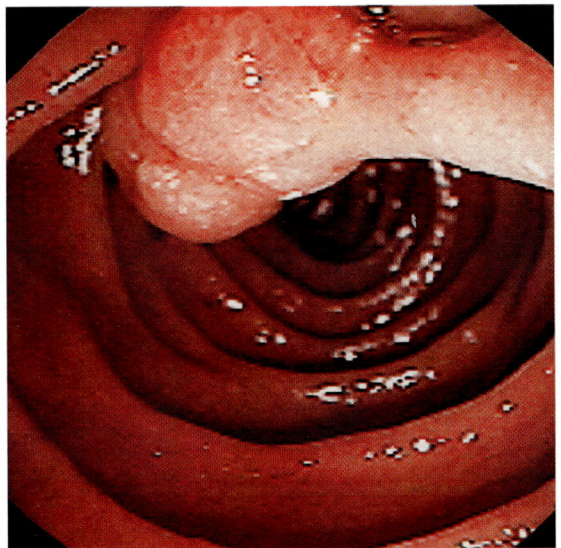

Figure 3-154: **Duodenum. Hyperplastic Polyp (of Gastric Type).** A multilobular pedunculated polyp extending from the apical portion of the duodenal bulb. The stalk appears similar to the head of the polyp.

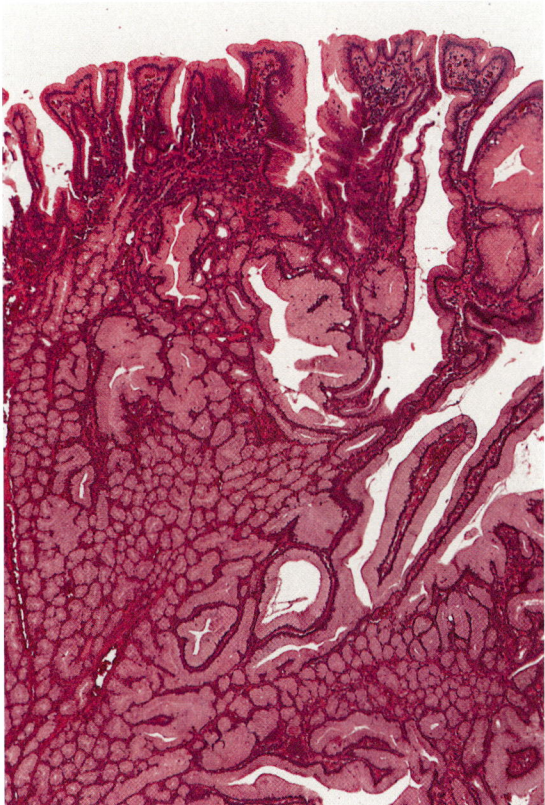

Figure 3-155: **Duodenum. Hyperplastic Polyp (of Gastric Type).** Heterotopic antral mucosa with tortuous elongated foveolae (foveolar hyperplasia).

INFLAMMATORY FIBROID POLYP

- Morphology .... Pale spindle cells with eosinophils expand the submucosa and infiltrate, and eventually ulcerate, the mucosa. The eosinophils are an intrinsic part of the process but vary in intensity. Mucosal biopsies of inflammatory fibroid polyps have been confused with eosinophilic enteritis. Small blood vessels are evenly distributed and typically have a concentric, perivascular, onion-skin orientation of fibrous cells, or are sclerotic. With intussusception, the deeper lesional tissue may infiltrate the muscularis propria.

- Endoscopic features .... Generally located within the jejunum or ileum, they are submucosal in appearance, often solitary, large, and pedunculated, but smaller sessile nodules may be encountered.

- Clinical features .... Abdominal pain, nausea and vomiting due to intussusception, GI blood loss secondary to mechanical irritation of the involved and surrounding mucosa. These benign, tumorlike lesions can occur at any age.

- Differential diagnosis ...... Histologic: Eosinophilic enteritis, stromal tumors.

    Endoscopic: Other polyps, submucosal neoplasms.

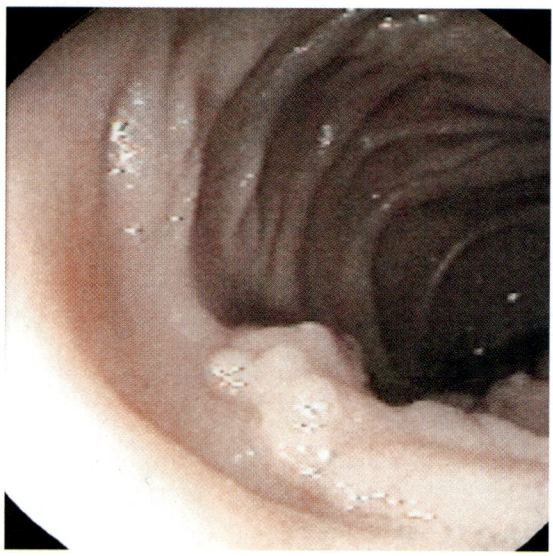

Figure 3-156: **Jejunum. Inflammatory Fibroid Polyp.** A cluster of minute polyps or nodules seen during push enteroscopy. The mucosa is intact.

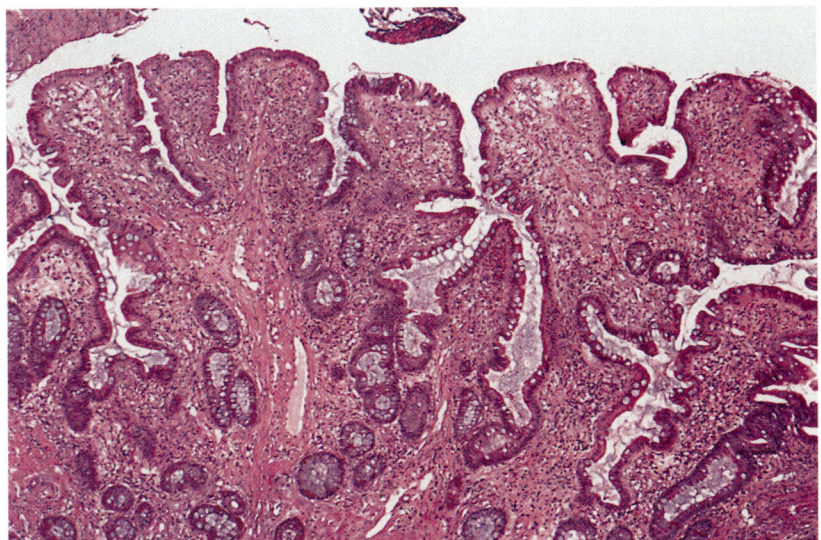

Figure 3-157: **Small Intestine. Inflammatory Fibroid Polyp.** When the submucosal process extends into the mucosa, the villi are broad and distorted; crypts are long and tortuous.

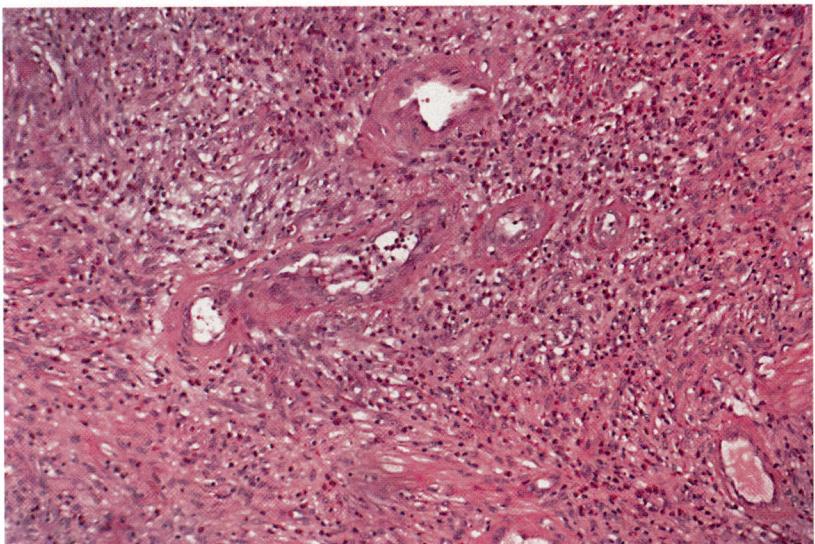

Figure 3-158: **Small Intestine. Inflammatory Fibroid Polyp.** Submucosa infiltrated by spindle cells with pale nuclei and interspersed eosinophils. Vessels are sclerotic.

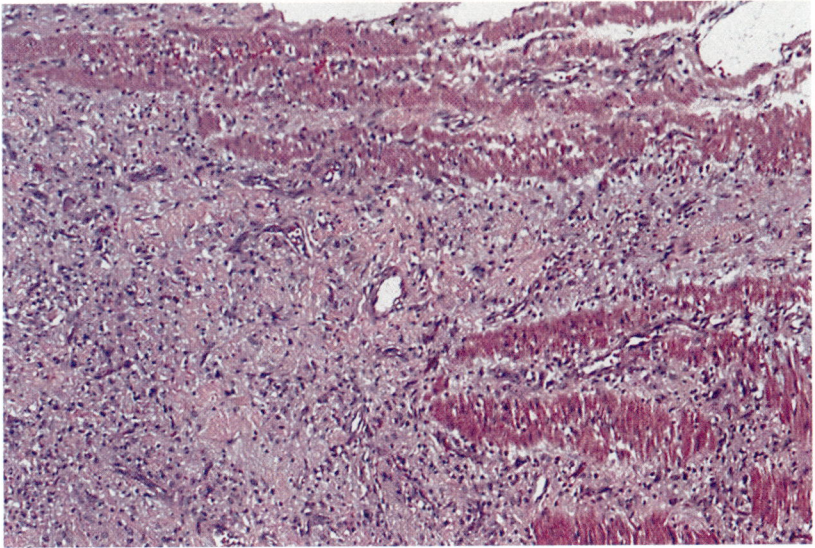

Figure 3-159: **Small Intestine. Inflammatory Fibroid Polyp.** The polyp stroma separates the muscularis propria, characteristic of small bowel rather than gastric lesions.

PEUTZ-JEGHERS POLYP

- Morphology .... Peutz-Jeghers polyps are hamartomas composed of well-organized mucosa on an arborizing muscular framework. The epithelium of the polyps is hyperplastic, but similar to the adjacent mucosa. Pseudoinvasive herniation occurs in about 10% of jejunal-ileal Peutz-Jeghers polyps and can simulate invasive mucinous adenocarcinoma. Pseudoinvasion appears to be related to intussusception and can be transmural.

- Endoscopic features .... Peutz-Jeghers polyps are often multiple and scattered throughout the small intestine. They vary from small sessile polyps to large pedunculated lesions that are friable and bleed spontaneously.

- Clinical features .... Occult and overt GI blood loss, recurrent small intestinal obstruction secondary to intussusception.

- Differential diagnosis ...... Histologic: Adenomas and carcinomas when there is pseudoinvasion.

    Endoscopic: Any mucosal polyp.

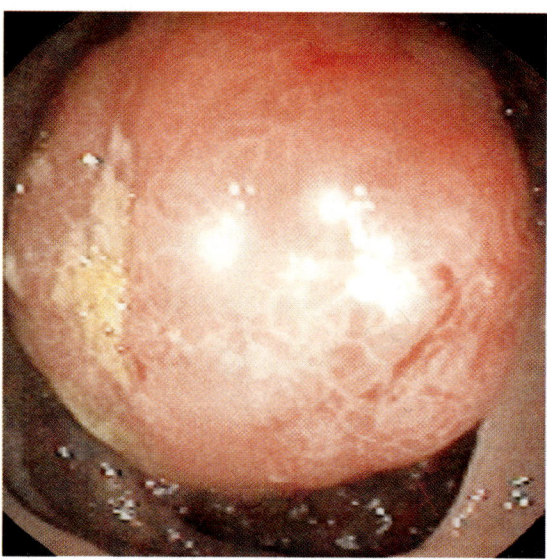

Figure 3-160: **Jejunum. Peutz-Jeghers Polyp.** Large hemorrhagic polyp nearly fills the bowel lumen.

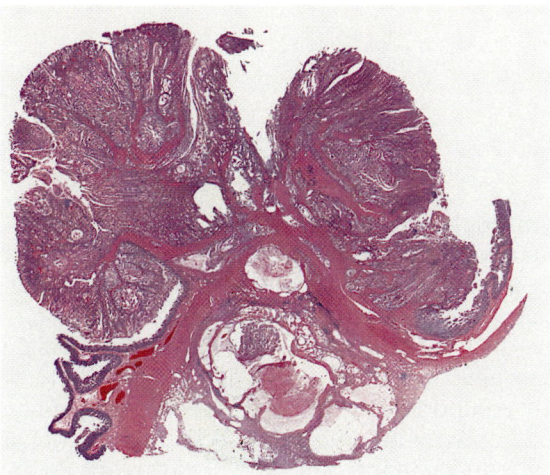

Figure 3-161: **Small Intestine. Peutz-Jeghers Polyp with Pseudoinvasion.** Cystic structures in muscularis propria and mesentery beneath a typical Peutz-Jeghers polyp.

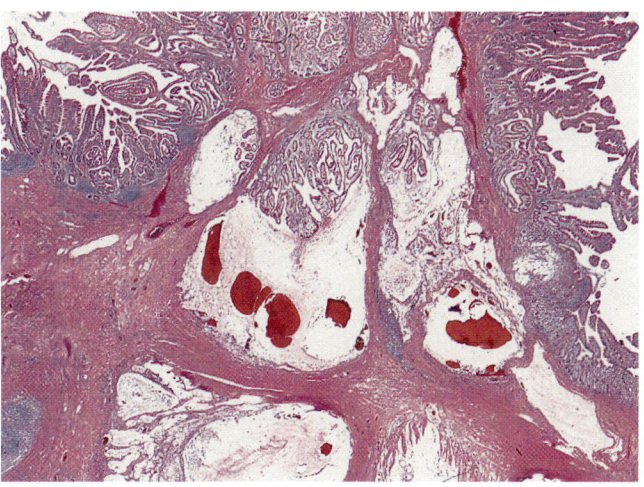

Figure 3-162: **Small Intestine. Peutz-Jeghers Polyp.** Cystic structures contain displaced small bowel mucosa, mucin, and hemorrhage.

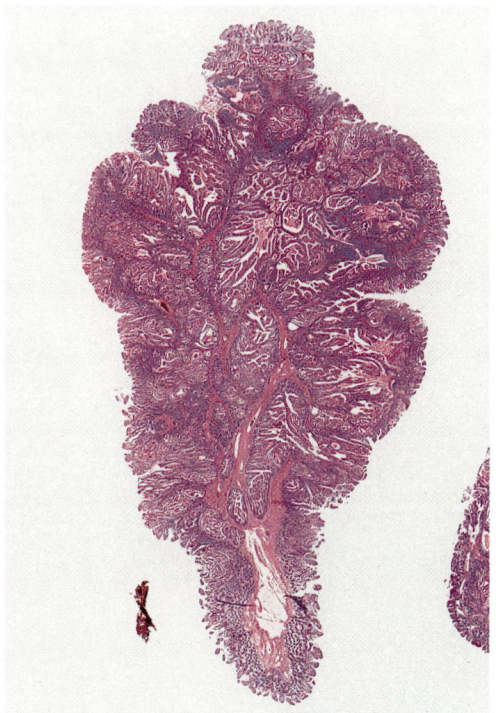

Figure 3-163: **Small Intestine. Peutz-Jeghers Polyp.** Arborizing smooth muscle covered by proliferative small bowel-type mucosa.

PANCREATIC HETEROTOPIA

- Morphology .... Pancreatic heterotopia occurs throughout the small bowel. In the distal small bowel it is most often found in a Meckel diverticulum. In the duodenum it forms a submucosal mass with a central dimple which is the duct opening. Small biopsies usually are not deep enough to detect the heterotopic pancreatic tissue, but may obtain the duct that is lined by cells indistinguishable from gastric foveolar cells. There are 3 histologic forms of pancreatic heterotopia defined by the pancreatic components present. In order of frequency, they are (1) pancreatic ducts admixed with smooth muscle (myoepithelial hamartoma), (2) pancreatic ducts and acinar tissue, and (3) pancreatic ducts, acinar tissue, and endocrine islets.

- Endoscopic features .... Pancreatic heterotopia (pancreatic rest) in the duodenum appears as a small submucosal nodule with a characteristic central depression or dimple.

- Clinical features .... None. These are typically incidental findings.

- Differential diagnosis ...... Endoscopic: Other submucosal masses.

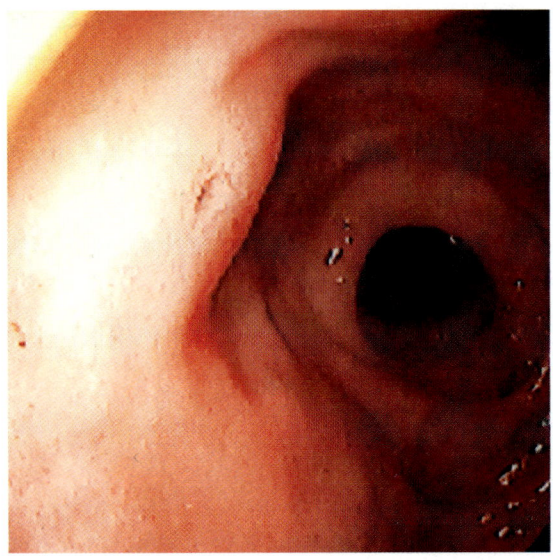

Figure 3-164: **Duodenum. Pancreatic Heterotopia.** A small nodule in the duodenal bulb contains a minute central depressed area. The nodule was soft to probing.

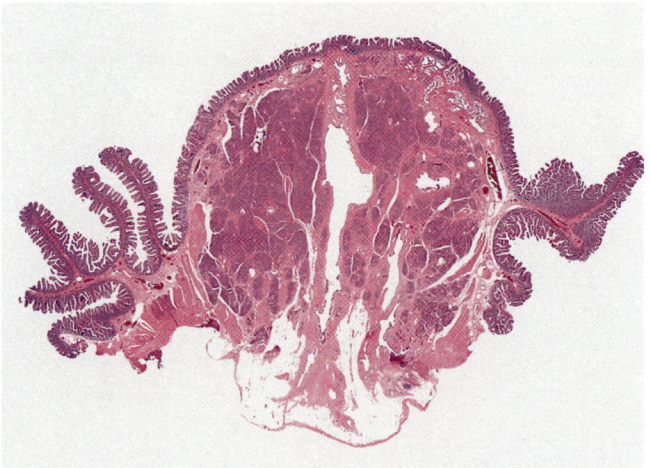

Figure 3-165: **Duodenum. Pancreatic Heterotopia.** Submucosal mass of pancreatic tissue bulges into lumen. Centrally located, longitudinally sectioned duct extends toward the surface.

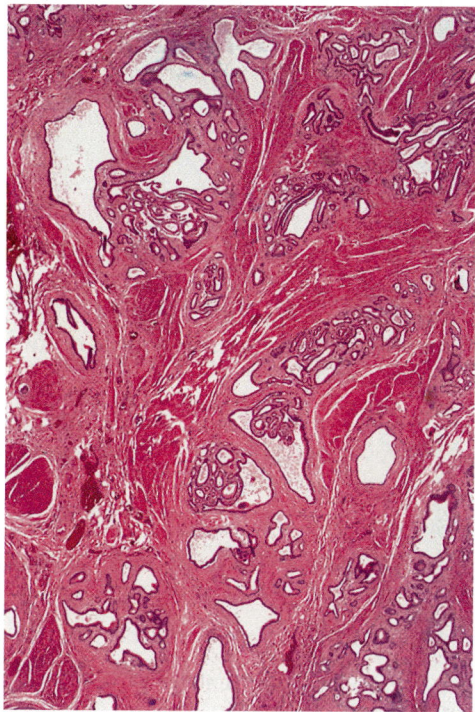

Figure 3-166: **Duodenum. Pancreatic Heterotopia.** Submucosal mass composed of clusters of pancreatic ducts separated by smooth muscle (myoepithelial hamartoma).

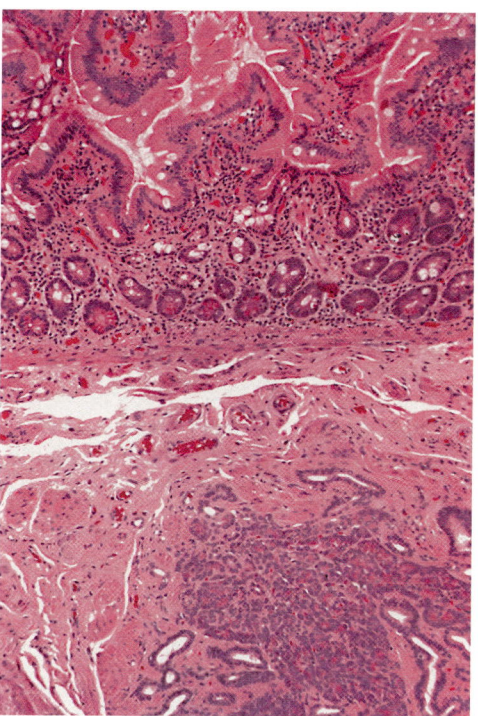

Figure 3-167: **Duodenum. Pancreatic Heterotopia.** Pancreatic ducts and acinar tissue beneath the mucosa.

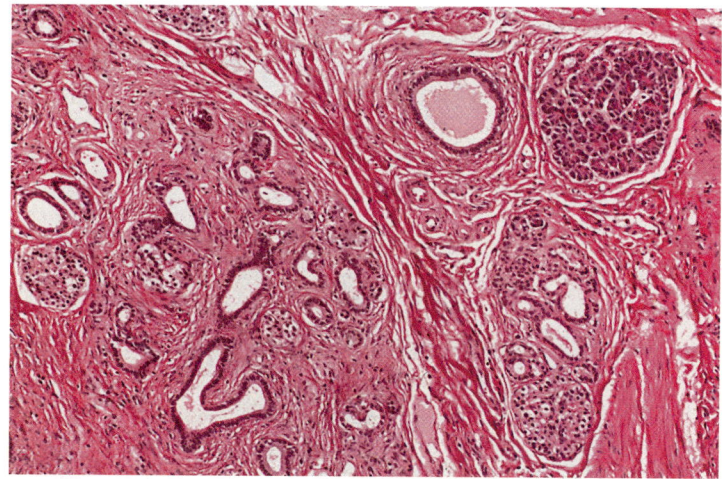

Figure 3-168: **Duodenum. Pancreatic Heterotopia.** All components (ducts, acini, islets) are present.

GANGLIOCYTIC PARAGANGLIOMA

- Morphology .... Rare submucosal tumors usually of the periampullary duodenum; may extend into the mucosa. There are several patterns: ribbon, trabecular, insular, and spindled with rare to numerous ganglion cells. They resemble carcinoids. They generally behave in an indolent manner, but may infiltrate locally and have rarely metastasized to regional lymph nodes. Positive for chromogranin, S-100 protein, and GFAP.

- Endoscopic features .... Encountered during endoscopy of the duodenum and jejunum, this lesion is indistinguishable from any other exophytic neoplasm. Larger lesions can be friable and ulcerated, and may bleed spontaneously.

- Clinical features .... Acute intermittent gastrointestinal bleeding and bleeding of obscure origin are the most common presentations of symptomatic gangliocytic paragangliomas. Some patients have abdominal discomfort.

- Differential diagnosis...... Histologic: Carcinoid tumor, ganglioneuroma, neurofibroma.

    Endoscopic: Any mucosal-submucosal neoplasm.

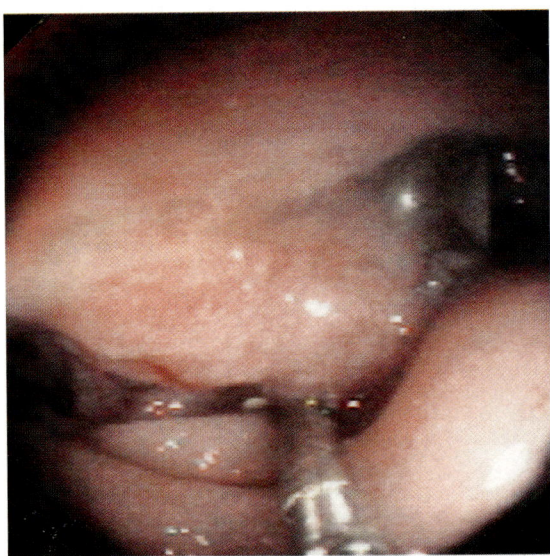

Figure 3-169: **Jejunum. Gangliocytic Paraganglioma.** In the center of the photograph, deep pink, nodular tissue with an irregular surface is probed with a biopsy forceps. To the left there is a small amount of blood. This lesion, located on the mouth of a jejunal diverticulum, was encountered during push enteroscopy.

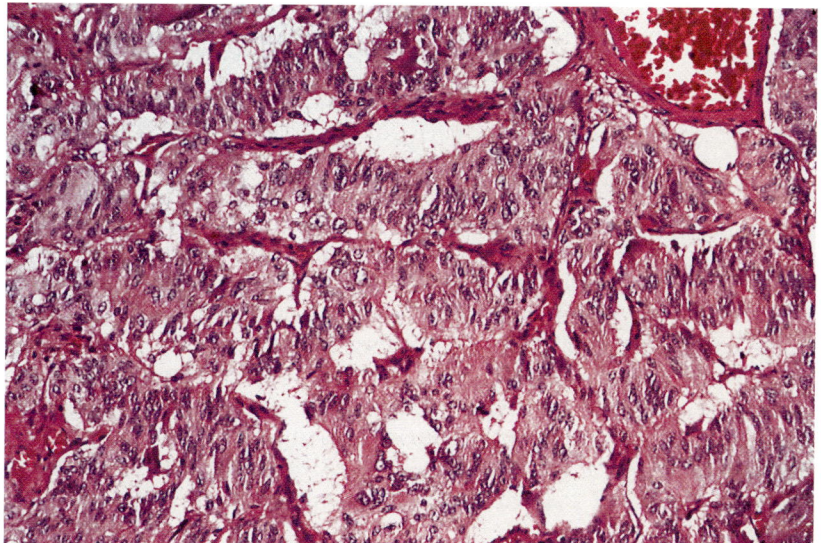

Figure 3-170: **Duodenum. Gangliocytic Paraganglioma.** Ribbons of uniform epithelial cells with abundant amphophilic cytoplasm and round to oval nuclei.

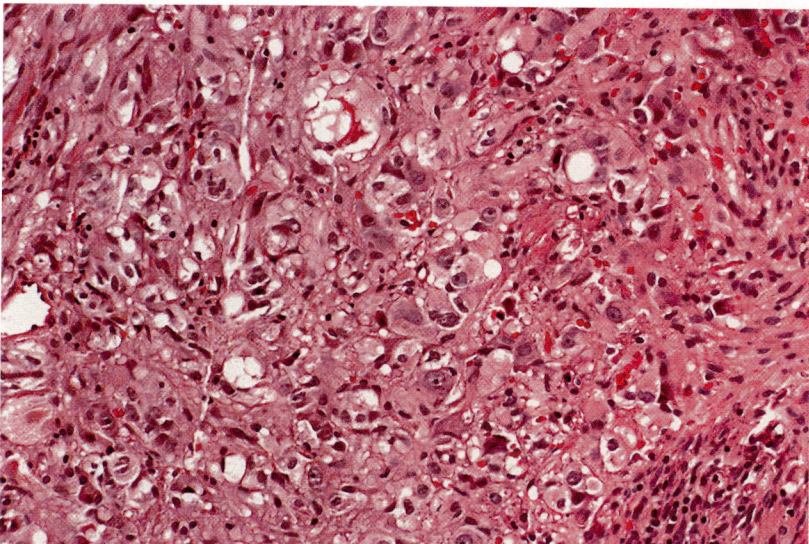

Figure 3-171: **Duodenum. Gangliocytic Paraganglioma.** Numerous ganglion cells interspersed with nests of epithelioid cells and spindle (Schwann) cells.

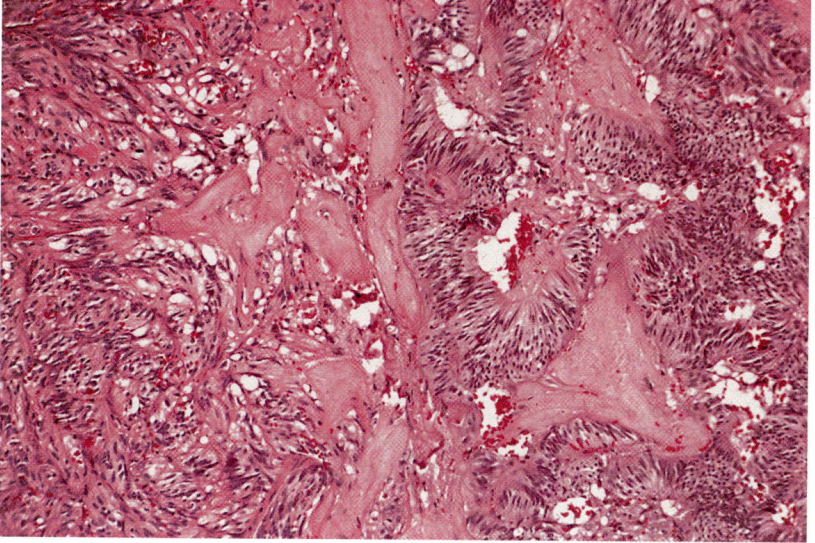

Figure 3-172: **Duodenum. Gangliocytic Paraganglioma.** Ribbons of cells separated by hyalinized stroma.

SCHWANNOMA

- Morphology .... Schwannomas of the small intestine are benign spindle cell neoplasms that should be distinguished from histologically similar, often malignant, gastrointestinal stromal tumors and smooth muscle neoplasms. While the typical pattern of schwannomas in soft tissues may be present (e.g., compact and palisaded spindle cell fascicles alternating with loose edematous tissue infiltrated by small lymphocytes, hyalinized thick-walled vessels), usually it is not. In the digestive tract these tumors have a characteristic rim of lymphoid follicles at the periphery, a useful identifying marker. Immunostains for S-100 protein are strongly and diffusely positive and help to separate schwannomas from other gastrointestinal stromal tumors.

- Endoscopic features .... The schwannoma is a submucosal nodular mass with a propensity for central ulceration. More often encountered in the duodenum than distally.

- Clinical features .... Gastrointestinal bleeding if ulcerated. May be associated with von Recklinghausen disease.

- Differential diagnosis ...... Histologic: Gastrointestinal stromal tumors, smooth muscle tumors.

    Endoscopic: Any submucosal tumor or tumorlike lesion.

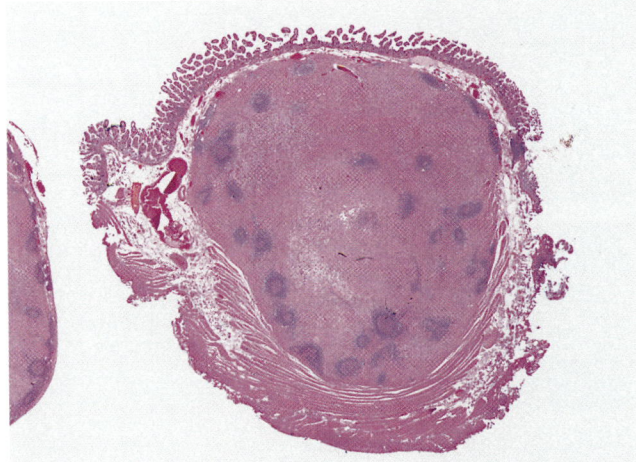

Figure 3-173: **Small Intestine. Schwannoma.** Submucosal spindle cell neoplasm with surrounding and interspersed lymphoid follicles.

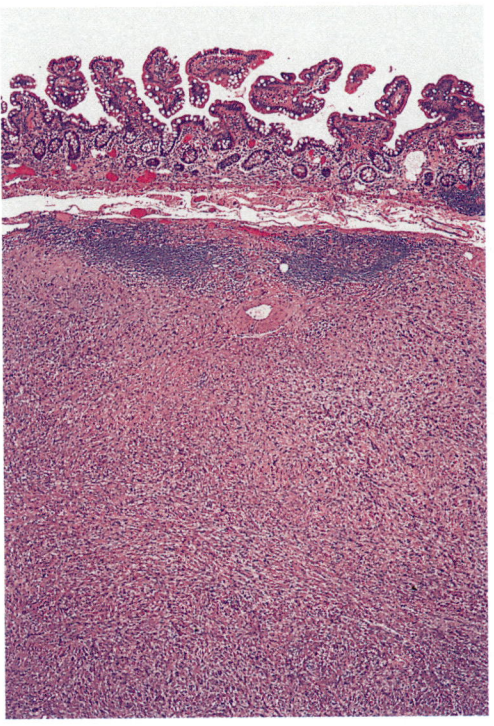

Figure 3-174: **Small Intestine. Schwannoma.** Submucosal spindle cell neoplasm. Lymphoid follicles help distinguish this from other stromal tumors. S-100 protein was diffusely and strongly positive immunohistochemically.

NEUROFIBROMA

- Morphology .... Very rare in the small intestine, this benign tumor is located in the submucosa, extends into the mucosa, and is composed of widely separated bland spindle cells in a wavy pink background of cell cytoplasm and collagen fibers. Focal staining for S-100 in the context of light microscopic features confirms the diagnosis.
- Endoscopic features .... Submucosal mass or nodule with or without ulceration in the duodenum or ileum. Some may extend into the mucosa and resemble other mucosal polyps.
- Clinical features .... None, or occult GI blood loss. May be isolated, nonsyndromatic, or associated with von Recklinghausen disease, especially if multiple or plexiform.
- Differential diagnosis...... Histologic: Paraganglioma, stromal tumors such as schwannoma and leiomyoma.

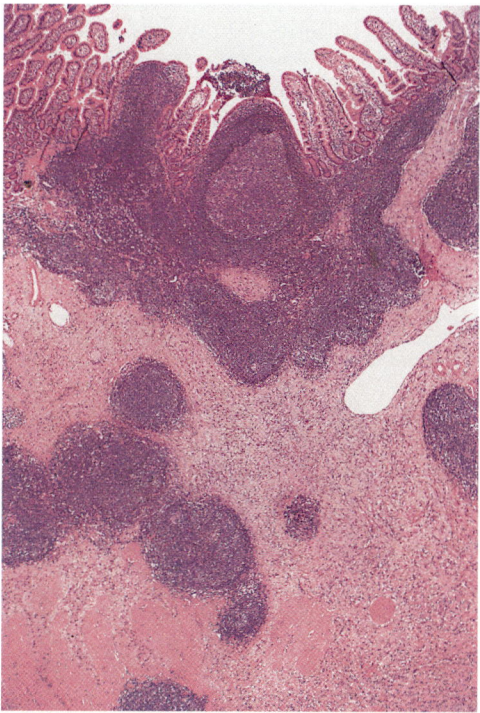

Figure 3-175: **Ileum. Neurofibroma.** Submucosa expanded by pink paucicellular infiltrative stromal cells with lymphoid follicles.

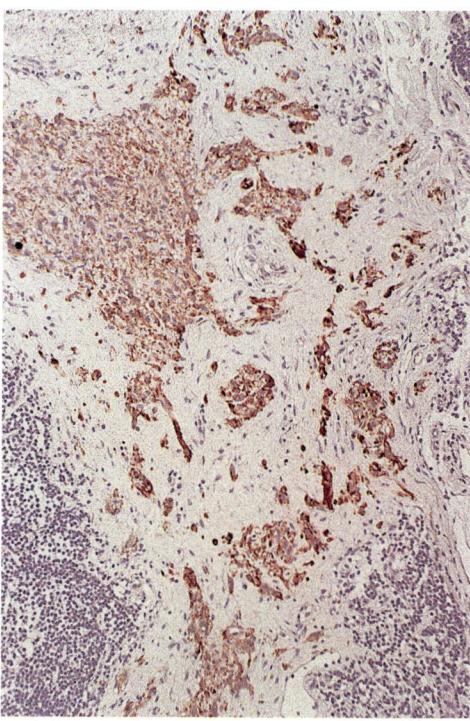

Figure 3-176: **Small Intestine. Neurofibroma.** Strong focal S-100 protein staining in bland spindle cells supports Schwann cell differentiation and contrasts with "wall-to-wall" S-100 protein positivity of schwannomas.

CARCINOID TUMOR

- Morphology .... Carcinoid tumor is a term applied to low-grade neuroendocrine tumors. They are composed of uniform cells with amphophilic cytoplasm, round nuclei, and inconspicuous nucleoli and are arranged in nests, ribbons, cords, glands, and trabeculae. Mitotic figures are scarce. More aggressive atypical or intermediate-grade carcinoid tumors have increased numbers of mitotic figures and sometimes areas of necrosis. Large carcinoids elicit a desmoplastic response that causes kinking of the bowel wall and symptoms of obstruction. Psammoma bodies are a feature of somatostatin-producing periampullary tumors; subnuclear eosinophilic granules are often seen in those producing serotonin. Serotonin production is most common in ileal (and appendiceal) carcinoids and gastrin is more common in duodenal carcinoids. All carcinoids have metastatic potential, however, those less than 2 cm typically behave indolently. The carcinoid syndrome occurs in cases with liver metastasis.

- Endoscopic features .... Often multiple, small intestinal carcinoids are submucosal nodules and masses that are usually yellow. In the duodenum, a small submucosal nodule located in the duodenal bulb is typical. In the ileum, they are generally larger and may ulcerate.

- Clinical features .... Most common in middle-aged patients. Duodenal carcinoids may cause obstruction or symptoms due to peptide secretion. Distal small bowel carcinoids cause obstructive symptoms such as abdominal pain, and vomiting due to kinking from mesenteric involvement. Ulcerated ileal carcinoids cause acute, episodic, or occult gastrointestinal bleeding.

- Differential diagnosis...... Histologic: Primary or metastatic carcinoma.

    Endoscopic: Heterotopic pancreas, stromal tumors, neurofibromas, lipomas.

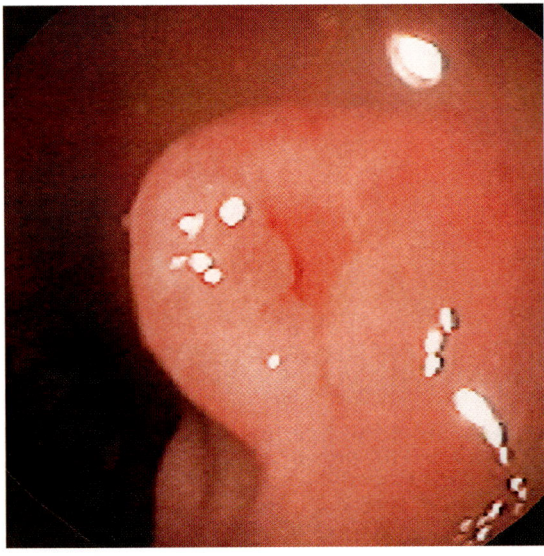

Figure 3-177: **Duodenum. Carcinoid Tumor.** Small irregular mucosal nodule in the duodenal bulb with a centrally depressed area.

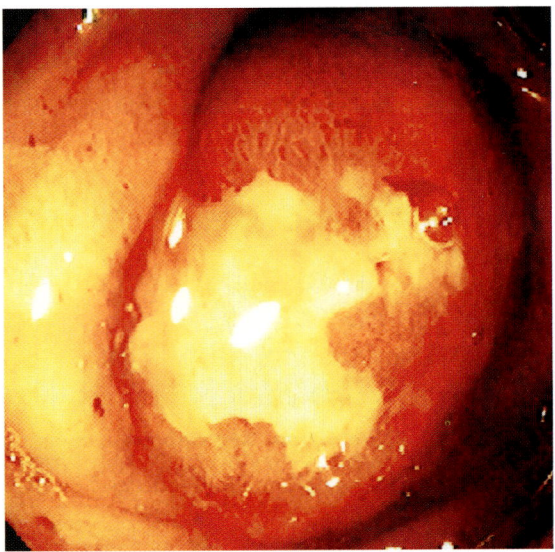

Figure 3-178: **Ileum. Carcinoid Tumor.** Ulcerated, hemorrhagic, submucosal polyp in terminal ileum.

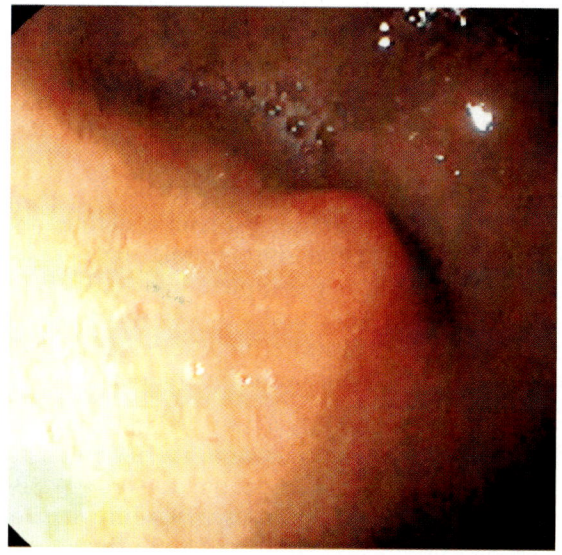

Figure 3-179: **Small Intestine. Carcinoid Tumor.** Diminutive duodenal bulb submucosal nodule.

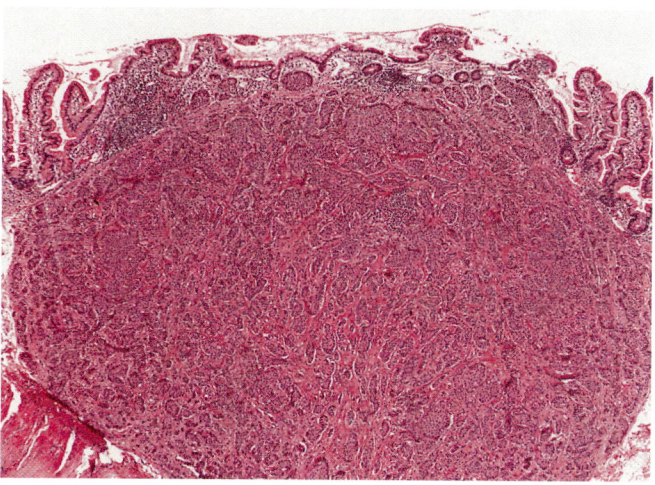

Figure 3-180: **Small Intestine. Carcinoid Tumor.** Well-demarcated tumor fills submucosa and extends into the atrophic, compressed mucosa with flattened villi.

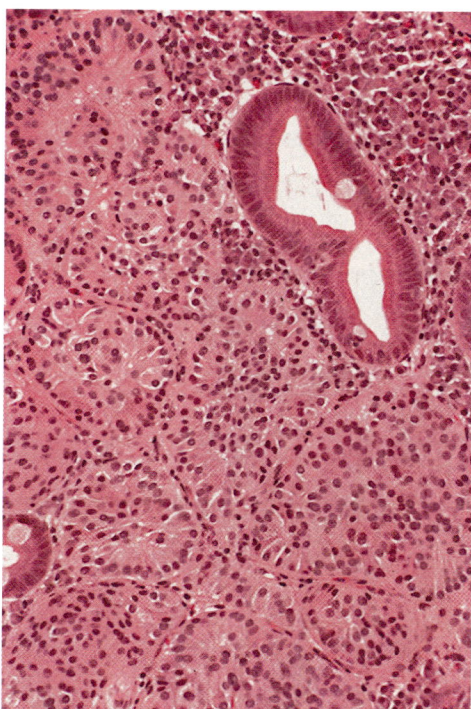

Figure 3-181: **Small Intestine. Carcinoid Tumor.** Bland, uniform, polygonal cells in nests in lamina propria.

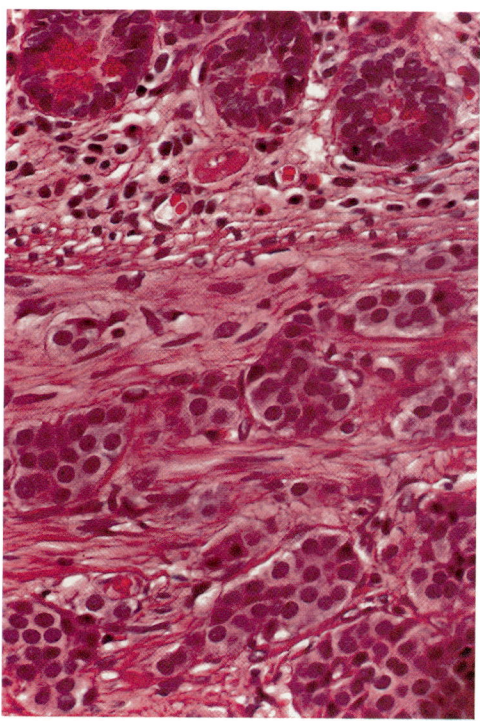

Figure 3-182: **Small Intestine. Carcinoid Tumor.** Nests of amphophilic cells with round nuclei and inconspicuous nucleoli separated by a fibrous stroma.

ADENOMA

- Morphology — Adenomas are, by definition, dysplastic. Low-grade dysplasia is defined as nuclear stratification confined to the base of the epithelium. High-grade dysplasia is characterized cytologically by either complete loss of nuclear polarity or anaplastic nuclear changes, or architecturally by low-grade cytology with architectural complexity, e.g., cribriform structure, back-to-back crypts. Small intestinal adenomas are most common in the duodenum.

- Endoscopic features — When small, they typically have a white surface, a feature that may be striking. When large, the polyps are erythematous and multilobulated, similar to large sessile colonic adenomas. In familial adenomatous polyposis syndrome, they are usually multiple, sometimes numerous, pale white, sessile polyps, which may lie on the tops of the circular folds or carpet the entire mucosa (Fig. 3-189). Large villous adenomas are sessile, friable, and may ulcerate, a feature favoring malignancy.

- Clinical features — Large sporadic adenomas are associated with ulceration and occult GI blood loss. If sufficiently large, they may obstruct. Adenomas of the small intestine in patients with FAP syndrome are asymptomatic. The discovery of a duodenal adenoma in a young patient should raise the possibility of familial adenomatous polyposis.

- Differential diagnosis — Endoscopic: Small polyps: other mucosal polyps and heterotopias. Large villous polyps: carcinoma and lymphoma.

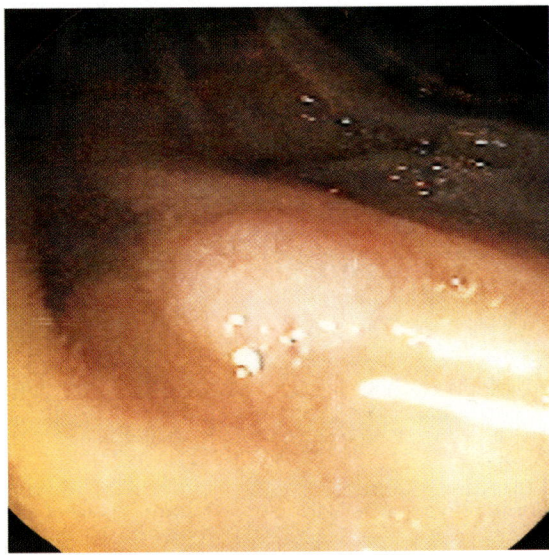

Figure 3-183: **Jejunum. Tubular Adenoma.**
Diminutive sessile polyp in the jejunum encountered during push enteroscopy for GI bleeding of obscure origin.

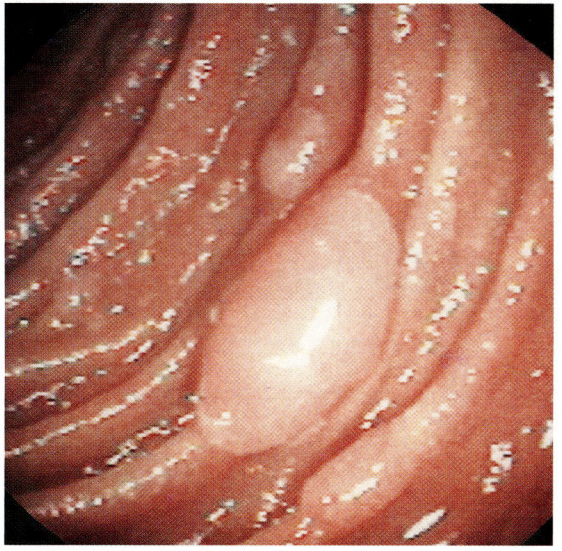

Figure 3-184: **Duodenum. Tubular Adenomas.** Multiple sessile polyps on the circular folds in a patient with familial adenomatous polyposis. The polyps are smooth. There is whitish coloration to the margins of the largest polyp.

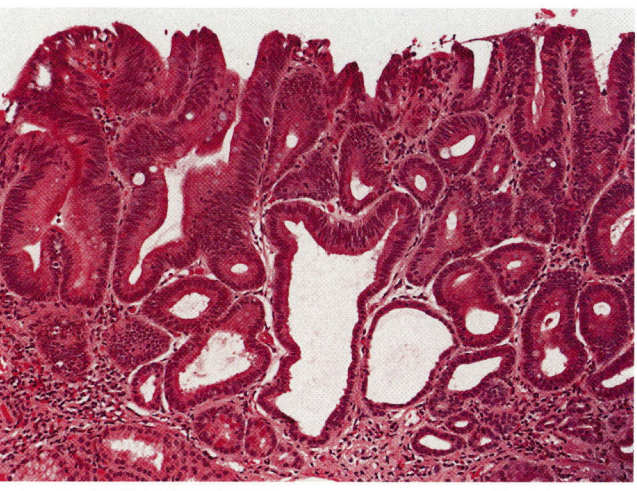

Figure 3-185: **Small Intestine. Tubular Adenoma.** Dysplastic cells line crypts and the flattened surface.

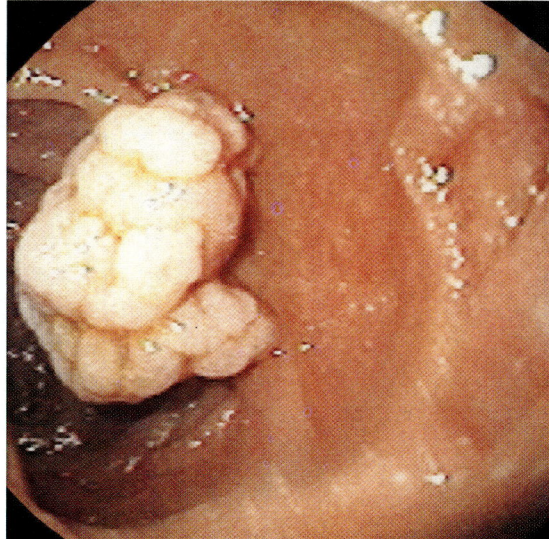

Figure 3-186: **Duodenum. Tubulovillous Adenoma.** A large, pale whitish, sessile neoplasm in the post-bulbar duodenum.

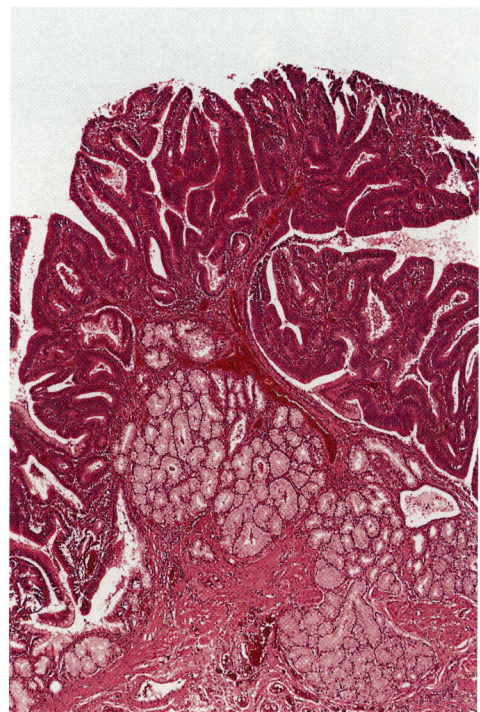

Figure 3-187: **Duodenum. Tubulovillous Adenoma.** Dysplastic cells line crypts and villi.

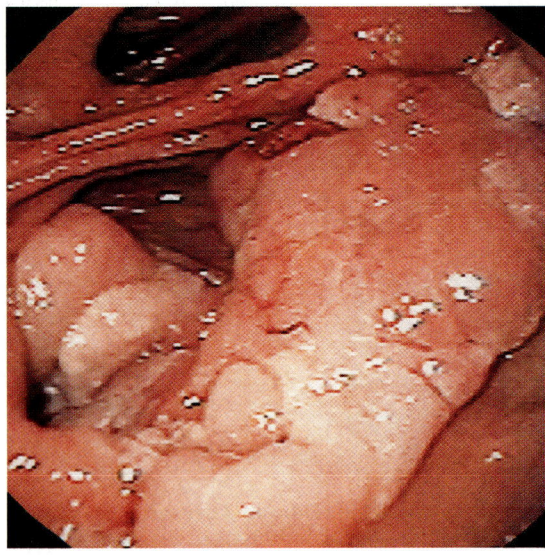

Figure 3-188: **Duodenum. Tubulovillous Adenoma.** Large sessile polyp in the postbulbar duodenum along the margin of, and extending into, a large diverticulum around the papilla of Vater (periampullary adenoma). The polypoid tissue has an irregular surface and a characteristic whitish appearance in some areas.

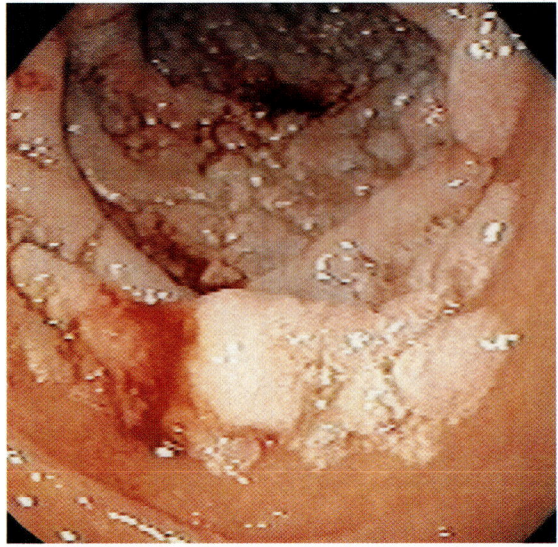

Figure 3-189: **Duodenum. Villous Adenoma.** Sessile neoplasm with an irregular, white, nodular surface carpets and circumferentially involves a segment of the postbulbar duodenum. Although not ulcerated, spontaneous bleeding is evident.

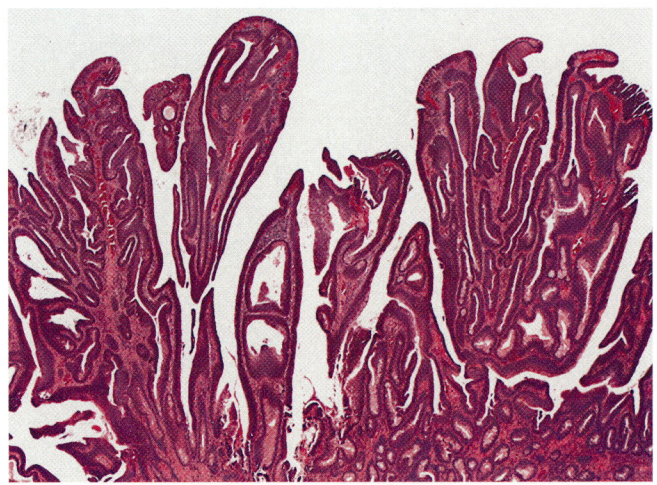

Figure 3-190: **Small Intestine. Villous Adenoma.** Dysplastic epithelium with villous architecture.

AMPULLARY ADENOMA

- Morphology .... Adenomas arise in the ampulla, in periampullary duodenal mucosa, or in the transition zone between the two. It is neither possible nor necessary to determine the point of origin from biopsy specimens. Dysplastic epithelium may grow into periampullary accessory glands that are normally mingled with muscle and connective tissue and mimic invasive carcinoma. Invasion is often focal, therefore, a biopsy which shows only adenoma does not necessarily exclude adenocarcinoma.

- Endoscopic features .... Ampullary adenomas have a wide range of presentations. In very early stages there may be a subtle polypoid change involving the papilla of Vater, coarsening its appearance. Especially in familial adenomatous polyposis, the adenomatous tissue may extend inferiorly below the papilla in a triangular "goatee" distribution. With more advanced growth, the papilla becomes disfigured, enlarged, or replaced with variegated white and pink polypoid tissue, which extends into the duodenal hood surrounding the papilla as well. With further progression, the polypoid tissue extends onto the duodenal mucosa and the duodenal hood. The endoscopic definition for this latter situation is that of a periampullary adenoma with polypoid changes involving the papilla and surrounding duodenum within 2 cm of the papilla.

- Clinical features .... Sporadic ampullary adenomas may present with unexplained abdominal pain, episodic pancreatitis, and cholestasis. Syndromatic patients with familial adenomatous polyposis and variants are predisposed to develop ampullary adenomas, which are asymptomatic until the advanced stage when the biliary system or pancreas becomes obstructed.

- Differential diagnosis ...... Histologic and endoscopic: Periampullary carcinoma. Following liver transplantation, there may be exuberant overgrowth of **reactive tissue at the** papilla or sphincterotomy site, resembling an adenoma.

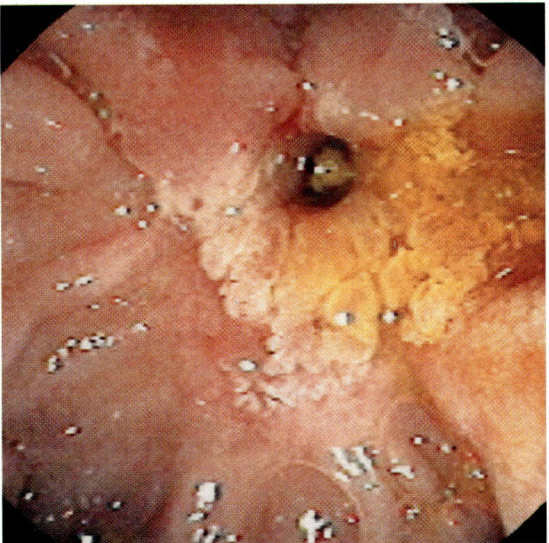

Figure 3-191: **Ampulla of Vater. Tubular Adenoma.** Sessile polypoid tissue with irregular margins surrounds the common bile duct orifice in a patient who had a prior transduodenal excision of a periampullary adenoma with sphincteroplasties of the pancreatic and bile ducts. Bile covers the mucosa, which in areas is variegated white and deep pink. The pancreatic duct opening, indistinct in this view, is located below the common bile duct terminus at the margin of the distal extension of the polyp.

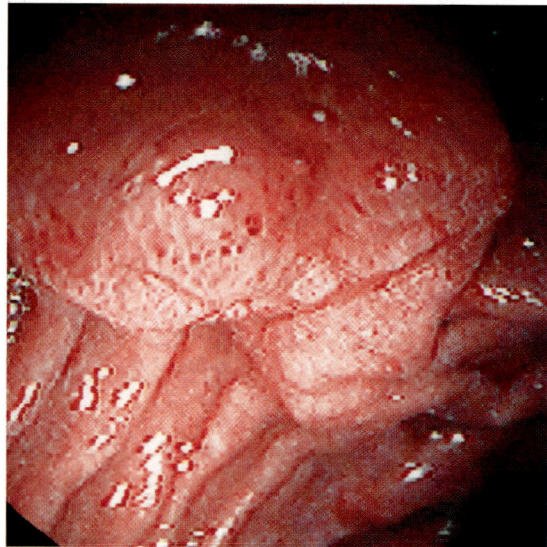 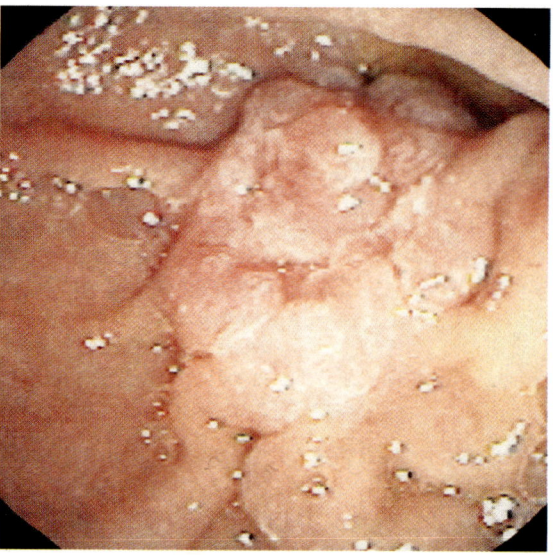

Figure 3-192: **Ampulla of Vater. Tubular Adenoma.** Periampullary adenoma with polypoid changes involving the papilla and overlying duodenal hood. The polypoid tissues have coarse, irregular surface features and blur the boundaries between the papilla and the duodenal hood. The polyp extends distally in a "goatee" fashion. There is a small area of spontaneous bleeding.

Figure 3-193: **Ampulla of Vater. Tubular Adenoma.** Periampullary adenoma in a patient with familial adenomatous polyposis syndrome. The papilla and surrounding duodenal tissues are grossly polypoid with irregular surface features and coloration characteristic of adenomas in this location.

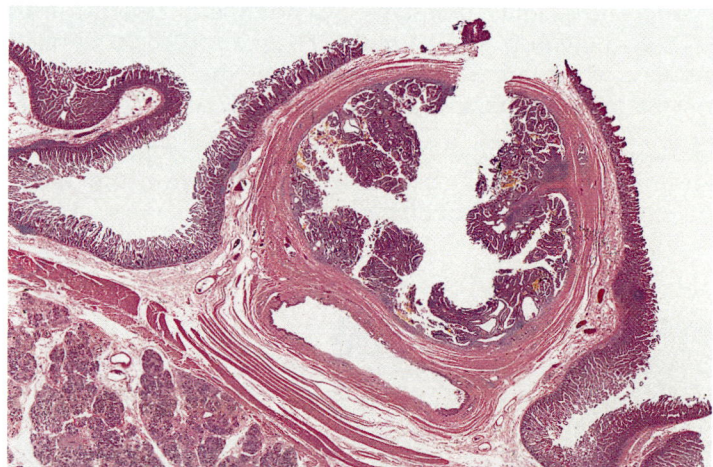 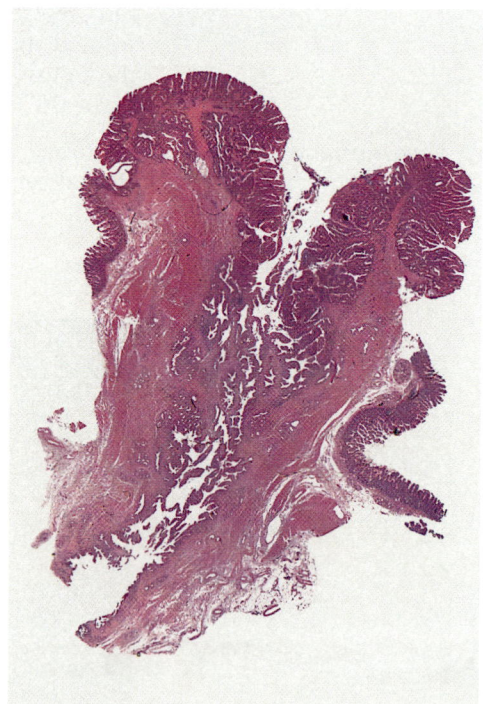

Figure 3-194: **Ampulla of Vater. Tubular Adenoma.** Ampullary adenoma. Dysplastic epithelium with villous architecture lines ampulla. Duodenal mucosa is normal.

Figure 3-195: **Ampulla of Vater. Tubular Adenoma.** Ampullary/periampullary adenoma. Dysplastic epithelium involves ampullary ostium and duodenal mucosa.

ADENOCARCINOMA

- Morphology .... Adenocarcinoma primary in the small intestine is uncommon. It usually arises in a background of chronic inflammation, as in celiac sprue, Crohn, and protein-losing enteropathy, or from sporadic adenomas or adenomas in polyposis syndromes, e.g., familial adenomatous polyposis and hamartomatous polyposis syndromes. It may be impossible to distinguish primary adenocarcinoma from metastatic disease without evidence of a preexisting adenoma or predisposing chronic inflammatory process.

- Endoscopic features .... Adenocarcinoma of the duodenum is often detected in advanced stages, when it becomes large and obstructing. Most are exophytic, polypoid, and ulcerated; they may be focal or circumferential.

- Clinical features .... Gastrointestinal bleeding of obscure origin, unexplained abdominal pain, partial small bowel obstruction.

- Differential diagnosis ...... Histologic and endoscopic: Primary versus metastatic adenocarcinoma. Endoscopic: Adenoma, other malignancies such as melanoma, lymphoma, or sarcoma.

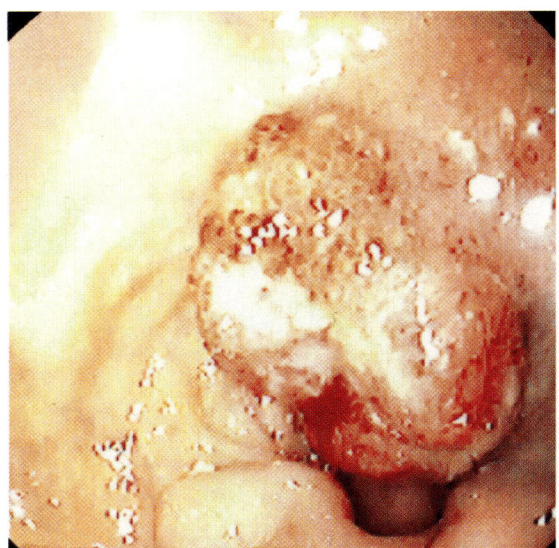

Figure 3-196: **Duodenum. Adenocarcinoma.** Polypoid, ulcerated, spontaneously bleeding neoplasm. The surface is irregular, hard to palpation, and bleeds briskly with contact. These features, in addition to the color changes and stenotic lumen seen in the distance, suggest malignancy.

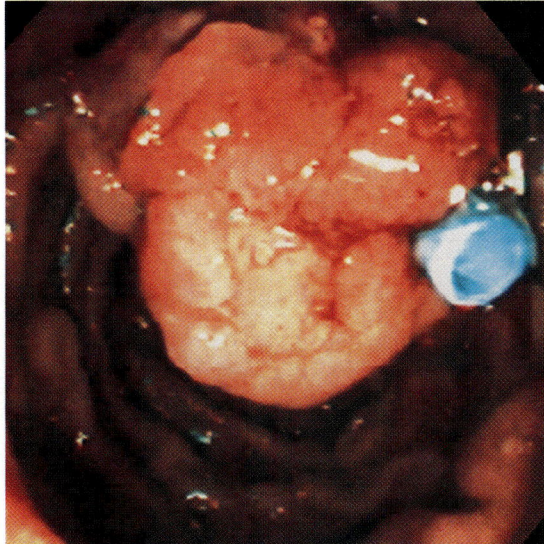

Figure 3-197: **Ampulla of Vater. Adenocarcinoma.** Complete replacement of the papilla and surrounding periampullary tissues with a large polypoid neoplasm extending well into the duodenal lumen. The tumor is firm and friable. A plastic biliary stent has been placed through the tumor into the common bile duct to decompress the obstructed biliary tree.

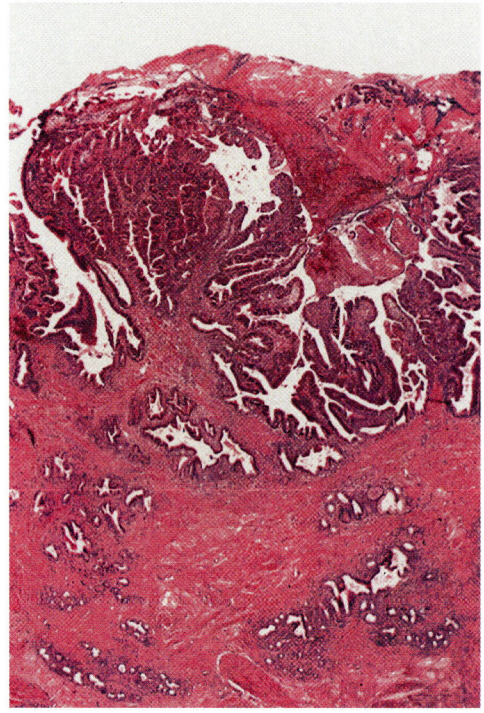

Figure 3-198: **Ampulla of Vater. Adenocarcinoma.** Irregular, well-differentiated glands invade periampullary stroma. Remnant of adenoma. Uniform, regularly spaced accessory glands are deep to the invasive carcinoma.

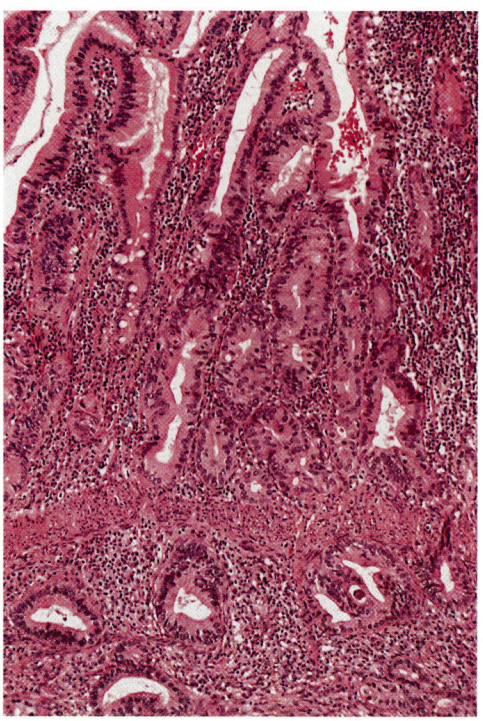

Figure 3-199: **Terminal Ileum. Adenocarcinoma.** Well-differentiated adenocarcinoma in an area of active Crohn's disease.

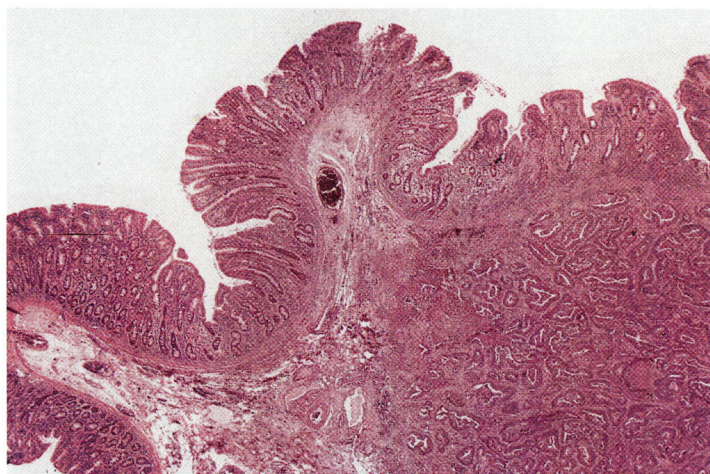

Figure 3-200: **Duodenum. Adenocarcinoma.** Invasive adenocarcinoma in patient with celiac sprue. The adjacent mucosa is flat and inflamed, features typical of sprue.

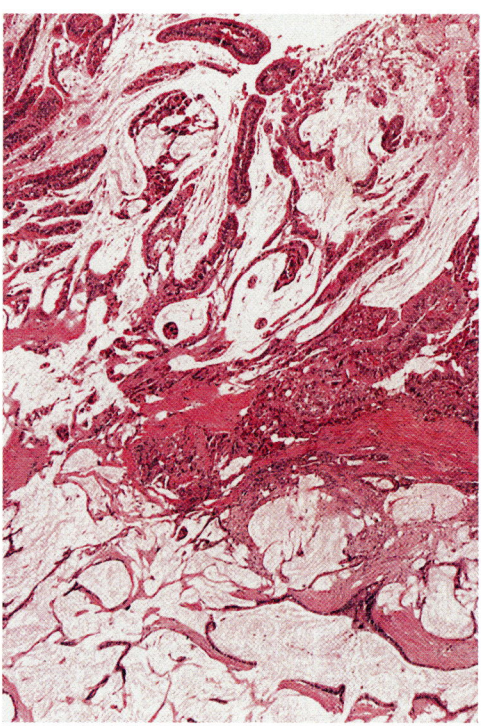

Figure 3-201: **Duodenum. Mucinous Adenocarcinoma.** Well-differentiated tumor cells float in pools of mucin.

MALIGNANT LYMPHOMA

- Morphology — The gastrointestinal tract is the most common site of primary extranodal lymphoma. On mucosal biopsy it may be difficult or impossible to diagnose lymphoma because of the small size of the specimen, and because inflammation is a normal component of intestinal mucosa. The majority of lymphomas, whether primary or secondary, are B-cell lymphomas. MALT lymphoma (extranodal marginal zone lymphoma of mucosa-associated lymphoid tissue) is associated with foci of epithelial destruction by small lymphocytes. MALT lymphoma may evolve into large cell lymphoma. T-cell lymphoma of the gastrointestinal tract is less common, but is a known complication of celiac sprue. It has also been associated with lymphocytic colitis. Often there is only thickening of the mucosal folds endoscopically and ulcer without a well-defined mass.

  Follicular lymphoma (follicle center cell lymphoma) may involve the gastrointestinal tract and appear as submucosal polyps. On small biopsy specimens it may be mistaken for lymphoid hyperplasia or Peyer patches. The lack of germinal centers and presence of monotonous small cleaved lymphocytes are helpful features. Immunostains help to confirm the diagnosis.

- Endoscopic features — Lymphoma involving the small intestine may be nodular or polypoid and is the color of the surrounding mucosa. There may be distinct nodules that range up to 5 mm. These can coalesce and become heaped up forming large tumors. The infiltrate can be more diffuse, efface the circular folds, and cause mucosal thickening, friability, spontaneous bleeding, and ulceration. In patients with sprue, lymphoma may be subtle, as demonstrated in Fig. 3-202. T-cell lymphomas may have the appearance of an ulcerative jejunoileitis (Fig. 3-203).

- Clinical features — Patients present with vague abdominal pain, weight loss, anorexia, or symptoms of obstruction. Small intestinal lymphomas account for nearly half of the malignancies in patients with celiac sprue, usually occurring many years after the diagnosis of sprue. Symptoms include weight loss, diarrhea, and abdominal pain. Bleeding and bowel perforation may also occur. Ulcerative jejunitis may be an inflammatory complication of sprue, a manifestation of lymphoma, or a separate entity, which involves multiple deep ulcers of the jejunum and ileum. Symptoms include bleeding, malabsorption, perforation, and obstruction.

- Differential diagnosis — Large cell, marginal (MALT), mantle, and follicular lymphoma. Histologic and endoscopic: Lymphoid hyperplasia, Peyer patches.

  Endoscopic: Any submucosal tumor, Crohn's disease, lymphoid hyperplasia due to agammaglobulinemia, AIDS enteropathy, viral gastroenteritis.

  Enteropathy-associated T-Cell lymphoma. Histologic and endoscopic: T-cell lymphoma versus ulcerative jejunitis.

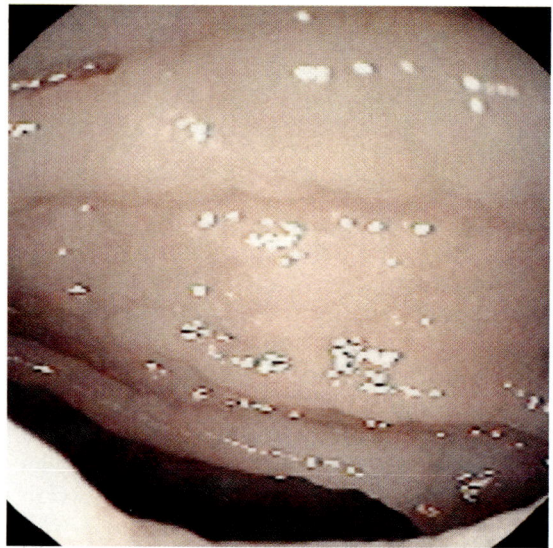

Figure 3-202: **Jejunum. Enteropathy-Associated T-Cell Lymphoma.** Jejunal mucosa without villi. There is flattening and thickening of the circular folds (upper). Below this the mucosa appears thickened and slightly nodular. The patient is known to have celiac sprue.

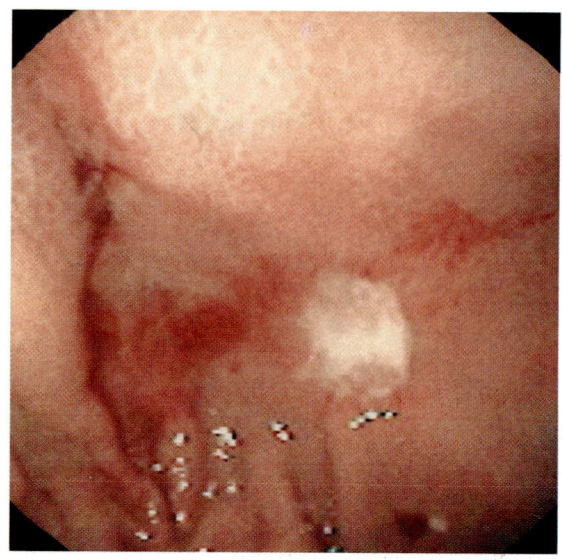

Figure 3-203: **Duodenum. Enteropathy-Associated T-Cell Lymphoma.** Disrupted and effaced circular folds. There is ulceration and gross thickening of the mucosa with a fine reticular pattern (upper area).

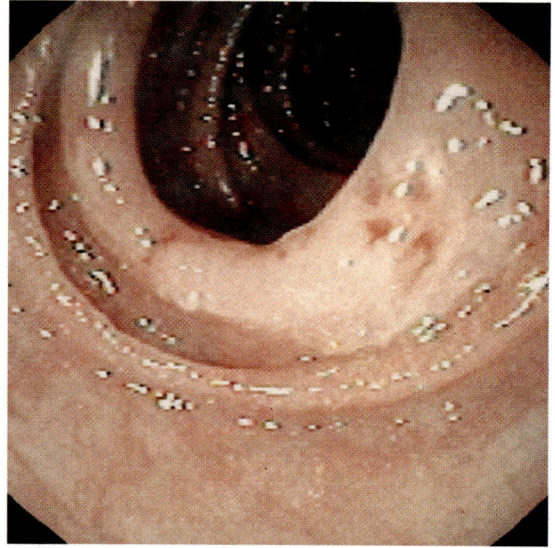

Figure 3-204: **Jejunum. Enteropathy-Associated T-Cell Lymphoma.** A circular fold within the jejunum is thickened with sessile polypoid changes and several areas of spontaneous bleeding. The coloration of the polypoid area differs from that of the surrounding mucosa.

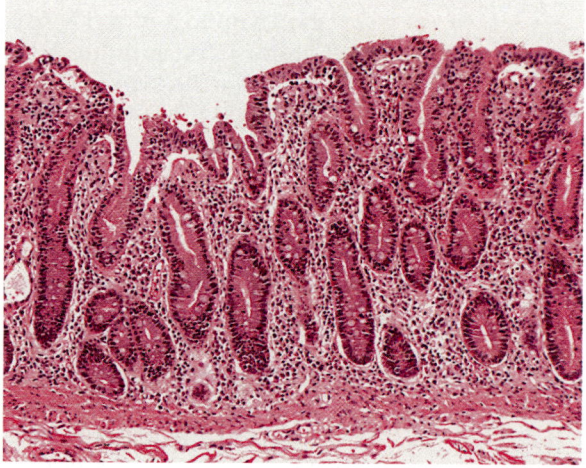

Figure 3-205: **Jejunum. Celiac Sprue.** Complete villous atrophy, crypt hyperplasia, and increased numbers of intraepithelial lymphocytes. Same patient as Fig. 3-207.

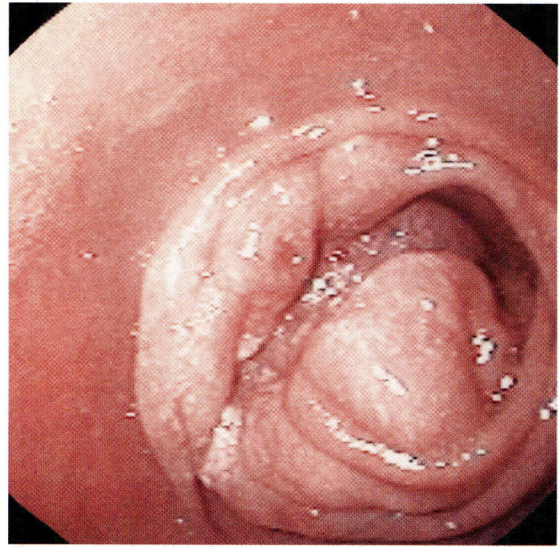

Figure 3-206: **Duodenum. Malignant Lymphoma.** In the apical portion of the duodenal bulb, a polypoid lesion compromises the lumen and coarsens the mucosa. There is a small area of mucosal hemorrhage and, in the cleft occupying the central portion of the photograph, there may be mucosal disruption by lymphoma or an ulcer.

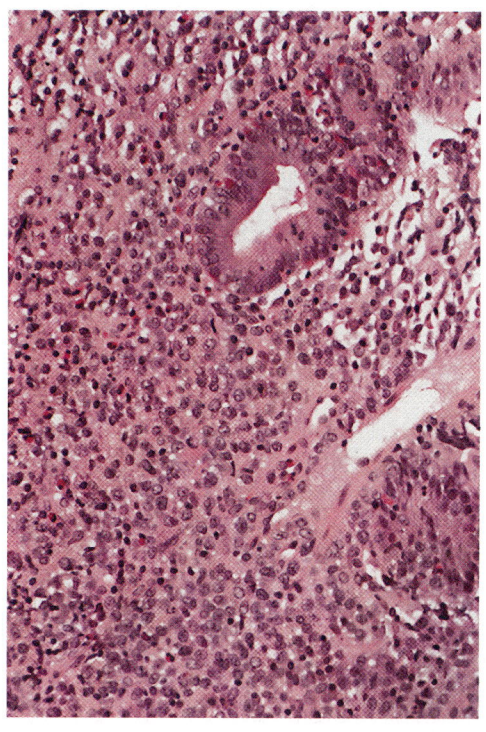

Figure 3-207: **Jejunum. Enteropathy-Associated T-Cell Lymphoma.** Same celiac sprue patient as in Fig. 3-205, with malignant, monotonous lymphoid infiltrate in lamina propria. Positive for T-cell markers.

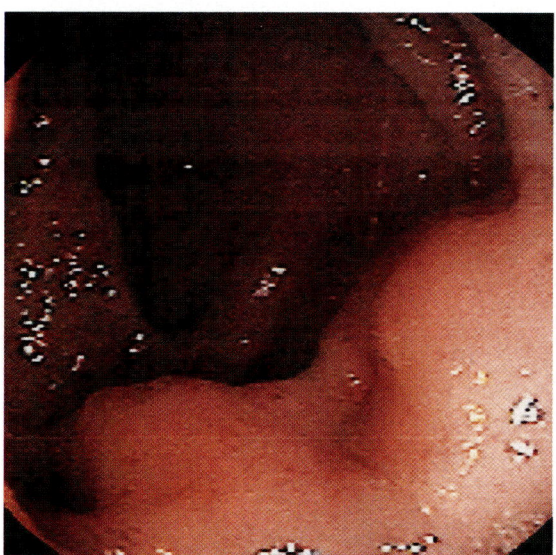

Figure 3-208: **Ileum. Malignant Lymphoma.** A firm, submucosal nodular mass in the terminal ileum.

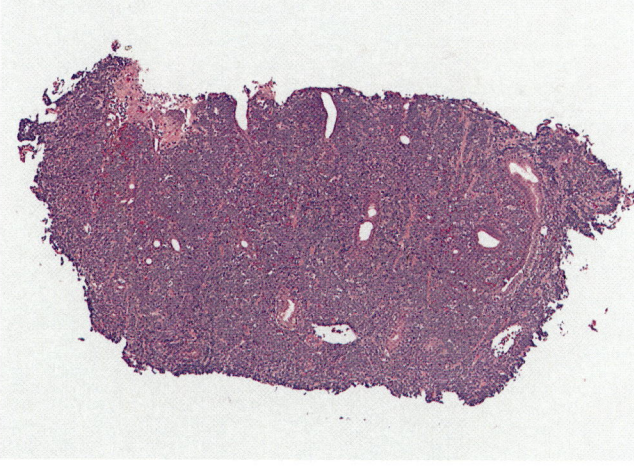

Figure 3-209: **Small Intestine. Malignant Lymphoma.** Low power of mucosal biopsy specimen with dense lymphoid infiltrate. Villi are absent, few crypts remain.

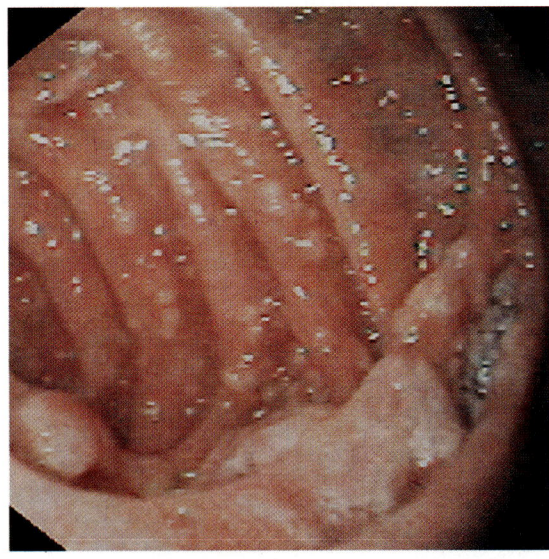

Figure 3-210: **Duodenum. Malignant Lymphoma, Follicle Center Cell.** Multiple minute, whitish nodules in the distal duodenum. In the lower portion of the photograph, there is an irregular, pale, sessile polypoid area with larger nodules nearby.

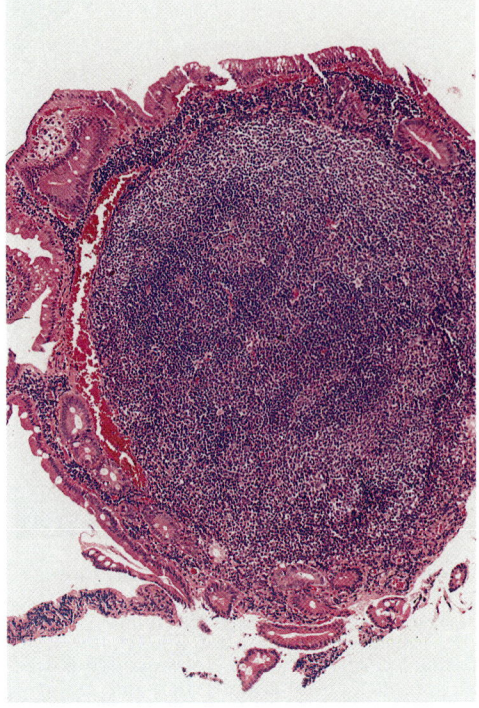

Figure 3-211: **Duodenum. Malignant Lymphoma, Follicle Center Cell.** Submucosal lymphoid nodule composed of small cleaved lymphocytes in the follicle center.

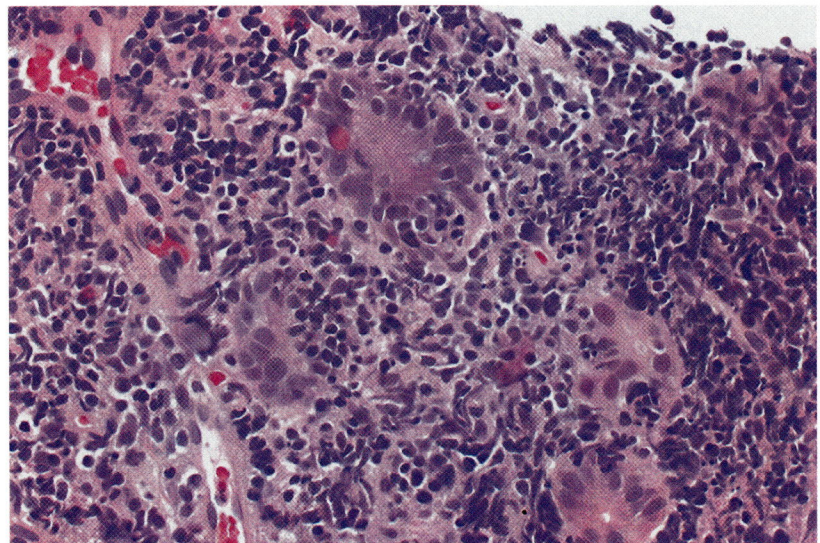

Figure 3-212: **Small Intestine. Malignant Lymphoma.** Small monotonous lymphocytes infiltrate and destroy crypt epithelium (lymphoepithelial lesion), suggestive of extranodal marginal zone lymphoma (MALT).

SMOOTH MUSCLE/STROMAL TUMORS

- Morphology .... Smooth muscle/stromal tumors of the small intestine resemble those of the stomach, but appear to have a greater malignant potential. It is difficult to predict the behavior of these tumors. The presence of any mitotic activity and a size greater than 2 cm should suggest potential malignancy. Features associated with malignancy include an infiltrative growth pattern, ulceration, and necrosis. Mucosal biopsy may be too superficial for diagnosis.

- Endoscopic features .... Sarcomas of the small intestine are generally large. They may infiltrate the bowel wall, distort the luminal architecture, thicken and efface the circular folds, and produce a thickened, edematous mucosa that is friable and ulcerated. The tumor is usually dark, erythematous, or beefy red with coarse surface features.

- Clinical features .... Abdominal pain, small intestinal obstruction, and when ulceration is present, GI bleeding of obscure origin.

- Differential diagnosis ...... Histologic: Schwannoma, hyperplasia of muscularis mucosae, neurofibroma, leiomyoma.

    Endoscopic: Metastatic tumor, lymphoma.

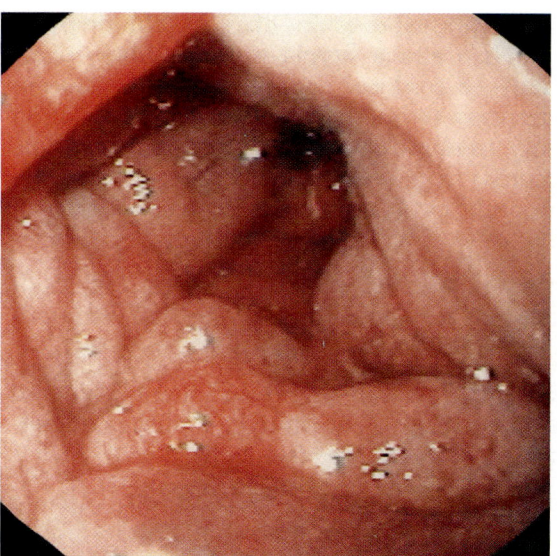

Figure 3-213: **Jejunum. Gastrointestinal Smooth Muscle/Stromal Tumor.** The lumen is compromised by marked thickening and crowding of the circular folds. The mucosa is erythematous and mottled with multiple pinpoint areas of hemorrhage with ulceration (bottom of photograph).

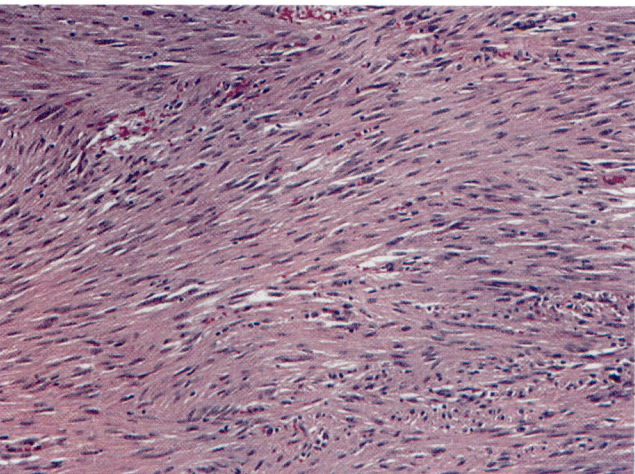

Figure 3-214: **Small Intestine. Malignant Gastrointestinal Smooth Muscle/Stromal Tumor.** Interlacing fascicles of spindle cells with eosinophilic cytoplasm and blunt-ended nuclei resemble smooth muscle.

BENIGN VASCULAR NEOPLASMS

- Morphology .... Hemangiomas differ from ectasias and telangiectasias in that they form a discrete, circumscribed, submucosal mass. They are uncommon and are capillary, cavernous, or a mixture of both. Capillary hemangiomas are usually asymptomatic and of little clinical significance. Cavernous hemangiomas may be larger and may bleed, obstruct, or cause intussusception. Superficial biopsies of angiosarcomas may be indistinguishable from hemangiomas or granulation tissue. In AIDS patients a vascular tumor should be considered Kaposi sarcoma until proven otherwise.

- Endoscopic features .... Endoscopically, hemangiomas are discrete, blue to purple, well-circumscribed sessile or nodular lesions that vary in size from several millimeters to several centimeters. They are frequently multiple.

- Clinical features .... Refractory overt and/or occult gastrointestinal bleeding.

- Differential diagnosis ...... Histologic and endoscopic: Granulation tissue, vascular ectasia over vascular malformations or other tumors, angiosarcoma, Kaposi sarcoma.

VASCULAR MALIGNANCIES

- Morphology .... Angiosarcoma and Kaposi sarcoma are uncommon in the intestine. They occur in older individuals, persons exposed to toxins like vinyl chloride, and in immunosuppressed individuals. Cellular atypia may be subtle; these lesions are easily missed entirely or confused with granulation tissue or benign hemangioma. Close attention to nuclear size, shape, and variation and to macronucleoli is necessary. Immunostains help to distinguish spindle cell-predominant vascular sarcomas from other stromal sarcomas. Red cell extravasation and round eosinophilic cytoplasmic inclusions are features of Kaposi sarcoma.

- Endoscopic features .... Angiosarcoma and Kaposi sarcoma appear as discrete, deep red nodules or sessile polypoid lesions. The margins are well-delineated from the surrounding normal mucosa.

- Clinical features .... Gastrointestinal bleeding, overt and of obscure origin. Abdominal pain and intussusception. In some cases the patient is known to be immunocompromised (HIV, AIDS) and has Kaposi cutaneous involvement.

- Differential diagnosis ...... Histologic: Granulation tissue, reactive fibroblast proliferations, vascular tumors, melanoma, other spindle cell or epithelioid sarcomas.

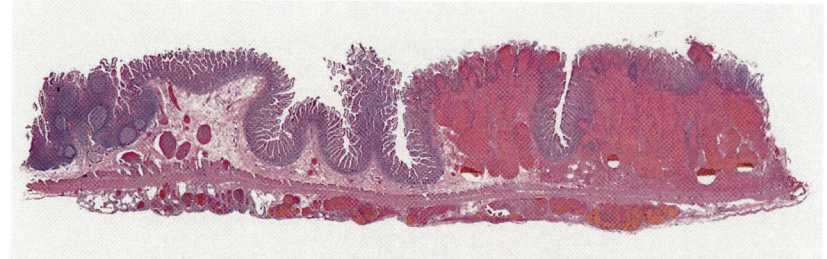

Figure 3-215: **Small Intestine. Cavernous Hemangioma.** Compact collection of dilated, thin-walled blood vascular spaces in submucosa and mucosa.

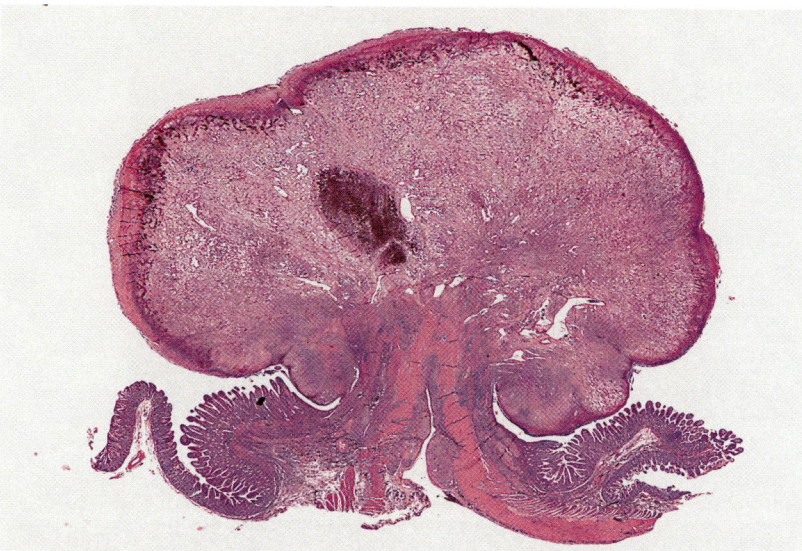

Figure 3-216: **Small Intestine. Capillary Hemangioma.** Cellular, pale, lobulated, submucosal mass forming a stalked polyp. Muscularis propria is pulled into stalk.

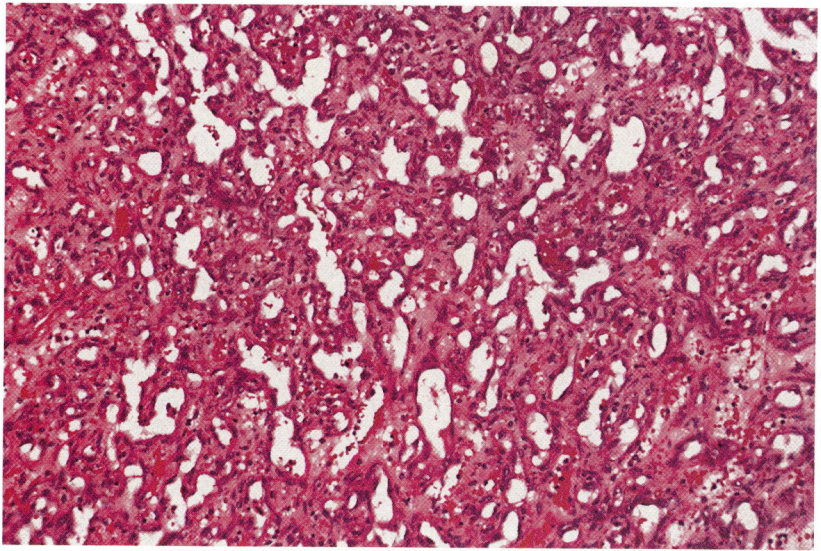

Figure 3-217: **Small Intestine. Capillary Hemangioma.** Cellular neoplasm composed of elements with bland uniform nuclei forming capillary spaces.

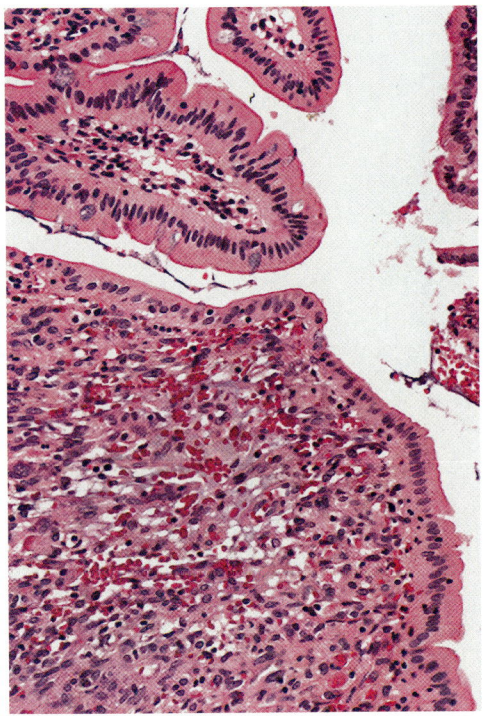

Figure 3-218: **Small Intestine. Angiosarcoma.** Villus expanded by cellular proliferation of endothelial cells, some with lumens, others with collapsed vascular channels.

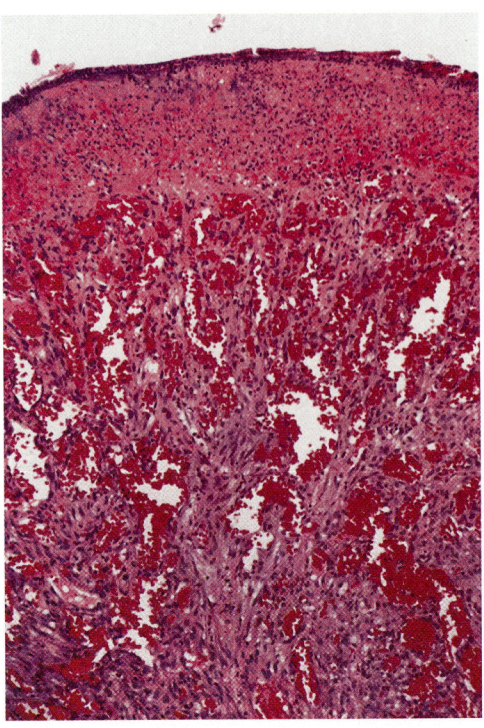

Figure 3-219: **Small Intestine. Angiosarcoma.** Vascular polyp with eroded surface. Large, dilated blood vascular spaces overshadow intervening fascicles of spindle cells.

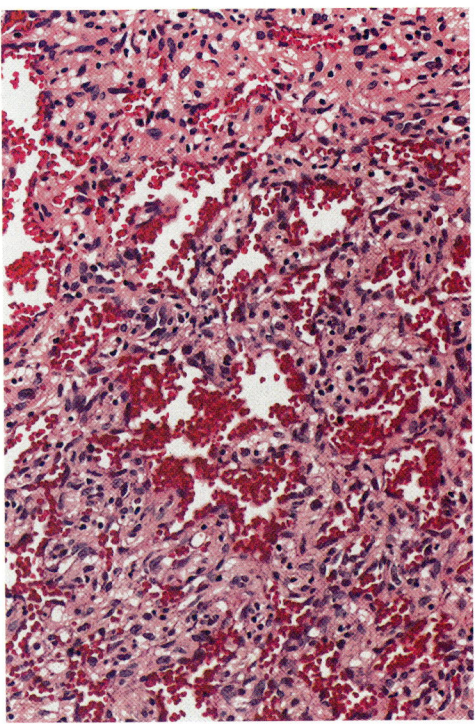

Figure 3-220: **Small Intestine. Angiosarcoma.** Large, irregular, anastomosing vascular spaces in cellular endothelial neoplasm. Endothelial nuclei are large and mildly atypical.

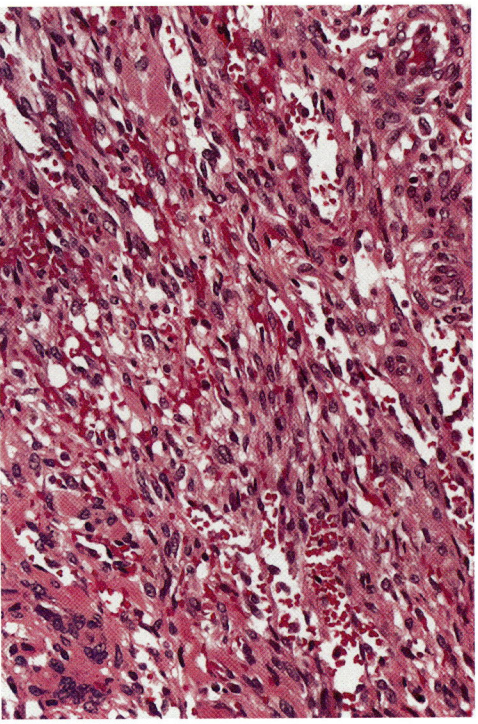

Figure 3-221: **Small Intestine. Kaposi Sarcoma.** Fascicle of spindle cells with atypical nuclei. Red cell extravasation and poorly formed vascular channels suggest Kaposi sarcoma.

LYMPHANGIOMA

- Morphology .... These tumors are composed of numerous dilated submucosal lymphatics filled with lymph. The discrete nature of lymphangioma distinguishes it from the diffuse lymphangiectasias due to obstruction and congenital lymphangiectasia.
- Endoscopic features .... The lymphangioma is a submucosal nodule. The surface may appear hemorrhagic and contain dilated vascular elements. The lesions are small (< 1 cm) and cystic.
- Clinical features .... Incidental finding.
- Differential diagnosis ...... Histologic and endoscopic: Vascular malformation.

    Endoscopic: Lipoma, other submucosal nodule.

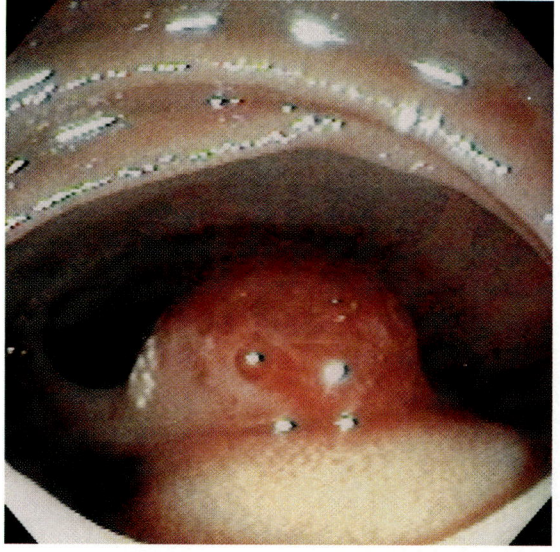

Figure 3-222: **Jejunum. Lymphangioma.** Discrete, raised, hemorrhagic, spontaneously bleeding nodule with scant blood at base. Push enteroscopy in patient with GI bleeding of obscure origin.

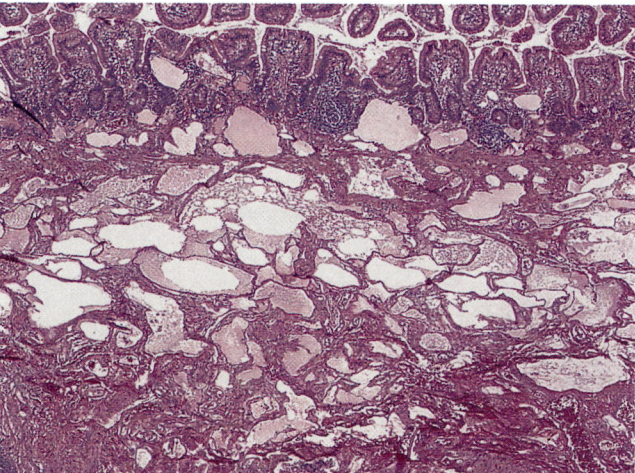

Figure 3-223: **Duodenum. Lymphangioma.** Numerous dilated, thin-walled vascular spaces filled with pink proteinaceous material.

METASTATIC TUMORS

- Morphology .... It may not be possible to distinguish metastatic from primary adenocarcinoma unless a remnant of adenoma is found. Signet-ring cell carcinomas can be primary in the small intestine, but are more likely to originate in stomach or breast, where they commonly metastasize to the gastrointestinal tract. Metastatic melanoma is not uncommon and mimics undifferentiated carcinoma. Pleomorphic large cell lymphomas may mimic both carcinoma and melanoma. Often, primary site can not be determined by histologic examination alone. Panels of immunostains combined with histologic features and statistical prevalence sometimes allow an educated guess.

- Endoscopic features .... Tumors metastasize through the blood stream or grow into the bowel from a contiguous site. In the former situation, the tumors are polypoid or exophytic and often ulcerated. The neoplastic tissue is distinct from surrounding normal mucosa, is darker with irregular surface features, and is firm and bleeds on contact.

- Clinical features .... GI blood loss anemia, abdominal pain, small intestinal obstruction.

- Differential diagnosis ...... Histologic and endoscopic: Primary versus metastatic carcinoma, melanoma, sarcoma, lymphoma.

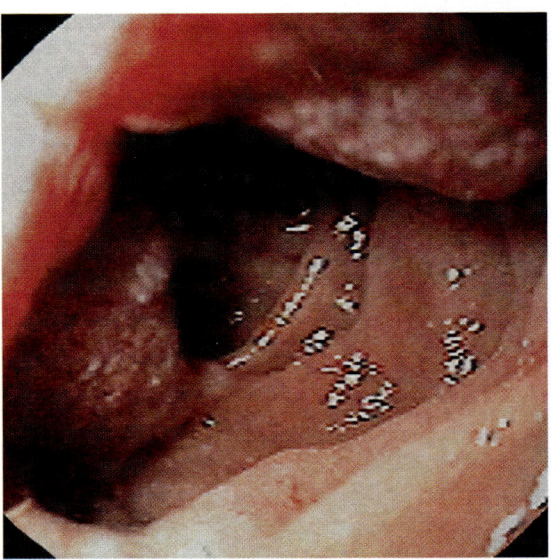

Figure 3-224: **Duodenum. Metastatic Pancreatic Adenocarcinoma.** A friable, beefy red neoplasm occupies half the circumference of the postbulbar duodenum at the level of the papilla of Vater. The surface is coarsened and irregular. The duodenal lumen is partially compromised.

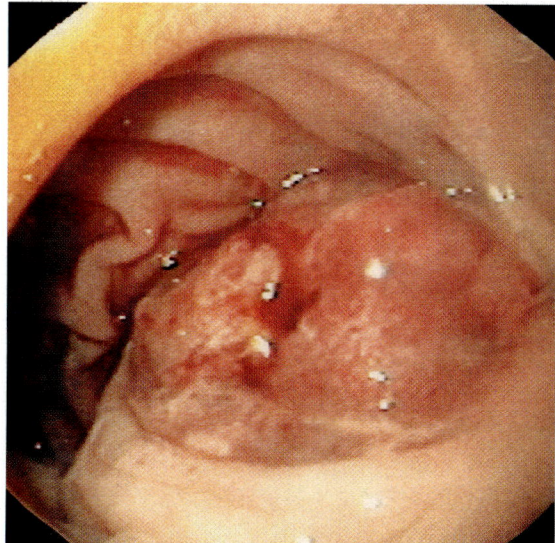

Figure 3-225: **Duodenum. Metastatic Pancreatic Adenocarcinoma.** A firm, dark, hemorrhagic neoplasm (center) protrudes into the postbulbar duodenum. The tumor appears to arise from an intramural or extramural position. There is a ring of duodenal mucosa with a smooth margin adjacent to the malignant-appearing tumor, resulting in an area that bulges into the duodenal lumen.

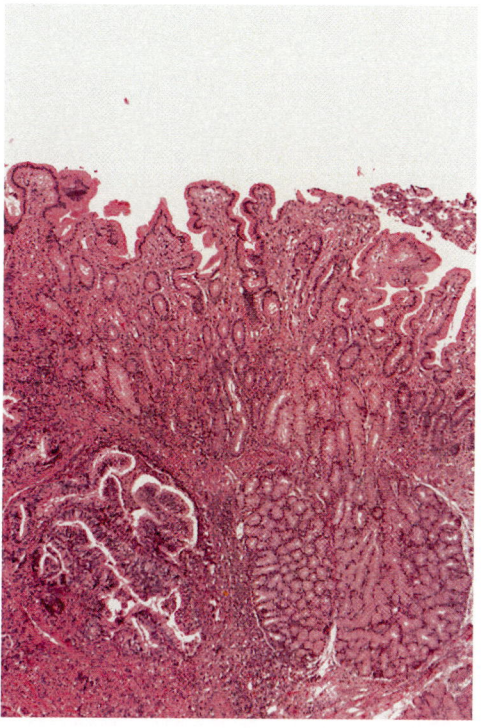

Figure 3-226: **Duodenum. Metastatic Pancreatic Adenocarcinoma.** Papillary carcinoma, adjacent to Brunner gland, undermines the mucosa.

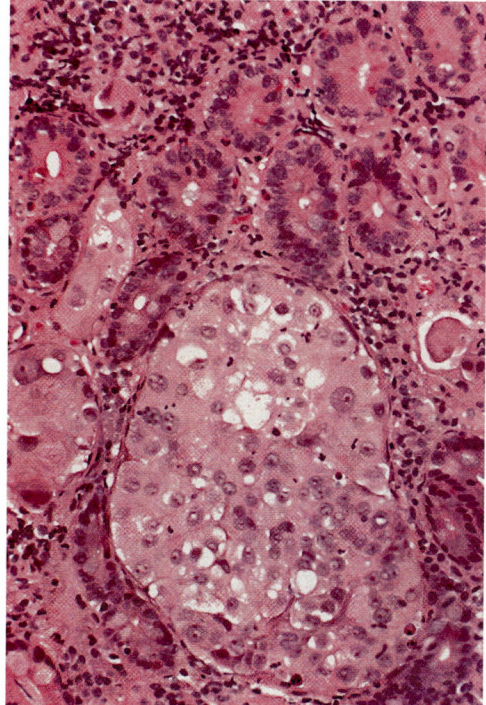

Figure 3-227: **Duodenum. Metastatic Endometrial Adenocarcinoma.** Adenocarcinoma, probably in lymphatics, infiltrates mucosa.

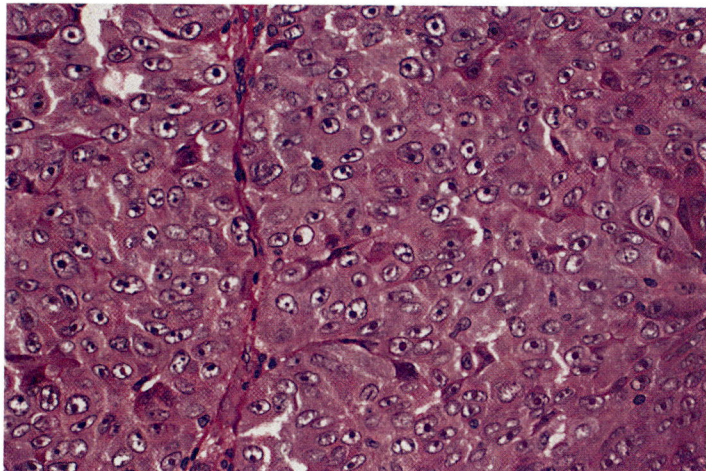

Figure 3-228: **Small Intestine. Metastatic Malignant Melanoma.** Large epithelioid cells with prominent nucleoli, without visible melanin resemble carcinoma or large cell lymphoma. S-100 protein and HMB-45 were positive.

CHAPTER 4

LARGE INTESTINE

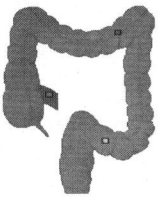

Endoscopic examination	280
Histology	281
Normal large intestine	282
Patterns of injury	289
Insufflation artifact (pseudolipomatosis)	293
Histiocyte infiltrates	294
Near-normal colonic mucosa with pathogenic organisms	296
Specific infectious agents	298
Parasites	301
Acute colitis	303
Pseudomembranous colitis	306
Ischemia	307
Radiation injury	310
Active chronic destructive colitis	312
Dysplasia and adenocarcinoma in ulcerative colitis	318
Dysplasia-associated lesion/mass (DALM)	318
Crohn's colitis	321
Adenocarcinoma arising in Crohn's disease	321
Granulomatous colitis	325
Chronic nondestructive colitis	329
Eosinophilic colitis	331
Graft-versus-host disease	332
Diversion colitis	334
NSAID ileocolitis/ulcers	335
Melanosis coli	337
Diverticular disease	338
Stricture/anastomosis	342
Vascular lesions	344
Hemorrhoids/varices	349
Vasculitis	351
Fibrosing colopathy	353
Amyloidosis	354
Dysmotility syndromes	356
Lymphoid hyperplasia	357
Pneumatosis coli	359
Endometriosis	361
Inverted appendix	362
Rectal prolapse syndrome and inflammatory cloacogenic polyp	363
Barium granuloma and oleogranuloma	367
Hypertrophied anal papilla/skin tag	369
Inflammatory polyps	370
Hyperplastic polyp	373
Combined adenoma/hyperplastic polyp	376
Serrated adenoma	376
Juvenile polyp	379
Peutz-Jeghers polyp	381
Cowden syndrome	383
Ganglioneuroma	384
Cronkhite-Canada polyps	386
Granular cell tumor	387
Lipoma	388
Lipohyperplasia of ileocecal valve	388
Adenomas	391
Adenoma with pseudoinvasion	395
Familial adenomatous polyposis	397
Flat adenoma	399
Adenocarcinoma arising in an adenoma	401
Adenocarcinoma	403
Carcinoma variants	406
Mucinous adenocarcinoma	406
Signet-ring cell and small cell carcinomas	406
Recurrent adenocarcinoma	409
Metastatic tumors	410
Carcinoid tumor	412
Smooth muscle/stromal tumors	414
Kaposi sarcoma	416
Malignant lymphoma	417
Malignant melanoma	419
Squamous lesions	421

ENDOSCOPIC EXAMINATION

Complete visualization of the large intestine can be difficult, especially passage of the endoscope through the sigmoid colon and intubation of the ileum. The various topographic regions are recognized by a combination of features including lumen size and shape, distribution of haustral folds, and specific landmarks, e.g., the appendiceal orifice and ileocecal valve (Figs. 4-1 to 4-12).

Although the mucosa is visualized during passage of the endoscope, critical inspection occurs during withdrawal. Normal findings should be described, e.g., salmon-colored mucosa, orderly mucosal folds, a visible submucosal vascular pattern, and lymphoid nodules in the rectum, cecum, or terminal ileum. These nodules are a distinctive feature of the terminal ileum, especially in younger patients. The contrast between a pale lymphoid nodule and the surrounding mucosa, the "red ring sign," can be confused with aphthous ulcers (Figs. 4-14, 4-15). Mucosal injury due to introduction of the endoscope (e.g., erythema, hemorrhage, and localized edema) may be seen on withdrawal and mistaken for lesions.

Interpreting erythema is important, as it usually implies congestion with or without inflammation. Small areas of erythema may resemble angiectasia, being differentiated by a discerning eye and high-resolution video endoscopy. Patchy erythema suggests mild acute colitis. Spontaneous bleeding and friability are often associated with inflammatory diseases.

The loss of mucosal folds, haustral markings, and submucosal vascular pattern suggests chronic destructive colitis, such as idiopathic inflammatory bowel disease. These findings may be segmental (Crohn's disease) or diffuse (ulcerative colitis). The colonic mucosa of lymphocytic or collagenous colitis, where crypts are not destroyed, appears normal.

It is important to sample normal and abnormal areas to correlate endoscopic and histologic patterns. Surveillance biopsies for dysplasia should be taken from all areas of the bowel, avoiding active inflammation, as these are difficult to interpret. Sessile, erythematous, villous, or flat nodular lesions should be sampled to rule out a dysplasia-associated lesion or mass (DALM) (Fig. 4-17).

Ulcers are described by their size, shape, depth, and distribution; these characteristics may suggest an etiology. In bleeding patients, deep discrete ulcers and thermally ulcerated polypectomy sites are closely examined for a visible vessel. Biopsies of ulcers should be taken from the edge, unless CMV or a submucosal process such as lymphoma is suspected. In such cases, biopsy samples from the base may be more informative.

Neoplasms are described as polyps or masses, either mucosal or submucosal. Polyps are sessile or pedunculated, and are characterized as diminutive (< 5mm), small (up to 1 cm), or large (> 1 cm). They may be smooth, nodular, or villous. Villous polyps have an irregular carpetlike or cerebriform surface (Fig. 4-16). Malignant lesions are sessile or exophytic, localized or circumferential, and often are firm, friable, and ulcerated. Neoplasms are sampled with pinch avulsion-type biopsy forceps. Mucosectomy is an evolving method that allows complete removal of sessile lesions less than 2 cm in diameter. Saline is injected submucosally to isolate and elevate the lesion allowing the lesion to be snared directly or aspirated into a suction cylinder on the tip of the endoscope.

HISTOLOGY

Colonic crypts are uniform, straight, and parallel, and extend to the muscularis mucosae (Fig. 4-18). The crypt base is composed of small, immature, basophilic cells with scant cytoplasm. These differentiate into goblet, absorptive, and endocrine cells and, in the right colon, Paneth cells (Figs. 4-21, 4-23). Mitotic activity is usually confined to the crypt base. Epithelial cells normally undergo apoptosis and slough at the crypt surface. In early regeneration following mucosal injury, the epithelial cells appear immature and mitoses may extend to the crypt surface. In chronic mucosal injury, the crypts are often irregular and unevenly spaced and the crypt bases are located above the muscularis mucosae. The presence of Paneth cells in the left colon is considered an indicator of chronic mucosal injury. Spotty crypt epithelial apoptosis is abnormal; it is associated with viral infections, immunodeficiency, and graft-versus-host disease.

A single layer of myofibroblasts forms a sheath surrounding the crypts. The sheath functions as an attachment site for perpendicular muscle fibers that extend from the muscularis mucosae (Fig. 4-22). These fibers anchor and order the mucosa. Under prolonged tension, the muscle fibers hypertrophy and are a useful indicator of mucosal prolapse. In early ischemia, crypt epithelium sloughs away from the myofibroblastic sheath. The resulting preservation of the crypt outline is a diagnostic feature of early ischemic colitis.

Plasma cells, eosinophils, histiocytes, and a few lymphocytes are normally concentrated in the upper third of the lamina propria and on low magnification have a bandlike appearance (Figs. 4-18 to 4-20). The deep lamina propria has fewer inflammatory cells and the crypts are closer together. Lymphoid follicles are located along the muscularis mucosae. Small T-lymphocytes are normally found within the crypt epithelium in a ratio of approximately 1 lymphocyte to 20 enterocytes. Macrophages are scattered throughout the mucosa and may contain mucin, pyknotic nuclear debris, and lysosomal breakdown products. Neutrophils in the lamina propria are an indication of pathologic rather than physiologic inflammation, as is the downward expansion of the normal superficial mucosal band of inflammatory cells. The type and distribution of the inflammatory cell infiltrate changes, over the course of several weeks, from predominantly neutrophilic to plasmacytic and from superficial to full thickness. It therefore can be useful in determining the duration of injury. Intraepithelial lymphocytosis occurs in immune reactions and is a characteristic feature of lymphocytic colitis.

At regular intervals the surface epithelium dips down to the muscularis mucosae, forming a mosaic of indentations known as innominate grooves. The crypts empty into the sides of the grooves, which accommodate mucosal expansion. Lymphoid follicles are often found at the groove base and form lymphoglandular complexes (a site of antigen processing). A biopsy of an innominate groove, especially if it includes a lymphoglandular complex, can be mistaken for the abnormal crypt branching and inflammation seen in chronic destructive colitis.

Submucosal arterioles extend into the mucosa and break into a network of capillaries just beneath the surface epithelium basement membrane. The capillaries collect into venules and descend into the submucosa. In acute inflammatory injury, neutrophils emerge from the capillary network, just beneath the surface epithelium. Chronic venous hypertension, whether discrete or generalized, is associated with vascular ectasia and sclerosis of mucosal vessels.

NORMAL LARGE INTESTINE

- Morphology .... Uniform, evenly spaced crypts that reach the muscularis mucosae characterize normal colonic mucosa (Fig. 4-18). Inflammatory cells are usually concentrated in the upper third of the lamina propria and consist of plasma cells, eosinophils, macrophages (muciphages), and occasional lymphocytes (Fig. 4-19). In oblique sections, the crypts appear as evenly spaced, circular structures, with inflammatory cells concentrated towards the surface (Fig. 4-20). Normal physiologic inflammation lacks neutrophils and varies significantly between individuals; it is often more prominent in the cecum. A mild degree of chronic inflammation is a normal finding and should not lead to a pathologic diagnosis. Neutrophils are never normal; they are a marker of colitis. Increased mononuclear cells, with or without epithelial proliferation, may indicate previous injury, however, they should be considered as a nonspecific reactive change. Muciphages may be normal or represent prior epithelial injury. They are found anywhere in the mucosa, especially in the distal colon, where goblet cells are more frequent and trauma more likely.

- Endoscopic features .... The rectum is a straight tube (Fig. 4-1). After the rectosigmoid angle, the sigmoid colon is smaller in caliber and the haustral folds more irregularly spaced (Fig. 4-2). The descending colon is again straight and has fewer haustral folds than the sigmoid colon, but may be indistinguishable from the proximal sigmoid. The splenic flexure is angulated and sometimes transmits the blue hue of the adjacent spleen (Fig. 4-3). The lumen of the transverse colon is larger than that of the descending colon, and is organized into a series of triangular-shaped haustral folds (Fig. 4-4). It may be straight or loop toward the pelvis before it reaches the angle of the hepatic flexure, where the darker color of the adjacent liver is evident (Fig. 4-5). The lumen of the ascending colon is quite large, with fairly well-organized and sometimes triangular folds (Figs. 4-6, 4-7). The cecum is delineated by the first and most prominent haustral fold, which contains the ileocecal valve (Figs. 4-8, 4-9). The appearance of the valve ranges from slitlike to rounded and smooth. The haustral fold pattern of the cecum resembles a crow's foot. The appendiceal orifice is located at the base of the crow's foot.

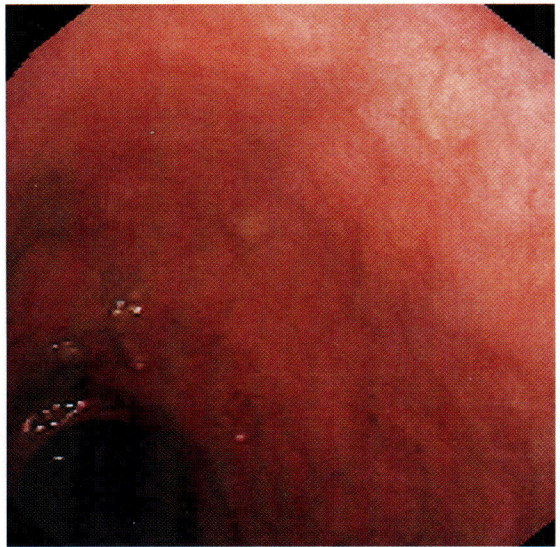

Figure 4-1: **Rectum. Normal.** Normally distended rectum.

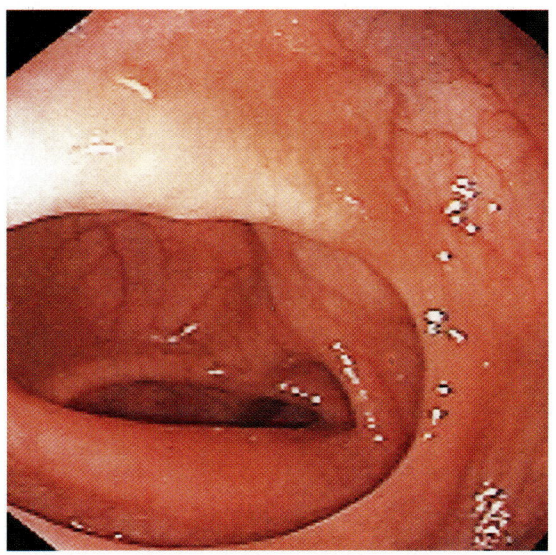

Figure 4-2: **Colon, Sigmoid. Normal.** Angulation and variation in the shape and form of haustral folds.

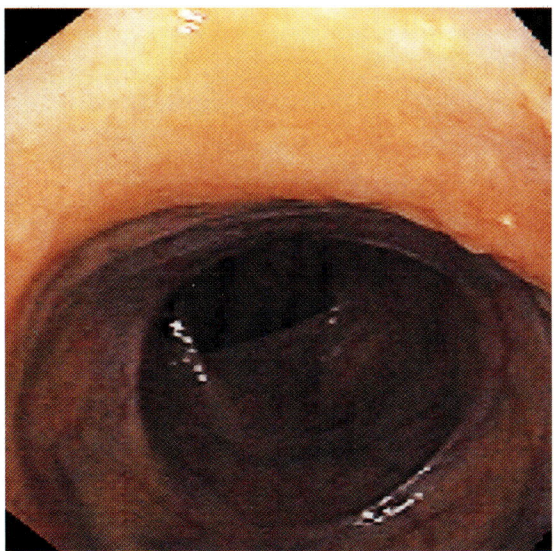

Figure 4-3: **Colon, Splenic Flexure. Normal.** Typical-appearing blue coloration at the splenic flexure.

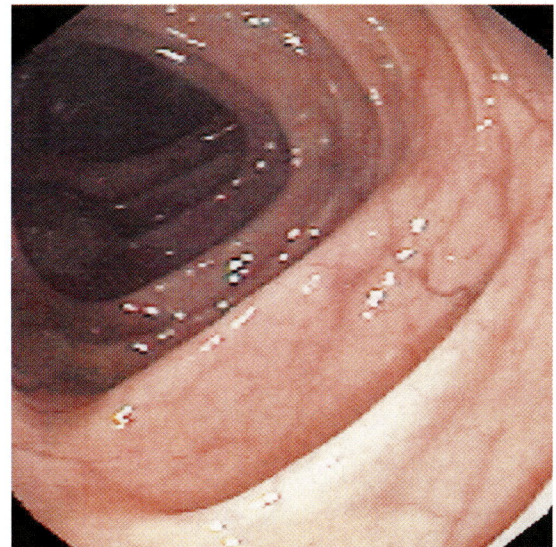

Figure 4-4: **Colon, Transverse. Normal.** Typical triangular haustral configuration of the transverse colon.

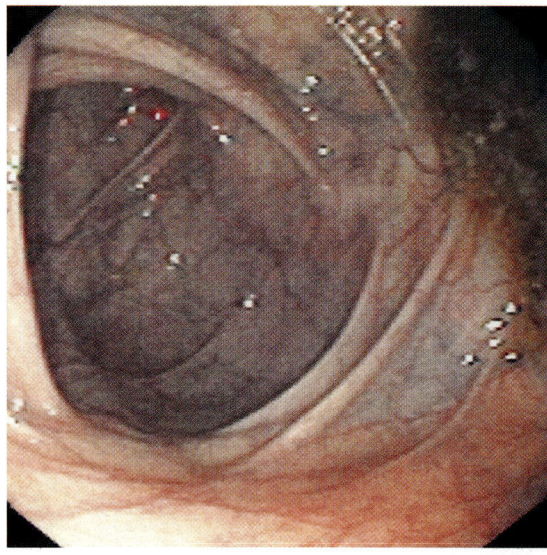

Figure 4-5: **Colon, Hepatic Flexure. Normal.** Slight bluish coloration typical of the hepatic flexure.

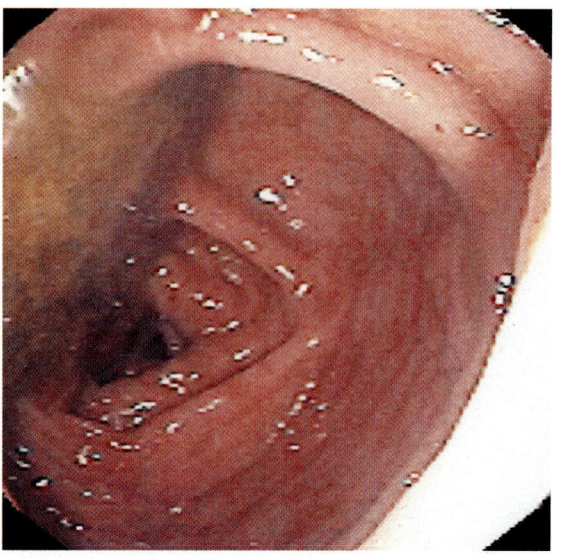

Figure 4-6: **Colon, Ascending. Normal.** The distinctive triangular haustral folds of the transverse colon may be present. The lumen is larger than in the transverse or sigmoid colon.

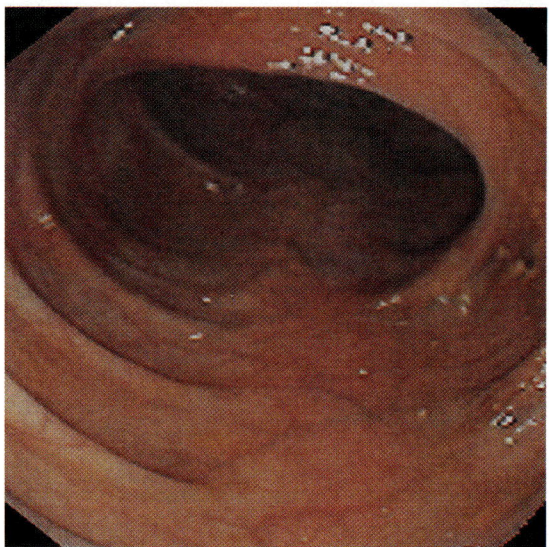

Figure 4-7: **Colon, Ascending. Normal.** Wide lumen and well-spaced haustral folds.

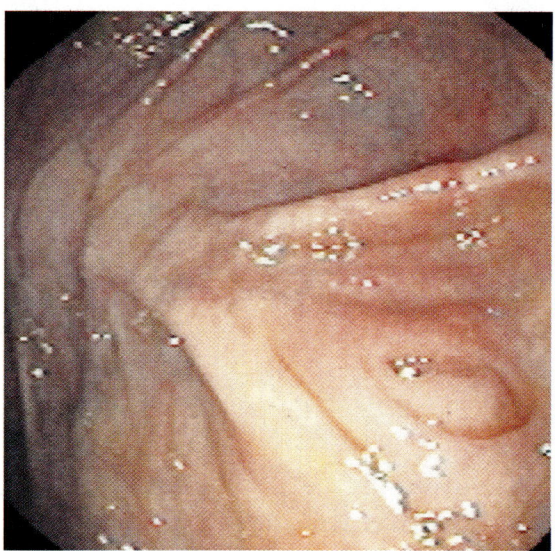

Figure 4-8: **Cecum. Normal.** Cecum with appendiceal orifice and view of the "crow's foot" appearance of the haustral folds.

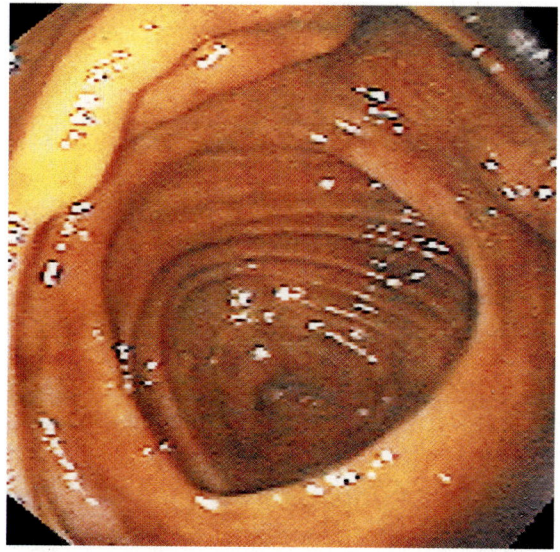

Figure 4-9: **Cecum and Ileocecal Valve. Normal.** View looking into the cecum. Characteristic landmarks of the appendiceal orifice and ileocecal valve (upper left). Typical smooth, round, fish-mouthed appearance of the ileocecal valve.

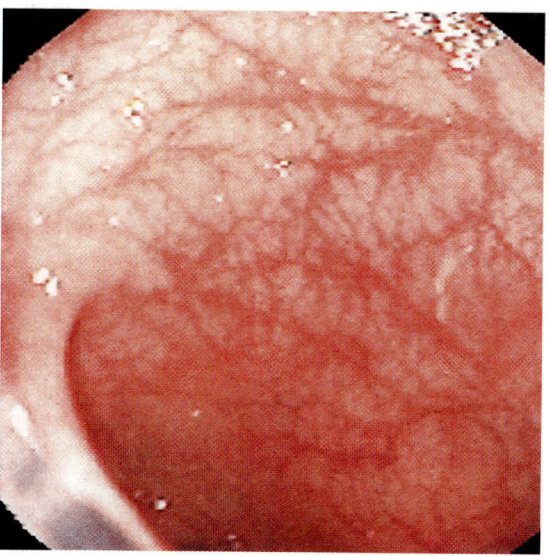

Figure 4-10: **Rectum. Normal.** Normal rectal vascular pattern.

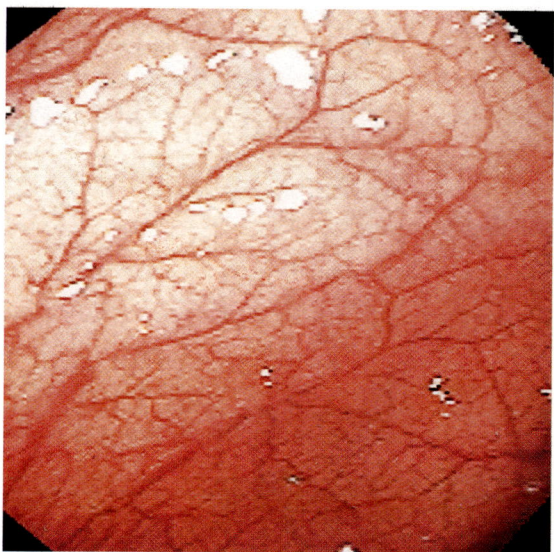

Figure 4-11: **Colon, Transverse. Normal.** Normal arborizing pattern of submucosal vessels.

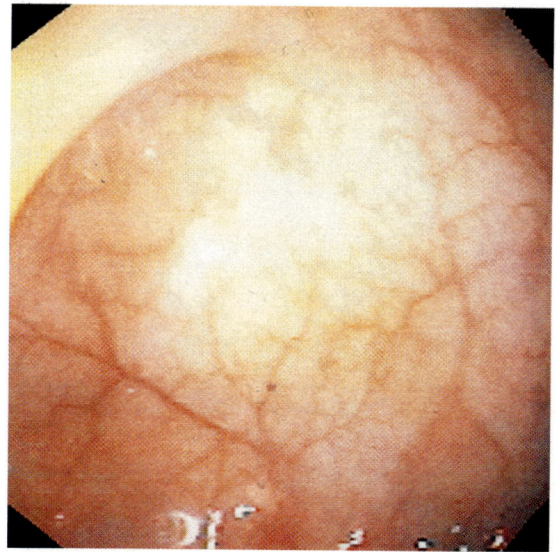

Figure 4-12: **Cecum. Normal.** Normal cecal vascular pattern.

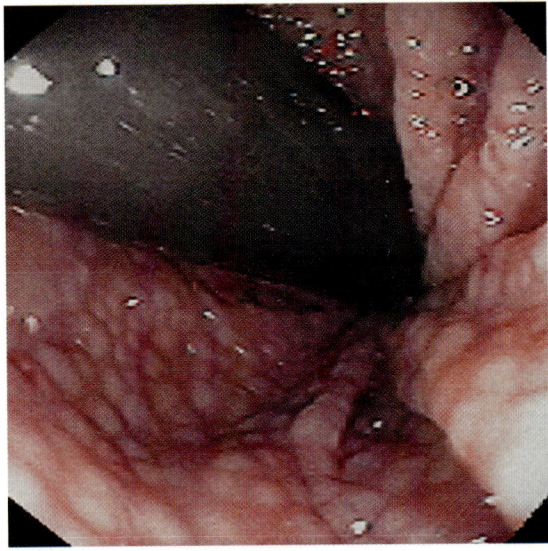

Figure 4-13: **Rectum. Normal.** Multiple lymphoid nodules seen during retroflexion.

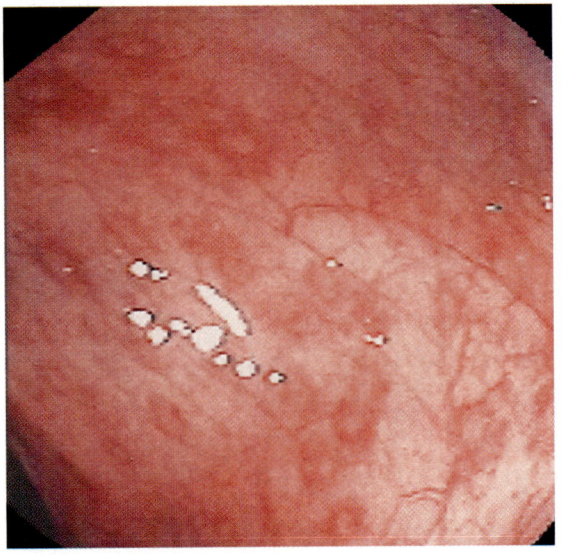

Figure 4-14: **Rectum. Normal.** Red ring sign around lymphoid nodules.

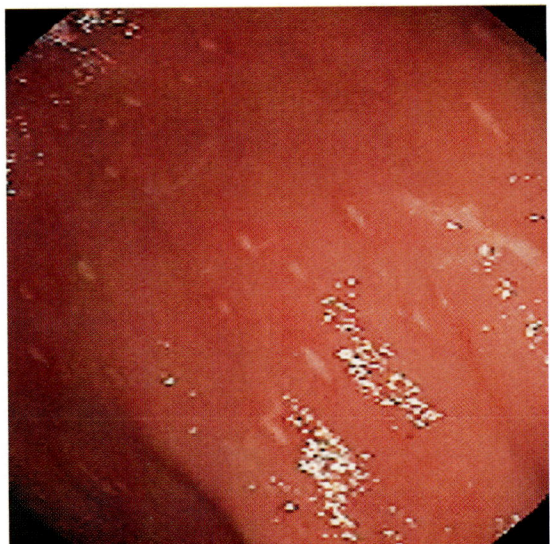

Figure 4-15: **Terminal Ileum. Crohn's Disease.** Aphthous ulceration of Crohn's disease within the terminal ileum.

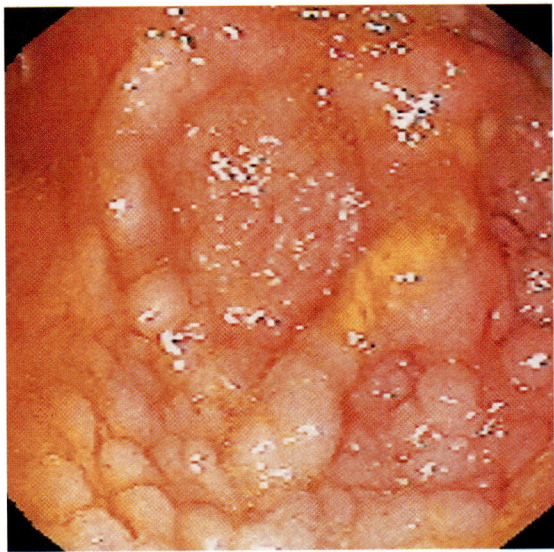

Figure 4-16: **Cecum. Villous Adenoma.** Sprawling, sessile, cecal polyp with villous appearance consisting of innumerable tightly packed nodules.

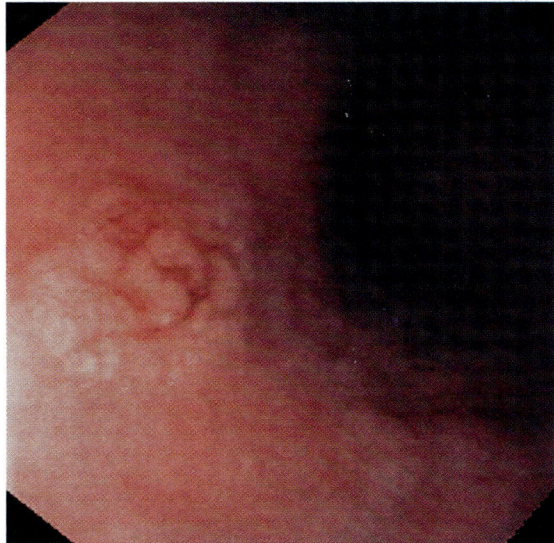

Figure 4-17: **Rectum. Polyp in Ulcerative Colitis.** Sessile, atypical-appearing polyp in a patient with long-standing colitis. Possible DALM.

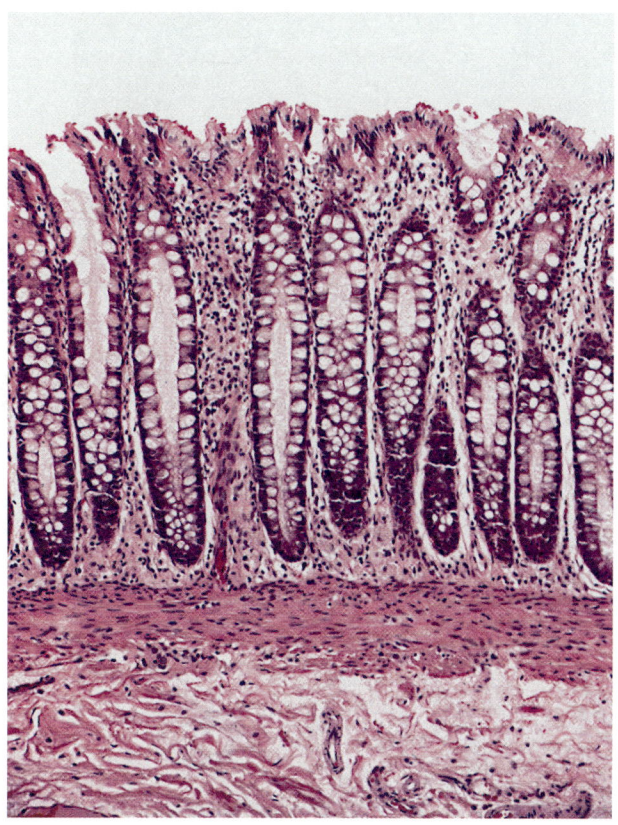

Figure 4-18: **Colon. Normal Mucosa.** Straight, parallel, uniform crypts, evenly spaced, with base near muscularis mucosae. Nuclear crowding in the proliferative zone at the crypt base. Normal physiologic inflammation. Muciphages at base.

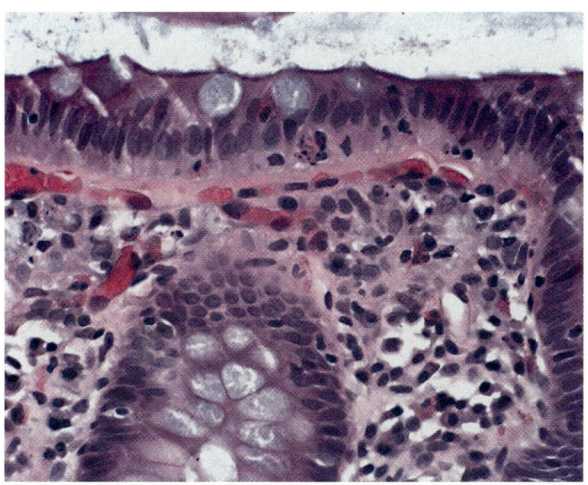

Figure 4-19: **Colon. Normal Mucosa.** Scattered intraepithelial lymphocytes (T cells). Apoptotic cells and debris in the epithelium and surface lamina propria. Capillary network just beneath the basement membrane. Inflammatory cells (plasma cells, eosinophils, lymphocytes, and histiocytes) predominate in the upper lamina propria.

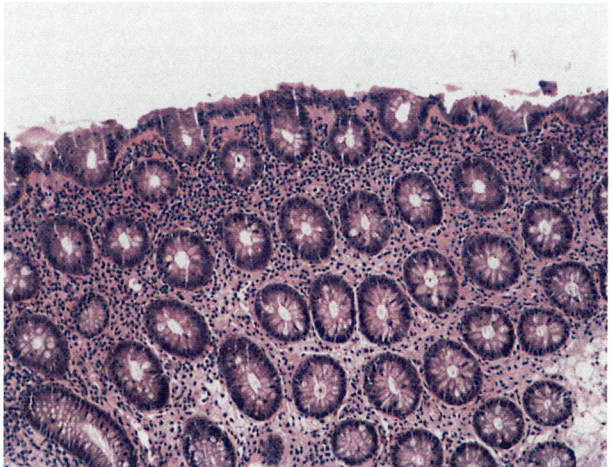

Figure: 4-20: **Colon. Normal Mucosa.** Inflammatory cell density greater near the surface.

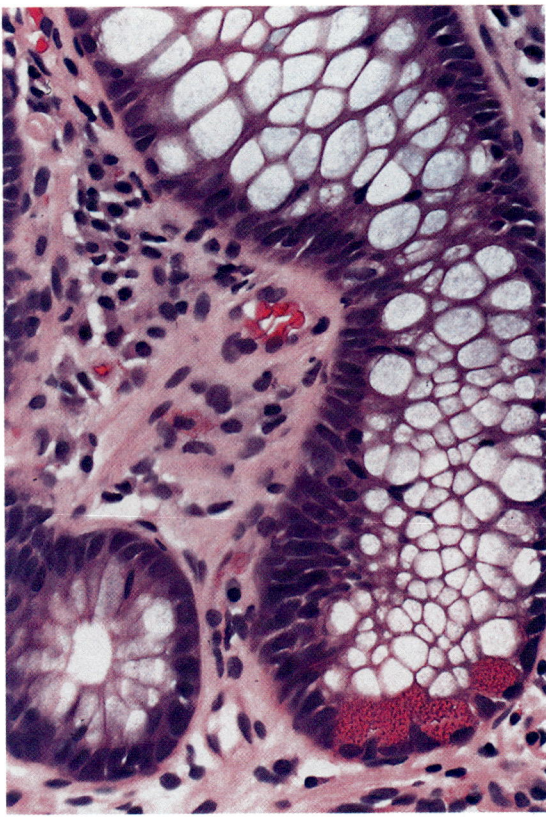

Figure 4-21: **Colon. Normal Mucosa.** Paneth cells with large, supranuclear eosinophilic granules.

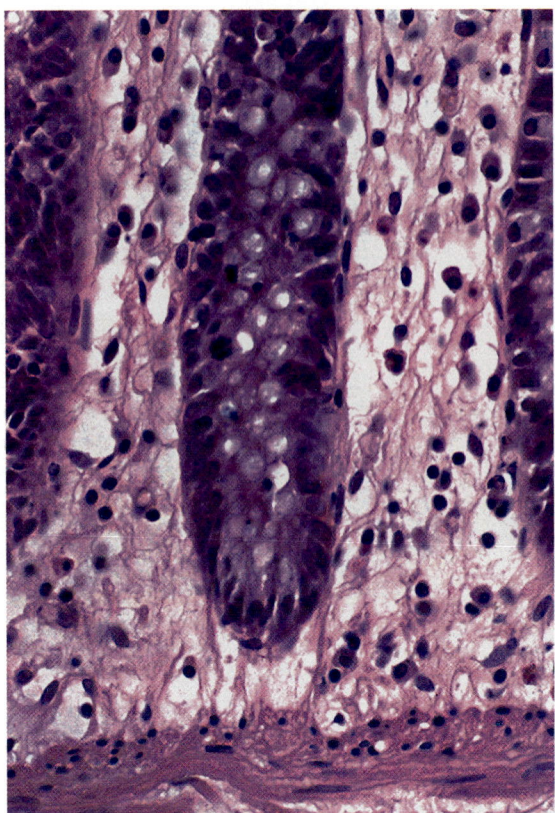

Figure 4-22: **Colon. Normal Mucosa.** Smooth muscle fibers extend from muscularis mucosae and attach to pericryptal myofibroblasts. Lymphatic channels just above muscularis mucosae. Sparse inflammatory infiltrate at crypt base.

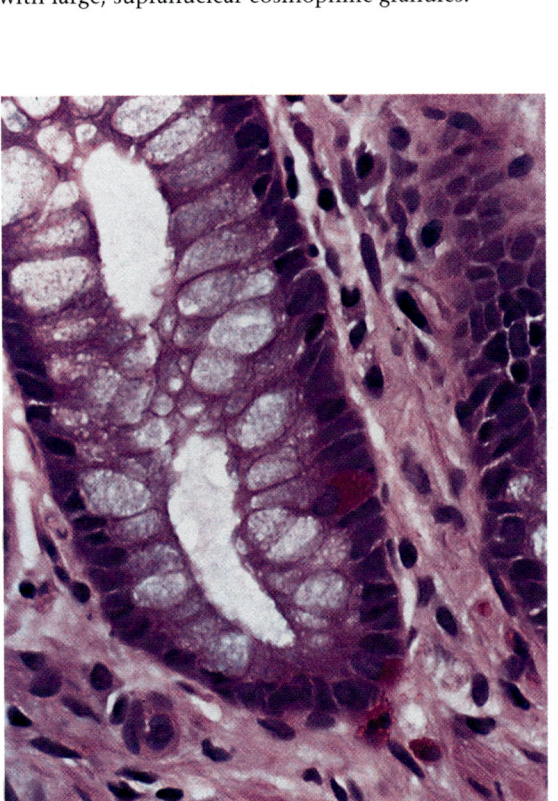

Figure 4-23: **Colon. Normal Mucosa.** Endocrine cells with small, subnuclear eosinophilic granules. Perpendicular smooth muscle cells between crypts. Spindled pericryptal myofibroblasts surround crypts.

PATTERNS OF INJURY

The colorectal mucosa reacts to injury in a limited number of ways. Histologic patterns are not specific, but reflect pathogenesis, severity, and duration. Clinical diagnosis requires clinicopathologic correlation, facilitated by a close working relationship between gastroenterologist and pathologist. (See Tables 4-1 and 4-3.)

The common histologic reaction patterns are: (1) acute colitis, (2) acute colitis with ischemic features, including punctate pseudomembranous and well-developed ischemic patterns, (3) chronic crypt destructive colitis, and (4) chronic noncrypt destructive colitis (Table 4-1).

Sequence of Inflammation

Neutrophils enter the mucosa first, emerge from the postcapillary venule, and persist throughout the course of the active inflammatory process. The presence of neutrophils in the lamina propria is a reliable objective marker of pathologic inflammation. The majority of inflammatory cells remain in the upper lamina propria (normal zonation pattern) during the first week. Mononuclear cells, mainly plasma cells, increase in the upper lamina propria during the second week. By the third week, the inflammatory infiltrate spreads into the deep lamina propria. It takes about 4 weeks to develop significant basal plasmacytosis, which persists for the duration of the disease. If crypts are destroyed and enough time has elapsed (3 to 4 weeks), crypt regeneration appears as distorted and branched crypts. The presence of basal plasmacytosis and/or crypt regeneration can indicate a chronic process (duration of more than 4 weeks).

Acute Colitis

Acute, self-limited colitis usually resolves within 3 weeks. There is neutrophilic inflammation in the lamina propria, less often in the crypts, and early crypt epithelial proliferation. If the process persists for several weeks, there may be an increase in mononuclear cells; however, most cells remain in the upper mucosa or are just beginning to spread into the depths. Branching crypts are not seen.

Acute Colitis with Ischemic Features

Acute colitis with superimposed ischemic features is characterized by crypt and surface epithelial necrosis, with preservation of crypt outlines, and eruption of mucin and fibrinoinflammatory exudate onto the surface. The *pseudomembranous pattern* is a mild or early pattern of injury, with punctate distribution characterisitic of pseudomembranous colitis. The *ischemic pattern* denotes more severe or prolonged injury. There is widespread epithelial necrosis, vascular thrombosis, and extravasation of blood and fibrin into the lamina propria.

Chronic Destructive Colitis

In chronic destructive colitis, mononuclear inflammatory cells extend into the deep lamina propria, and there is crypt architectural distortion and branching. This pattern, while characteristic of idiopathic chronic inflammatory bowel disease, is not specific.

Chronic Nondestructive Colitis

Chronic nondestructive colitis is characterized by chronic inflammation extending deep without crypt distortion. The particular pattern, lymphocytic or collagenous colitis, is defined by additional features, such as increased intraepithelial lymphocytes and the presence or absence of thickened collagen beneath the surface epithelium.

Other Patterns

Less common inflammatory patterns are listed in Table 4-2.

Table 4-1. Diagnostic Features and Etiologies of Common Histologic Patterns

Common Histologic Patterns	Diagnostic Histologic Features	Etiologies & Clinical Associations
Acute colitis	Neutrophils predominate. Mononuclear cells confined to upper lamina propria. No crypt branching.	Self-limited infection *C difficile* Drug reaction
Acute mucosal injury with punctate pseudomembranes: pseudomembranous colitis	Neutrophils predominate. Other features include edema, focal surface epithelial necrosis, pseudomembranes, and dilated cysts with flattened epithelium.	Early ischemia *C difficile* Verotoxic *E coli* 0157:H7 Drug reaction
Acute mucosal injury: ischemic colitis	Neutrophils predominate. Other features include edema, hemorrhage, thrombi, and epithelial necrosis with preservation of crypt outlines.	Hypovolemia/low-flow states Verotoxic *E coli* 0157:H7 *Shigella* verotoxin Vasculitis/vasculopathy Drug reaction
Chronic crypt destructive colitis	Predominantly mononuclear inflammatory infiltrates with basal plasmacytosis; neutrophils persist. Cryptitis, crypt destruction, and branching crypts. Inactive phase characterized by empty, distorted lamina propria, crypt branching, and Paneth cell metaplasia.	Ulcerative colitis Crohn's colitis Indeterminate colitis Prolonged enteric infections Uncommon chronic systemic, venereal, or parasitic infections Drug reaction Diverticular disease-associated colitis Diversion colitis Idiopathic proctitis
Chronic noncrypt destructive colitis	Mononuclear cells predominate. Basal plasmacytosis, neutrophils persist. Intraepithelial lymphocytes increased. Subepithelial collagen in collagenous colitis.	Lymphocytic colitis Collagenous colitis Drug reaction

Table 4-2. Diagnostic Features and Etiologies of Less Common Histologic Patterns

Less Common Histologic Patterns	Diagnostic Histologic Features	Etiologies & Clinical Associations
Eosinophilic colitis	Eosinophilic infiltrates with or without crypt destruction	Food allergy Drug allergy Parasitic infestation Idiopathic eosinophilic enteritis Hypereosinophilic syndrome Vasculitis
	Pericryptal eosinophils, basal band of mast cells	Pericryptal eosinophilic enterocolitis
Graft-versus-host/immune suppression pattern	Mononuclear cells predominate in lamina propria. Crypt apoptosis and lymphocytic infiltration of crypts.	Graft-versus-host Viral infections Immunosuppression
Chronic mucosal prolapse	Variable combinations of ischemic change, erosions, ulcers, epithelial regeneration/hyperplasia (polyps), hypertrophic smooth muscle fibers, fibrosis, and displacement of epithelium into the submucosa	Occult rectal prolapse Prolapse in other locations Chronic mechanical trauma
Portal hypertensive colopathy	Mucosal capillaries and venules prominent with thickened sclerotic walls; venular ectasia	Portal hypertension due to cirrhosis, hepatic arteriovenous fistula, portal vein or tributary obstruction
Nonspecific ulcer of the colon	Isolated ulcer with granulation tissue base; epithelial regeneration on edge but no colitis in surrounding mucosa	Drug reaction, particularly NSAIDs Vasculitis Cytomegalovirus Stercoral ulcers

Table 4-3. Histologic Patterns of Particular Infections and Drugs

Histologic Patterns	Infectious Agents	Drugs and Chemicals
Normal/near-normal mucosa	Spirochetosis Enteroadherent E coli Cryptosporidium Cholera	Narcotics, phenothiazines, vincristine, atropine, other anticholinergics, ganglionic blocking agents, tricyclic antidepressants
Acute colitis	Common enteric pathogens: Yersinia, Shigella, Salmonella, Campylobacter, Aeromonas. Toxin-producing bacteria: C difficile, Staphylococcus, others. Viruses: cytomegalovirus, herpesvirus. Parasites: Cryptosporidium	Bisacodyl, NSAIDs, hypertonic enemas, methyldopa, deferoxamine (promotes Yersinia infection)
Acute mucosal injury with punctate pseudomembranes: pseudomembranous colitis	Toxin-producing bacteria: C difficile, E coli 0157:H7, others	Antibiotics
Acute mucosal injury: ischemic colitis	Toxin-producing bacteria: E coli 0157:H7, Shigella, Clostridium, others	Estrogen, cocaine, ergotamine amphetamines, digitalis, vasopressin, methysergide, NSAIDs, salicylates, potassium chloride, Kayexalate, hyperosmolar solutions, glutaraldehyde, chemotherapeutic agents (promote neutropenic colitis)
Chronic crypt destructive colitis	Common enteric bacteria: Campylobacter, Shigella, Aeromonas, Yersinia. Venereal agents: syphilis, Chlamydia. Systemic bacterial infections: tuberculosis. Fungi: Histoplasma, Cryptococcus, Coccidioides, Candida. Parasites: ameba	NSAIDs
Chronic noncrypt destructive colitis: lymphocytic and collagenous colitis		NSAIDs, Cyclo 3 Fort, carbamazepine
Eosinophilic colitis	Helminths	Gold, alpha-methyldopa, carbamazepine flucytosine, methotrexate, azathioprine, L-tryptophan, sulfasalazine, NSAIDs, salicylates
Solitary or multiple idiopathic ulcer	Cytomegalovirus	NSAIDs, potassium chloride, steroids, oral contraceptives

INSUFFLATION ARTIFACT (PSEUDOLIPOMATOSIS)

- Morphology .... Characterized by clear (air) spaces of varying size in the mucosa and submucosa, resembling fat cells. The lack of nuclei, focal nature, and intramucosal location distinguish this from adipose tissue.
- Endoscopic features .... Insufflation artifact is often misinterpreted as an abnormal finding. It is rarely encountered, but is more likely seen in a prolonged, difficult examination. It is typically reported as a localized exudate. The term *leukoplakia* has been used to describe this finding; however, leukoplakia has a precancerous connotation at other sites and is best avoided.
- Clinical features .... None.
- Differential diagnosis ...... Histologic: Lipoma, xanthelasma (rare).

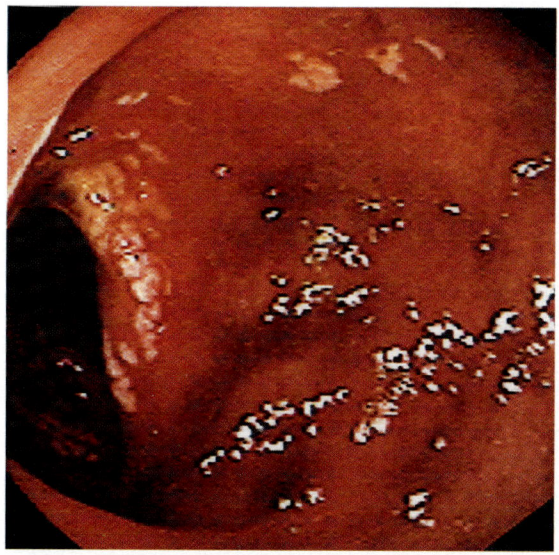

Figure 4-24: **Colon, Ascending. Insufflation Artifact (Pseudolipomatosis).** Distinctive cluster of minute, white plaques that are resistant to washing, suggesting a lesion other than an exudate.

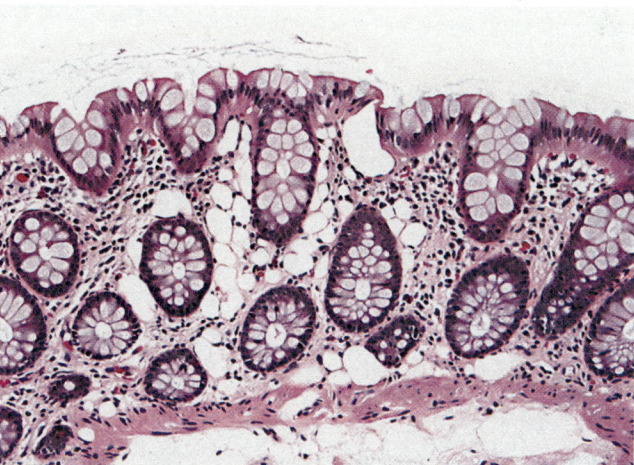

Figure 4-25: **Colon. Insufflation Artifact (Pseudolipomatosis).** Empty spaces in the lamina propria resemble fat.

HISTIOCYTE INFILTRATES

- Morphology .... *Muciphages* can be a normal finding or an indication of previous epithelial injury. *Melanosis* may be due to ingestion of anthraquinone laxatives, but is also seen in chronic inflammatory conditions due to the accumulation of lysosomal breakdown products. *Lipid-filled histiocytes* are seen in conditions where there is interruption of enterohepatic circulation of bile, in chronic inflammatory conditions, and as a drug effect (cyclosporine).

- Endoscopic features .... Melanosis is evident as a gray-brown mucosal discoloration that may highlight uninvolved lymphoid follicles. Xanthelasma appears as diffusely distributed yellow-white dots or flecks. Muciphages are not visible.

- Clinical features .... Chronic constipation, inflammatory bowel disease, immunosuppressive therapy with cyclosporine.

- Differential diagnosis...... Histologic: Histiocytes sometimes resemble signet-ring cells; however, the nucleus is usually one third the size of signet-ring cell carcinoma nuclei and lacks their large macronucleoli. Whipple disease and *Mycobacterium avium-intracellulare* infection produce histiocytic infiltrates with eosinophilic or foamy cytoplasm.

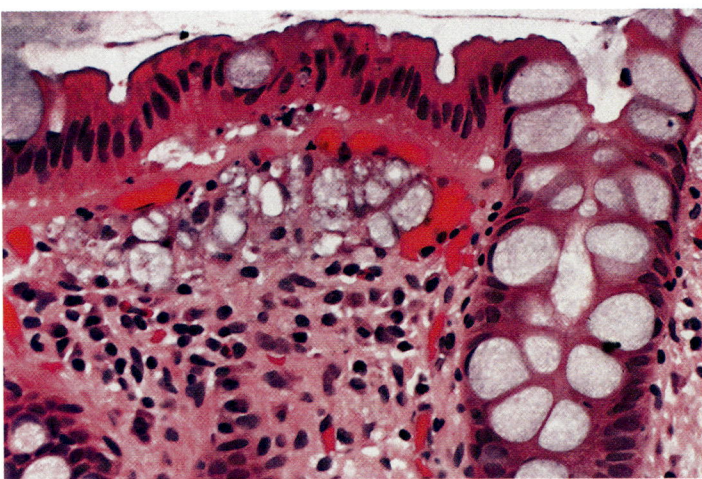

Figure 4-26: **Colon. Muciphages**. Macrophages distended with mucin beneath the surface epithelium. PAS with diastase was positive.

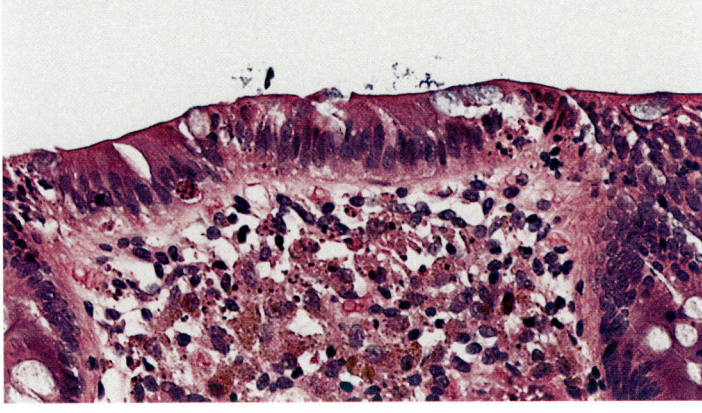

Figure 4-27: **Colon. Melanosis**. Histiocytes contain pigment and nuclear debris.

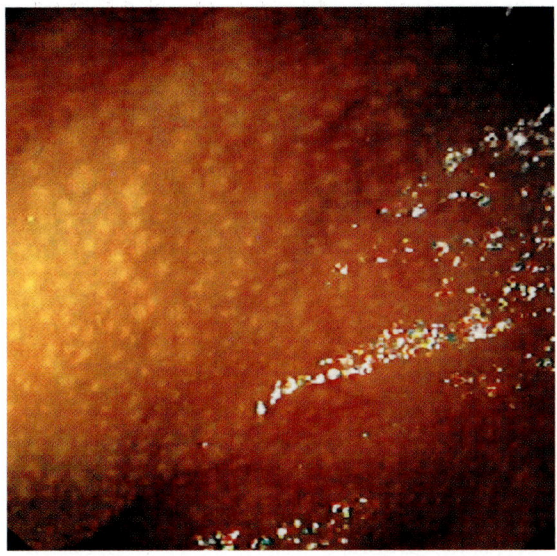

Figure 4-28: **Colon, Ascending. Muciphages.** Diffusely distributed raised miliary white spots. Background mucosa is dark, possibly due to excessive pigmentation (melanosis).

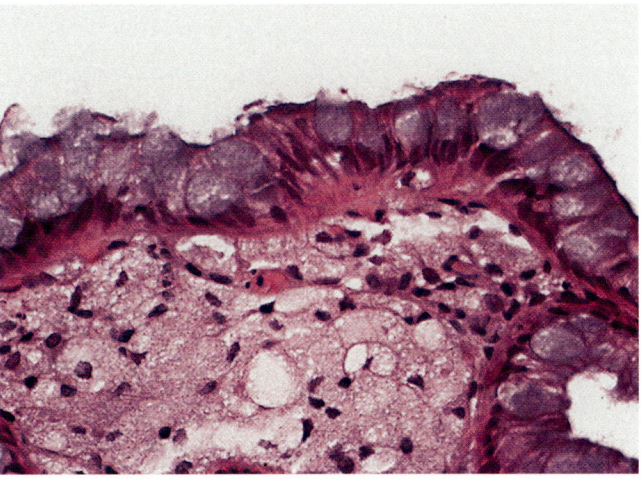

Figure 4-29: **Colon. Lipophages.** Finely vacuolated, lipid-filled histiocytes. Requires fresh-tissue fat stain. PAS with diastase was negative.

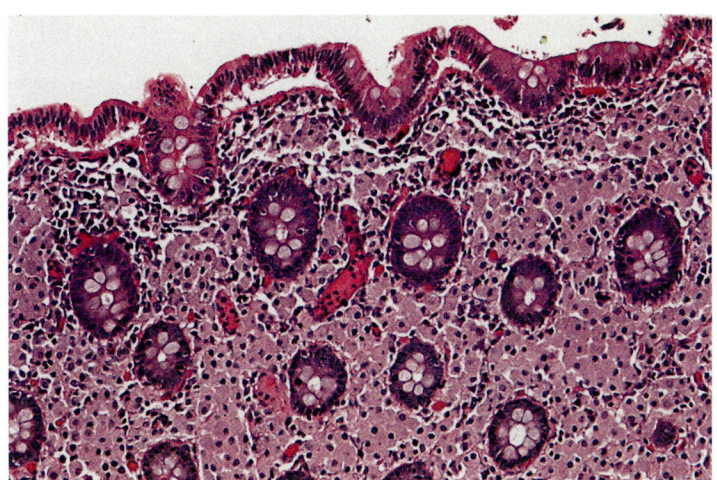

Figure 4-30: **Cecum. *Mycobacterium avium-intracellulare*.** Histiocytes with dense eosinophilic cytoplasm. PAS and acid-fast stains were positive for bacteria.

NEAR-NORMAL COLONIC MUCOSA WITH PATHOGENIC ORGANISMS

- Morphology .... Careful inspection of the surface (and crypt) epithelium at higher magnification is necessary to diagnose infections that cause little or no tissue reaction.
- Endoscopic features .... Although pathogenic bacteria cause acute inflammatory findings with erythema, erosions, ulcerations, and exudate, the examples shown here are associated with endoscopically normal appearances.
- Clinical features .... May cause watery diarrhea.
- Differential diagnosis ...... Histologic: Mucus "blobs" resemble cryptosporidia, but are more variable in size and shape and less distinct. A darkly blue-stained brush border may be confused with spirochetosis. Microvilli are shorter and uniform and produce a refractile line when the condensor is lowered.

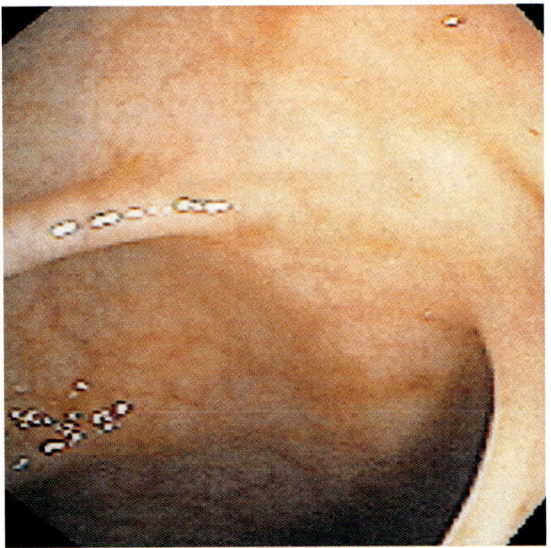

Figure 4-31: **Colon, Sigmoid. Cryptosporidiosis.** Nonspecific erythema, surrounding mucosa appears normal.

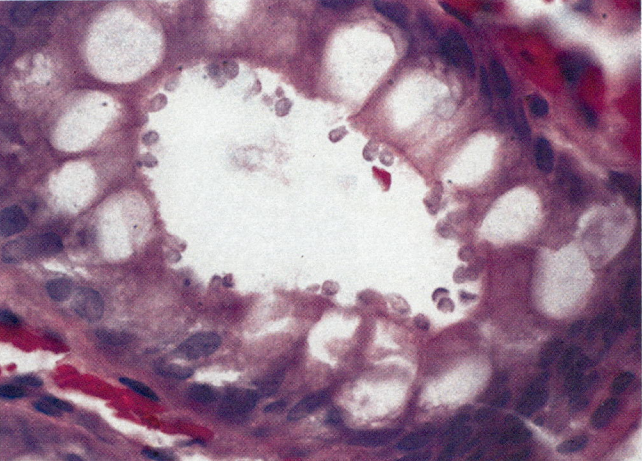

Figure 4-32: **Colon. Cryptosporidiosis.** Distinct, small, round hematoxylinophilic bodies attached to crypt epithelium.

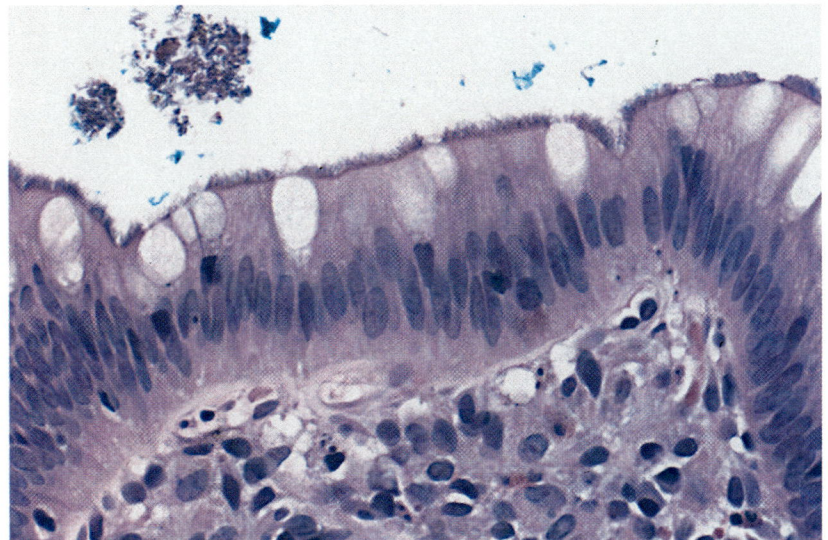

Figure 4-33: **Colon. Spirochetosis.** A wispy, basophilic, hairlike mat of spirochetes covers the epithelial surface.

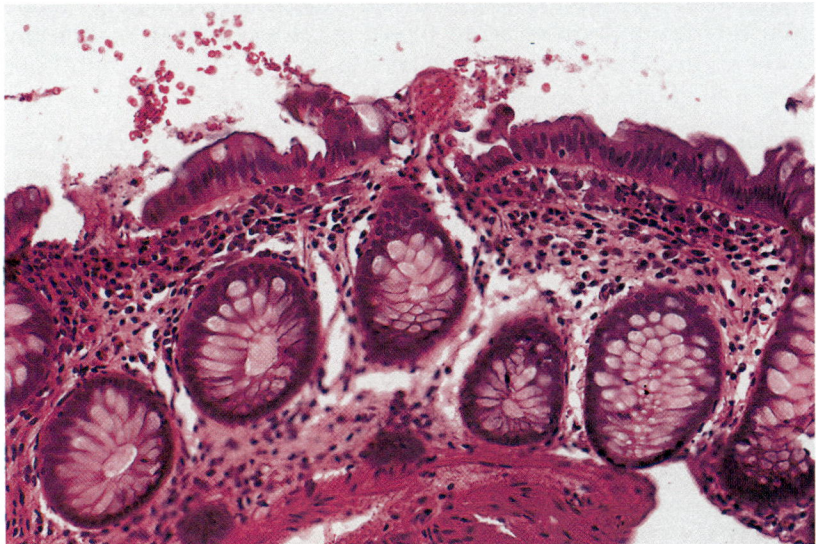

Figure 4-34: **Colon. Enteroadherent *E coli*.** Large bacterial rods cling to the surface epithelium. Small focal erosions.

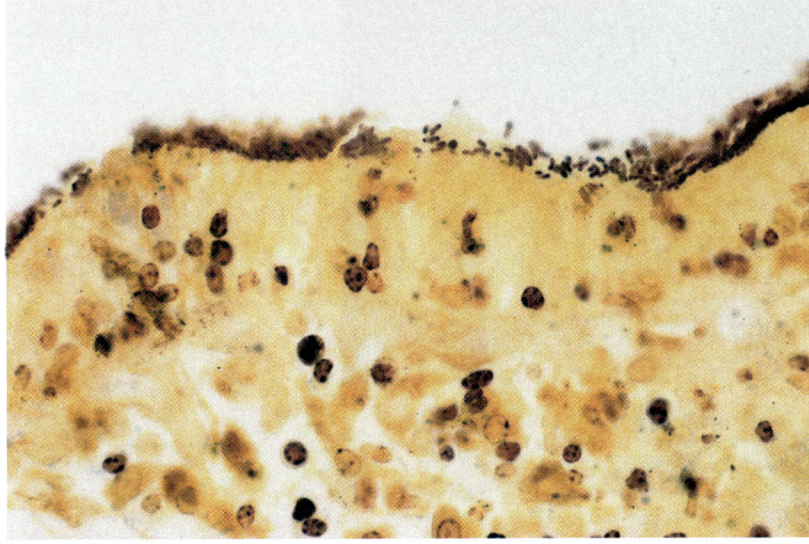

Figure 4-35: **Colon. Enteroadherent *E coli*. Warthin-Starry.**

SPECIFIC INFECTIOUS AGENTS

- Morphology .... *Cytomegalovirus* infects colonic endothelial and stromal cells more commonly than epithelial cells. There may be large, discrete ulcers or diffuse colitis. *Herpes* infection is most commonly found in the anorectal area, and rarely involves other colonic sites. The virus infects epithelial nuclei, eliciting minimal inflammatory response. *Microsporidia* typically infect the epithelium of the small intestine, and, when the infection is severe, histiocytes at other sites. They should be differentiated from intrahistiocytic organisms with similar morphology, e.g., histoplasma and leishmania. *Amebae* may cause chronic crypt destructive colitis and resemble ulcerative colitis or Crohn's disease on biopsy.

- Endoscopic features .... *Cytomegalovirus* produces colitis with features indistinguishable from infectious or idiopathic ulcerative colitis, or discrete ulcers deep enough to erode intramural arteries and cause acute bleeding. *Herpes* infection typically involves the anorectal area, with edema and discrete or coalescing aphthous ulcers.

  Microsporidia and other intrahistiocytic organisms produce nonspecific endoscopic changes, or none at all.

- Clinical features .... Diarrhea, abdominal pain, hematochezia, and anorectal pain (herpes).

- Differential diagnosis ...... Histologic: *Cytomegalovirus*, bizarre stromal cells.

  Endoscopic: Acute colitis, Crohn's disease, solitary rectal ulcer syndrome.

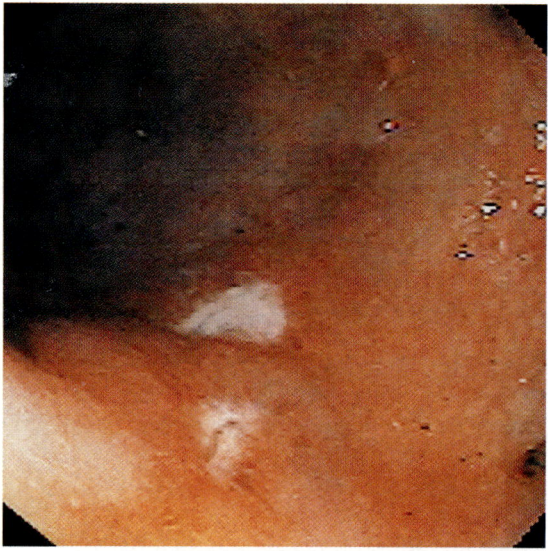

Figure 4-36: **Colon, Sigmoid. Cytomegalovirus Infection.** Two discrete, relatively clean-based, smooth-margined ulcers. The larger one appears to be deeper. The mucosa surrounding the smaller ulcer seems thickened.

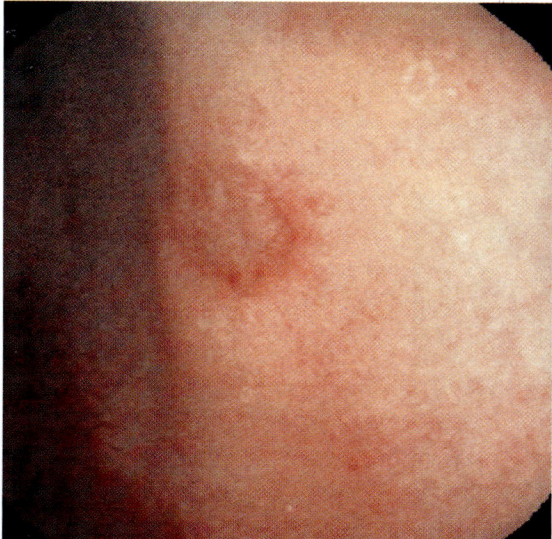

Figure 4-37: **Colon, Sigmoid. Cytomegalovirus Infection.** Discrete ulcer with smooth margin and clean base.

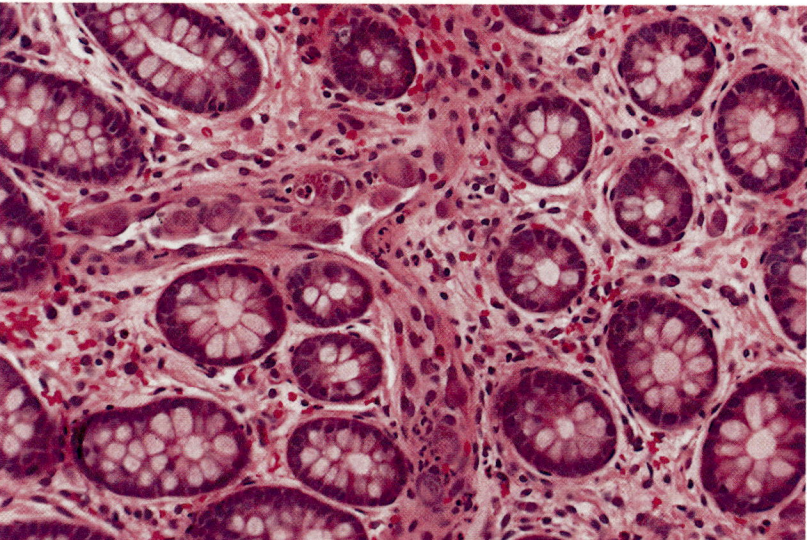

Figure 4-38: **Colon. Cytomegalovirus Infection.** Cytomegalovirus inclusions in endothelial cells.

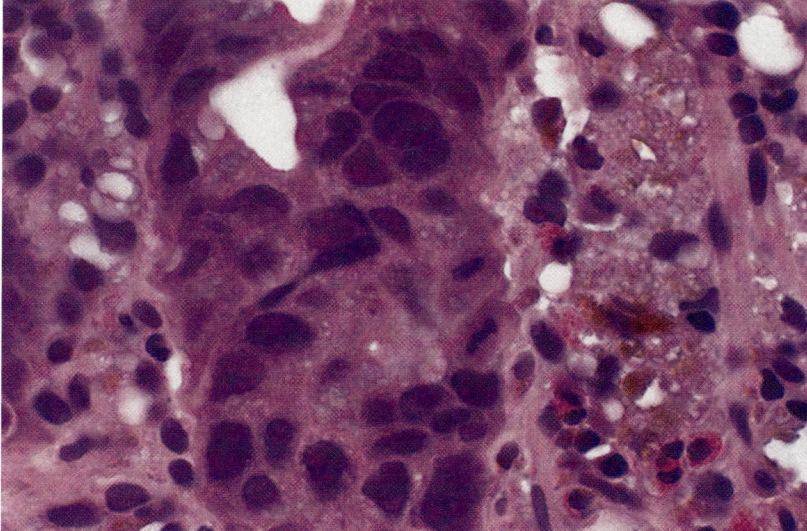

Figure 4-39: **Colon. Herpesvirus Infection.** Multinucleated epithelial cells with nuclear molding, and eosinophilic inclusions.

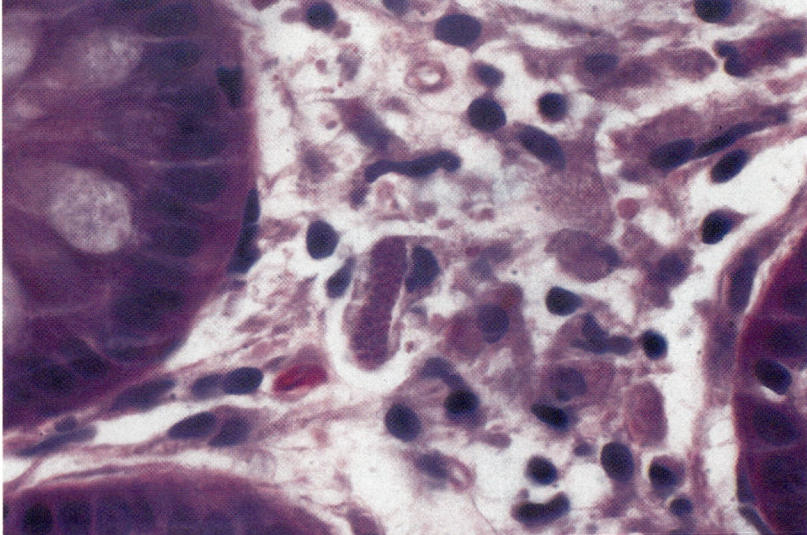

Figure 4-40: **Colon. Microsporidiosis.** Histiocytes filled with microsporidia in patient with severe microsporidial infection in the small intestine.

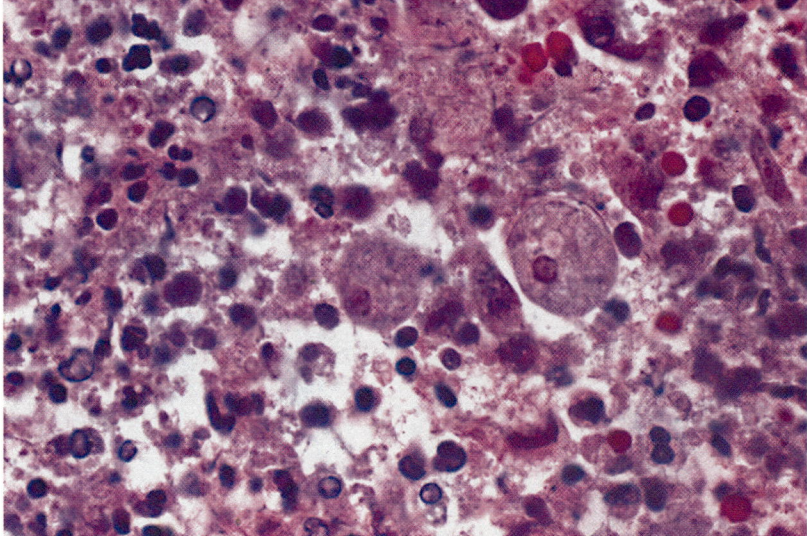

Figure 4-41: **Colon. Amebic Colitis.** Amebae in ulcer.

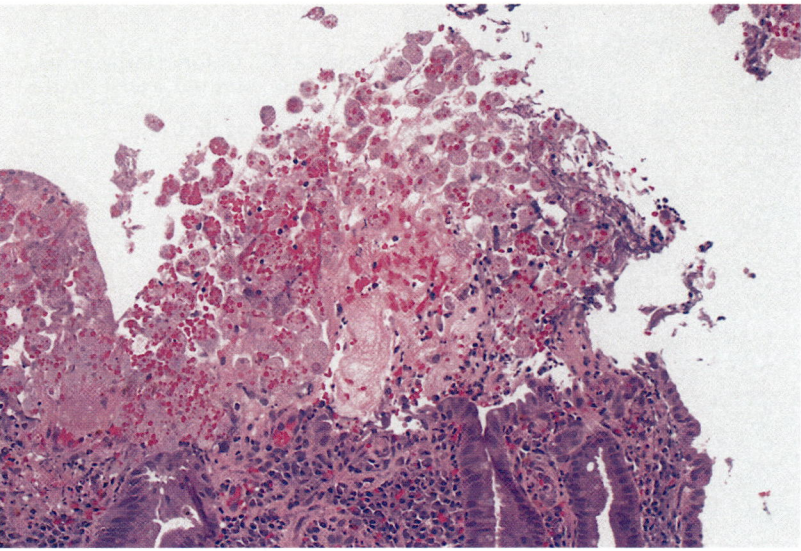

Figure 4-42: **Colon. Amebic Colitis.** Amebae overlying eroded mucosa.

PARASITES

- Morphology .... Parasites may attach to the luminal surface with no mucosal reaction, or penetrate the mucosa and cause an eosinophilic inflammatory reaction.

- Endoscopic features .... Worms are usually encountered incidentally, especially in endemic areas. Large worms such as ascarides and tapeworms may protrude from the ileocecal valve.

    Amebic infections produce minute punctate erosions in the left colon or impressive inflammatory changes in the right colon accompanied by edema and narrowing of the lumen.

    Most parasites cause no distinctive mucosal findings.

- Clinical features .... Nonspecific abdominal pain, bloating and gas, weight loss, iron deficiency anemia.

- Differential diagnosis ...... Histologic: Seeds and starch grains ("lentils") are frequently mistaken for parasites. Prominent cell walls and an external layer that often has a spiny coat distinguish seeds from parasites.

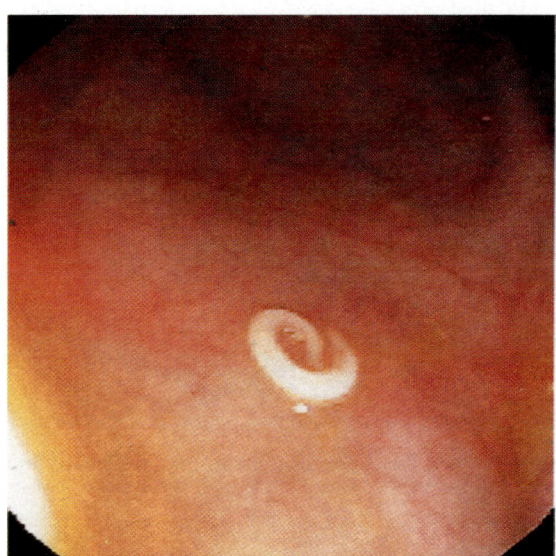

Figure 4-43: **Cecum. *Trichuris trichiura* (Whipworm).** The size and appearance of this worm suggest *Trichuris trichiura* (whipworm) infection.

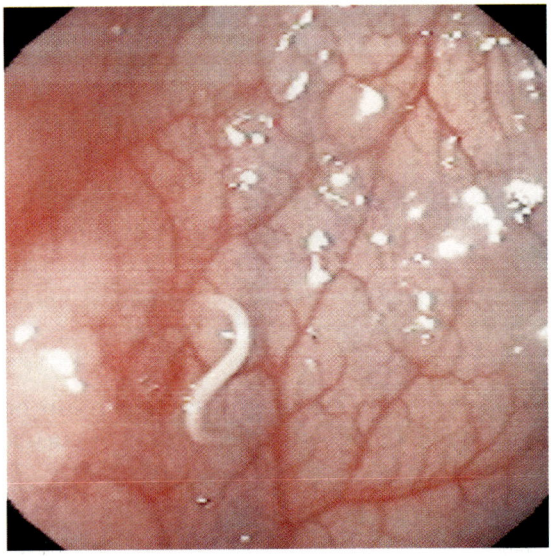

Figure 4-44: **Colon, Transverse. Parasite, Probably** *E vermicularis* **(Pinworm).** Small S-shaped worm approximately 1 cm in length.

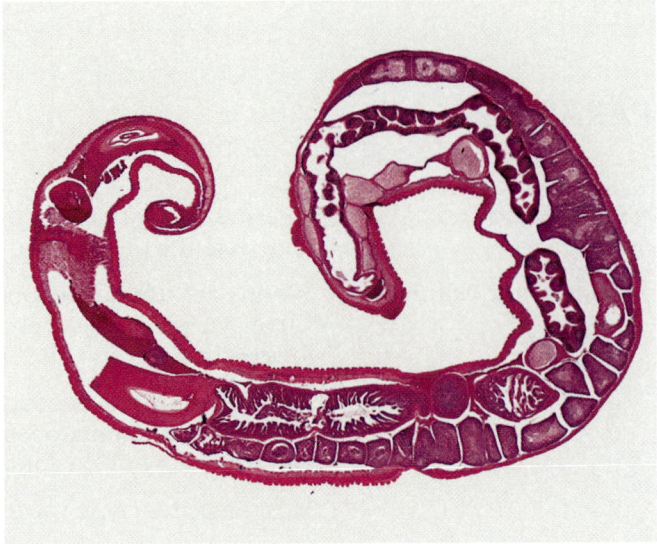

Figure 4-45: **Colon.** *E vermicularis.*

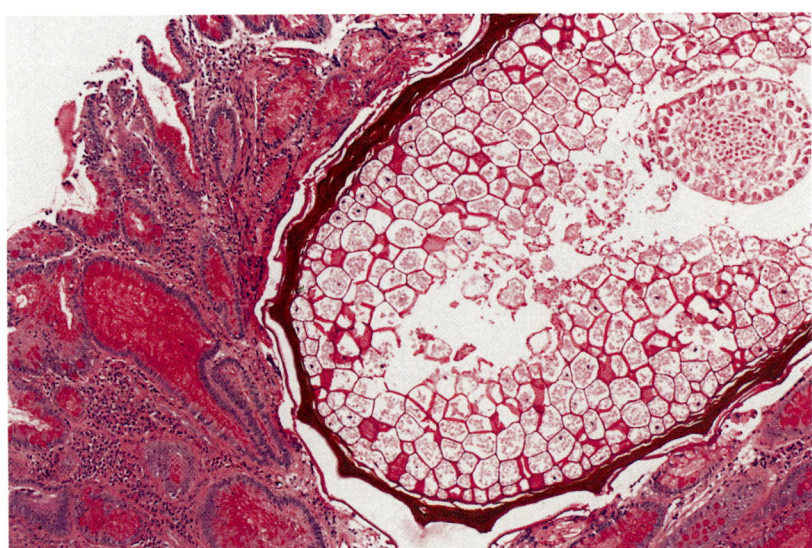

Figure 4-46: **Colon. Seed Embedded in Adenoma.** Cell walls and spiny outer coat characterize this seed and distinguish seeds from parasites. PAS.

ACUTE COLITIS

- Morphology .... In acute infectious colitis, neutrophils mainly infiltrate lamina propria. Cryptitis and crypt abscesses, if present, are usually a minor component. Crypt architecture is normal; there is no evidence of prior crypt destruction and regeneration. Congestion and surface erosion are common. Focal neutrophilic inflammation is a feature of aphthous erosions. The mononuclear cell population is normal or only slightly increased.

- Endoscopic features .... Acute inflammation causes focal patchy or segmental erythema, mucosal friability, mucosal hemorrhage, ulceration, and erosion. Acute bacterial colitis can produce patchy erythema, discrete ulceration, and erosions ranging from aphthous-type (1 to 2 mm diameter) to larger lesions (2 to 5 mm diameter) scattered throughout the colon. There may be thickening of the haustral folds and mucosa with luminal narrowing.

- Clinical features .... Diarrhea, pain (cramping or generalized and constant), urgency and tenesmus, hematochezia, and, with a bacterial infection, fever. In toxic presentations, there may be severe abdominal pain accompanied by tenderness either localized in the lower quadrants or generalized, suggestive of peritonitis.

- Differential diagnosis ...... Etiologic: Bacterial infections; toxin-producing bacteria (e.g., *C difficile*), and drugs (NSAIDs). Acute or toxic phase of idiopathic inflammatory bowel disease may be clinically or histologically indistinguishable from these causes.

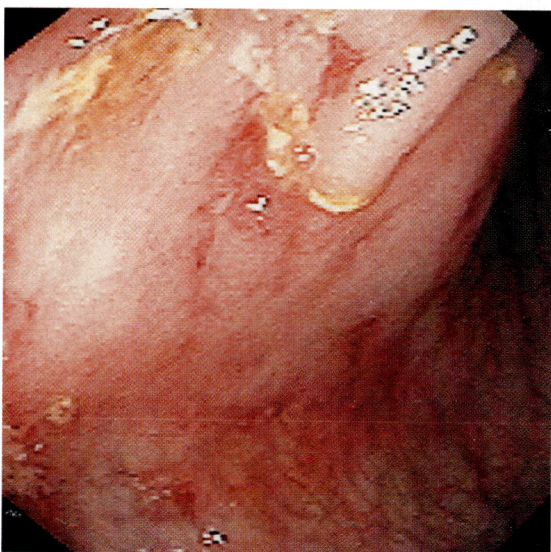

Figure 4-47: **Colon, Hepatic Flexure. Acute Colitis.** Shallow ulceration with erythematous borders on the edge of a haustral fold. The surrounding mucosa appears normal.

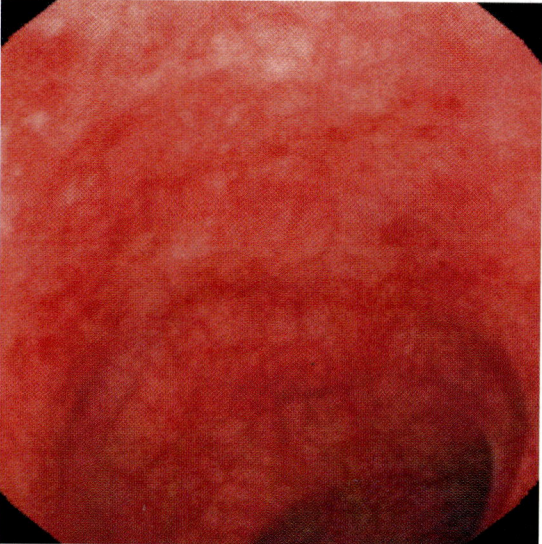

Figure 4-48: **Colon, Sigmoid. Acute Colitis.** Segment with patchy and punctate erythema. Suggestion of minute erosions in some of the larger erythematous patches (upper left).

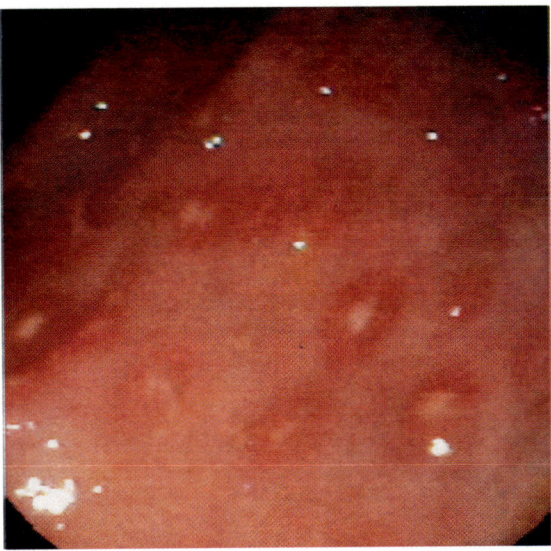

Figure 4-49: **Colon, Sigmoid. Acute Colitis with Erosions.** Multiple minute, shallow, aphthous erosions with erythematous borders.

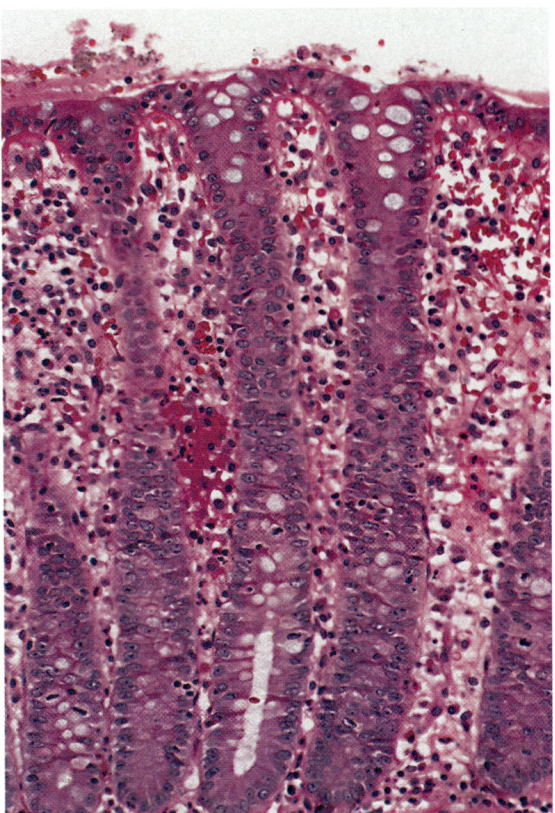

Figure 4-50: **Colon. Acute Colitis.** A small number of neutrophils in the lamina propria; a few in the epithelium. Mononuclear cells appear in normal numbers and distribution. Crypts are proliferative with decreased mucin.

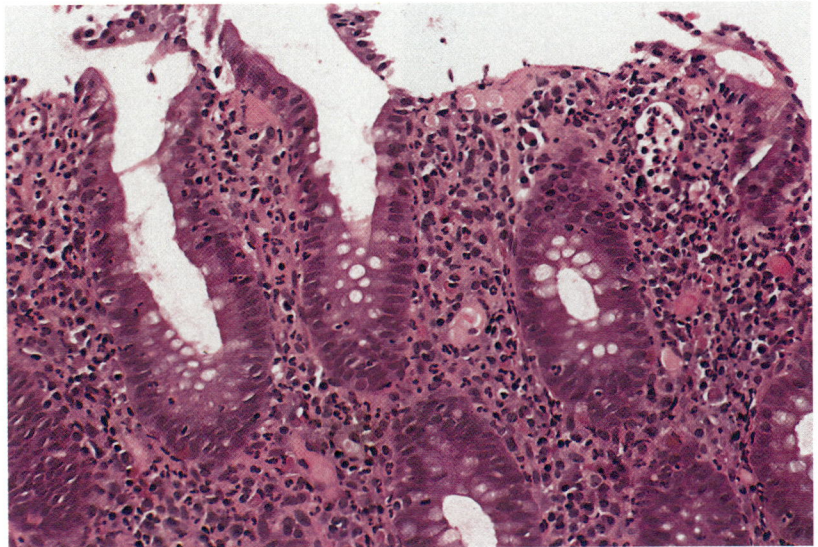

Figure 4-51: **Colon. Acute Colitis.** Numerous neutrophils, but normal numbers of mononuclear cells.

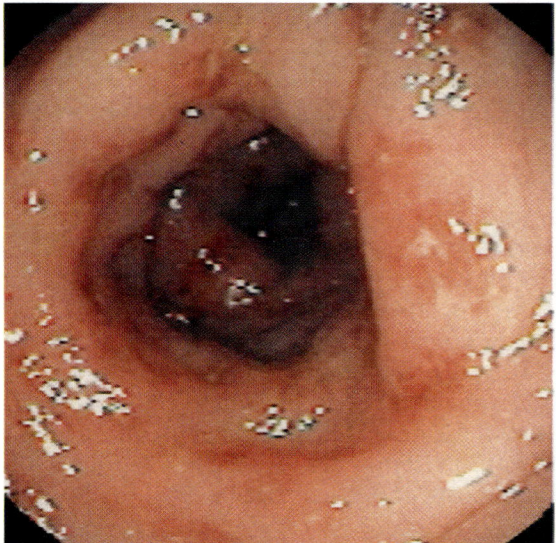

Figure 4-52: **Colon, Transverse. Acute Colitis with Erosions.** Multiple erosions with irregular erythematous borders. Suggestion of edema; thickening of haustral folds and minimal narrowing of the lumen.

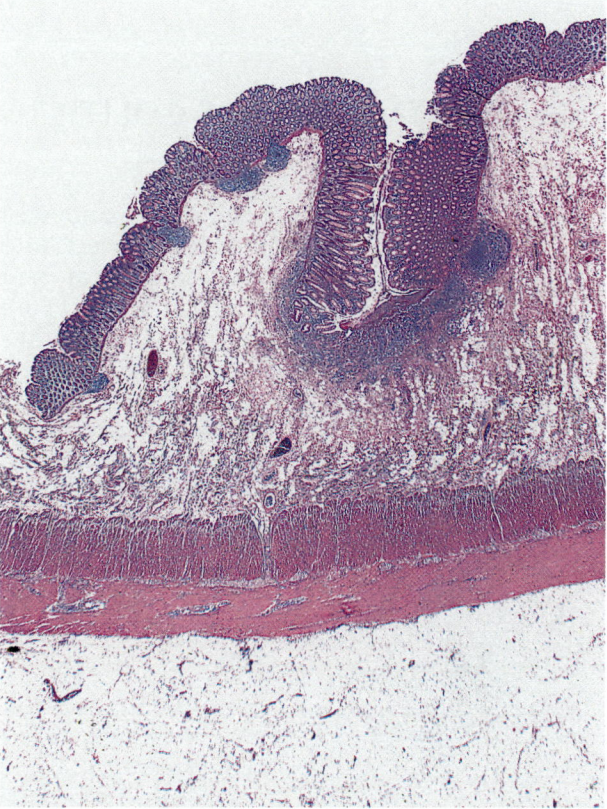

Figure 4-53: **Colon. Focal Acute Crohn's Colitis with Aphthous Erosion.** Shallow erosion and inflammation over a lymphoid follicle. Surrounding mucosa normal. Submucosa very edematous. Early lesion of Crohn's disease.

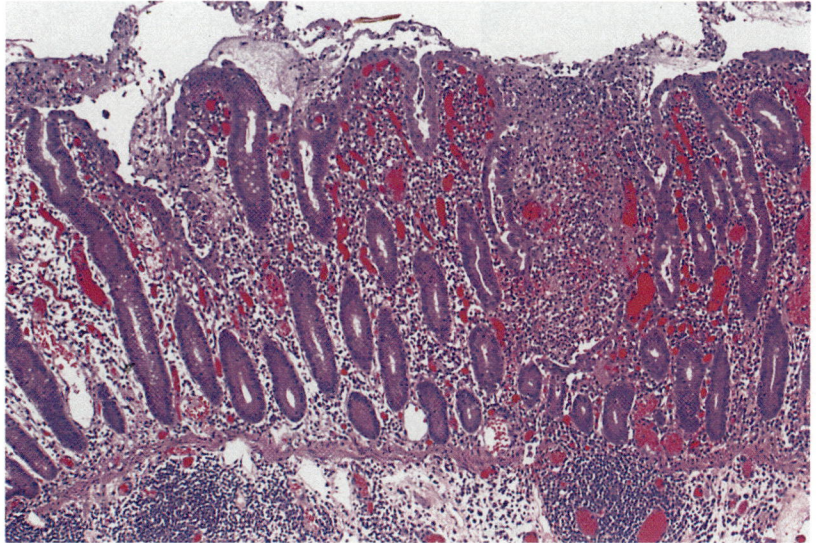

Figure 4-54: **Colon. Acute Salmonella Colitis.** Neutrophilic inflammation with crypt abscess and erosion, but overall preservation of crypt architecture. Marked congestion. Evenly spaced crypts remain close to the muscularis mucosae.

PSEUDOMEMBRANOUS COLITIS

- Morphology .... Pseudomembranous colitis due to *C difficile* is typically a mild, superficial, and multifocal process, but it can develop into an ischemic/toxic picture. *C difficile* may also cause an acute colitis indistinguishable from other common self-limited infections. Subacute or incompletely suppressed disease may result in an acute inflammatory reaction, in spite of a chronic relapsing clinical course. In resolving or partially treated disease, pseudomembranes may be absent, and isolated dilated crypts lined by attenuated epithelium containing few neutrophils are the only finding. Although the histologic pattern of pseudomembranous colitis is characteristic of *C difficile*, it may also be seen as a result of early or mild ischemia, other bacterial toxins, or a drug reaction.

- Endoscopic features .... Discrete, rounded collections of adherent, white-to-yellow exudate can coalesce into large swatches. Lesions are most common in the rectum but can occur throughout the colon. *C difficile* colitis may not produce the characteristic pseudomembranous exudate, but rather appear as an acute colitis of any cause.

- Clinical features .... Diarrhea and, occasionally, urgency and tenesmus. Antibiotics have been most commonly taken orally; however, in hospitalized patients, they are administered intravenously. Fungal infections may cause pseudomembranous colitis. These patients are typically hospitalized and debilitated, and may be immunosuppressed.

- Differential diagnosis...... Etiologic: Early ischemia, bacterial toxins, drug reaction. The full-blown pattern of pseudomembranous colitis is more often an effect of weak bacterial toxins than early ischemia.

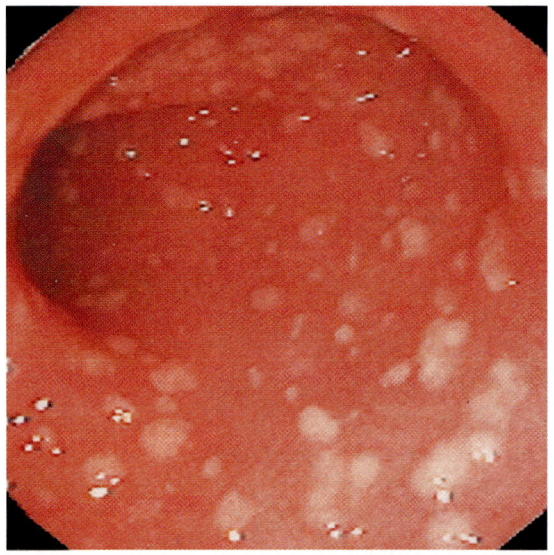

Figure 4-55: **Rectum. Pseudomembranous Colitis.** Discrete, glistening, yellow-white patches of adherent exudate, some coalescing, scattered throughout the mucosa.

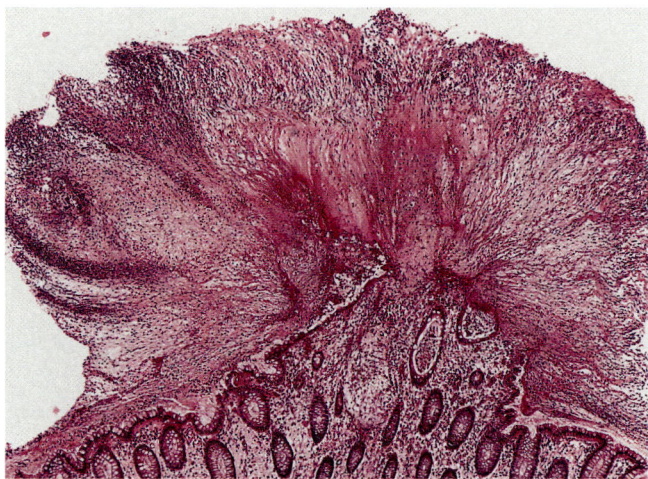

Figure 4-56: **Colon. Pseudomembranous Colitis.** Superficial acute colitis with surface epithelial necrosis and extravasation of mucin, neutrophils, and fibrinous exudate in a volcanic fashion onto the surface mucosa. This is the classical appearance of *C difficile* colitis.

ISCHEMIA

- **Morphology** .... Pseudomembranous and ischemic patterns may overlap, e.g., a severe *C difficile* lesion may resemble ischemia histologically and endoscopically. A healing reaction of 4 or more weeks duration resembles the healing reaction of chronic crypt destructive colitis. A relative lack of inflammation may distinguish between chronic or healing ischemic injury and chronic destructive colitis, but in the absense of acute ischemic changes, the distinction may be impossible. Marked submucosal edema is characteristic of ischemia but is not seen on biopsy. Edema may evolve to fibrosis and segmental strictures indistinguishable from Crohn's disease.

- **Endoscopic features** .... Ischemic colitis due to large vessel disease is segmental and frequently involves the sigmoid to the midtransverse colon, a distribution helpful in endoscopic diagnosis. Ischemic changes proximal to the midtransverse colon occur with verotoxin-producing *E coli* infections. If vascular in origin, however, they imply occlusion of the superior mesenteric artery and require urgent intervention with angiography as well as surgery. Rectal ischemia is unusual because of the dual blood supply, but ischemia due to bacterial toxins or rectal prolapse occurs. Endoscopic findings of mild colonic ischemia of any cause include patchy erythema, mucosal hemorrhage, and edema. Moderate ischemic changes produce submucosal hemorrhage ("thumbprinting" seen on x-ray) and ulcers that may be shallow, irregular, and, in some cases, longitudinal, suggesting the possibility of Crohn's disease. Ulcers may also be focal and deep. In severe ischemia, bowel necrosis, seen endoscopically, results in loss of identifiable mucosa, with extensive exudative ulceration and possibly a blackened or dusky hue.

- **Clinical features** .... Abrupt onset of crampy abdominal pain, often localized to the left abdomen, followed by diarrhea with urgency and then hematochezia is typical and distinctive. Bleeding is usually minor, never severe. There is abdominal tenderness over the involved bowel segment. Peritoneal signs often develop, but usually resolve relatively quickly (24 to 48 hours). After abdominal aortic vascular surgery, ischemic colitis may be subtle and marked by postoperative diarrhea, without other signs or symptoms. Fever may be the only indication.

  Superior mesenteric artery occlusion produces typical, but more severe, symptoms and signs. Blood lactate levels are elevated. Embolic vascular occlusion may be recognized by peripheral findings in the lower extremity, especially the toes, due to showering of emboli.

- **Differential diagnosis** ...... Endoscopic: Acute bacterial colitis, idiopathic inflammatory bowel disease.

  Etiologic: Causes include hypovolemic/low-flow states, *E coli* 0157:H7, *Shigella* verotoxin, vasculitis/vasculopathy, thrombotic states, emboli, drug reactions.

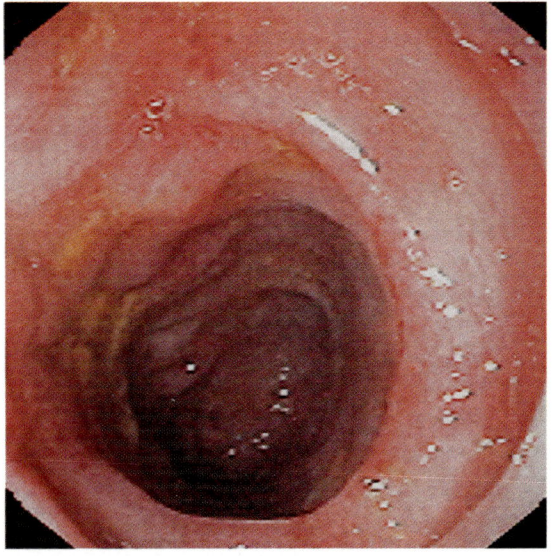

Figure 4-57: **Colon, Descending. Ischemia.** Patchy mucosal erythema. The haustral folds in the foreground appear thickened.

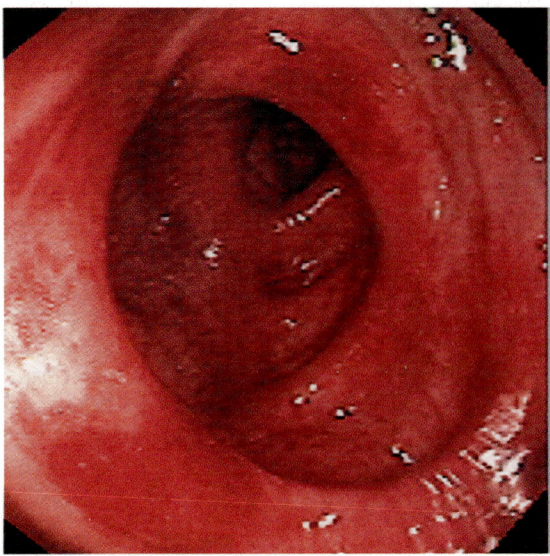

Figure 4-58: **Colon, Sigmoid. Ischemia.** Mucosal hemorrhage with multiple punctate areas of erythema or hemorrhage.

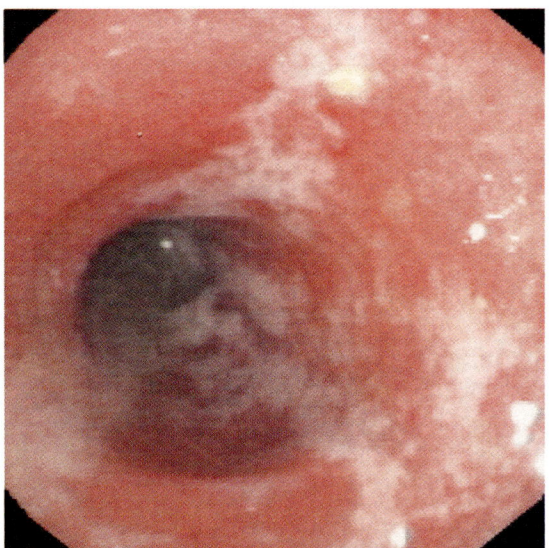

Figure 4-59: **Colon, Splenic Flexure. Ischemia.** Shallow, irregular, exudative ulceration with interspersed erythema.

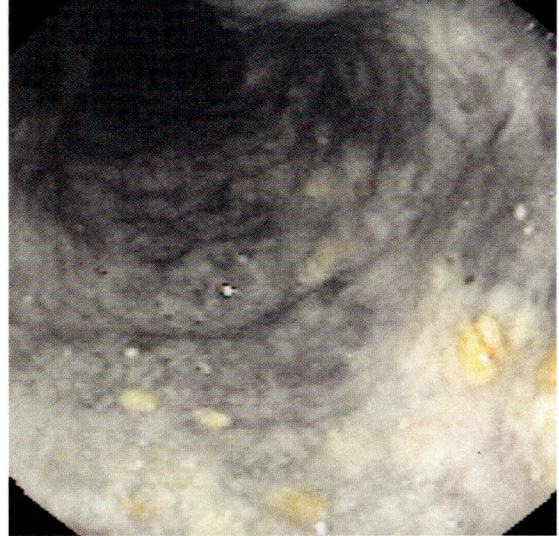

Figure 4-60: **Colon, Descending. Ischemia.** Necrotic bowel with extensive ulceration, exudate, and a dusky black background.

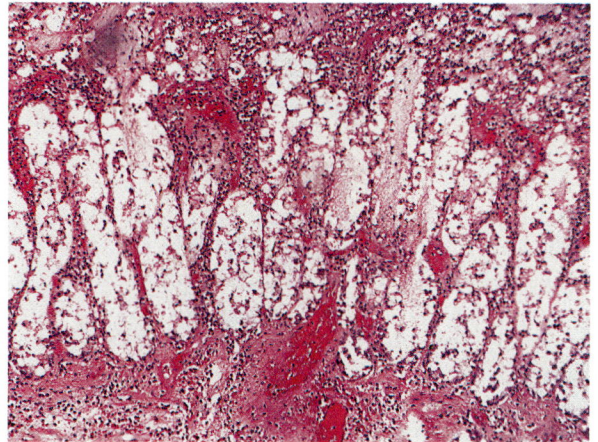

Figure 4-61: **Colon. Ischemia.** Dilated crypts, necrotic and sloughed crypt epithelium, inflammatory exudate, microvascular thromboses, and hemorrhage.

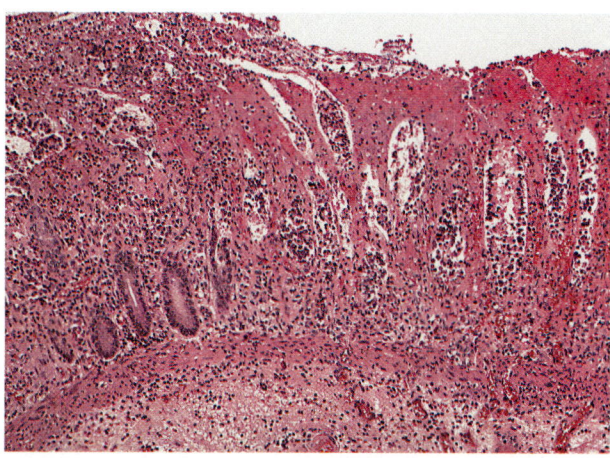

Figure 4-62: **Colon. Ischemia.** Fibrinoinflammatory exudate, surface and crypt epithelial necrosis with focal crypt preservation, fibrin extravasation in lamina propria, and fibrin thrombi in submucosal vessels.

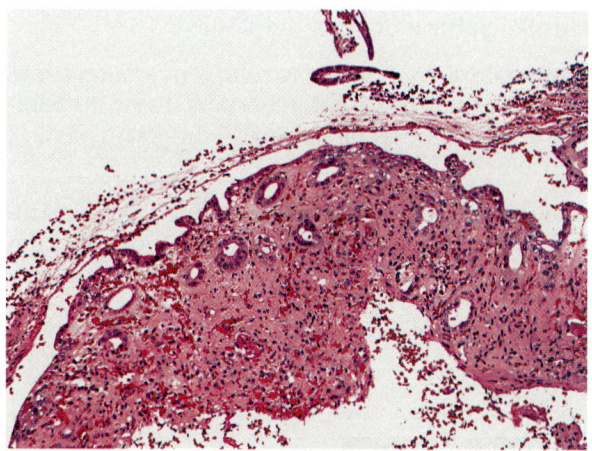

Figure 4-63: **Colon. Ischemia.** Thin, fibrinous exudate over surface. Shrunken crypts with attenuated epithelium. Paucicellular lamina propria filled with pink, proteinaceous fluid.

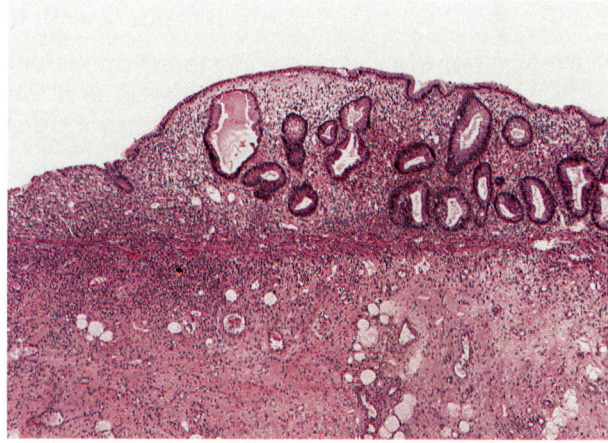

Figure 4-64: **Colon. Ischemic Pattern, 4 Weeks Duration.** Healing reaction: surface re-epithelialization, inflammation, crypt regeneration with branching and distortion near edge of ulcer. Edematous submucosa.

RADIATION INJURY

- Morphology — The histologic features of acute radiation injury are essentially those of ischemia, with or without radiation-induced cytologic changes. Included are nuclear and cytoplasmic enlargement and vacuolization, large macronucleoli, or subtle alterations in nuclear chromatin, similar to those of chemotherapy or folate deficiency. The mucosa in chronic radiation injury may be normal or fibrotic, with or without microvascular telangiectasia. The characteristic lesions of chronic radiation injury, submucosal vascular intimal hyperplasia and fibrosis, are seldom seen in biopsy specimens.

- Endoscopic features — Acute radiation injury causes edema, erythema, mucosal hemorrhage, spontaneous bleeding, erosions, ulceration, and exudate. Often the mucosa is granular. Massive submucosal edema may narrow the lumen.

    Chronic radiation injury causes mucosal pallor, friability, and innumerable angiectasias, which vary in size and shape. Unlike angiodysplasia, the individual lesions have a more irregular corkscrew vascular configuration, which contrasts with the fernlike pattern of angiodysplasia.

- Clinical features — Acute injury causes abdominal cramping, diarrhea with urgency, sometimes hematochezia, and, when the rectum is involved, tenesmus. Later, in addition to diarrhea and urgency, there may be rectal outlet bleeding with passage of blood and clots, and incontinence.

- Differential diagnosis — Histologic: Acute radiation injury is usually indistinguishable from inflammatory colitis or ischemia of other causes. The vascular lesions of radiation telangiectasia, angiodysplasia, portal hypertension, and scleroderma are identical. Radiation-induced cytomegaly can mimic cytomegalovirus, dysplasia, chemotherapy effect, folate deficiency, and malignancy.

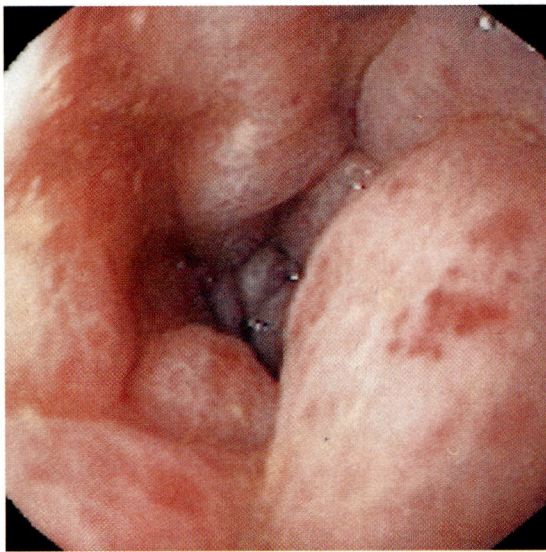

Figure 4-65: **Rectum. Acute Radiation Injury.** Marked edema with narrowing of the lumen in a patient receiving pelvic radiation.

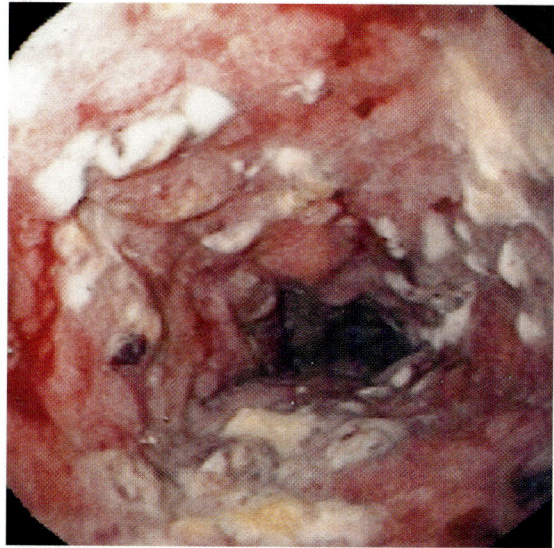

Figure 4-66: **Rectum. Acute Radiation Injury.** Diffuse edema, ulceration, exudates, granularity, loss of normal vascular pattern, and spontaneous bleeding.

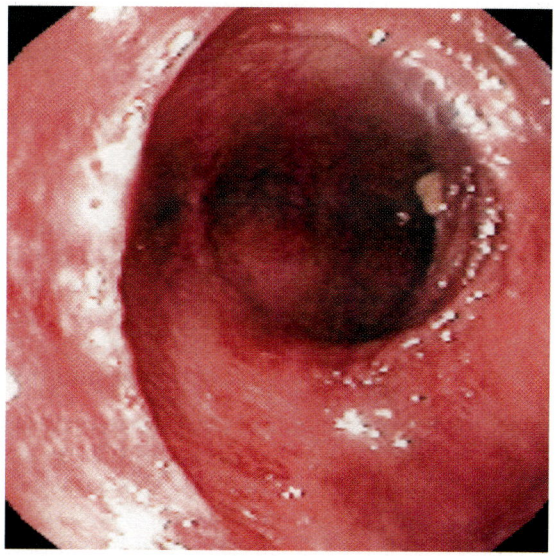

Figure 4-67: **Colon, Transverse. Acute Radiation Injury.** Mucosal granularity, diffuse erythema, punctate hemorrhages, spontaneous bleeding, and small, shallow ulcers.

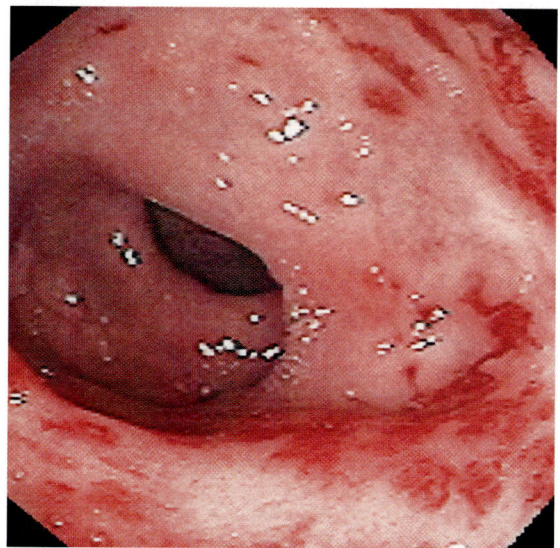

Figure 4-68: **Rectum. Chronic Radiation Injury.** Multiple angiectasias. Appearance, number, and distribution are characteristic of chronic radiation proctopathy. History of pelvic radiation.

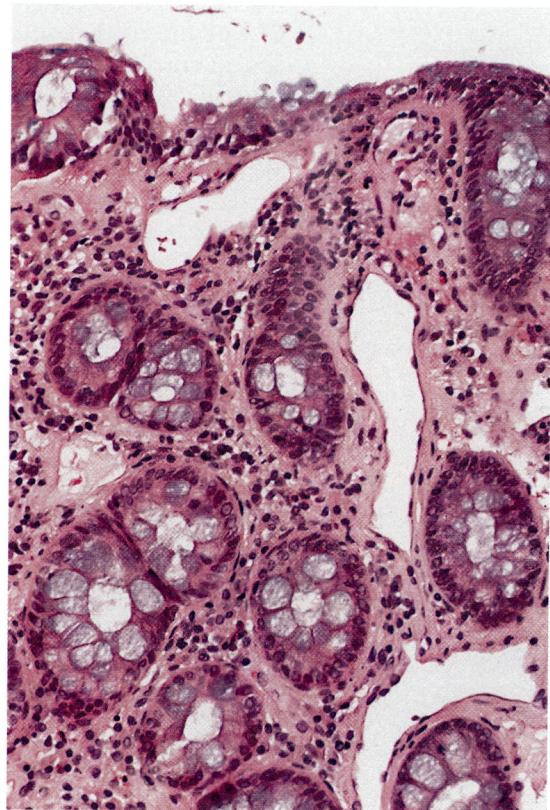

Figure 4-69: **Colon. Chronic Radiation Injury.** Ectatic sclerotic capillaries and venules in lamina propria; slight glandular distortion.

ACTIVE CHRONIC DESTRUCTIVE COLITIS

- Morphology .... This pattern of injury is characteristic of, but not specific for, chronic idiopathic inflammatory bowel disease. *Toxic colitis* is a complication of chronic ulcerative colitis, and of a number of other pathologic conditions affecting the colon, or it may occur de novo. In ulcerative colitis patients, infection may trigger the toxic colitis episode. Cytomegalovirus infection is an identifiable and treatable trigger in ulcerative colitis.

- Endoscopic features .... The spectrum includes erythema with loss of vascular pattern in the erythematous areas or widespread vascular pattern dropout, granularity, friability, spontaneous hemorrhage, shallow ulcers, and exudate. Ulcers are minute and focal, or large, shallow, and coalescing. The mucosa in inactive disease may be normal or appear damaged with scarring and thickening, bridging, cicatricial deformity, and pseudopolyps. Postinflammatory polyps and pseudopolyps may be isolated and infrequent or multiple, large, crowded, and heaped up, and may bridge the lumen. Severity should be estimated and distribution documented, since the latter has long-term implications regarding surveillance for dysplasia. Disease extending proximal to the splenic flexure is classified as pancolitis. The best strategy to distinguish Crohn's disease from ulcerative colitis is to take samples from areas of moderate disease intensity and normal areas, and then separately submit the biopsy specimens in order to document skip areas. A clinical diagnosis of Crohn's disease or ulcerative colitis assumes infection has been excluded.

- Clinical features .... Diarrhea, abdominal cramping, urgency, tenesmus, hematochezia, iron deficiency anemia, weight loss, fever. Extraintestinal signs and symptoms of active disease include erythema nodosum, arthritis, oral aphthous ulceration, scleritis, and pyoderma gangrenosum.

    New onset idiopathic inflammatory bowel disease presents acutely with bloody diarrhea, with or without weight loss and fever. In severe acute disease, there may be a toxic presentation with fever, anorexia, anemia, and profound bloody diarrhea. Fulminant acute disease may cause toxic megacolon. In chronic disease, bowel habits wax and wane depending upon the level of disease activity. Extraintestinal manifestations may precede or accompany flares.

- Differential diagnosis ...... Clinical and histologic: Ulcerative colitis; Crohn's disease; chronic enteric, systemic, venereal, or parasitic infections; ischemic injury; medication-induced colitis (NSAIDs); colitis associated with diverticular disease.

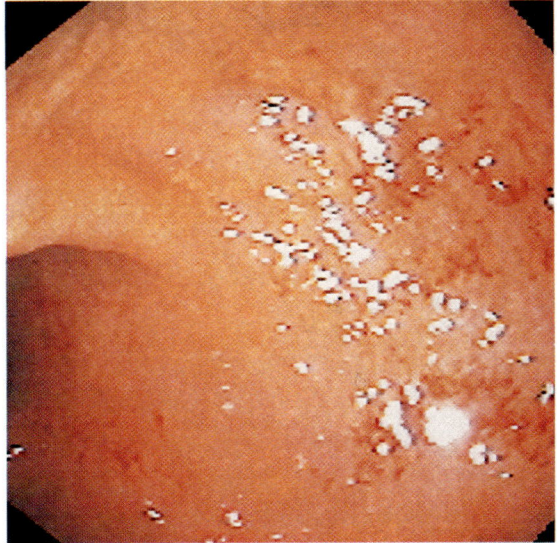

Figure 4-70: **Rectum. Active Chronic Destructive Colitis.** Minimal changes of inflammatory bowel disease; granularity and loss of normal vascular pattern. Irregular patches of erythematous mucosal hemorrhage (right).

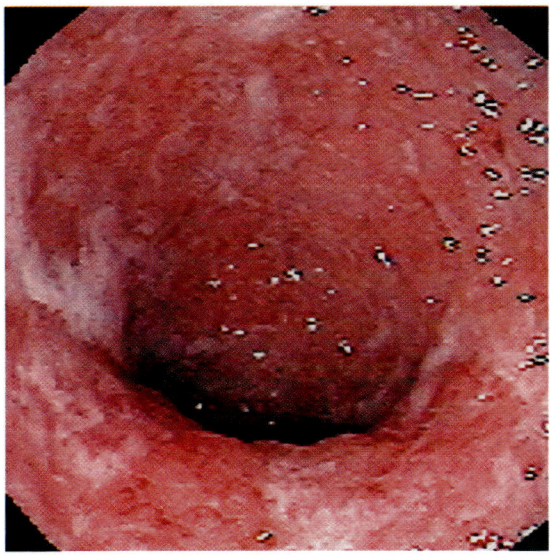

Figure 4-71: **Colon, Transverse. Active Chronic Destructive Colitis.** Panmucosal inflammation with loss of haustral folds and vascular pattern, diffusely scattered shallow ulcers, mucosal nodularity, granularity, and pinpoint areas of hemorrhage. Consistent with moderate to severe chronic inflammatory bowel disease.

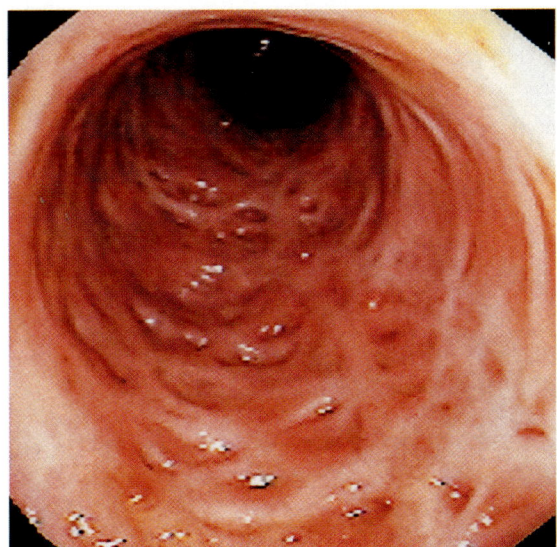

Figure 4-72: **Colon, Transverse. Active Chronic Destructive Colitis.** Prominent mucosal scarring with cicatricial mucosal bridges.

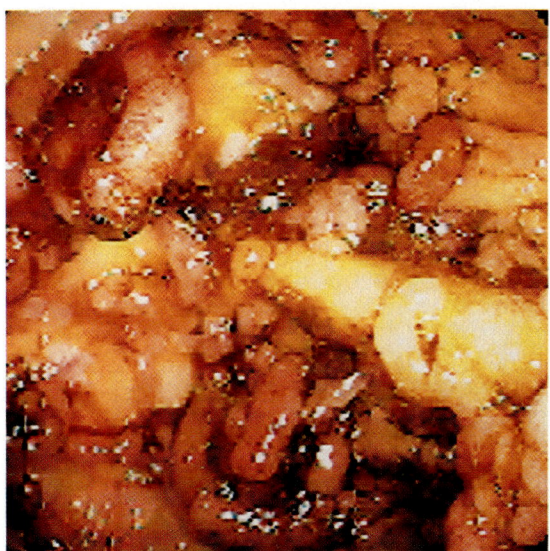

Figure 4-73: **Colon, Descending. Active Chronic Destructive Colitis.** Innumerable inflammatory polyps and pseudopolyps from diminutive sessile lesions to long, fingerlike structures.

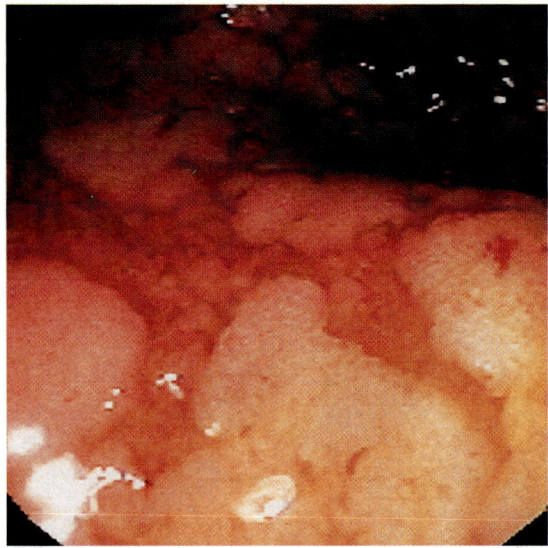

Figure 4-74: **Colon. Active Chronic Destructive Colitis.** Proximal colon with regenerative mucosa creating the appearance of "mucosal islands."

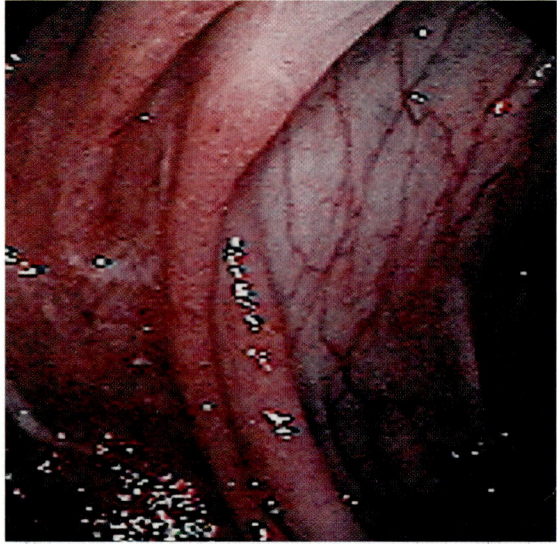

Figure 4-75: **Colon. Active Chronic Destructive Colitis.** Transition zone between active inflammation and normal mucosa. The active inflammation is highlighted by the loss of the vascular pattern, granularity, erythema, and some exudate.

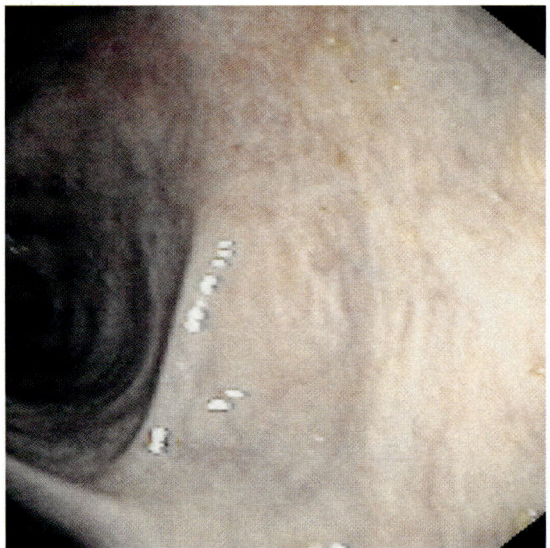

Figure 4-76: **Colon, Transverse. Chronic Destructive Colitis.** Quiescent colitis with mucosal pallor, loss of vascular pattern, and scarring (upper portion of photo).

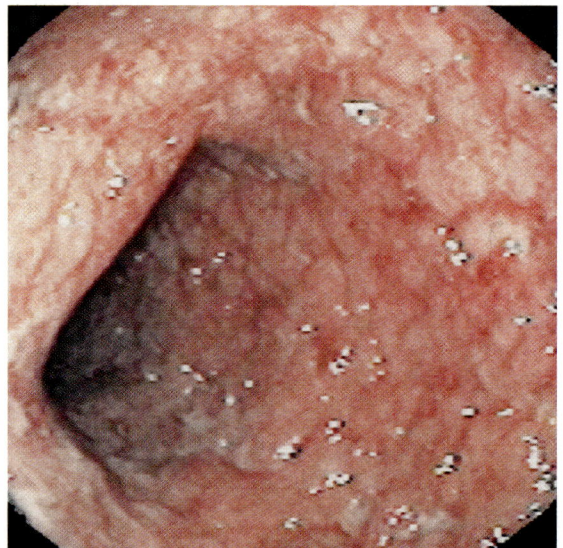

Figure 4-77: **Colon, Sigmoid. Active Chronic Destructive Colitis.** Active inflammation with granularity, hemorrhage, erythema, and microulceration. There is straightening of the lumen with haustral dropout as well.

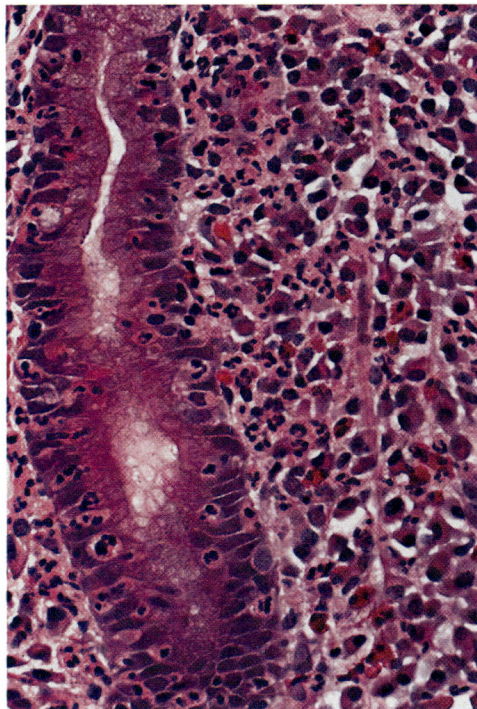

Figure 4-78: **Colon. Active Chronic Destructive Colitis.** Mononuclear cells and neutrophils fill the lamina propria and extend to the crypt base (basal plasmacytosis).

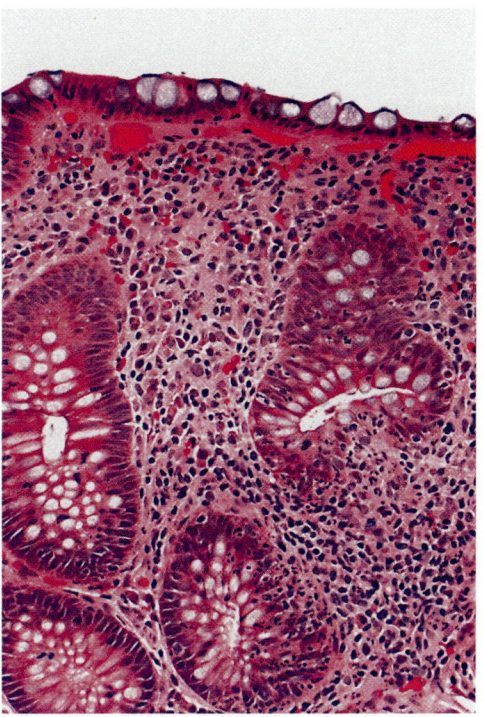

Figure 4-79: **Colon. Active Chronic Destructive Colitis.** Active cryptitis with focal crypt destruction and chronic inflammation. Normal surface epithelium, despite chronic destructive inflammation, favors Crohn's disease.

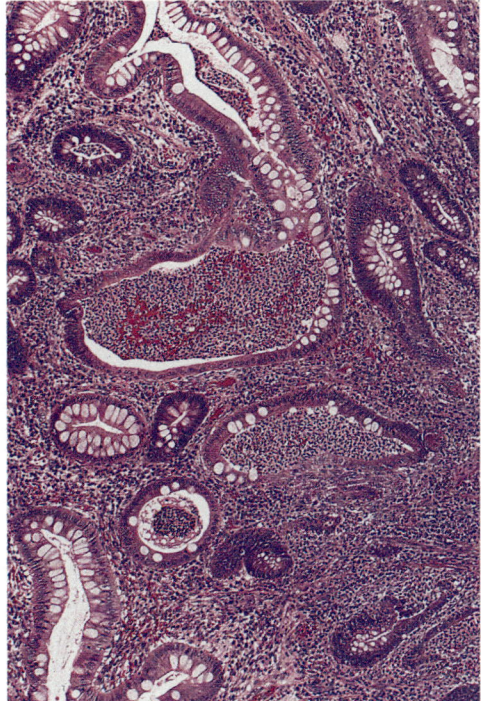

Figure 4-80: **Colon. Active Chronic Destructive Colitis.** Crypt abscesses and crypt destruction with architectural distortion characteristic of ulcerative colitis.

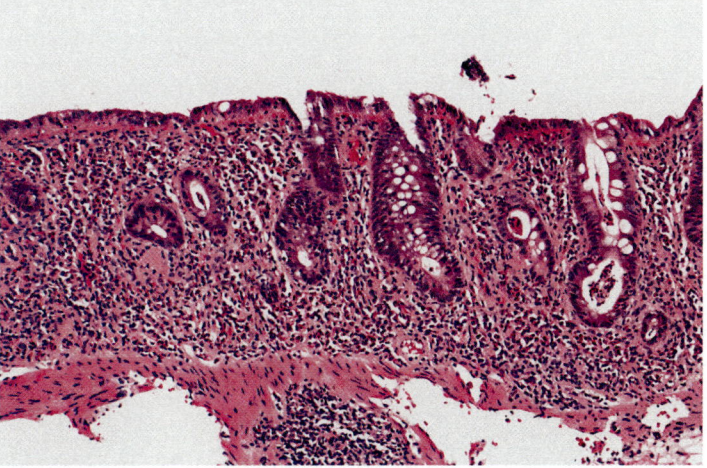

Figure 4-81: **Colon. Active Chronic Destructive Colitis.** Chronic inflammation and basal plasmacytosis; crypt dropout, regeneration, distortion, and separation from the muscularis mucosae.

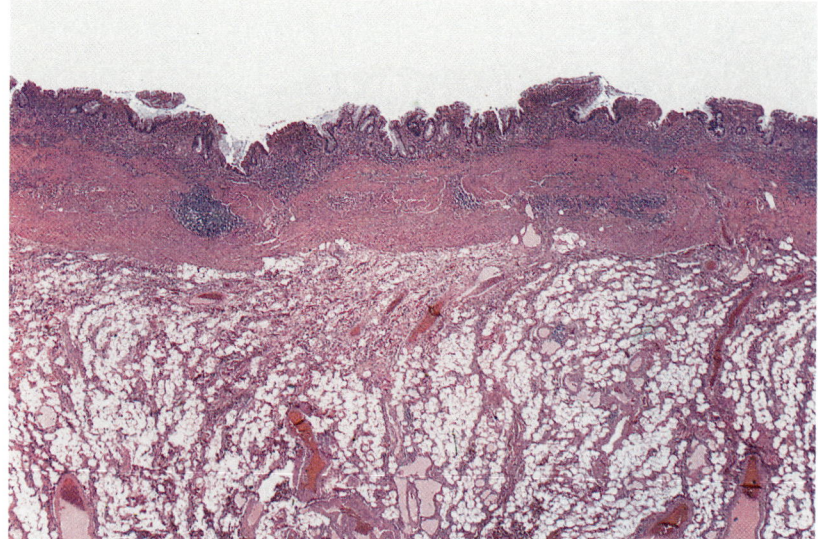

Figure 4-82: **Colon. Atrophic and Distorted Active Chronic Destructive Colitis (Ulcerative Colitis).** Diffuse atrophic and distorted mucosa with marked thickening of the muscularis mucosae. Submucosa not inflamed.

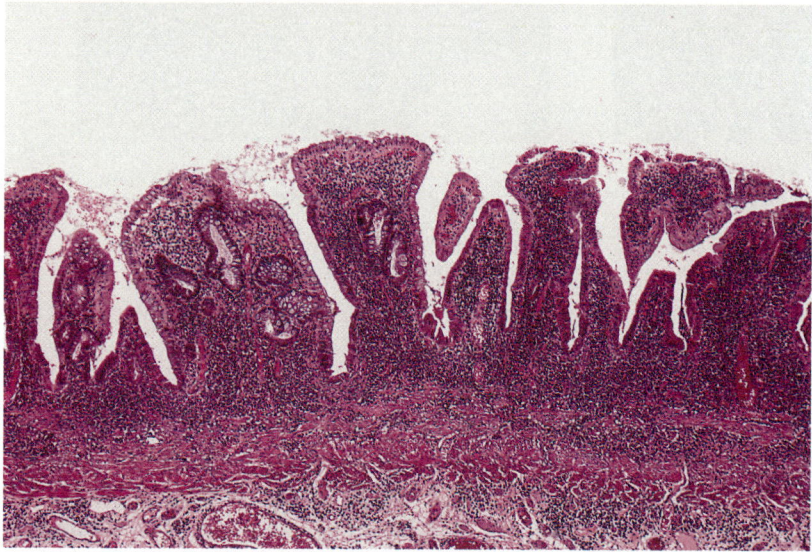

Figure 4-83: **Colon. Active Chronic Destructive Colitis (Ulcerative Colitis).** Villiform architecture due to chronic crypt destruction and regeneration. Thickened muscularis mucosae.

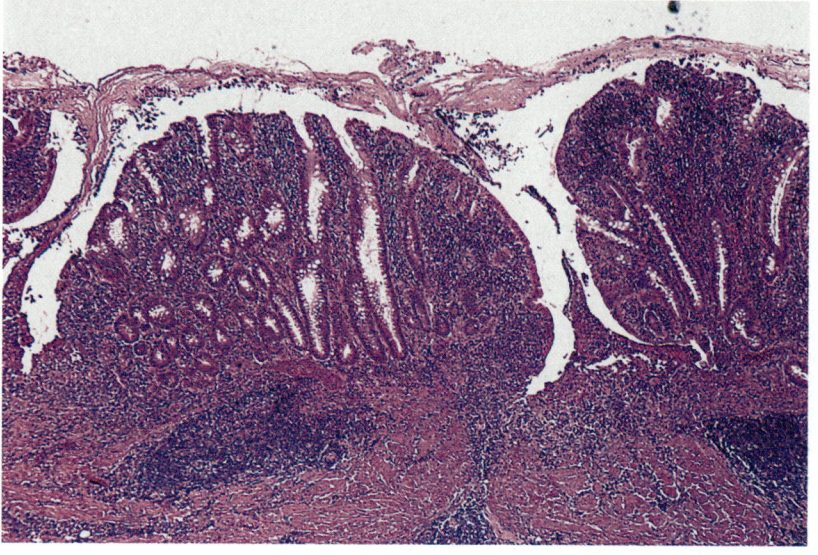

Figure 4-84: **Colon. Active Chronic Destructive Colitis.** Regenerating inflamed mucosa, atrophy, and pseudopolyp formation with ulcerated mucosa on either side of the "polyp."

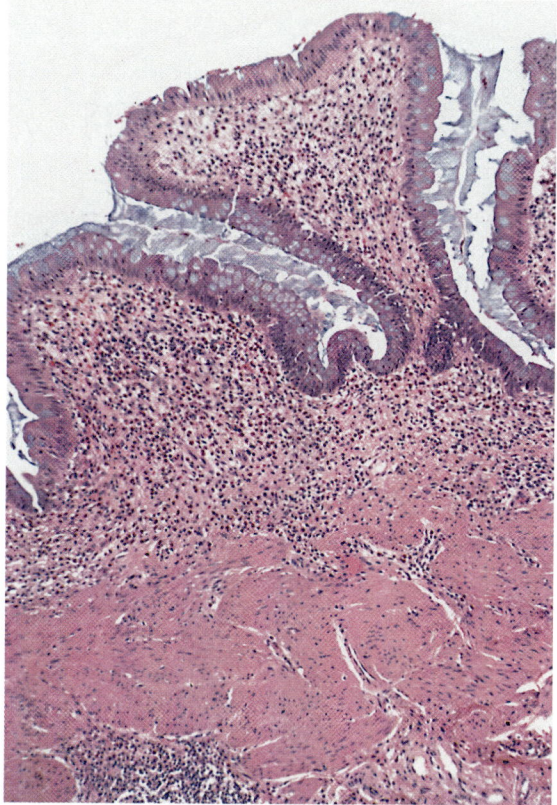

Figure 4-85: **Colon. Chronic Destructive Colitis.** Chronic mucosal inflammation, crypt distortion, without significant neutrophilic component.

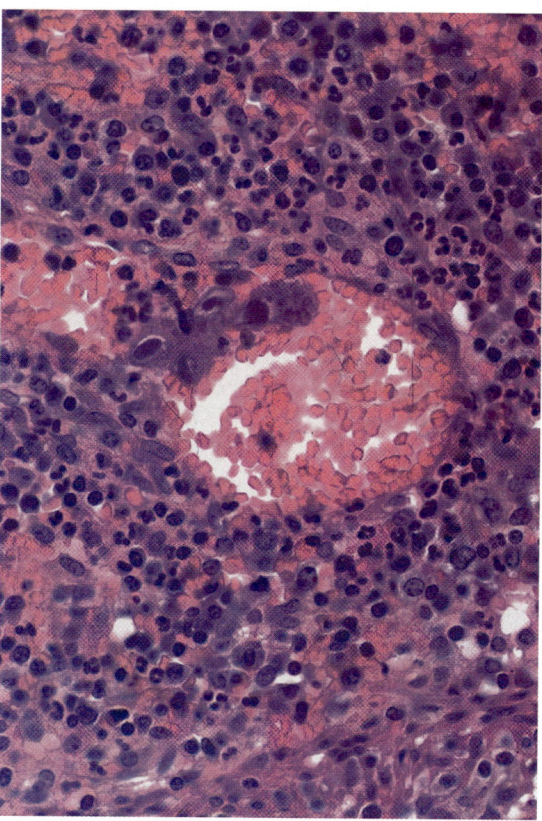

Figure 4-86: **Colon. Ulcerative Colitis and CMV.** Cytomegalovirus inclusions in endothelial cells of dilated venule surrounded by active chronic inflammation.

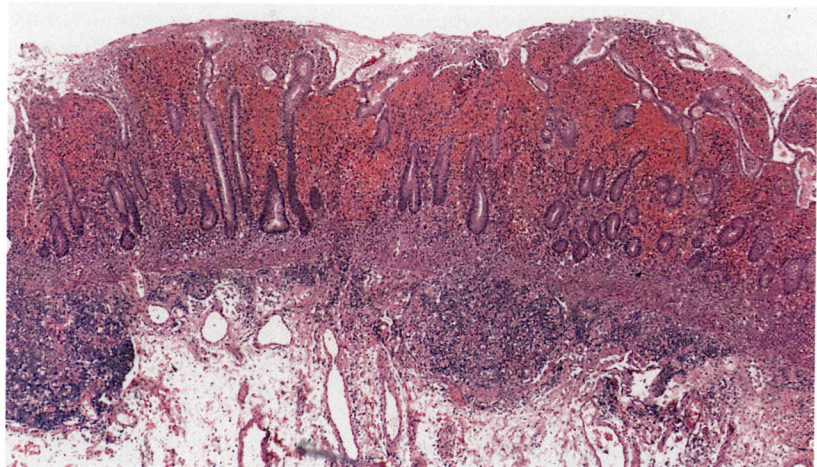

Figure 4-87: **Colon. Ulcerative Colitis.** Chronic crypt destructive colitis with hemorrhage.

DYSPLASIA AND ADENOCARCINOMA IN ULCERATIVE COLITIS

- Morphology .... Low-grade dysplasia has nuclear changes similar to those of an adenoma and nuclear stratification limited to the lower half of the epithelium. High-grade dysplasia has nuclear stratification extending to the luminal border of the epithelium and/or marked nuclear anaplasia. Crypts can be crowded, complex, or cribriform. Dysplasia begins at the crypt base or at the luminal surface; it may be isolated or multifocal. Dysplasia may be limited to cytologic changes in the crypt base in flat mucosa and be undetectable grossly, or have an irregular, nodular, or villous profile. Adenocarcinoma can arise beneath an area of flat, low-grade dysplasia.

- Endoscopic features .... Unless there is a dysplasia-associated lesion/mass, dysplasia is endoscopically inapparent. During surveillance, the endoscopist should sample areas that do not appear actively inflamed. Isolated small polyps should be removed completely for histologic examination.

- Clinical features .... Active or quiescent long-standing pancolitis.

- Differential diagnosis ...... Histologic: Reactive or regenerative atypia; adenocarcinoma.

DYSPLASIA-ASSOCIATED LESION/MASS (DALM)

- Morphology .... Dysplasia detected in surveillance biopsies is an indication of increased risk for development of invasive adenocarcinoma in the absence of a mass. When a mass is present, even if superficial biopsies show only low-grade dysplasia, the likelihood of invasive carcinoma beneath it is high. It can be difficult or impossible to distinguish a sessile adenoma from a DALM, particularly in the older (adenoma-prone) population. Features favoring adenoma: a lesion located well away from the area of colitis; a discrete nodule with a well-defined focus of dysplasia limited to the luminal surface; no evidence of crypt architectural distortion in biopsy samples from the adjacent mucosa or at the base of the polyp. Features favoring a DALM: patchy dysplasia; associated colitis, active or quiescent, in biopsy samples from the area; other areas of dysplasia in flat mucosa. DALM may arise in quiescent colitis.

- Endoscopic features .... The DALM most often presents as an isolated, irregular, sessile polyp; small (< 1 cm), discrete, or subtle, or large, sprawling, and similar to a villous adenoma.

- Clinical features .... Long-standing chronic ulcerative colitis.

- Differential diagnosis ...... Histologic and endoscopic: Adenoma.

  Endoscopic: Inflammatory polyp.

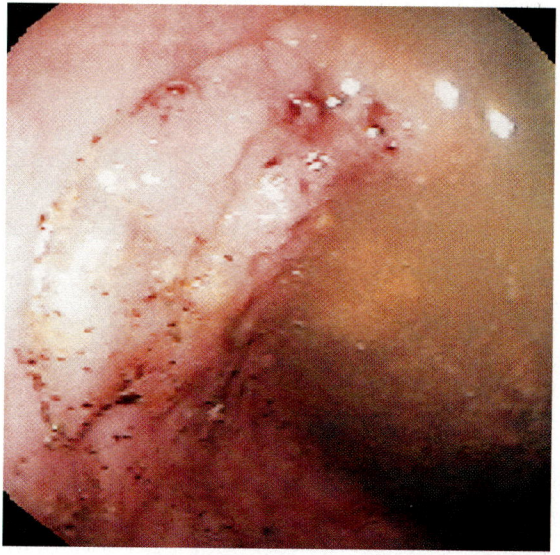

Figure 4-88: **Cecum. Dysplasia-Associated Lesion/Mass.** A subtle sessile polypoid lesion at the base of the cecum in long-standing active chronic ulcerative colitis. The left margin of the polyp and surface features are highlighted by altered blood.

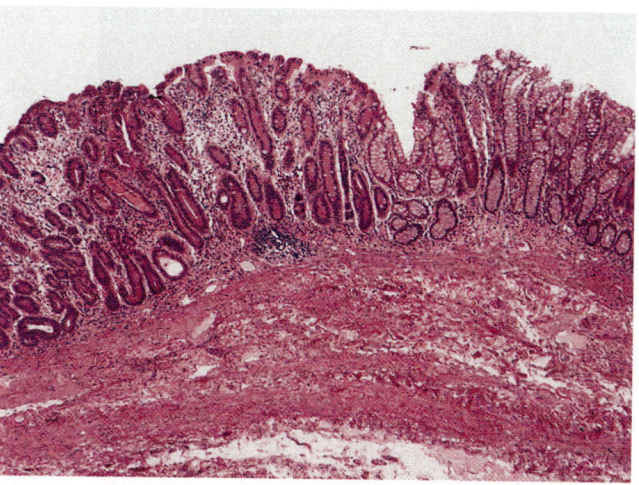

Figure 4-89: **Colon. Dysplasia in Ulcerative Colitis.** Low-grade basophilic atypical glands in flat mucosa of quiescent ulcerative colitis. Irregular distribution of affected glands distinguishes this from an adenoma.

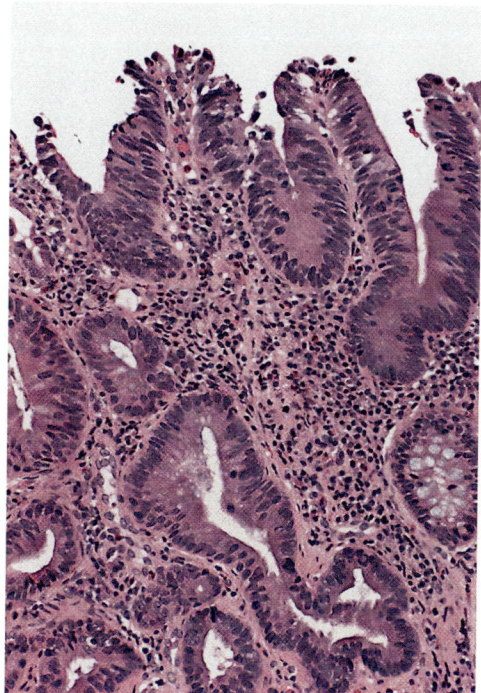

Figure 4-90: **Colon. High-Grade Dysplasia in Ulcerative Colitis.** Nuclear pleomorphism and stratification.

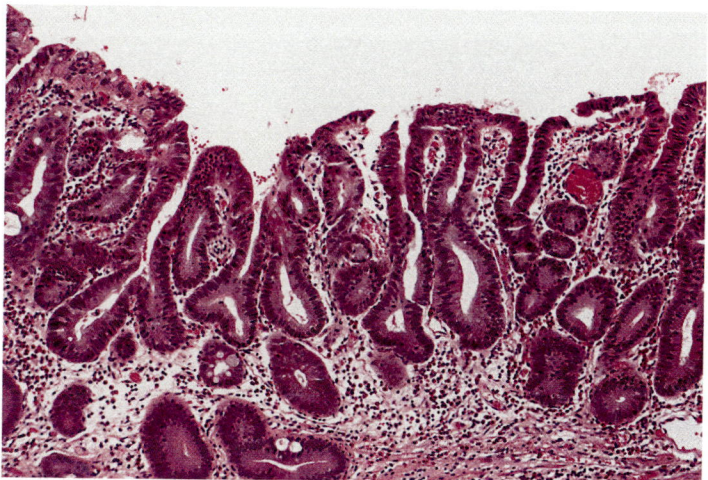

Figure 4-91: **Colon. Dysplasia in Ulcerative Colitis.** Dysplasia, focally high-grade, with piled-up nuclei extending to the luminal surface.

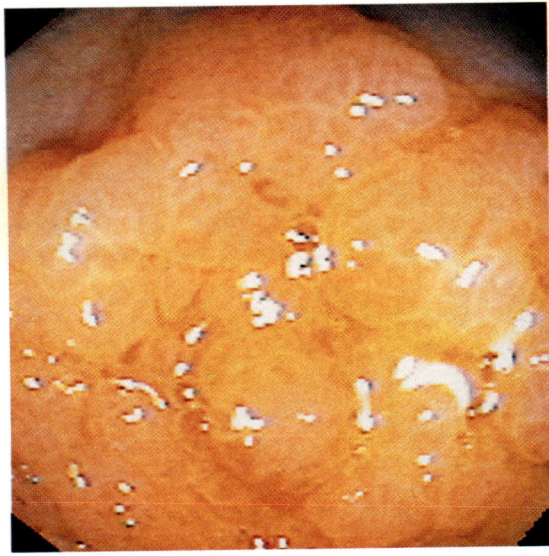

Figure 4-92: **Colon, Hepatic Flexure. Dysplasia-Associated Lesion/Mass.** Large polypoid lesion occupies nearly the entire photograph in a patient with long-standing ulcerative colitis.

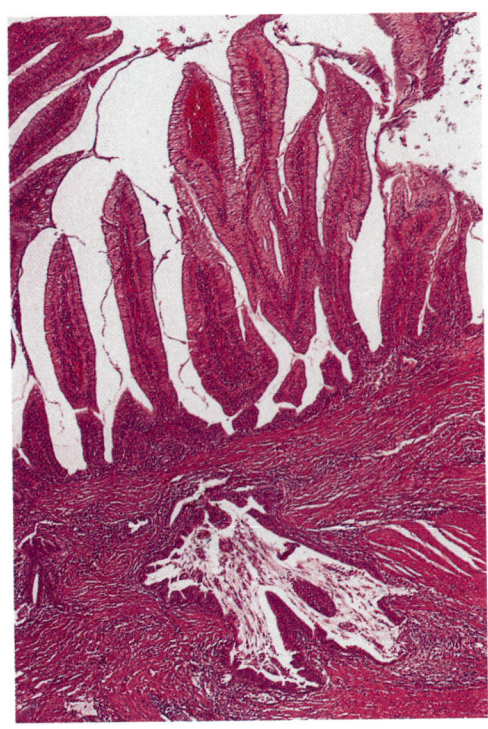

Figure 4-93: **Colon. Adenocarcinoma in Ulcerative Colitis.** Beneath the villiform dysplastic surface, angulated glands invade the wall.

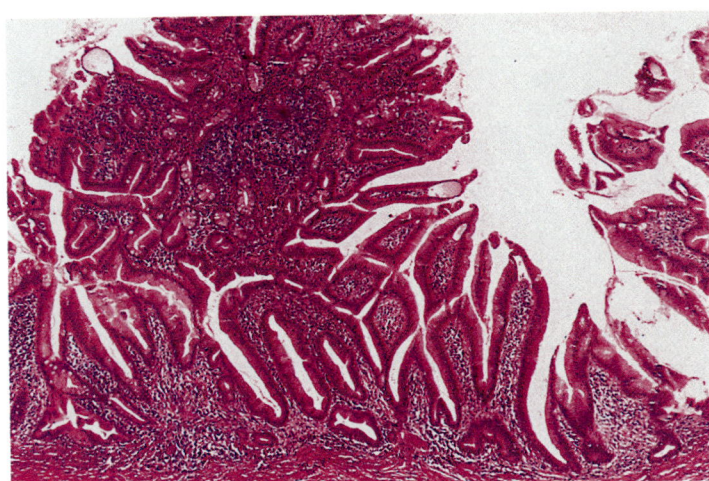

Figure 4-94: **Colon. Dysplasia-Associated Lesion/Mass.** Dysplastic villi forming a sessile mass that does not resemble a typical adenoma.

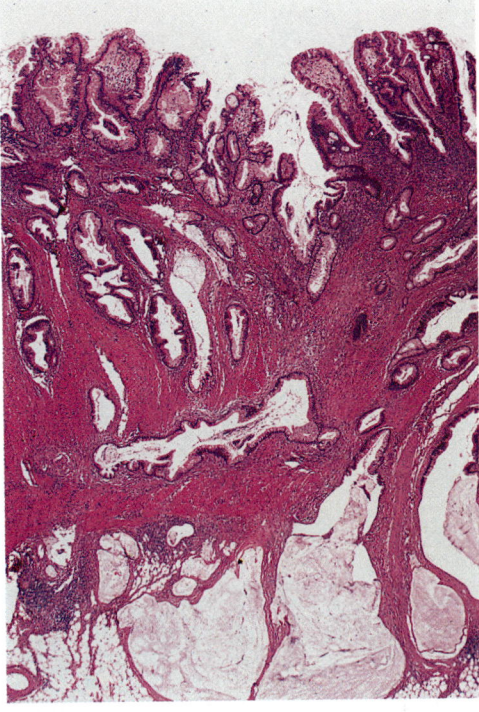

Figure 4-95: **Colon. Dysplasia-Associated Lesion/Mass with Adenocarcinoma.** Low-grade villous dysplasia over an invasive mucinous adenocarcinoma.

CROHN'S COLITIS

- Morphology .... Histologic features that suggest Crohn's over ulcerative colitis: skip areas; rectal sparing; variation in inflammatory intensity within and between biopsy specimens; normal surface epithelium, despite deep active chronic inflammation; discrete aphthous or fissuring ulcers; isolated cryptitis in areas of otherwise normal mucosa; epithelioid granulomas.

- Endoscopic features .... Aphthous ulcers are the earliest manifestations of Crohn's disease. They may precede symptoms by years. Crohn's ulcers are typically discrete and deep, involving normal or near-normal mucosa. Linear rake ulcers and cobblestoning (islands of mucosa separated by linear ulcers) are characteristic. Active Crohn's colitis is usually segmental, but panmucosal involvement occurs. Often, there is rectal sparing. In long-standing Crohn's disease, there can be significant deformity of the ileocecal area. Crohn's patients may present with perianal fistulas and exuberant perianal tags.

- Clinical features .... Diarrhea, weight loss, abdominal cramping, fever, anemia, perineal and perianal pain, purulent perianal discharge from fistulas.

- Differential diagnosis ...... Histologic and endoscopic: Ulcerative colitis; acute (e.g., *Yersinia*) and chronic (e.g., tuberculous, amoebic, venereal) infections; segmental chronic colitis associated with diverticular disease; segmental ischemic necrosis (chronic phase); and granulomatous colitis due to infections (tuberculous, fungal); drug reaction; sarcoidosis.

ADENOCARCINOMA ARISING IN CROHN'S DISEASE

- Morphology .... Adenocarcinoma complicates Crohn's disease less frequently than ulcerative colitis and usually arises in segments of active disease. The carcinoma may be deceptively low-grade.

- Endoscopic features .... Dysplasia in Crohn's disease is not visible. A mass or polypoid lesion should be viewed with suspicion for dysplasia and adenocarcinoma. Adenocarcinoma may have the usual appearance, or be found in deeply ulcerating Crohn's disease.

- Clinical features .... Adenocarcinomas tend to arise from long-standing active disease. They are often responsible for refractory symptoms or an apparent flare in quiescent disease.

- Differential diagnosis ...... Histologic: Sporadic adenocarcinoma.

    Endoscopic: Crohn's disease.

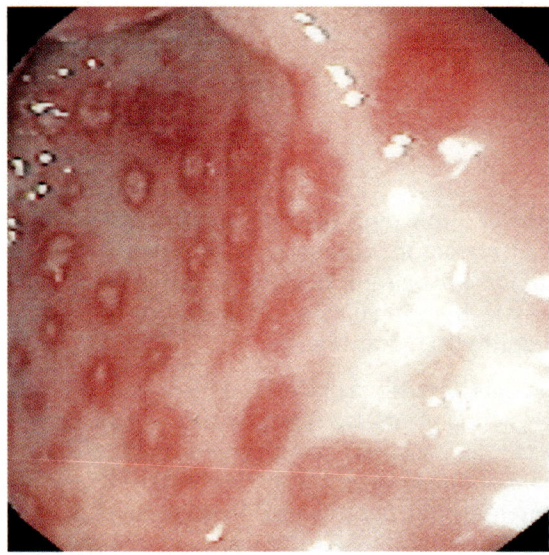

Figure 4-96: **Colon, Sigmoid. Crohn's Colitis** Multiple small, aphthous erosions (1 to 2 mm) with erythematous rims.

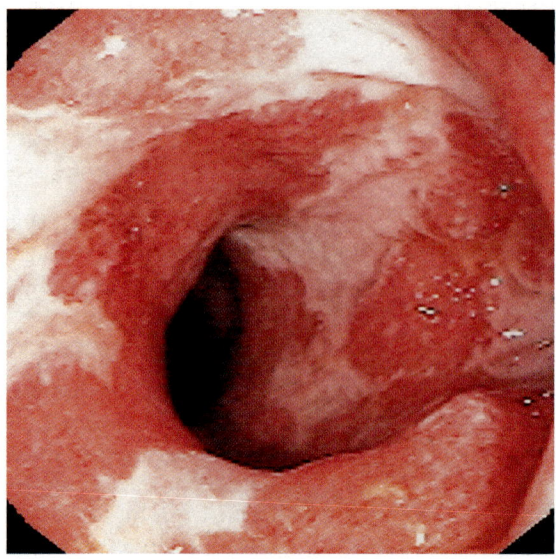

Figure 4-97: **Colon, Sigmoid. Crohn's Colitis.** Segmental colitis with discrete ulcers. The ulcers are linear with serpiginous margins ("rake" ulcers).

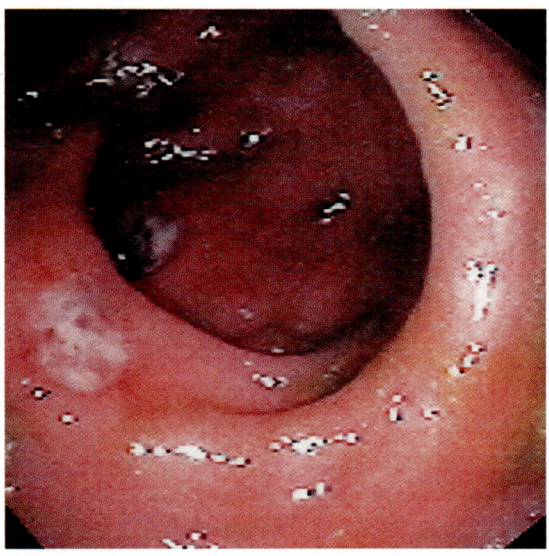

Figure 4-98: **Colon, Sigmoid. Crohn's Colitis.** Two discrete ulcers with minimal surrounding inflammatory change.

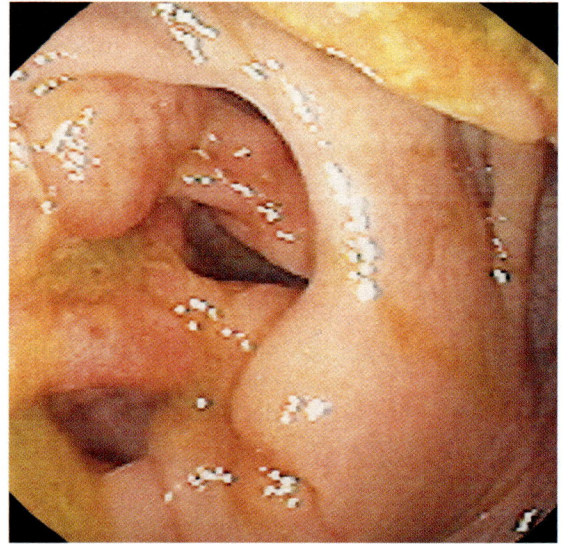

Figure 4-99: **Cecum. Crohn's Colitis.** Marked deformity of the cecum.

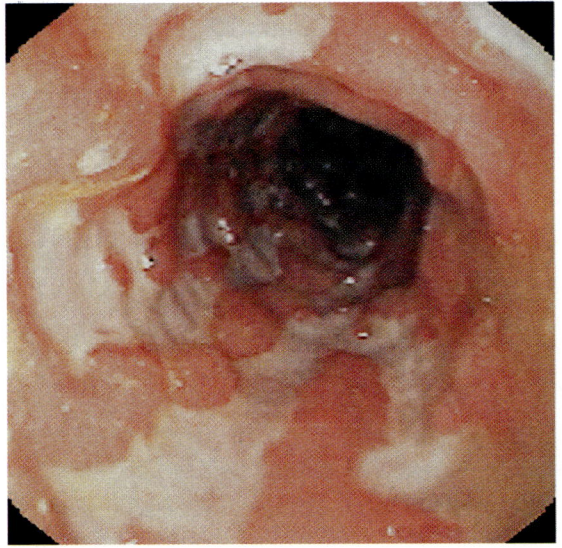

Figure 4-100: **Colon, Splenic Flexure. Crohn's Colitis.** Typical "rake" ulcers.

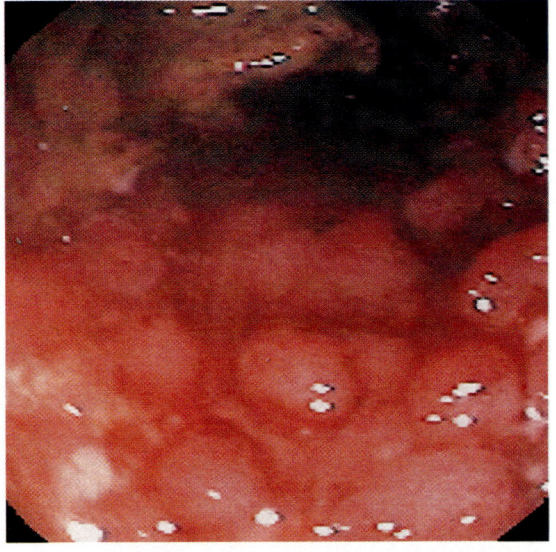

Figure 4-101: **Colon, Sigmoid. Crohn's Colitis.** Cobblestone pattern: islands of mucosa separated by fissuring ulceration.

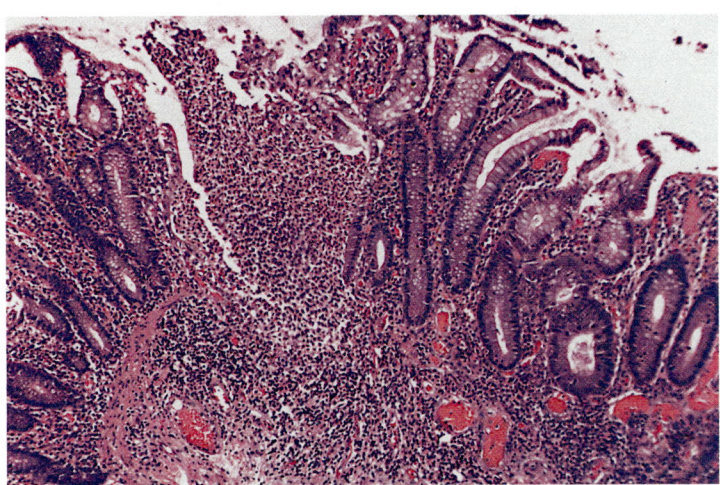

Figure 4-102: **Colon. Crohn's Colitis.** Aphthous ulcer over lymphoid nodule.

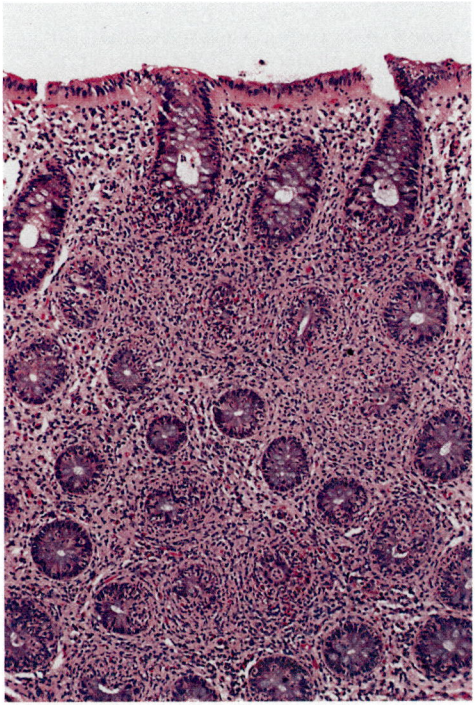

Figure 4-103: **Colon. Crohn's Colitis.** Isolated foci of cryptitis favor Crohn's over ulcerative colitis.

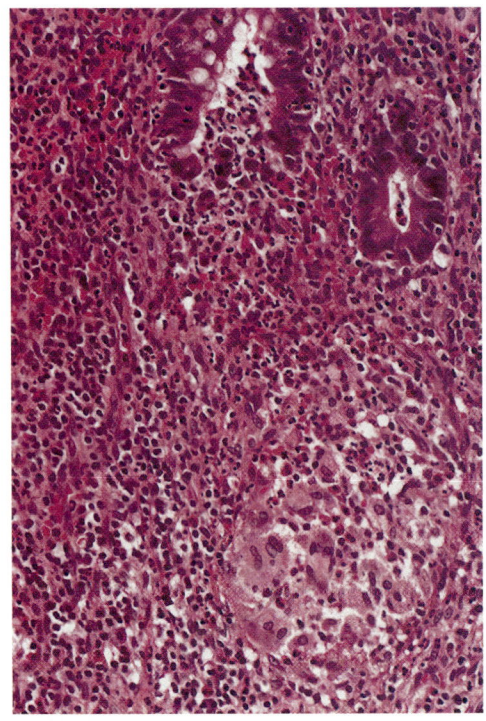

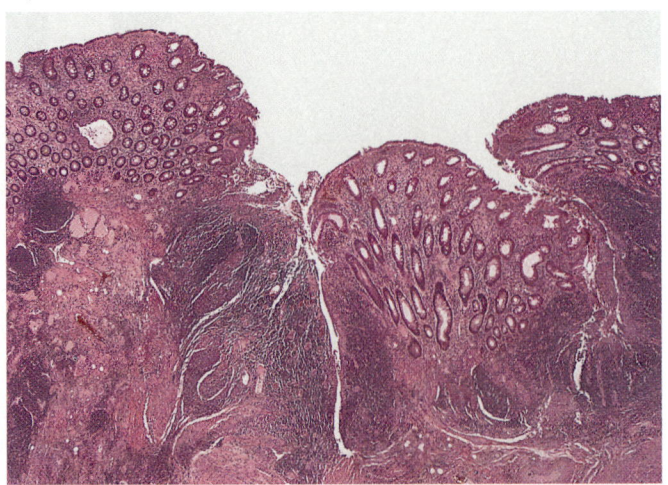

Figure 4-105: **Colon. Crohn's Colitis.** Fissures separated by relatively normal mucosa; lymphoid hyperplasia with granulomas.

Figure 4-104: **Colon. Crohn's Colitis.** Ill-defined granuloma in active chronic crypt destructive colitis.

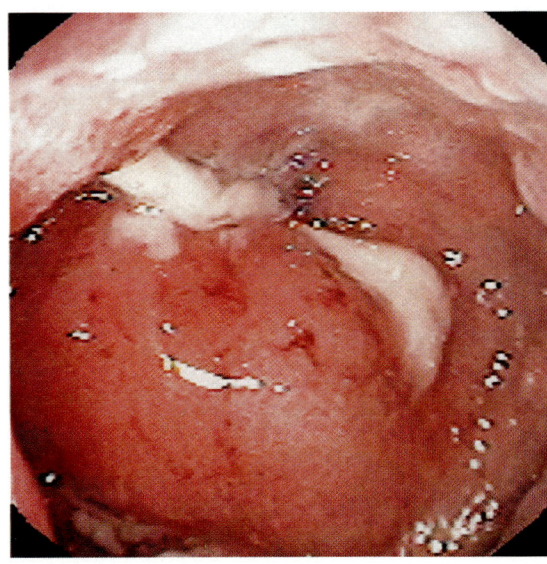

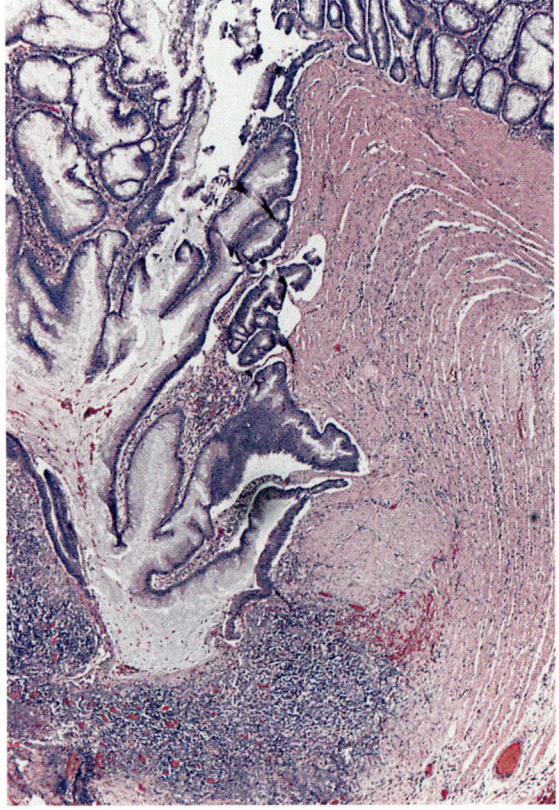

Figure 4-106: **Rectum. Adenocarcinoma Arising in Crohn's Disease.** Ulceration (upper) and an ulcerated mass with exudate (center).

Figure 4-107: **Colon. Adenocarcinoma Arising in Crohn's Disease.** Well-differentiated adenocarcinoma.

GRANULOMATOUS COLITIS

- Morphology .... Granulomas do not usually have disease-specific features, but combinations of features make some diagnoses more likely than others. Tuberculous granulomas are characteristically caseating and associated with circumferential ulcers and subsequent narrow diaphragm strictures similar to those produced by NSAIDs. Although caseation necrosis is characteristic of tuberculosis, noncaseating granulomas often occur. Stains for organisms are more frequently negative than positive. The granulomas of disseminated histoplasmosis are discrete and epithelioid, or vaguely granulomatous collections of yeast-filled histiocytes in the base of an ulcer. *Yersinia* granulomas are typically centered in lymphoid follicles and often contain neutrophils. Schistosome ova lodge in stroma or venules, where they may induce a localized granuloma, with little other reaction. Sarcoid granulomas are not usually associated with inflammation and are found in endoscopically normal mucosa.

- Endoscopic features .... Discrete ulceration, normal intervening mucosa, diffuse segmental inflammation with mucosal granularity, friability, spontaneous bleeding, and exudate. Patchy erythema without ulceration. Granulomatous diseases such as Crohn's, yersiniosis, and tuberculosis most commonly involve the terminal ileum and proximal colon.

- Clinical features .... *Crohn's disease* is a chronic disorder with variable levels of activity. Active disease causes diarrhea and often weight loss, a result of disease activity, and edema and narrowing of the bowel, which cause low-grade chronic obstruction. Nausea and abdominal bloating are features of mild, incomplete obstruction. *Yersinia* infection presents as an acute infectious syndrome. *Tuberculosis* and *histoplasmosis* are chronic diseases. All cause diarrhea. *Sarcoidosis* commonly involves the gut, but is usually an incidental finding in patients with known history of sarcoidosis.

- Differential diagnosis ...... Histologic: Crohn's disease, granulomatous enteric and disseminated infections (*Yersinia*, tuberculosis, fungal), sarcoidosis, drug reactions.

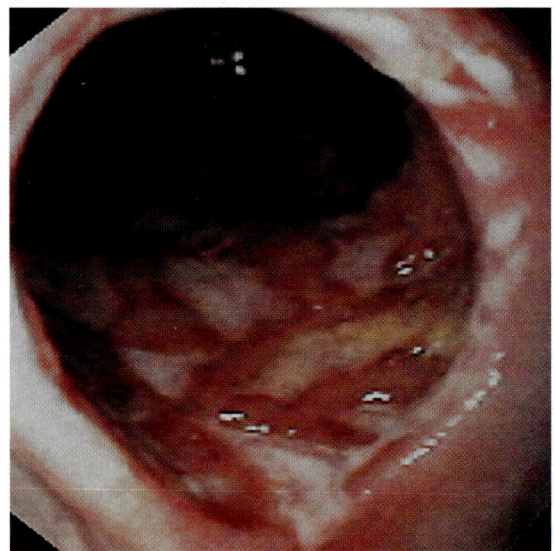

Figure 4-108: **Terminal Ileum. Crohn's Ileitis.** Discrete ulceration with normal mucosa between the ulcers.

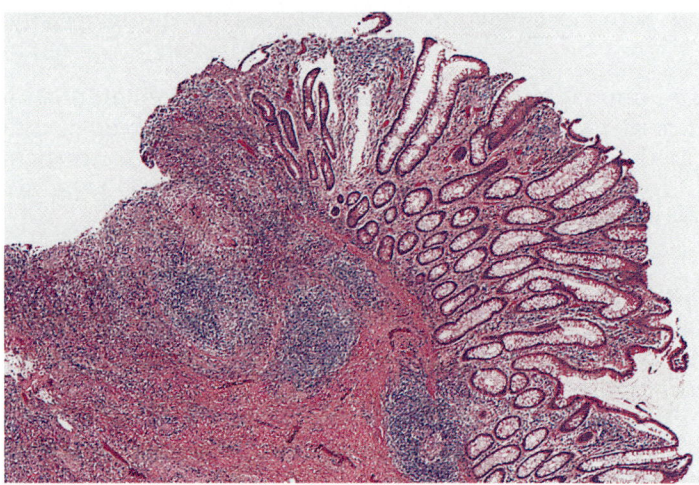

Figure 4-109: **Colon. Crohn's Colitis.** Typical Crohn's ulcer with granulomas and lymphoid hyperplasia.

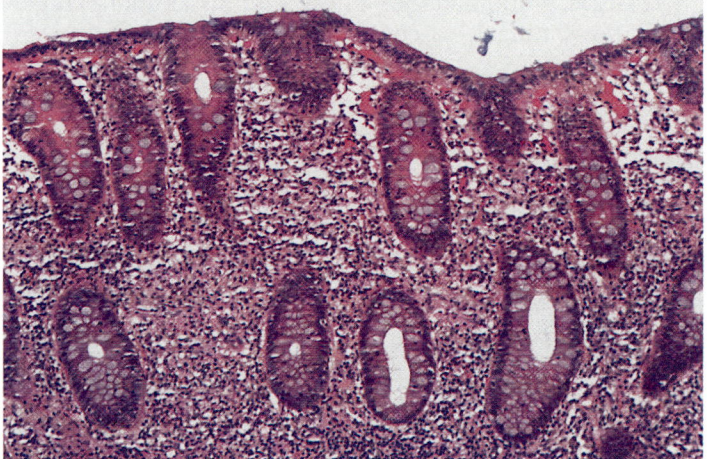

Figure 4-110: **Colon. Histoplasma.** Poorly defined granulomatous inflammation in disseminated histoplasmosis.

CHRONIC NONDESTRUCTIVE COLITIS

- Morphology .... Lymphocytic and collagenous colitis share common features, suggesting a relation between them. Both are characterized by an increased chronic inflammatory infiltrate in the lamina propria, with normal crypt architecture and increased intraepithelial lymphocytes. The distinguishing feature is the presence or absence of a collagen band beneath the surface epithelium/capillary network. There are qualitative differences as well; in collagenous colitis, there are fewer intraepithelial lymphocytes and more surface epithelial damage. Crypt abscesses are rare in lymphocytic or collagenous colitis. Usually, collagenous and lymphocytic colitis are more severe in the right than the left colon, and rectal sparing is not uncommon. Biopsy samples from the sigmoid and rectum, therefore, may not be sufficient for diagnosis. Occasionally, both collagenous and a superimposed crypt destructive colitis resembling Crohn's disease may be present.

- Endoscopic features .... Mucosa usually appears normal. The most common alteration is patchy erythema, typically located in the left colon.

- Clinical features .... Abrupt, refractory, watery diarrhea, often associated with weight loss.

- Differential diagnosis ...... Histologic: Acute, self-limited colitis versus lymphocytic colitis; ischemia versus collagenous colitis. Oblique tissue sections can accentuate the thickness of the subepithelial collagen band and be mistaken for collagenous colitis. Lack of associated colitis (increased lamina propria inflammation) prevents this misinterpretation.

    Clinical: Celiac sprue, hypersensitivity to foreign antigens in the fecal stream, drug reaction, autoimmune process.

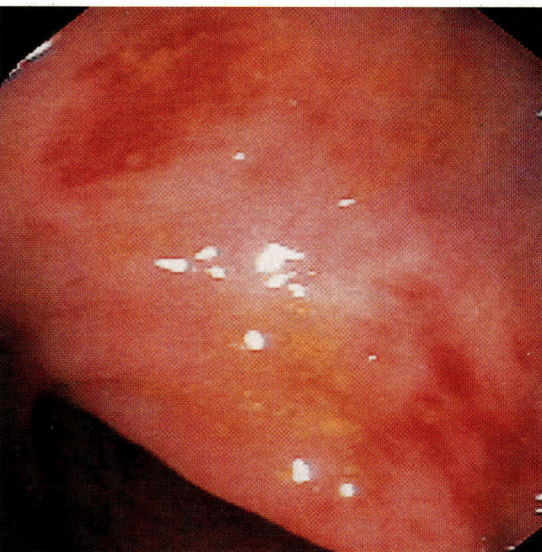

Figure 4-117: **Colon, Sigmoid. Lymphocytic Colitis.** Patchy, nonspecific erythema.

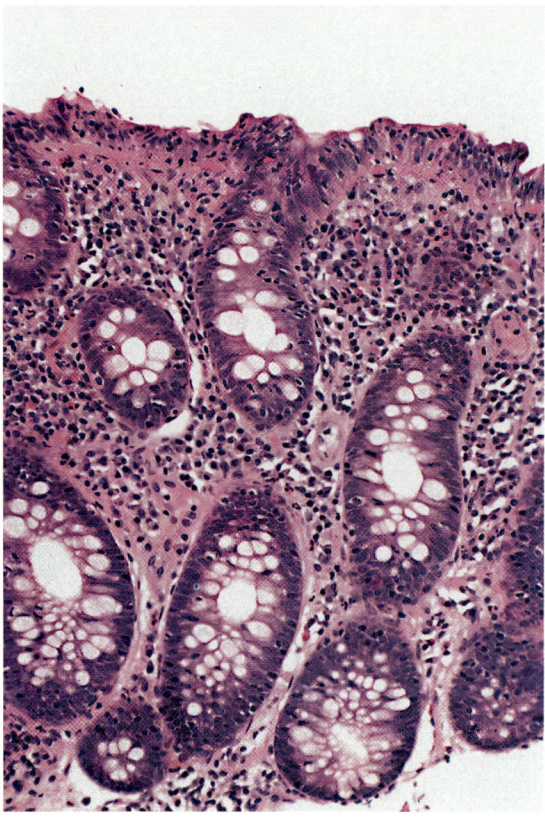

Figure 4-118: **Colon. Lymphocytic Colitis.** Chronic colitis without crypt destruction or distortion and with increased intraepithelial lymphocytes.

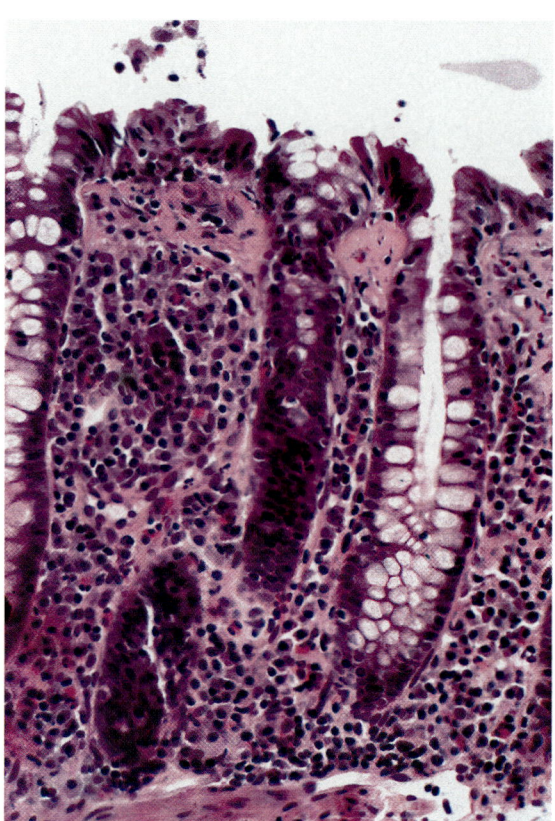

Figure 4-119: **Colon. Collagenous Colitis.** Chronic colitis with surface epithelial damage, increased intraepithelial lymphocytes, and thick subepithelial collagen band.

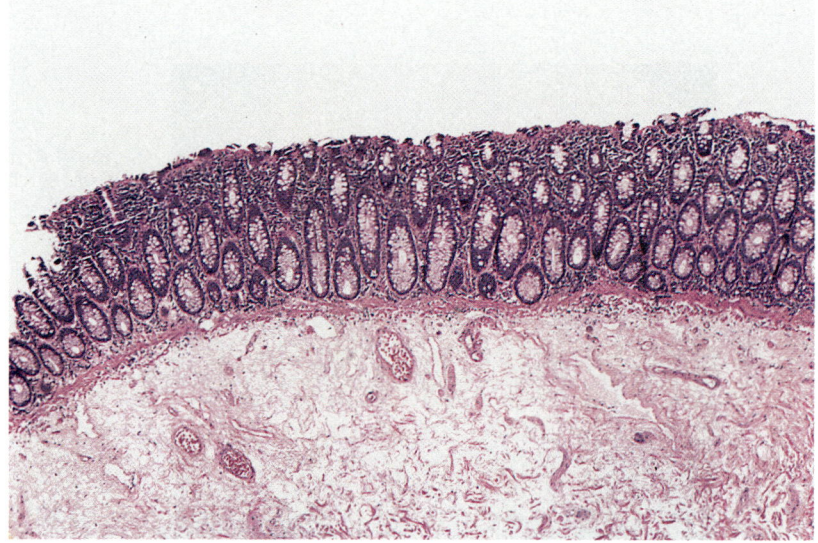

Figure 4-120: **Colon. Collagenous Colitis.** Chronic colitis, normal architecture, surface epithelial sloughing, subepithelial collagen band, marked submucosal edema.

EOSINOPHILIC COLITIS

- Morphology .... Increased eosinophils with no significant increase in other inflammatory cell types is diagnostic. Crypt destruction, if present, is usually minimal. Eosinophilic enteritis may involve submucosa and muscularis propria, with or without mucosal involvement, which is often patchy and may be segmental. Eosinophils infiltrate the deep mucosa, where they are not normally found in significant numbers. Eosinophils will be increased in any chronic inflammatory process; therefore, unless eosinophils are overwhelmingly dominant, the diagnosis cannot be made.
- Endoscopic features .... Mucosa may be normal. In severe disease, there are nonspecific inflammatory changes consisting of erythema and ulceration. Extensive sampling will improve diagnostic yield.
- Clinical features .... Diarrhea.
- Differential diagnosis ...... Idiopathic inflammatory bowel disease, infectious colitis, drug reaction.

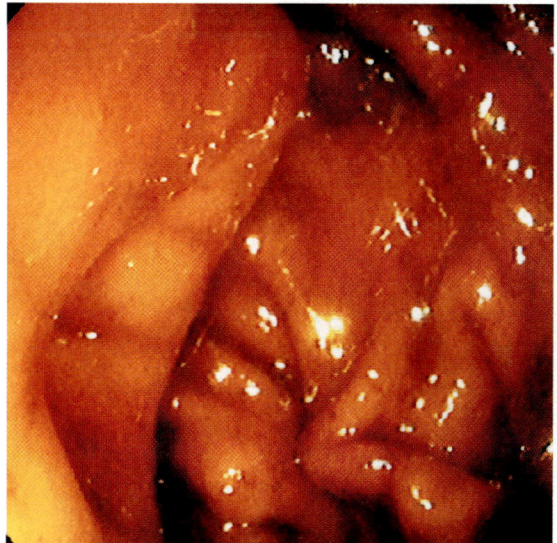

Figure 4-121: **Cecum. Eosinophilic Colitis.** Prominent ileocecal valve that is firm to probing.

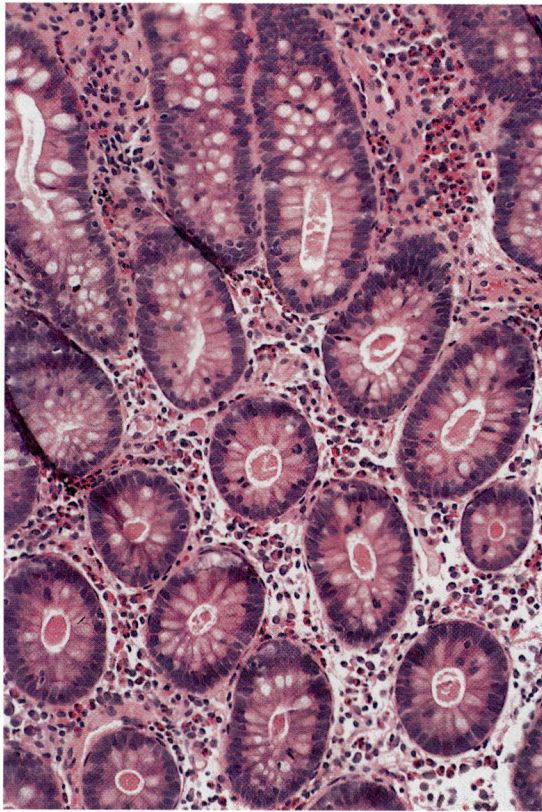

Figure 4-122: **Colon. Eosinophilic Colitis.** Eosinophils are increased, but lamina propria is only slightly expanded. No crypt architectural distortion.

GRAFT-VERSUS-HOST DISEASE

- Morphology .... The diagnostic pattern includes a bandlike lymphocytic infiltrate in the lamina propria, lymphocytic infiltration of the crypts, and crypt epithelial apoptosis. In more advanced cases, crypt epithelium may slough extensively. Chronic graft-versus-host disease may lack characteristic features, showing only atrophy. The process is usually patchy.

- Endoscopic features .... Patchy or diffuse inflammatory changes with ulceration, exudate, mucosal edema, friability, spontaneous bleeding, and sloughing of the mucosa.

- Clinical features .... Abdominal pain, diarrhea, fever, and, in some instances, hematochezia.

- Differential diagnosis ...... Histologic: Immunosuppressed states and autoimmune disease; idiopathic inflammatory bowel disease, unless diagnostic features are specifically sought.

  Clinical: Opportunistic infections.

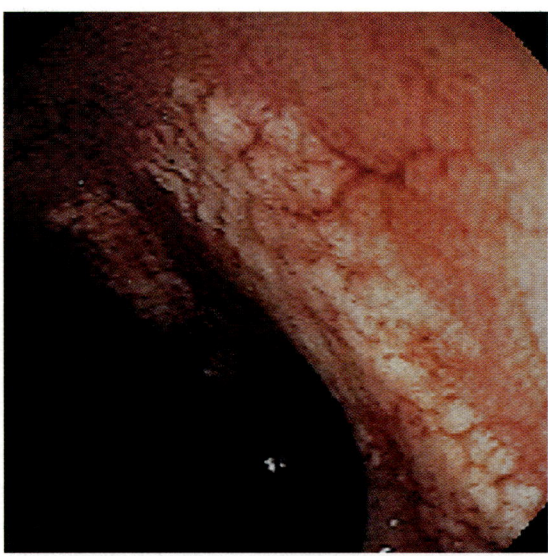

Figure 4-123: Colon, Transverse. Graft-Versus-Host Disease. Atypical white plaques. There is accentuation of the mucosal pit pattern (honeycomb) suggesting mucosal edema.

NSAID ILEOCOLITIS/ULCERS

- Morphology .... Nonsteroidal anti-inflammatory drugs (NSAIDs) cause nonspecific acute and active chronic inflammation, ulcers, and diaphragm strictures. Ulcers are discrete, sometimes multifocal, and occur in normal mucosa. Narrow, circumferential ulcers produce diaphragm strictures. Ischemia seems to be the major pathogenic mechanism. In the absence of characteristic ulcers, nonspecific inflammation resembles Crohn's disease, especially in the terminal ileum.

- Endoscopic features .... NSAID-induced ulcers are chronic, discrete, and associated with normal or minimally inflamed surrounding mucosa. The ulcers induce cicatricial scarring with the classic development of diaphragm strictures, first described in the terminal ileum but also found in the colon.

- Clinical features .... Iron deficiency anemia and chronic obstruction.

- Differential diagnosis ...... Endoscopic: Crohn's disease, CMV ulcers, ischemic ulcers, and ulcers of T-cell lymphoma. Circumferential ulcers, e.g., those of tuberculosis, can produce diaphragm strictures.

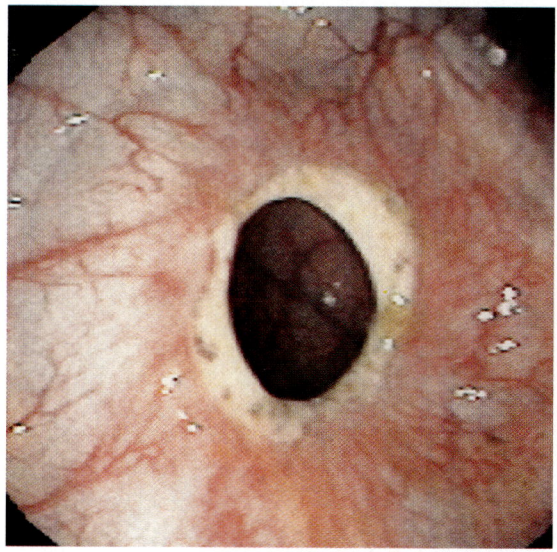

Figure 4-129: **Colon, Ascending. NSAID Stricture and Ulcer.** Distinctive diaphragm stricture. The rim of the stricture is ulcerated.

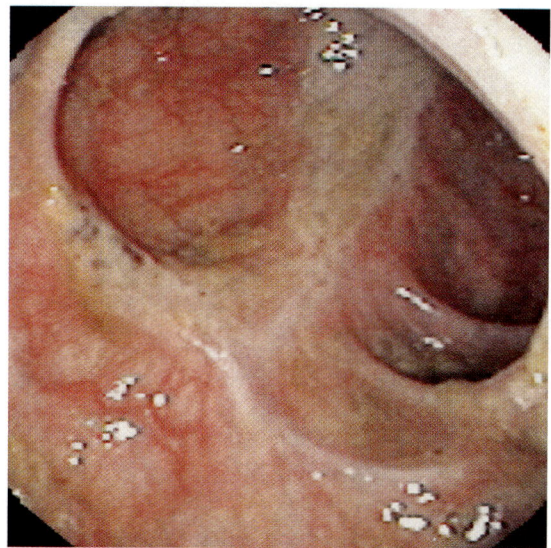

Figure 4-130: **Colon, Ascending. NSAID Ulcer.** Extensive ulceration with some cicatricial contraction of the mucosa and surrounding haustra.

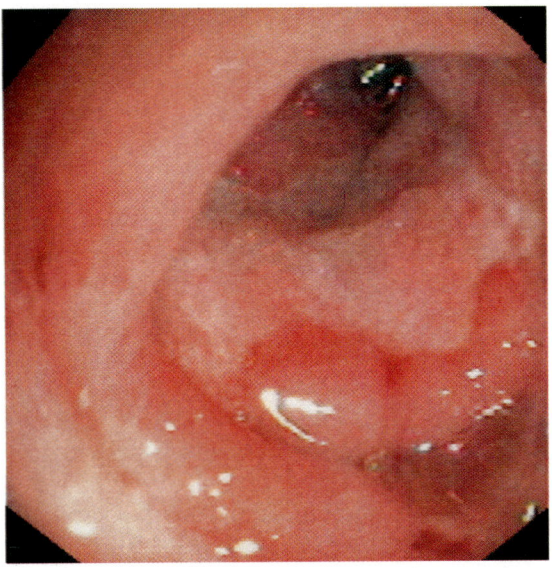

Figure 4-131: **Sigmoid. NSAID Ulcer.** Discrete ulcer with surrounding erythema and edema.

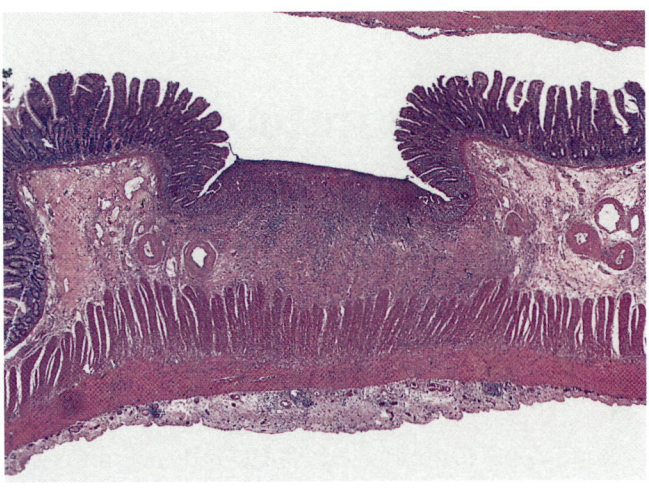

Figure 4-132: **Terminal Ileum. NSAID Ulcer.** Discrete ulcer, submucosal fibrosis, serosal reaction, adjacent normal mucosa.

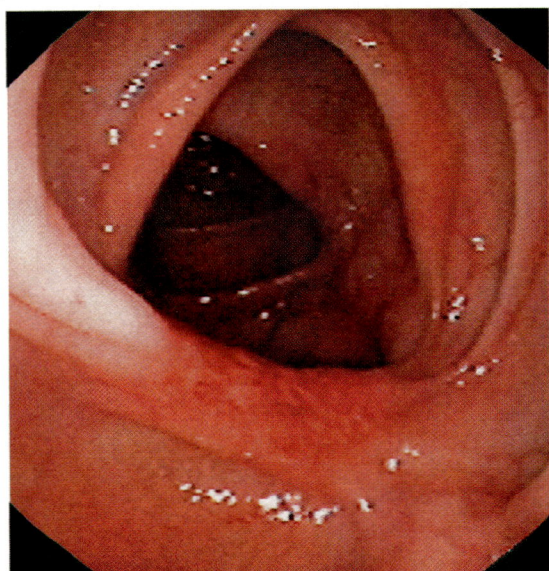

Figure 4-133: **Colon, Transverse. NSAID Ulcer.** Discrete ulcer on haustral fold. No other mucosal abnormalities.

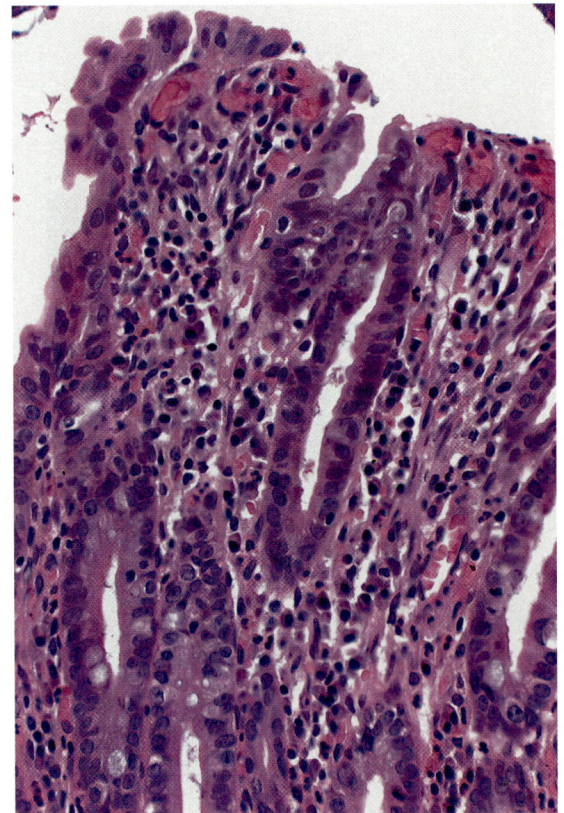

Figure 4-134: **Terminal Ileum. Active Ileitis.** Active chronic ileitis without specific features. NSAID user.

MELANOSIS COLI

- Morphology .... Macrophages contain brown lipofuscin and lysosomal debris.
- Endoscopic features .... Melanosis coli superimposed on innominate groove architecture can range in appearance from a subtle mosaic pattern to a deeply pigmented "leopard-skin" pattern; pigmentation varies.
- Clinical features .... Most patients have a history of chronic constipation and laxative use.
- Differential diagnosis ...... Etiologic: Anthraquinone laxatives, prolonged inflammatory conditions.

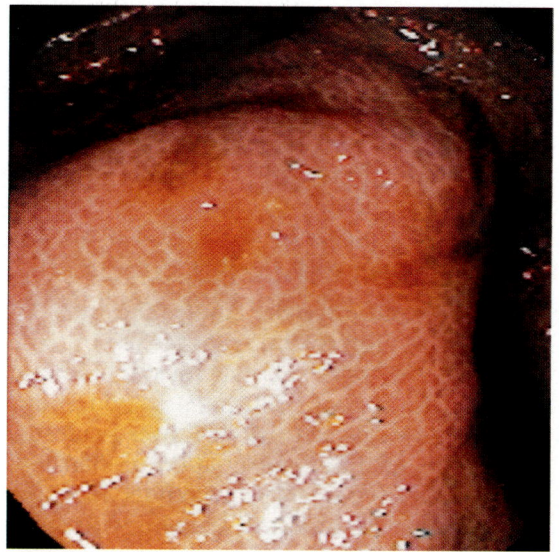

Figure 4-135: **Colon. Melanosis Coli**. Dark, leopard-skin mucosal appearance consistent with melanosis coli.

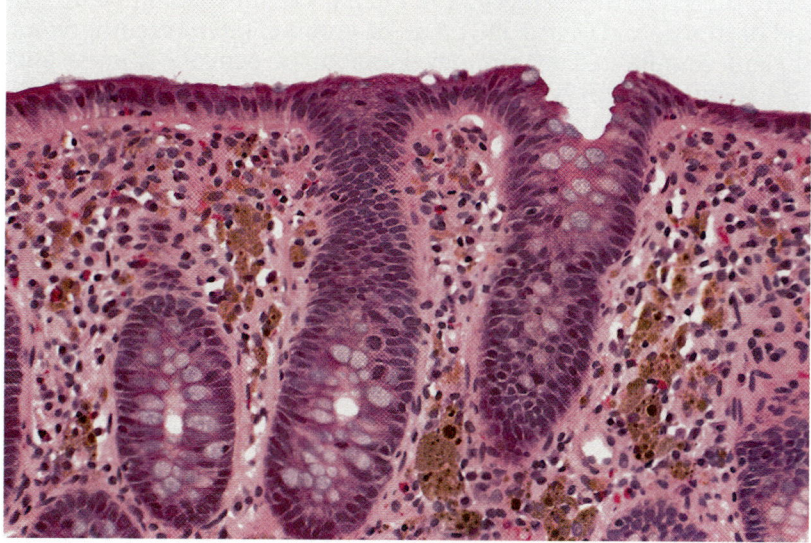

Figure 4-136: **Colon. Melanosis Coli**. Pigmented histiocytes in lamina propria. Glands appear normal.

DIVERTICULAR DISEASE

- Morphology .... Inflammation in diverticulitis usually surrounds the diverticulum. The ostium may be inflamed and polypoid. Occasionally, a segmental active chronic mucosal colitis, indistinguishable on biopsy from Crohn's disease, occurs. Proximal to a diverticular narrowing or stricture, as with any obstruction, there may be acute or active chronic inflammation with ulceration.

- Endoscopic features .... Diverticula appear as outpouchings from the colonic lumen. They vary from shallow depressions to large-mouthed structures. If inverted, they appear polypoid (Fig. 4-141); if they contain stool (Fig. 4-142) they can be greatly distended. There is often patchy and punctate mucosal erythema between diverticula, a feature that does not necessarily indicate diverticulitis (Fig. 4-143). Diverticulitis may be present without any luminal signs. When diverticula are concentrated in the sigmoid colon, bowel rigidity can impede passage of the endoscope and cause pain. Passage of the colonoscope into a segment with acute diverticulitis typically produces exquisite pain—a diagnostic feature. Acute diverticulitis may be limited to a few diverticula or may be segmental; luminal narrowing with mucosal edema can occur (Fig. 4-144). The involved segment of colon may be indistinguishable from acute ischemic injury because of mucosal hemorrhage and edema. Ulceration, however, is rare. In indolent or chronic diverticulitis, polypoid mucosal changes can simulate neoplasms, especially if ulcerated or with exudate.

- Clinical features .... Diverticula are common in the sigmoid colon in older adults. They may be diffusely scattered throughout the entire colon or limited to the left or right colon. Isolated right-sided diverticula are rare. Patients with symptomatic diverticular disease have abdominal pain that varies in intensity, duration, and onset. Most often pain is chronic and localized to the left lower quadrant. Patients may have normal bowel habits or suffer constipation or diarrhea. Abdominal examination may reveal easily palpable and tender loops of colon. Diverticulosis can cause sudden lower GI bleeding. Patients with acute diverticulitis experience an abrupt onset of severe abdominal pain, usually localized to the left lower quadrant or left flank, and often accompanied by fever and obstipation. Diverticulitis may be chronic, intermittently symptomatic, and complicated by the development of pericolic abscess and stricture. Patients typically do not have chronic anemia or chronic occult GI blood loss. As a general rule, young adults with symptomatic diverticulosis or diverticulitis, especially if complicated, will ultimately require surgery. In contrast, diverticulosis in older adults tends to be an incidental finding.

- Differential diagnosis ...... Histologic: Crohn's disease.

  Endoscopic: Ischemic colitis, infectious colitis in the setting of acute diverticulitis, carcinoma in the setting of cecal diverticulitis.

LARGE INTESTINE

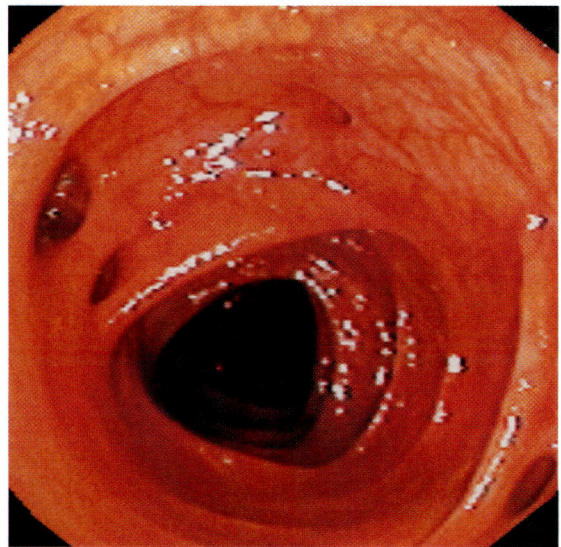

Figure 4-137: **Colon, Transverse. Diverticular Disease.** Scattered diverticular ostia of varying size and surrounding normal mucosa.

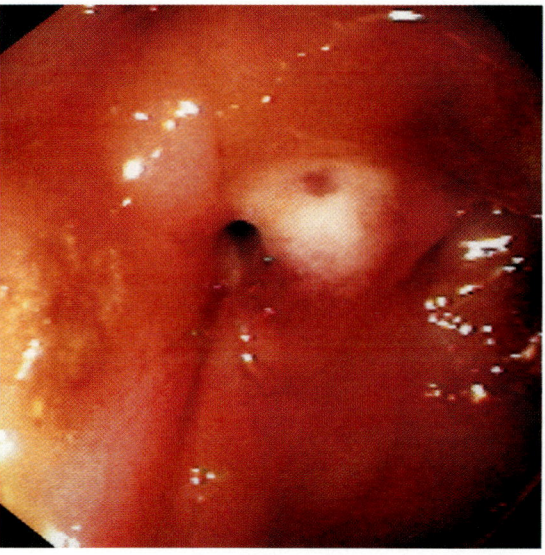

Figure 4-138: **Colon, Sigmoid. Diverticular Disease.** Edematous mucosa around ostium of a diverticulum. Mucosal hemorrhage and a yellow-white purulent or necrotic area to the right of the diverticulum.

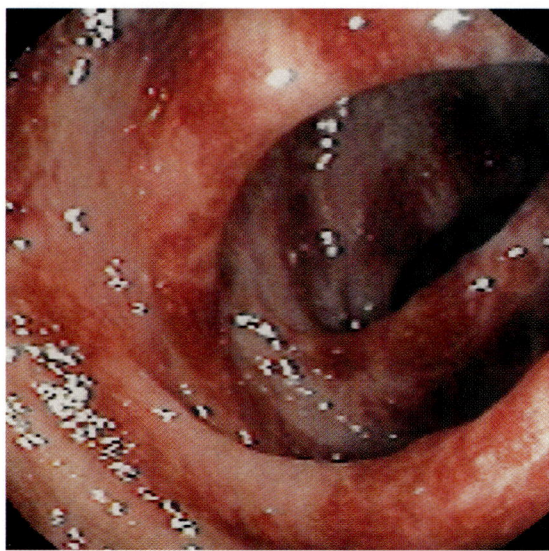

Figure 4-139: **Colon, Sigmoid. Diverticular Disease.** Scattered patches of dark erythematous mucosa (inflammation or hemorrhage). The dark appearance of the patches suggests that the acute phase has passed.

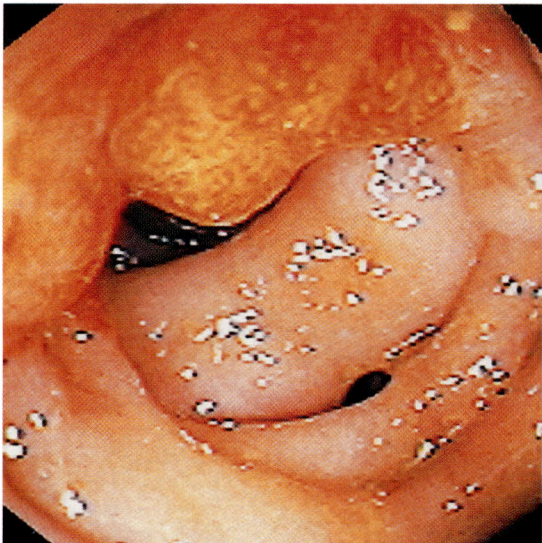

Figure 4-140: **Colon, Sigmoid. Diverticular Disease.** Polypoid mucosa in the upper portion of the photo with exaggeration of the honeycombed, innominate groove pattern suggests mucosal expansion by edema, chronic inflammation, or neoplasm. A small diverticulum is near the center.

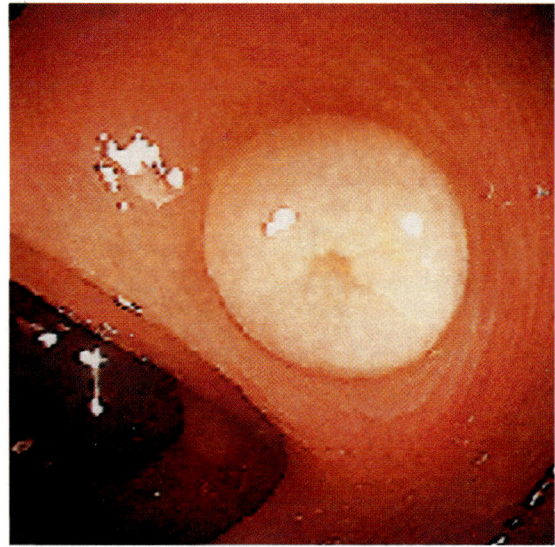

Figure 4-141: **Colon, Sigmoid. Diverticular Disease.** Inverted diverticulum.

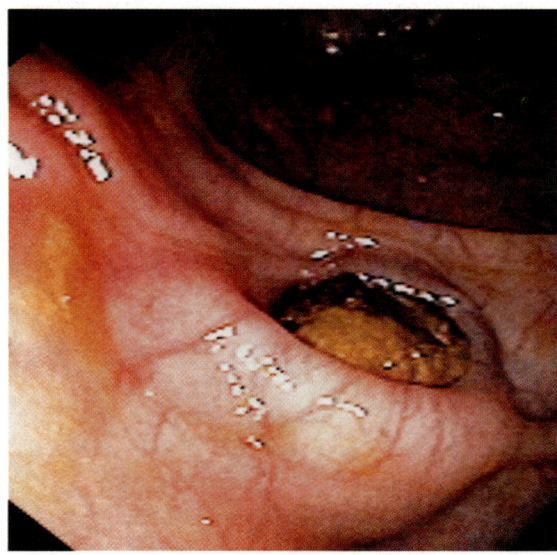

Figure 4-142: **Colon. Diverticular Disease.** Fecalith fills ostium and distends diverticulum.

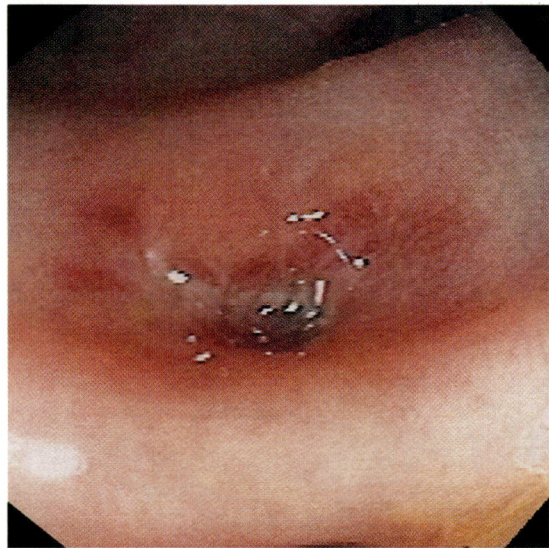

Figure 4-143: **Colon, Sigmoid. Diverticular Disease.** Punctate erythema around a diverticulum.

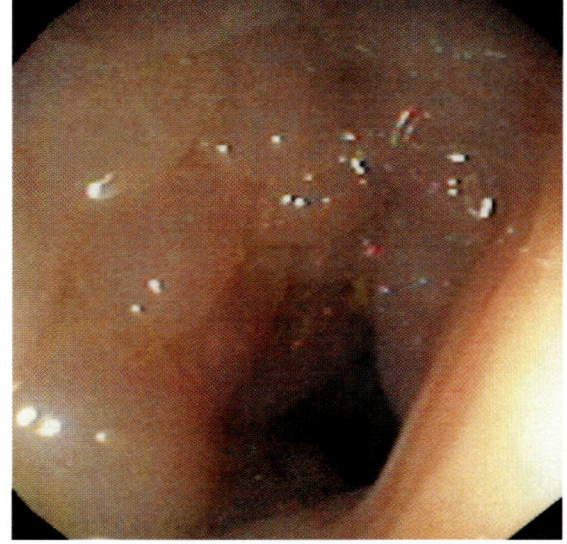

Figure 4-144: **Colon, Descending. Diverticular Disease.** Marked luminal narrowing and mucosal edema in acute diverticulitis.

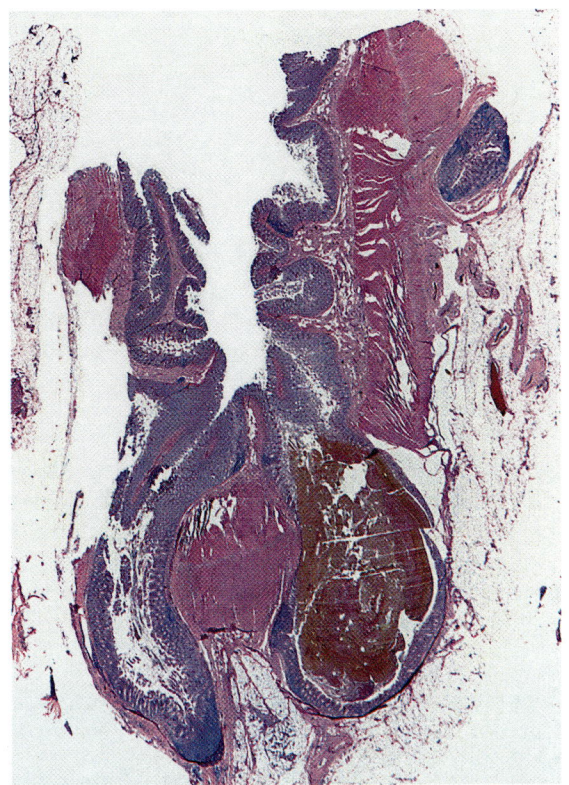

Figure 4-145: **Colon. Diverticular Disease.** Several diverticula extend through muscularis propria. One contains blood.

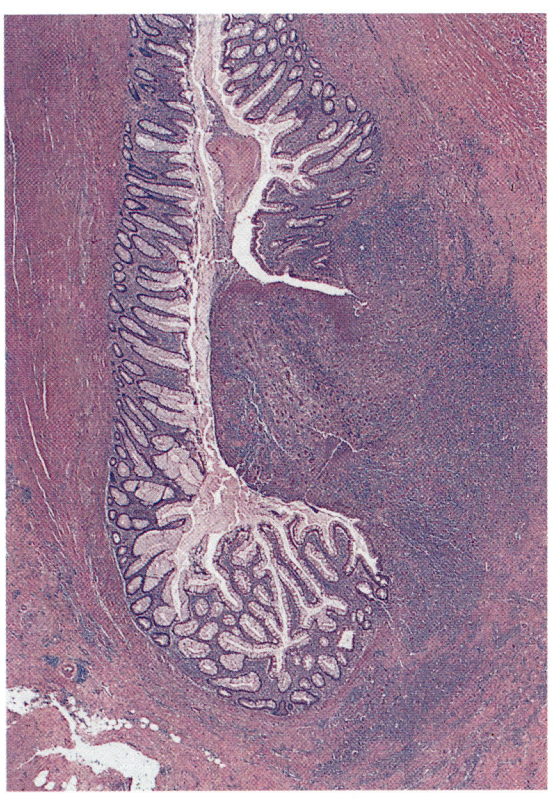

Figure 4-146: **Colon. Diverticular Disease.** Chronically inflamed diverticulum (diverticulitis) with ulceration and granulation tissue.

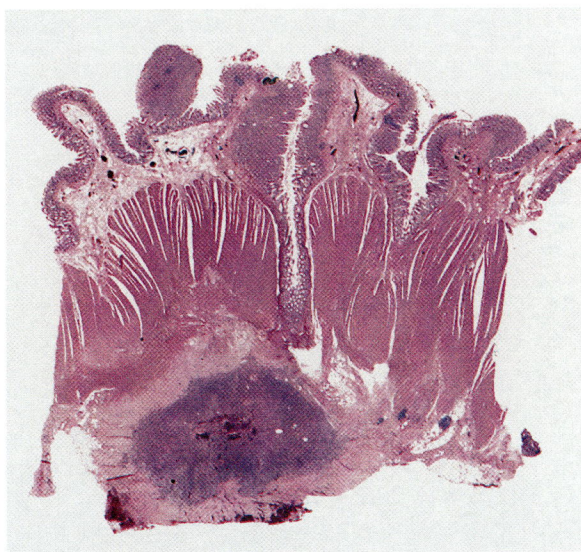

Figure 4-147: **Colon. Diverticular Disease.** Diverticulum overlying pericolic abscess.

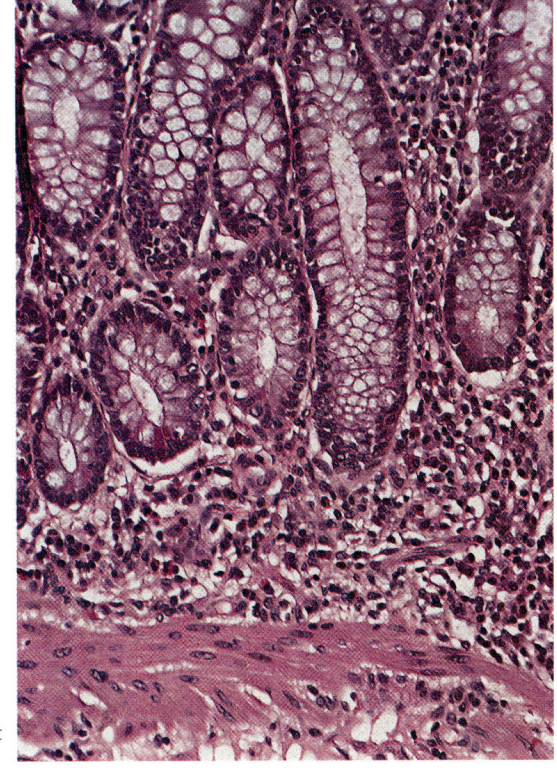

Figure 4-148: **Colon. Diverticular Disease.** Mild chronic colitis without evidence of crypt destruction.

STRICTURE/ANASTOMOSIS

- Endoscopic features .... Most anastomotic strictures are easily seen; however, this may not be the case in patients with remote colonic resections. Anastomoses following sigmoid resections are typically located 17 to 18 cm from the anal verge. Anastomoses may be constructed end-to-end, end-to-side, and side-to-side, with the last 2 varieties in ileocolonic anastomoses. Anastomoses appear as thickened ring deformities with subtle or obvious nodularity or polypoid mucosal changes. Chronic erosions and ulceration are most common with ileocolonic anastomoses. In the absence of inflammatory bowel disease, anastomotic strictures are most frequent after sigmoid resections. These strictures are presumed to be due to ischemia at the anastomotic site and are typically short and diaphragmlike or weblike. They are amenable to endoscopic balloon dilatation or, when refractory, are released by 1 to 3 radially placed cuts. Anastomotic strictures are common in inflammatory bowel disease, particularly Crohn's disease. Crohn's disease predictably recurs at, and just proximal to, an anastomosis.

    Nonanastomotic strictures may be sequelae of ischemic colitis or inflammatory bowel disease. Strictured areas in ulcerative colitis must be sampled for evidence of dysplasia and carcinoma.

- Clinical features .... Progressive constipation, obstipation, and obvious obstructive symptoms.
- Differential diagnosis ...... Endoscopic: Recurrent neoplasm, recurrent inflammatory bowel disease.

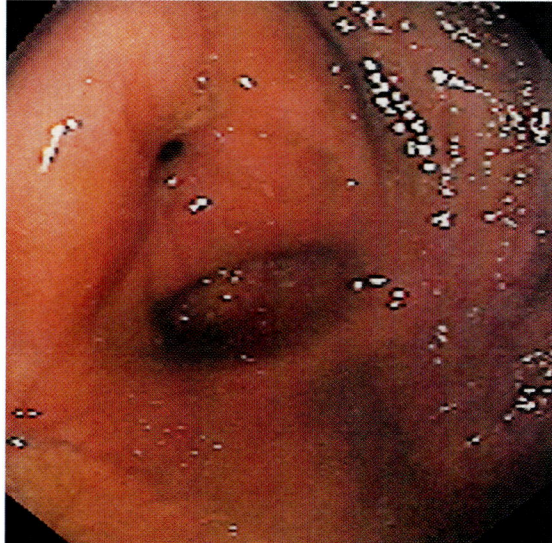

Figure 4-149: **Colon, Anastomosis. Stricture.** A high-grade ileocolonic anastomotic stricture.

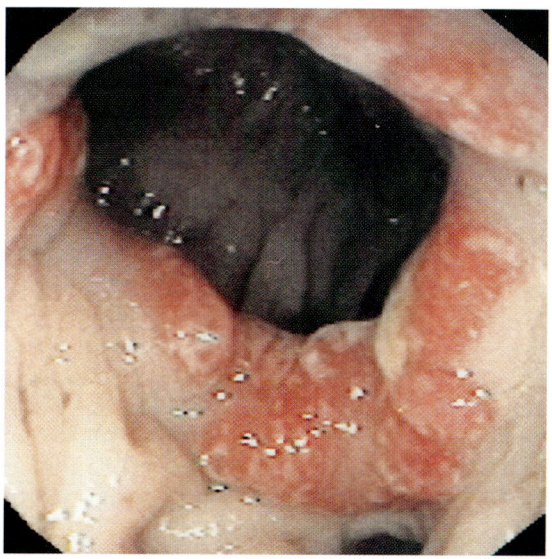

Figure 4-150: **Colon, Anastomosis. Stricture.** A colocolonic stricture with polypoid and chronic erosive mucosal changes. There is no compromise of the lumen.

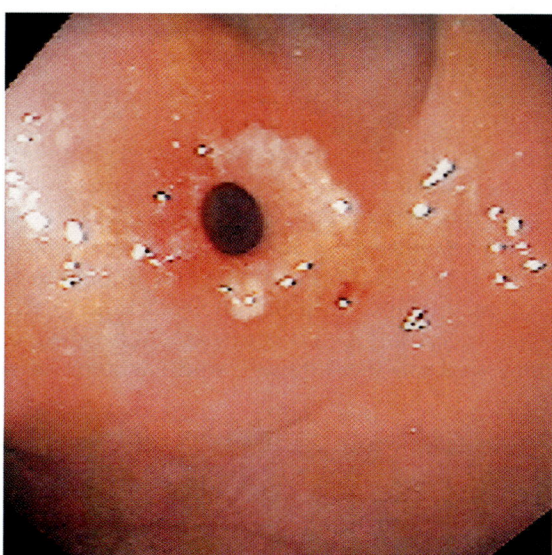

Figure 4-151: **Colon, Anastomosis. Stricture.** High-grade diaphragmlike stricture with pinpoint lumen and ulceration at rectosigmoid anastomosis.

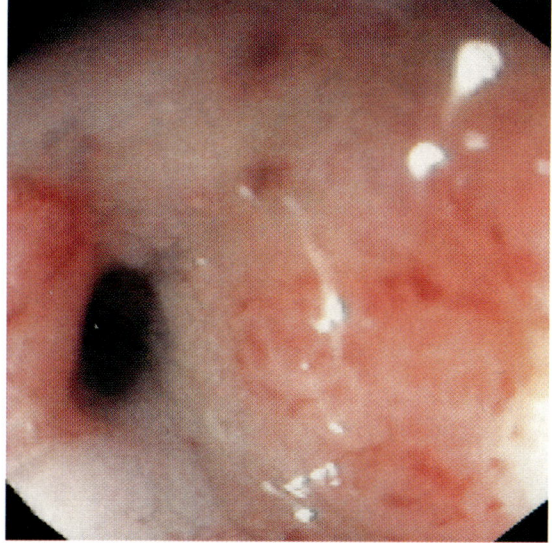

Figure 4-152: **Colon, Ascending. Stricture.** Stricture in a patient with long-standing ulcerative colitis. Active inflammation with pinpoint areas of hemorrhage, erythema, and loss of normal vascularity.

VASCULAR LESIONS

- Morphology .... Portal hypertensive colopathy due to cirrhosis or portal vein obstruction is accentuated in the right colon and often not apparent in the distal left colon because of the collateral circulation. The capillaries and venules are ectatic and sclerotic, and changes tend to be fairly uniform in appearance and distribution. Discrete telangiectasias are common as well. Telangiectasia and angiodysplasia usually cannot be distinguished on biopsy. Angiodysplasia is thought to be formed by local venous obstruction, with ectasia progressing from venule to capillary to arteriole. The different types of vascular malformations cannot be easily classified on biopsy. In all, the vessels are large, abnormal, and involve the submucosa. Arteriovenous malformations usually involve the full thickness of the bowel wall.

- Endoscopic features .... A wide range of vascular lesions is encountered in the colon. Venous blebs, or *phlebectasias*, are incidental findings in older patients. They are common in the distal colon. *Angiodysplasia* classically involves the cecum and ascending colon and gives rise to acute and chronic GI blood loss. These lesions rarely exceed 1 cm. Upon close inspection, they are dilated vascular structures. The lesions may be flat or slightly elevated and usually are not bleeding. Similar lesions may be seen in portal hypertensive gastropathy and Osler-Weber-Rendu syndrome (hereditary hemorrhagic telangiectasia). The angiectasias encountered in portal hypertension and the Osler-Weber-Rendu syndrome are often distributed throughout the entire colon. The angiectatic lesions of radiation proctopathy are more numerous and vary more in size. They are usually located in the distal rectum, but occasionally are found in the sigmoid colon. All of the preceding lesions appear to be mucosally based from the endoscopist's perspective. *Arteriovenous malformations* are transmural and composed of large, abnormal vessels that may involve the mucosa as grossly distorted and disorganized vessels and multiple angiectasias. A variety of luminal and mucosal appearances may be encountered, depending on the size of the lesion. *Hemangiomas* are focal, raised, nodular, blue or purple lesions.

- Clinical features .... Chronic GI blood loss anemia and overt lower GI bleeding with episodic hematochezia.

- Differential diagnosis ...... Endoscopic: Kaposi sarcoma, angiosarcoma.

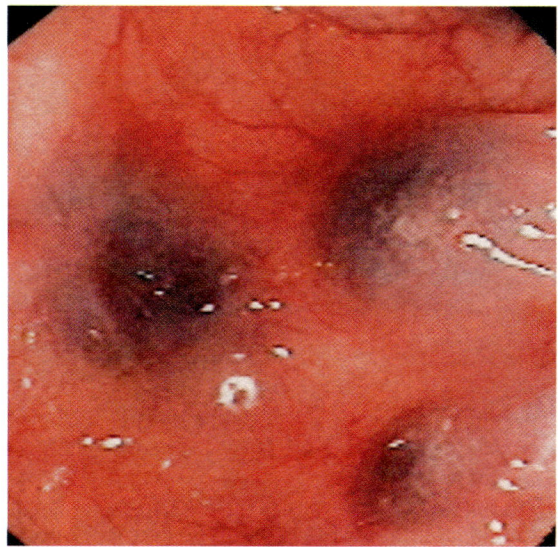

Figure 4-153: **Colon, Transverse. Phlebectasia.** Collection of venous ectasias, blue mucosal blebs.

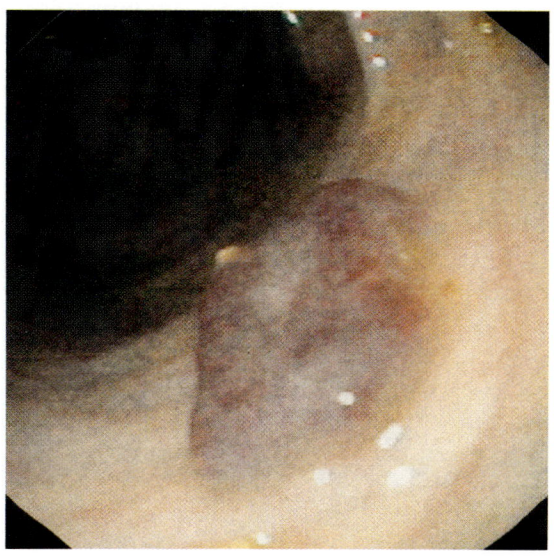

Figure 4-154: **Colon, Transverse. Hemangioma.** Raised, irregular, round, purple vascular lesion consistent with a small hemangioma in a patient with diffuse hemangiomatosis and chronic GI bleeding.

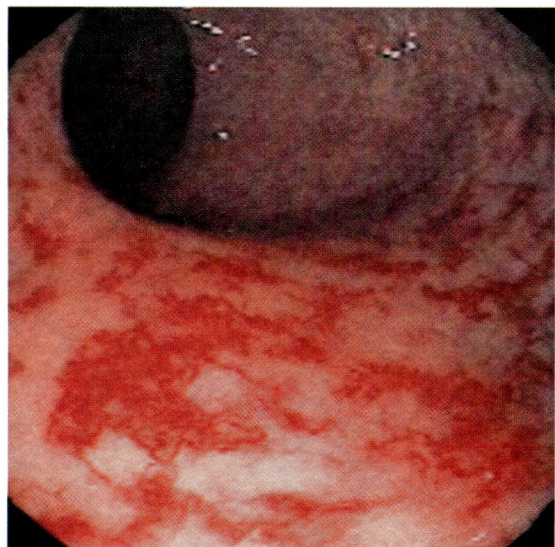

Figure 4-155: **Rectum. Angiectasia.** Numerous angiectatic lesions; a sequel of pelvic radiation (radiation proctopathy).

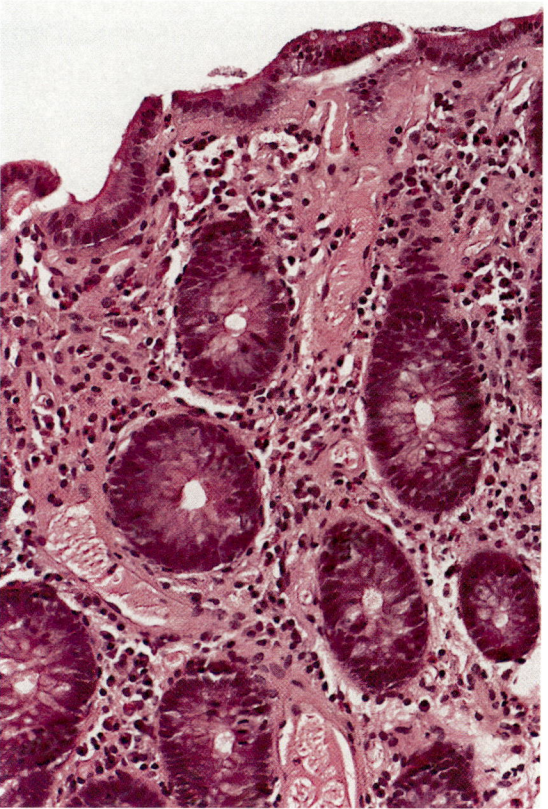

Figure 4-156: **Colon. Telangiectasia.** Focal, moderately ectatic, and minimally sclerotic venules.

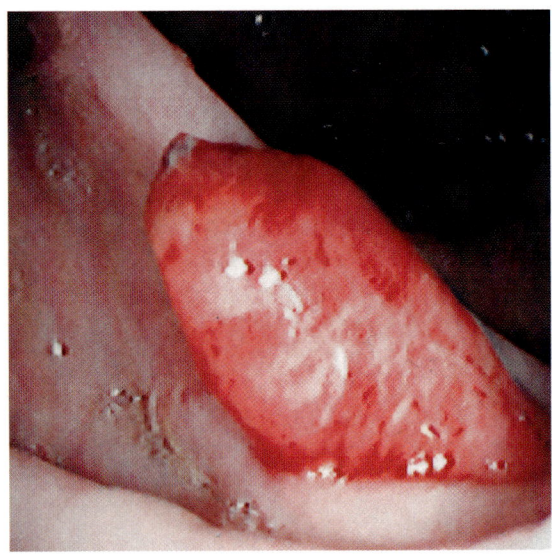

Figure 4-157: **Colon, Proximal Ascending. Vascular Malformation.** Atypical polyp with mucosal hemorrhage. A nipplelike protuberance at the tip of the polyp, possibly an exposed or visible vessel, in a patient who presented with massive lower GI bleeding.

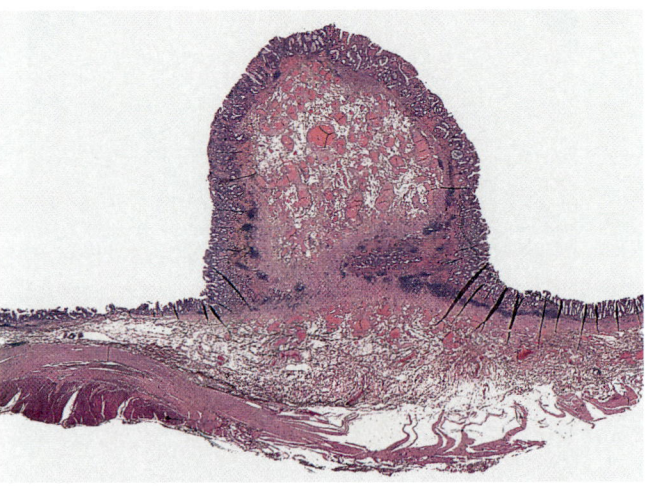

Figure 4-158: **Colon. Vascular Malformation.** Polypoid collection of abnormal vessels in the submucosa protrudes into the bowel lumen.

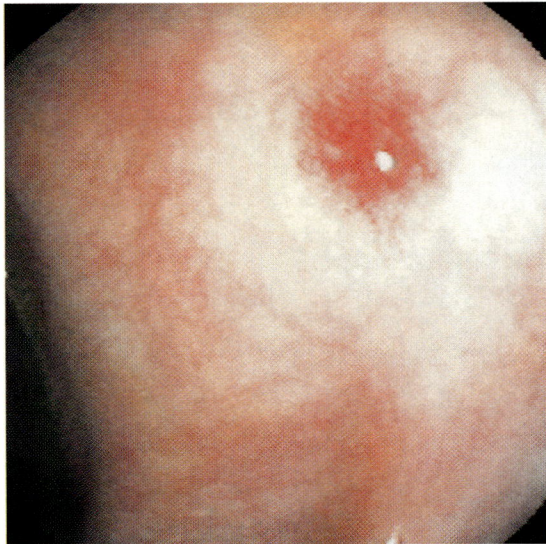

Figure 4-159: **Colon, Sigmoid. Angiectasia.** The lesion in the upper portion of the photo is discrete and contains a tight, radiating cluster of ectatic mucosal vessels; similar in appearance to cutaneous spider telangiectasia, in a patient with portal hypertension, portal hypertensive colopathy, and chronic iron deficiency anemia.

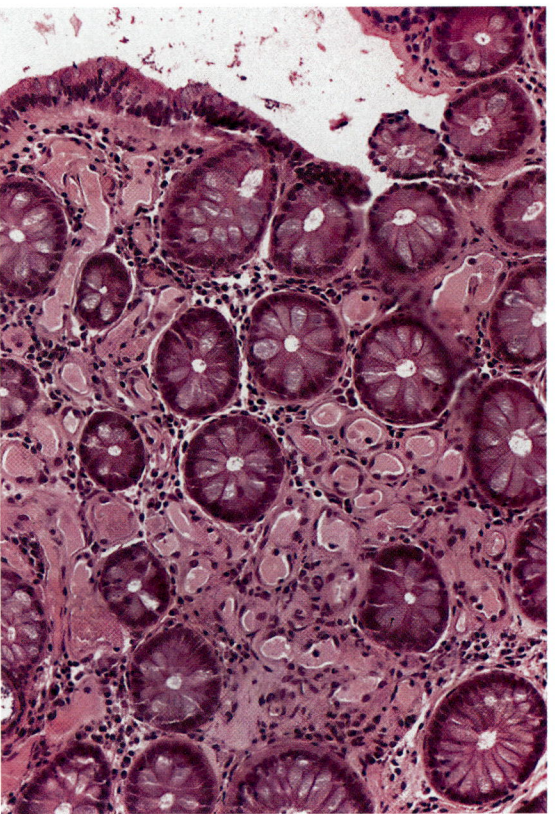

Figure 4-160: **Colon. Portal Hypertensive Colopathy.** Uniformly dilated and mildly sclerotic capillaries and venules in lamina propria. All vessels are involved equally.

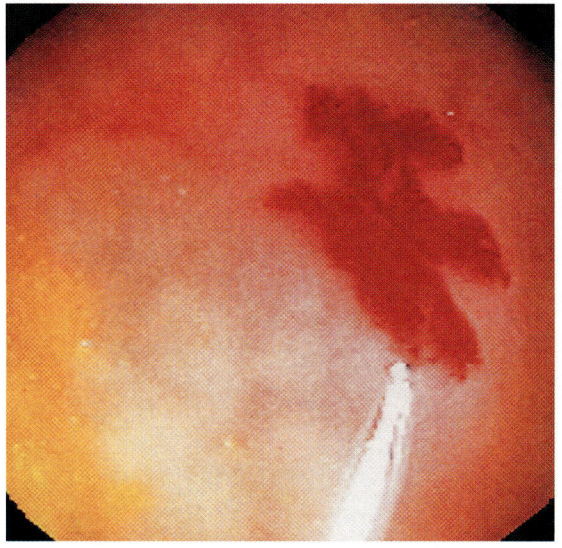

Figure 4-161: **Cecum. Angiectasia.** Discrete angiectatic lesion (angiodysplasia) is a bright red, irregularly shaped patch of ectatic vessels.

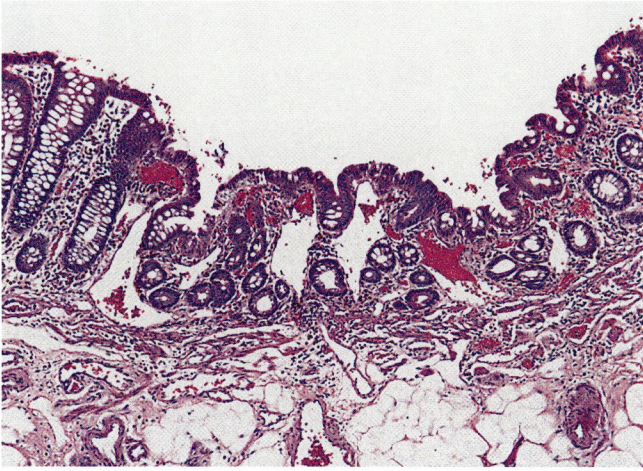

Figure 4-162: **Colon. Angiodysplasia.** Several dilated, thin-walled blood vessels disrupt mucosa.

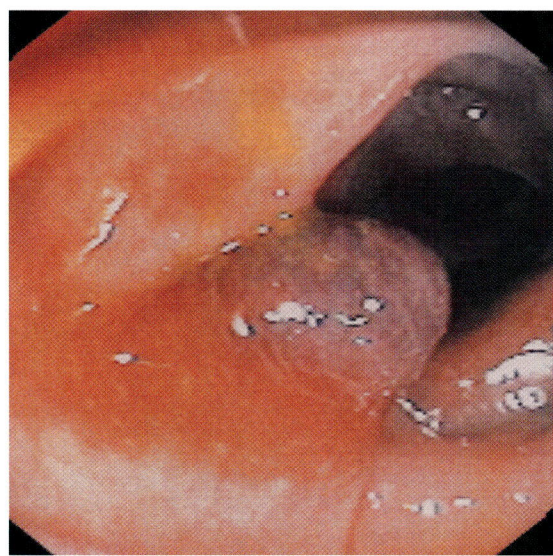

Figure 4-163: **Colon, Sigmoid. Vascular Malformation.** Atypical dark blue polyp that suggests a submucosal vascular component.

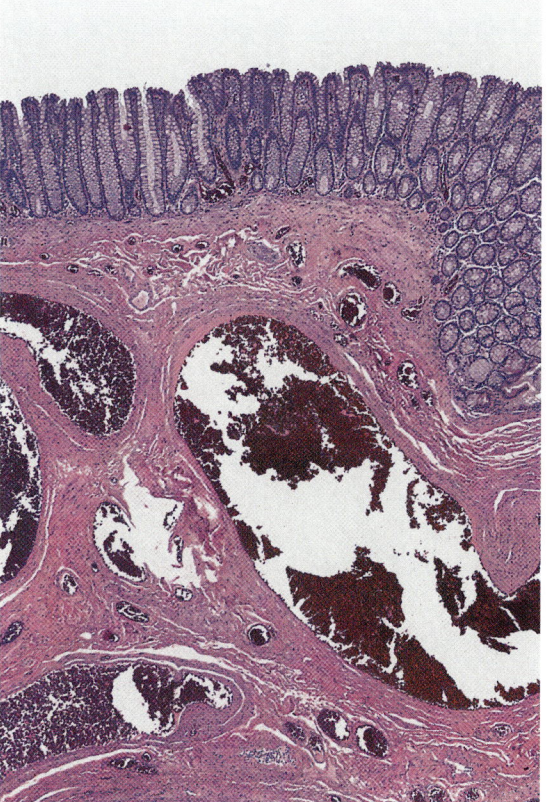

Figure 4-164: **Colon. Vascular Malformation.** Collection of large, irregularly arranged, dilated vessels within the submucosa.

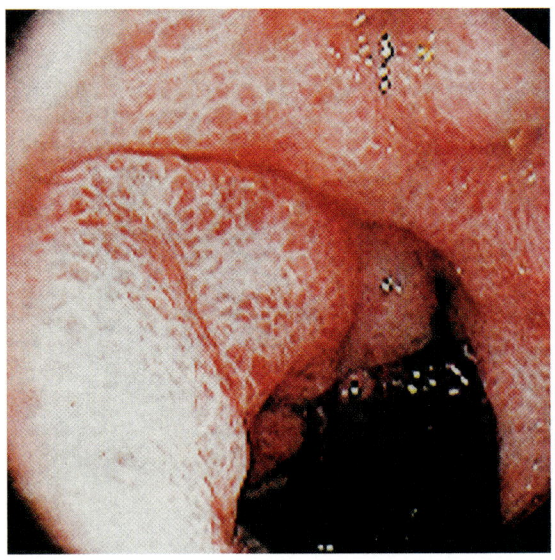

Figure 4-165: **Colon. Congestive Colopathy.** Edematous, erythematous mucosa with accentuated mosaic pattern. Mesenteric vein thrombosis; watery diarrhea for 6 months.

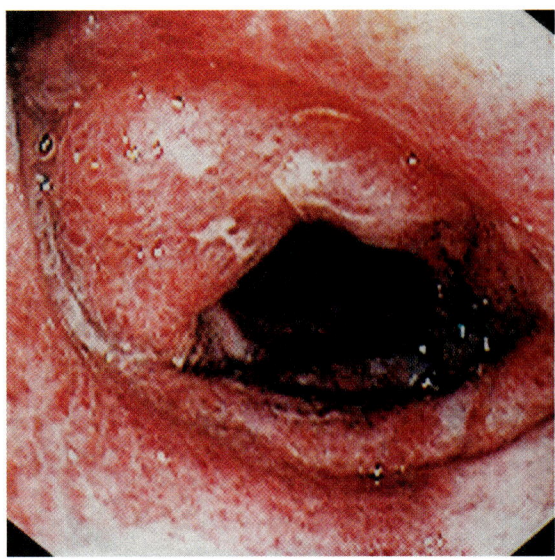

Figure 4-166: **Colon. Congestive Colopathy with Ischemic Erosions.** Area adjacent to Fig. 4-165 with white erosions and dusky red mucosa.

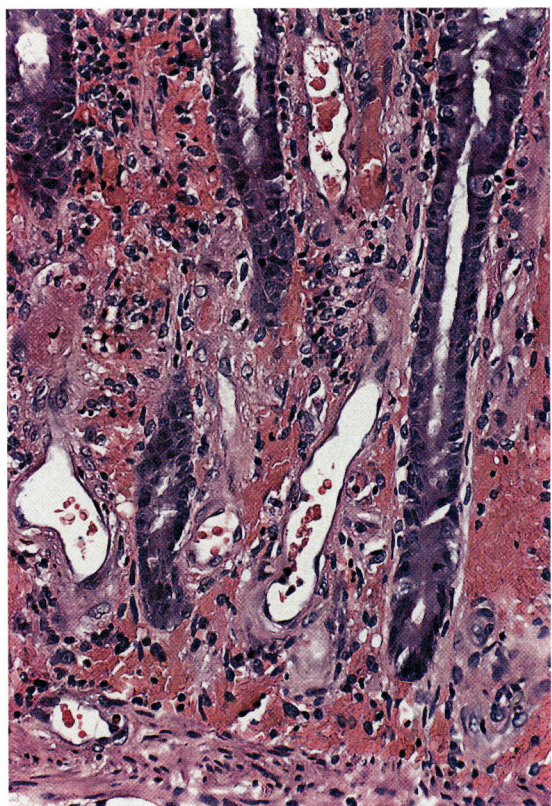

Figure 4-167: **Colon. Congestive Colopathy.** Engorged sclerotic capillaries and crypt degeneration. Same case as Fig. 4-165.

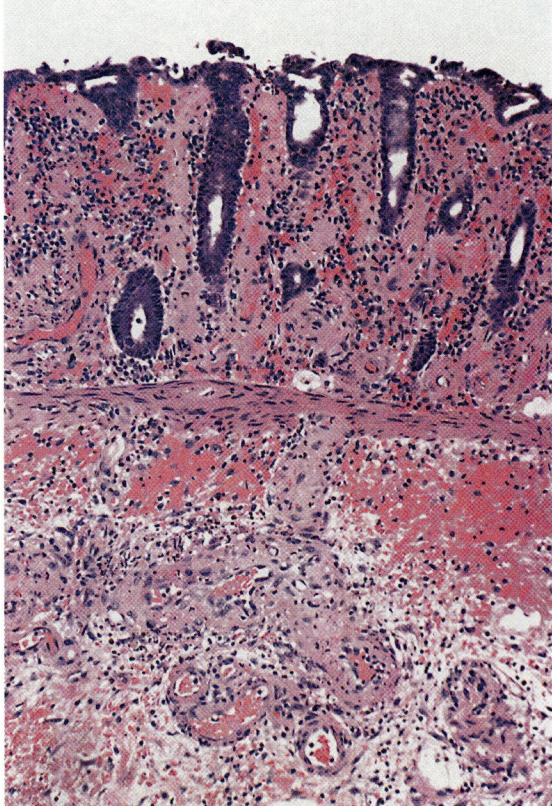

Figure 4-168: **Colon. Congestive Colopathy.** Mucosal and submucosal fibrosis, edema, congestion, hemorrhage, and crypt degeneration. Same case as Fig. 4-165.

HEMORRHOIDS/VARICES

- Morphology .... Large, dilated or thrombosed submucosal veins.
- Endoscopic features .... Internal hemorrhoids may be seen as the endoscope passes through the anal canal. On direct viewing with a flexible endoscope, hemorrhoids appear as large, erythematous, soft folds or cyanotic vascular cushions that encroach the lumen. Internal hemorrhoids are best seen during retroflexion.
- Clinical features .... Internal hemorrhoids present with rectal outlet bleeding. Rectal varices rarely bleed but when bleeding does occur, it is acute and voluminous, usually with multiple passages of blood and clot.
- Differential diagnosis ...... Endoscopic: Anal melanoma and mucinous adenocarcinoma of the anorectum. Rectal varices may be difficult to differentiate from prominent but clinically insignificant rectal venous patterns (Fig. 4-171).

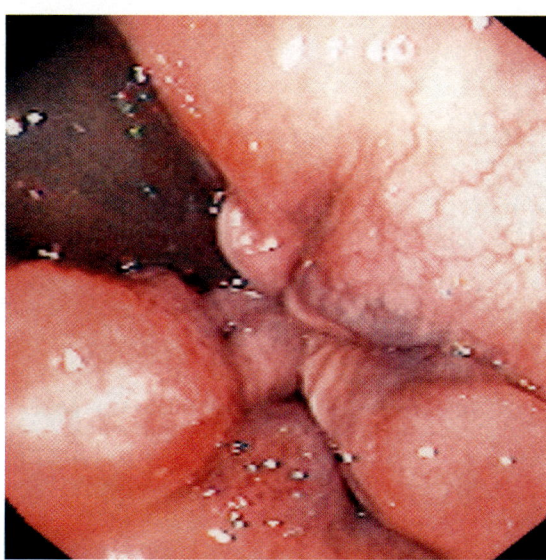

Figure 4-169: **Rectum. Hemorrhoids.** Retroflexed view of large vascular cushions consistent with internal hemorrhoids.

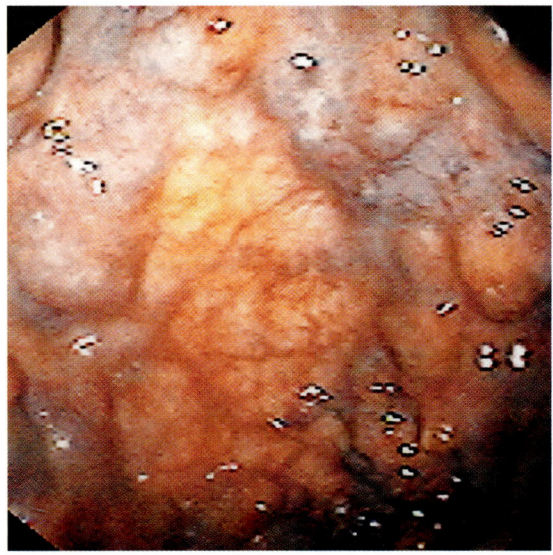

Figure 4-170: **Rectum. Varices.** Engorged, midrectal, tortuous veins in a patient with cirrhosis and known portal hypertension.

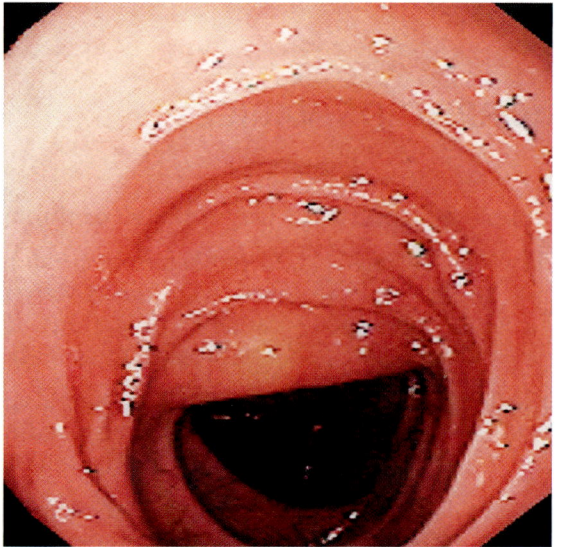

Figure 4-171: **Rectum. Varices.** Prominent submucosal venous pattern. In the distal rectum, there are raised, irregularly shaped venous varices. In the proximal rectum, the veins are prominent, engorged, and enlarged.

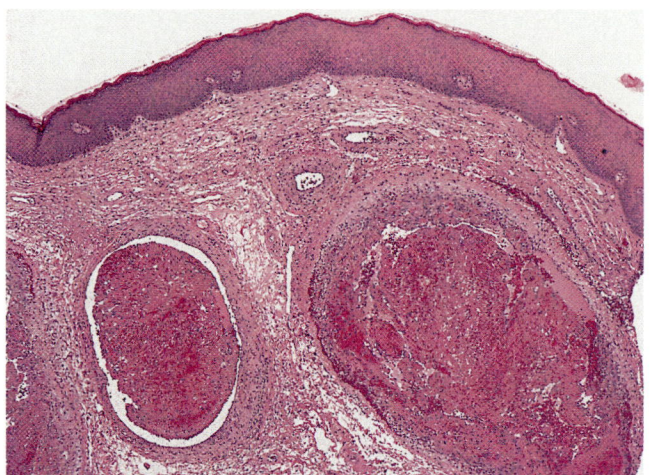

Figure 4-172: **Anal Area. Hemorrhoids.** Dilated, thrombosed, recanalized veins beneath squamous epithelium.

VASCULITIS

- Morphology .... Morphologic changes vary with disease process and size of vessels affected. Biopsy specimens are usually too superficial to fully evaluate vessels in the submucosa. Mucosal reaction is due to ischemia. Behcet syndrome may have discrete right-sided ulcers that are difficult to distinguish from Crohn's lesions.

- Endoscopic features .... Vasculitis can present as punctate erythema, wider patches of erythema, mucosal hemorrhage, and ulceration. Severe vasculitis results in colonic ischemia. If large vessels are involved, ischemic necrosis and sometimes megacolon, an ominous event, may follow.

- Clinical features .... Abdominal pain, abrupt or insidious, cramping or constant; diarrhea; uncommonly hematochezia and toxic megacolon. Patients with vasculitic involvement of the colon often have a history of vasculitis.

- Differential diagnosis ...... Histologic: Ischemic colitis of other causes; Crohn's disease, infectious colitis.

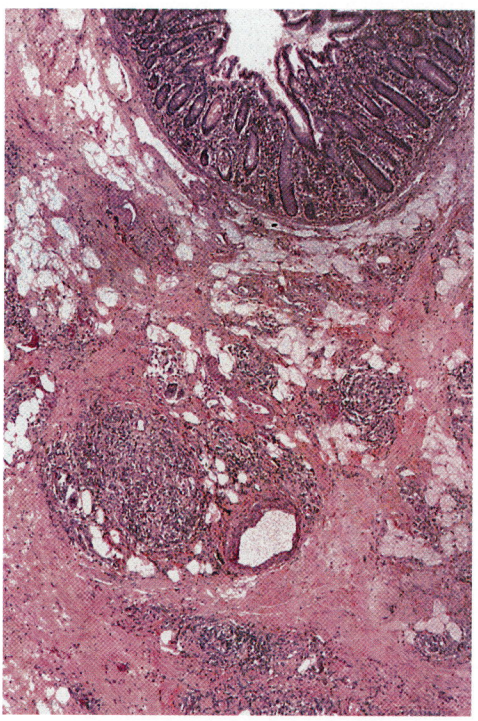

Figure 4-173: **Colon. Vasculitis.** Granulomatous inflammation involving submucosal veins.

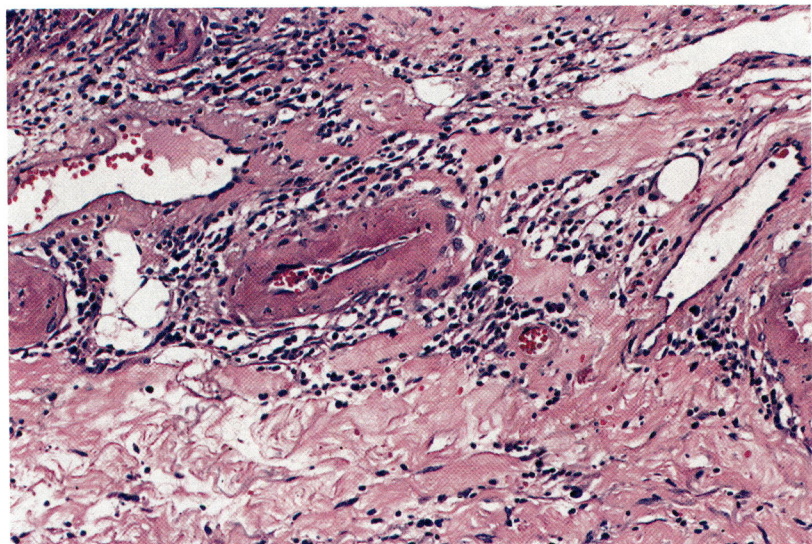

Figure 4-174: **Colon. Necrotizing Vasculitis.** Arteriole with fibrinoid necrosis and perivascular chronic inflammation.

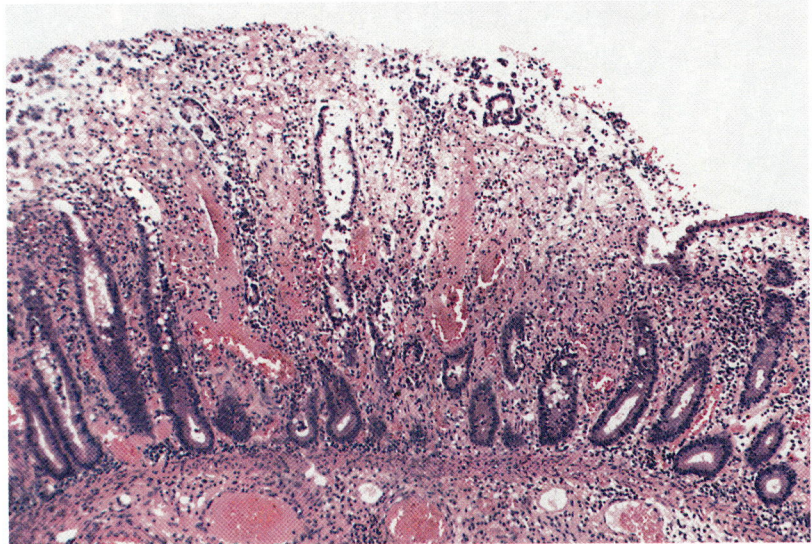

Figure 4-175: **Colon. Ischemic Necrosis Due to Vasculitis.** Superficial mucosal necrosis, with preservation of crypt outlines.

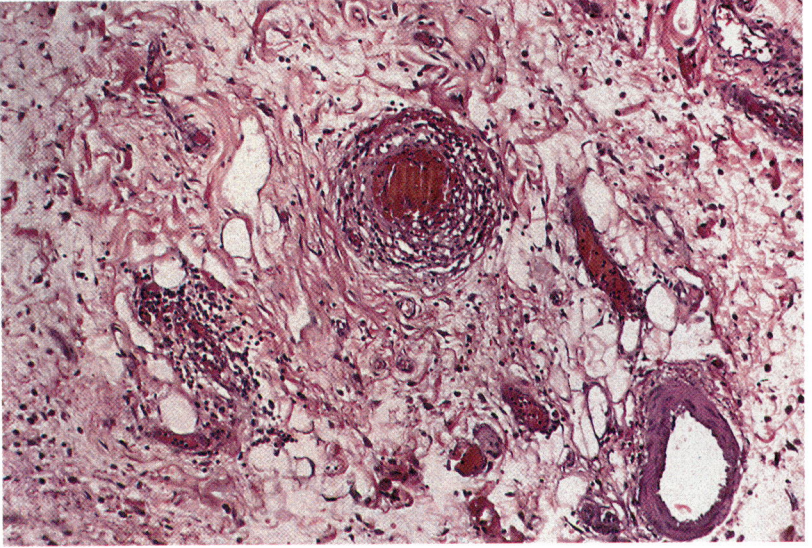

Figure 4-176: **Colon. Vasculitis and Amyloidosis.** Lymphocytic venulitis in submucosa. Hyalin wall of adjacent vessel typical of amyloid. Patient with rheumatoid arthritis and amyloidosis.

FIBROSING COLOPATHY

- Morphology .... Submucosal fibrosis may be missed on superficial biopsy. Mucosal changes include active chronic inflammation and increased numbers of eosinophils. Diagnosis requires the appropriate clinical setting of strictures in patients with cystic fibrosis who are on replacement pancreatic enzymes. The etiologic agent appears to be a material used to coat the medication.
- Endoscopic features .... Luminal narrowing with rigidity of the narrowed segment. The mucosa appears normal.
- Clinical features .... None or obstructive symptoms.
- Differential diagnosis ...... Histologic: Chronic colitis of idiopathic inflammatory bowel disease, chronic phase of ischemic colitis.

    Endoscopic: Stricture of other cause.

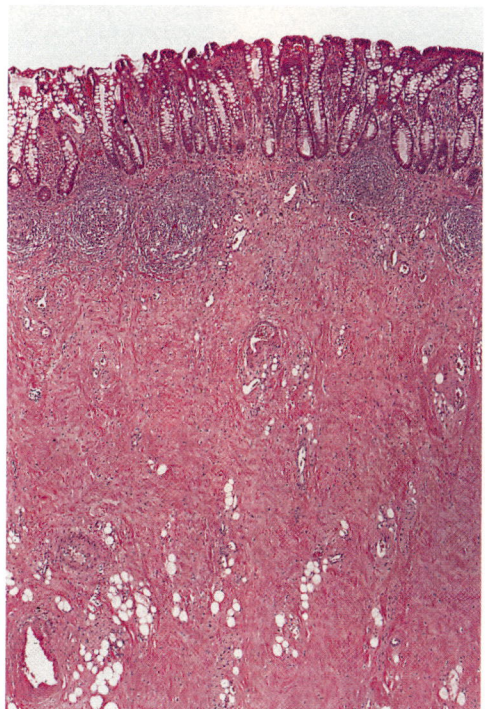

Figure 4-177: **Colon. Fibrosing Colopathy.** Strikingly uniform submucosal fibrosis. No inspissated, viscid mucus, typical of cystic fibrosis, in this patient treated with pancreatic enzymes for cystic fibrosis.

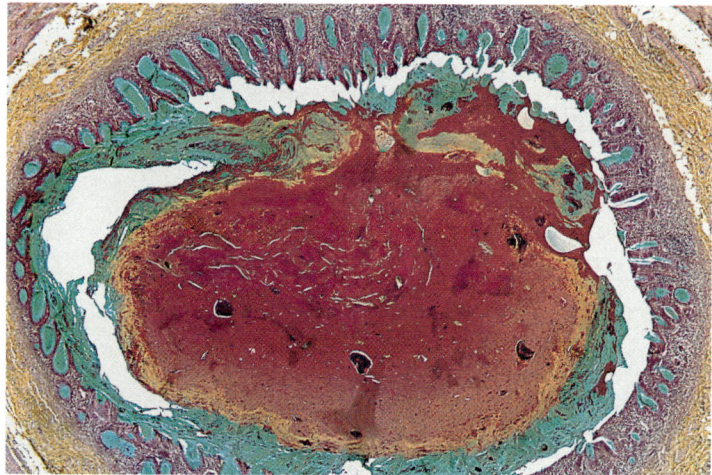

Figure 4-178: **Appendix. Cystic Fibrosis.** Inspissated mucus dilates glandular crypts and appendiceal lumen. Mild degree of submucosal fibrosis. (Movat)

AMYLOIDOSIS

- Morphology — Amyloid is most often found in the walls of submucosal vessels and is not usually seen in the mucosal vessels until late. Tent biopsies or jumbo forceps biopsies are more likely to provide diagnostic material. Superficial mucosal specimens lacking submucosa that do not demonstrate amyloid are inadequate to exclude the diagnosis. There are variations in distribution of amyloid. The common vessel wall pattern is seen in AA amyloidosis, i.e., amyloidosis of chronic disease, whereas preferential deposition in muscularis mucosae is more characteristic of AL amyloidosis, often associated with myeloma.

- Endoscopic features — The mucosa may be normal or may show erythema, mucosal hemorrhage, and, occasionally, ulcerated polypoid masses that appear malignant. The latter, when multiple throughout the colon, should raise strong suspicion for amyloidosis. The differential is with multicentric carcinoma.

- Clinical features — Patients may experience varying bowel habits and, in the presence of mass lesions, GI blood loss, either occult or overt, with episodic hematochezia. Patients usually have systemic symptoms of amyloidosis, especially orthostatic hypotension.

- Differential diagnosis — Histologic: Cautery artifact.

    Endoscopic: Acute infectious inflammation, carcinoma.

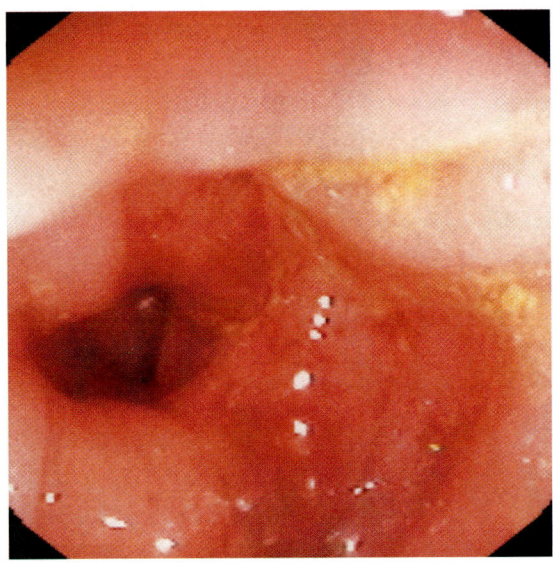

Figure 4-179: **Colon, Sigmoid. Amyloidosis.** The sigmoid is narrowed. Mucosa appears edematous, with patchy erythema.

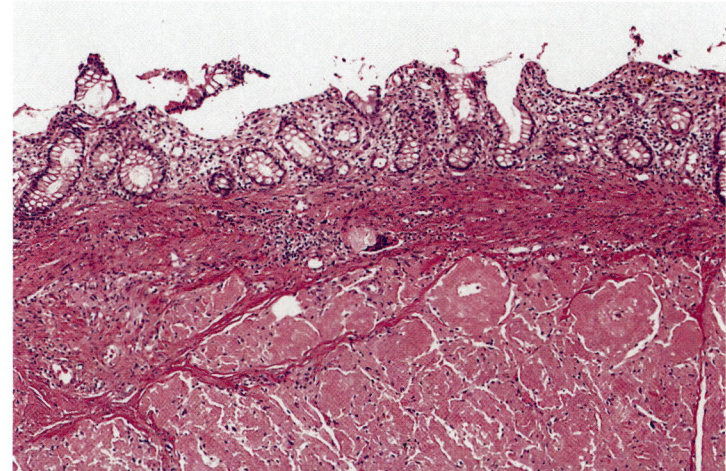

Figure 4-180: **Colon. Amyloidosis.** Massive deposition of homogeneous eosinophilic hyaline material in submucosal vessels and stroma.

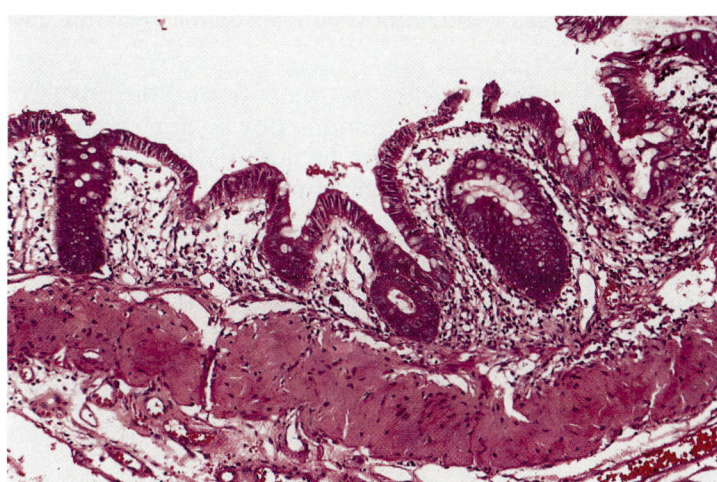

Figure 4-181: **Colon. Amyloidosis.** Homogenization of the muscularis mucosae by eosinophilic hyaline material. Vessels are normal.

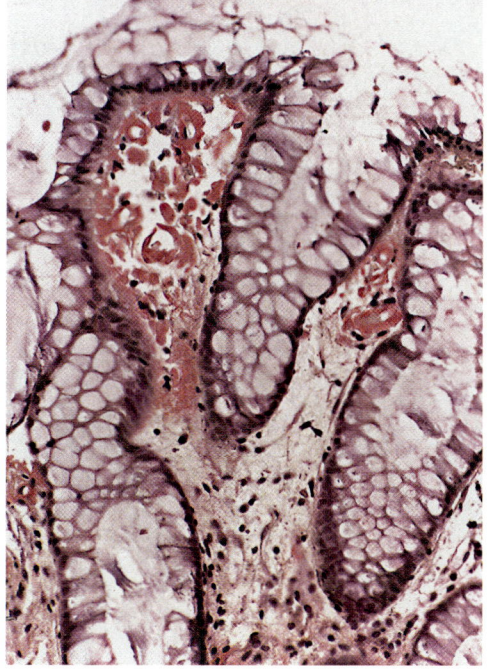

Figure 4-182: **Colon. Amyloidosis.** Eosinophilic hyaline material in superficial mucosal capillary walls.

DYSMOTILITY SYNDROMES

- Morphology .... Dysmotility is caused by a number of neural and muscular disorders. The cause is often elusive, and resection specimens often show no diagnostic abnormality. Mucosal biopsy specimens may be normal or nonspecifically inflamed, or, in scleroderma, may show mucosal vascular changes similar to portal hypertension. Diagnostic morphologic changes are seen in biopsy specimens from patients with Hirschsprung disease or amyloidosis, but resection specimens are necessary to demonstrate the inflammation of the myenteric plexus in paraneoplastic syndromes, muscular fibrosis of scleroderma, and muscle degenerative changes in hollow visceral myopathy.

- Endoscopic features .... Patients may develop very large or wide-mouthed diverticula. The mucosa appears normal.

- Clinical features .... Variable bowel habits, including delayed transit time, severe constipation, fecal impaction, and bowel obstruction. Colonoscopy is not commonly performed on patients with known scleroderma because of the increased risk of perforation secondary to the smooth muscle atrophy.

- Differential diagnosis ...... Etiologic: Abnormal bowel motility may be due to faulty neural transmission occurring anywhere between the brain and the bowel, or muscle dysfunction. Neural dysfunction may be caused by hormonal imbalance, diabetes, hypothyroidism, amyloidosis, paraneoplastic syndromes, and neuroganglionic developmental or degenerative disorders. Degenerative diseases of the muscularis propria include scleroderma, familial hollow visceral myopathy, and muscular dystrophy syndromes.

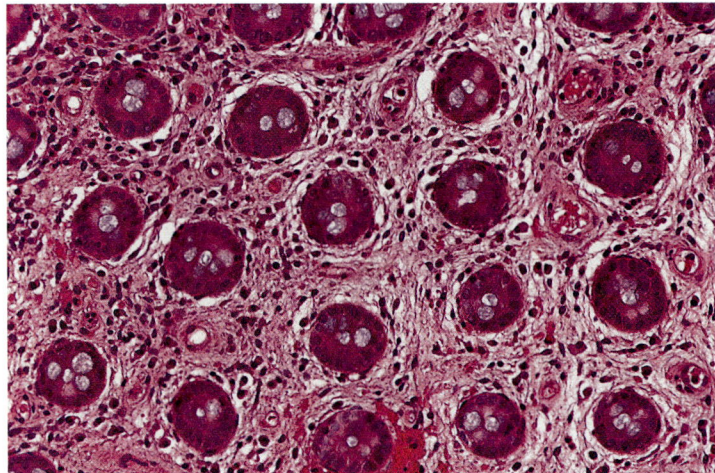

Figure 4-183: **Large Intestine. Scleroderma.** Venules and capillaries are prominent, slightly dilated, rigid, and thick-walled.

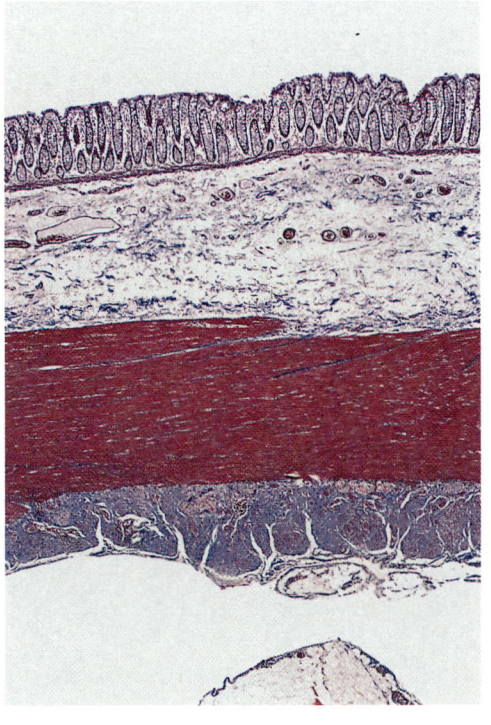

Figure 4-184: **Large Intestine. Hollow Visceral Myopathy.** Muscle atrophy and diffuse fibrosis (blue stained) of the outer layer of the muscularis propria. (Masson trichrome)

LYMPHOID HYPERPLASIA

- Morphology .... Reactive lymphoid aggregates have germinal centers, tingible body macrophages, and a well-defined mantle zone. Lymphoid nodules are usually prominent in the rectum, cecum, and terminal ileum. The amount of lymphoid tissue in the GI tract normally decreases with age. Diffuse or localized lymphoid hyperplasia in the ileum and rectum (rectal tonsil) is more common in children than in adults. Lymphoma involving the rectum is uncommon in the non-AIDS population.

- Endoscopic features .... Lymphoid hyperplasia typically consists of multiple minute (1 to 2 mm) to diminutive (2 to 5 mm) nodules. In the ileum of young patients, lymphoid nodules may be numerous, crowded, and heaped-up in Peyer patches.

- Clinical features .... Usually incidental. Common and numerous, especially in the ileum in diarrheal states.

- Differential diagnosis...... Endoscopic: Hyperplastic or adenomatous polyps, carcinoid tumor, acute colitis with erosions, lymphomatous polyposis (mantle cell lymphoma).

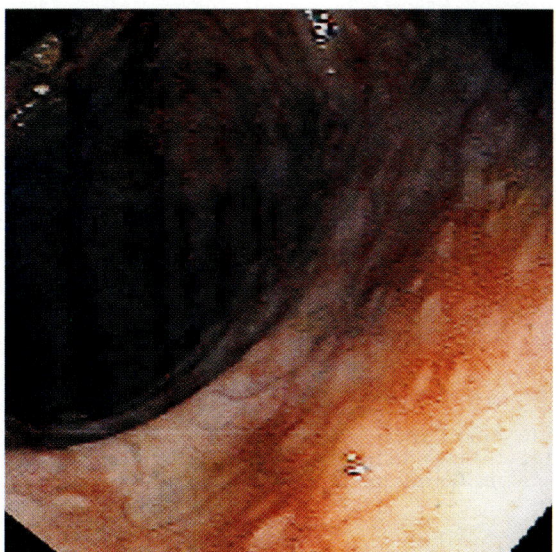

Figure 4-185: **Colon, Sigmoid. Lymphoid Hyperplasia.** Multiple nodules 1 to 2 mm in size. The erythema surrounding these minute nodules is typical.

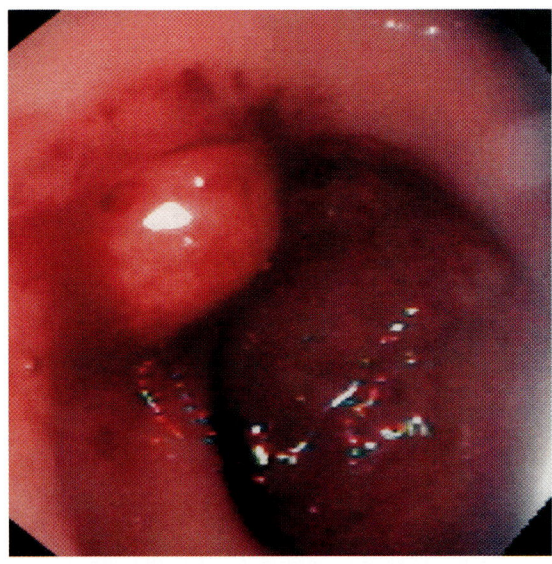

Figure 4-186: **Rectum. Lymphoid Hyperplasia.** Atypical rectal polyp with spontaneous bleeding and excessive friability.

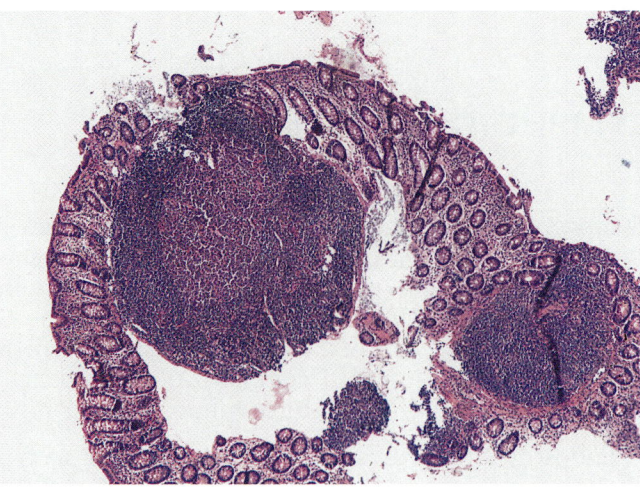

Figure 4-187: **Colon. Lymphoid Hyperplasia.** Reactive submucosal lymphoid aggregates beneath unremarkable colonic mucosa.

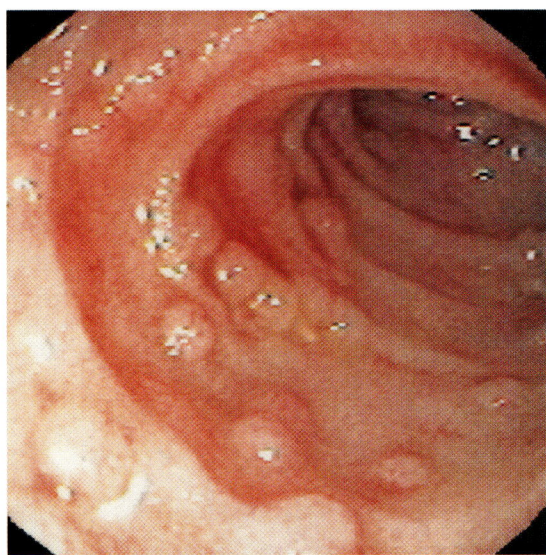

Figure 4-188: **Terminal Ileum. Lymphoid Hyperplasia.** Scattered diminutive nodules of the same color and appearance as the surrounding flat mucosa.

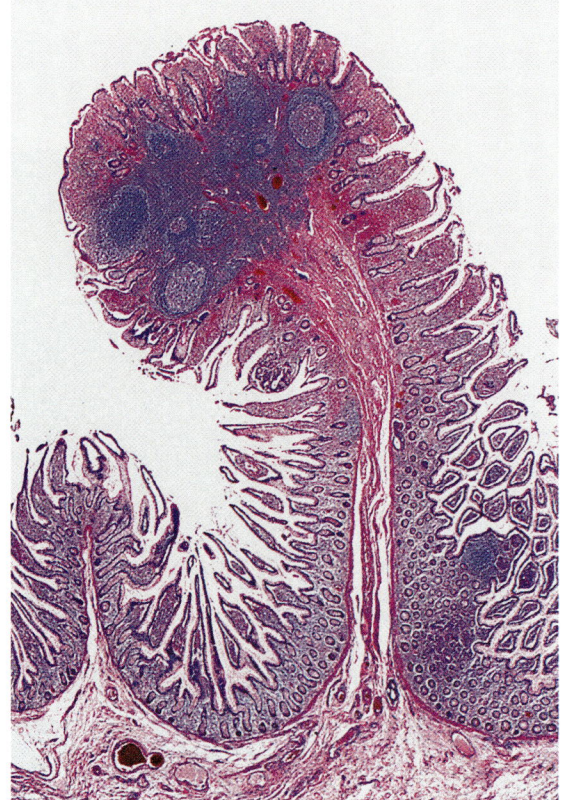

Figure 4-189: **Terminal Ileum. Lymphoid Hyperplasia.** Cluster of lymphoid follicles with germinal centers forming a polyp. Patient with cecal carcinoma.

PNEUMATOSIS COLI

- Morphology .... Air collects in the submucosa, forming dome-shaped polyps, and characteristically elicits a foreign-body giant cell reaction. Small biopsy samples are often too superficial to obtain diagnostic tissue. The presence of normal mucosa and a submucosal cyst wall with histiocytes on the edge suggest the diagnosis.

- Endoscopic features .... Patients with pneumatosis coli may or may not have symptoms. On endoscopic examination, there are multiple polyps or nodules covered by normal intact mucosa. The process can be quite impressive, as in Fig. 4-191. The diagnosis is obvious on radiologic examination and may be established by puncturing the cysts, resulting in deflation and flattening of the polyps. Being aware of this uncommon condition is the most important aspect of diagnosis.

- Clinical features .... Crampy discomfort when the rectum-sigmoid area is involved. Patients may have a history of obstructive pulmonary disease, duodenal ulcer, or necrotizing enteritis, particularly in the neonatal group. Localized segments of involvement proximal to the rectum may cause intussusception or, less commonly, obstructive symptoms due to the size and number of cysts.

- Differential diagnosis ...... Endoscopic: Polyposis syndromes.

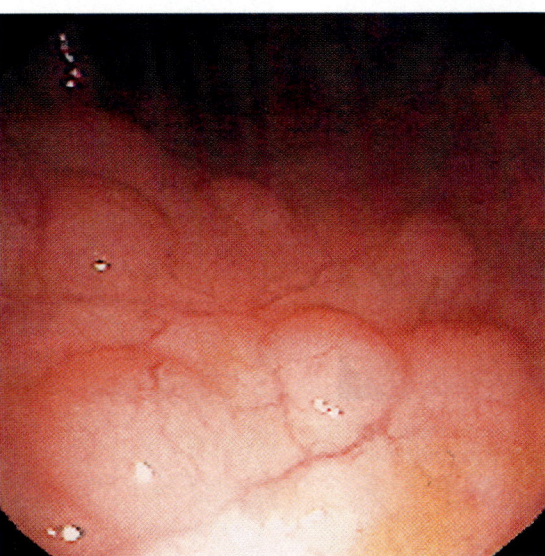

Figure 4-190: **Cecum. Pneumatosis Coli.** Multiple nodules covered by normal mucosa suggest a submucosal lesion.

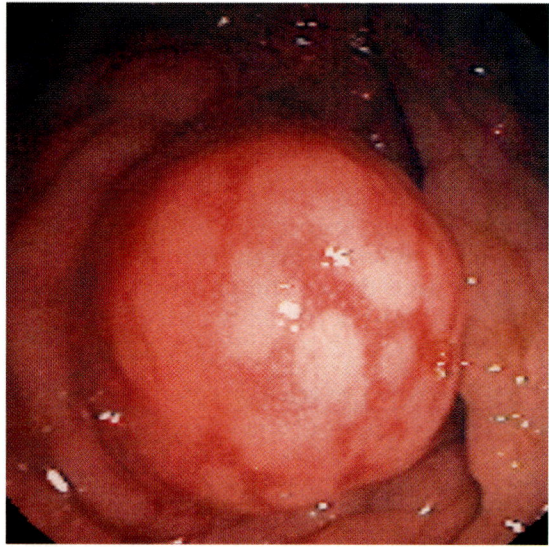

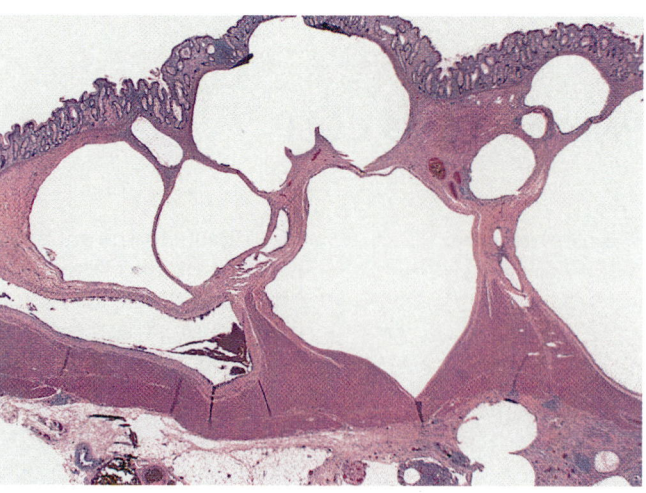

Figure 4-192: **Cecum. Pneumatosis Coli.** Cystic spaces, mainly submucosal, form mucosal nodules.

Figure 4-191: **Cecum. Pneumatosis Coli.** Giant submucosal air cysts distend the mucosa, exaggerating the mucosal groove pattern (honeycombing) and distorting the submucosal vascular network.

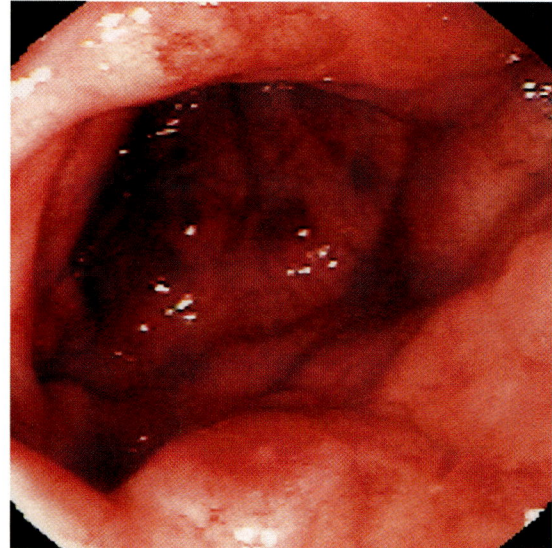

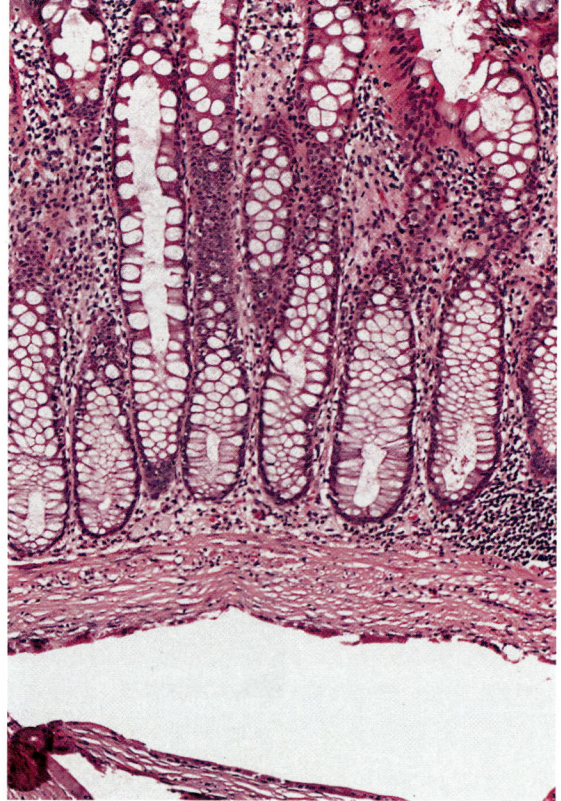

Figure 4-193: **Colon, Transverse. Pneumatosis coli.** Multiple soft, submucosal nodules. Needle puncture results in release of air bubbles.

Figure 4-194: **Colon. Pneumatosis Coli.** Submucosal cysts lined with histiocytes; often the only histologic clue to pneumatosis coli.

ENDOMETRIOSIS

- **Morphology** .... Common in the sigmoid colon, where it causes kinking or stricture, endometriosis involves the bowel wall and infrequently extends to the mucosa to produce a polyp (as illustrated). Histologic pattern will depend on proportion of glands and stroma and whether or not there is hemorrhage, fibrosis, or decidualization. Immunostains (cytokeratin 7, cytokeratin 20, estrogen receptor, and progesterone receptor) may be useful diagnostic adjuncts.

- **Endoscopic features** .... Extrinsic obstruction and stricture with intact mucosa is the most frequent finding.

- **Clinical features** .... Nonspecific abdominal pain, crampy lower quadrant pain, altered bowel habits, and hematochezia with mucosal involvement. A cyclic pattern of bleeding corresponding with menstruation may indicate the diagnosis.

- **Differential diagnosis** ...... Histologic and endoscopic: Adenocarcinoma.

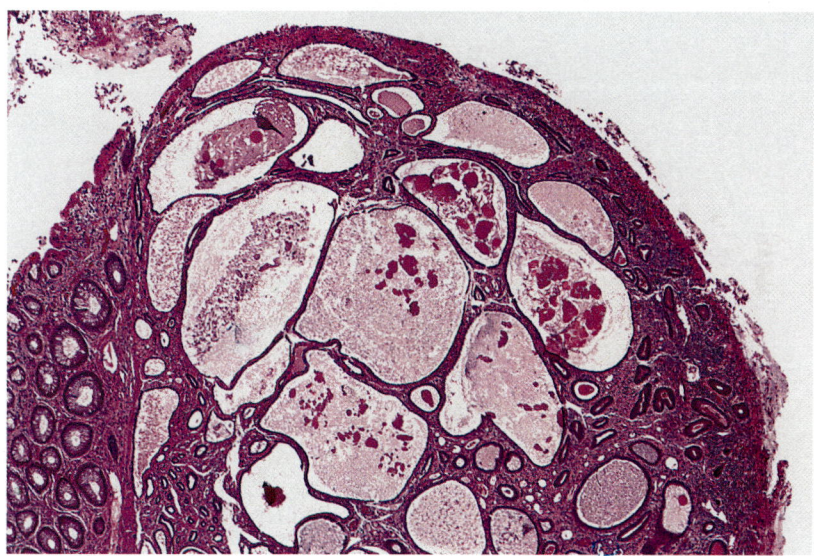

Figure 4-195: **Colon. Endometriosis.** Dilated and small dark glands and stroma distinctly different from colonic tissue occupy the mucosa. An uncommon occurence.

INVERTED APPENDIX

- Morphology .... On small biopsy specimens from a polyp in the cecum, normal mucosa with numerous lymphoid follicles suggests inverted appendix. Endometriosis may form a lead point if intussusception is the cause of inverted appendix.

- Endoscopic features .... The appendiceal orifice is located at the very base of the cecum, typically nestled between the distinctive "crow's feet." Whether the appendix is present or has been surgically removed, usually the appearance is that of a semilunar cleft, small opening, or diverticulum, in contrast to the prolapsing appearance in the figure.

- Clinical features .... When diseased, the appendix may prolapse into the cecal lumen due to obstruction, inflammation, and edema.

- Differential diagnosis ..... Endoscopic: Cecal adenoma. Location and characteristic surrounding semi-circular folds serve to distinguish an inverted appendiceal stump from an adenoma.

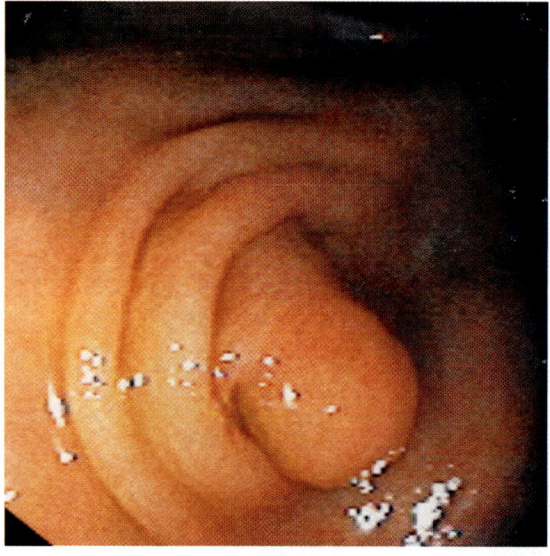

Figure 4-196: **Cecum. Inverted Appendix.** Inverted appendiceal stump prolapsing into the cecal lumen.

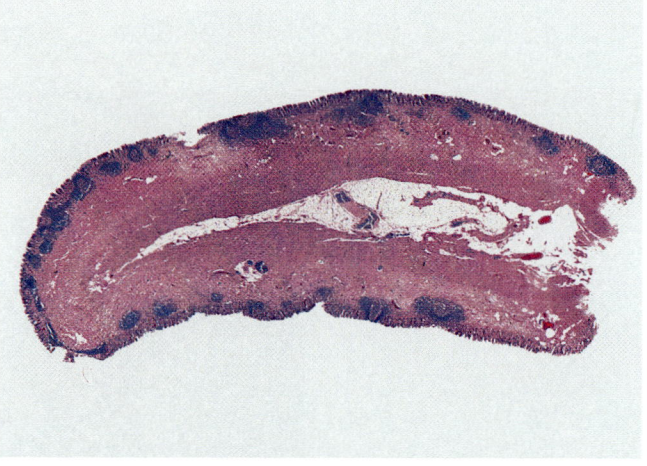

Figure 4-197: **Cecum. Inverted Appendix.** Numerous mucosal lymphoid follicles typical of appendiceal mucosa. All layers of appendiceal wall present but inverted. No obvious lead point.

RECTAL PROLAPSE SYNDROME AND INFLAMMATORY CLOACOGENIC POLYP

- Morphology .... Commonly located on the anterior wall of the rectum, there may be erythema and granularity, one or multiple ulcers, single or multiple polyps, and submucosal induration. The combination of histologic changes, i.e., epithelial hyperplasia, ischemic erosions, fibrin cap, ulceration, and, in particular, mucosal fibrosis and hypertrophy of mucosal smooth muscle cells, is characteristic. Inflammatory cloacogenic polyps and submucosal cysts (colitis cystica profunda) are components of the rectal prolapse syndrome.

- Endoscopic features .... In the absence of flagrant inducible prolapse, the rectal prolapse syndrome has no specific features. Diagnosis requires a high index of suspicion. Findings include solitary or multiple rectal ulcers, scarring, cicatricial contracture, prominent folds and ridges, solitary or multiple heaped-up polyps, and nodular mucosa of colitis cystica profunda. Polyps require removal for histologic diagnosis. Mucosal prolapse is typical at the anorectal junction, but also occurs in the sigmoid.

    Cloacogenic polyps present at the dentate line with or without associated hemorrhoids, and are sessile, erythematous, and friable. They differ from internal hemorrhoids, which are typically blue; anal papillae, which are pale yellow; and adenomas, which usually lack a fibrinous cap.

- Clinical features .... Obvious prolapse with straining, rectal outlet bleeding, perineal discomfort.

- Differential diagnosis ...... Histologic: Chronic ischemia, quiescent ulcerative colitis, hamartomatous polyps, adenocarcinoma, mucinous adenocarcinoma.

    Endoscopic: Crohn's disease, neoplasm.

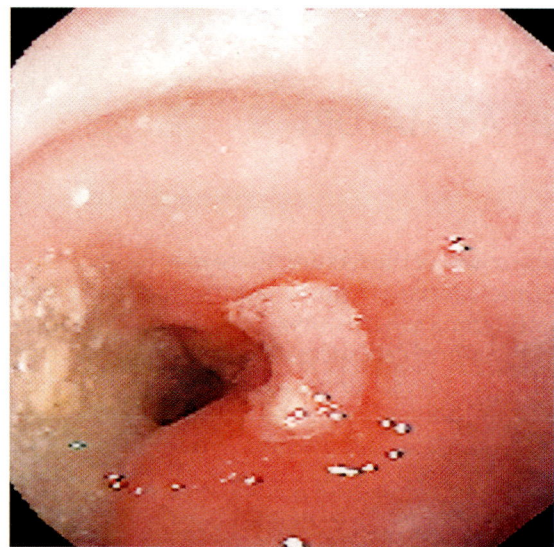

Figure 4-198: **Rectum. Rectal Prolapse.** Solitary rectal ulcer seen in the proximal rectum just distal to the rectosigmoid angle.

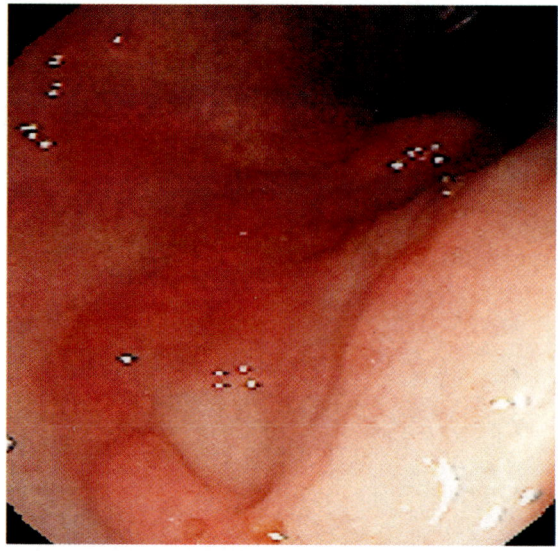

Figure 4-199: **Rectum. Rectal Prolapse.** Midrectal mucosal deformity consisting of erythematous nodular ridges, an area of mucosal depression, and the suggestion of cicatricial deformity to the right side of the depressed area. Overall, suggestive of hyperplastic tissue and scarring.

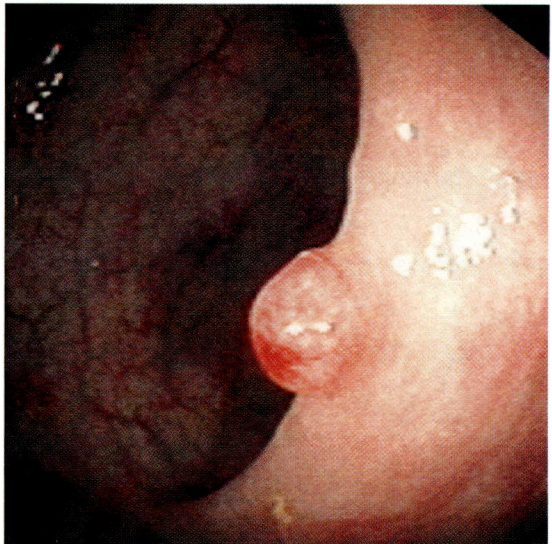

Figure 4-200: **Rectum. Rectal Prolapse.** Solitary diminutive rectal polyp located on a haustral fold. The polyp is friable and without distinguishing features.

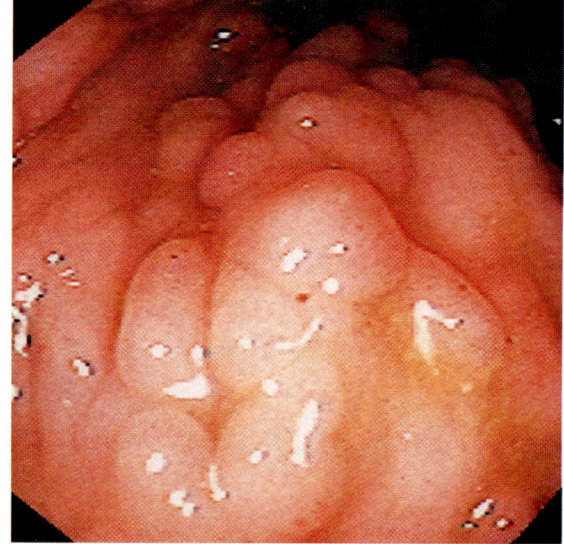

Figure 4-201: **Rectum. Rectal Prolapse.** Nodular polypoid mass covered by normal intact mucosa, suggestive of a submucosal process.

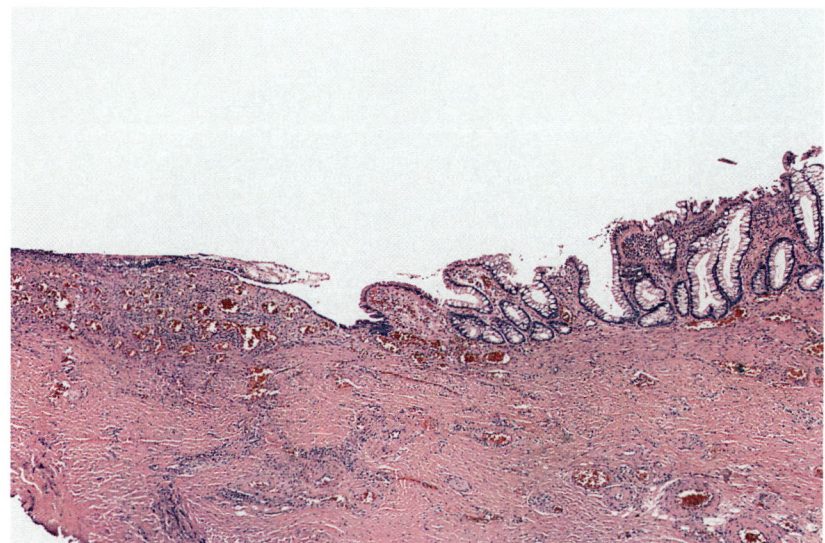

Figure 4-202: **Rectum. Rectal Prolapse, Ulcer.** Chronic ulcer, fibrotic mucosa and submucosa.

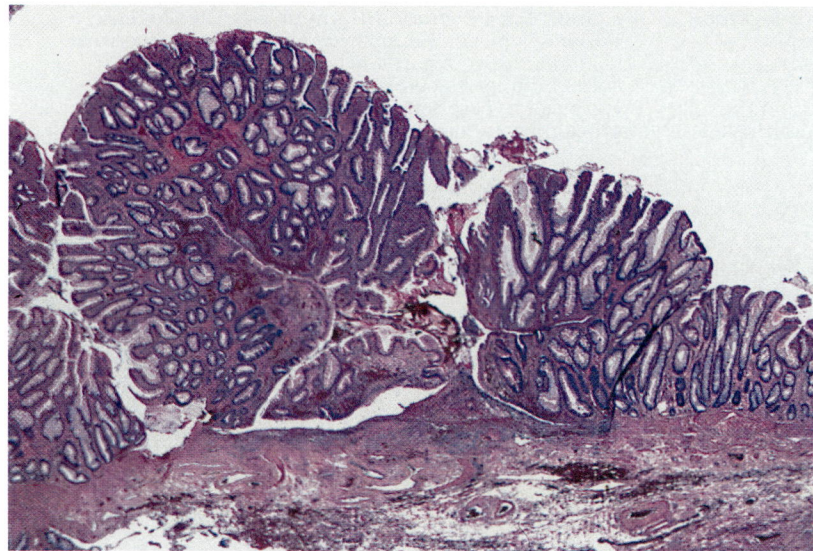

Figure 4-203: **Rectum. Rectal Prolapse, Polyp.** Hyperplastic polypoid mucosa in response to ulcer.

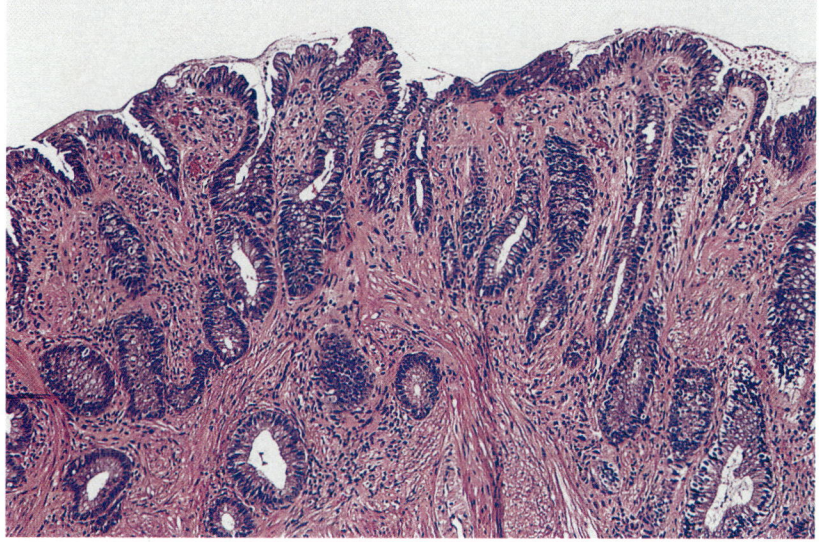

Figure 4-204: **Rectum. Rectal Prolapse.** Lamina propria replaced by fibromuscular stroma distorting glands.

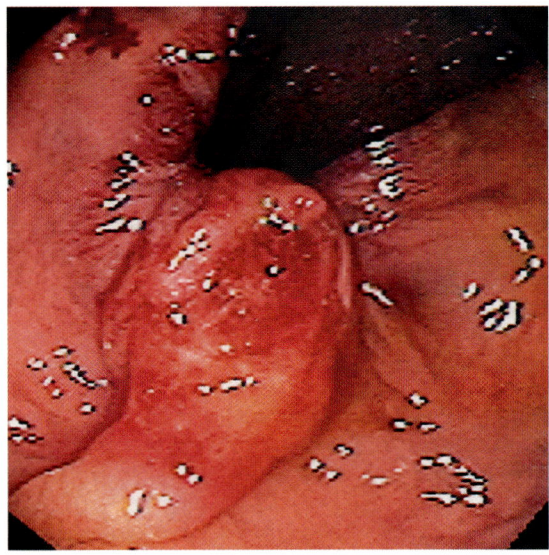

Figure 4-205: **Rectum. Inflammatory Cloacogenic Polyp.** Retroflexed view of the distal rectum demonstrating a large polyp resembling, but somewhat atypical for, a hemorrhoid. There is a mucosal ridge extending into the rectum from the dentate line. The overlying mucosa is hemorrhagic.

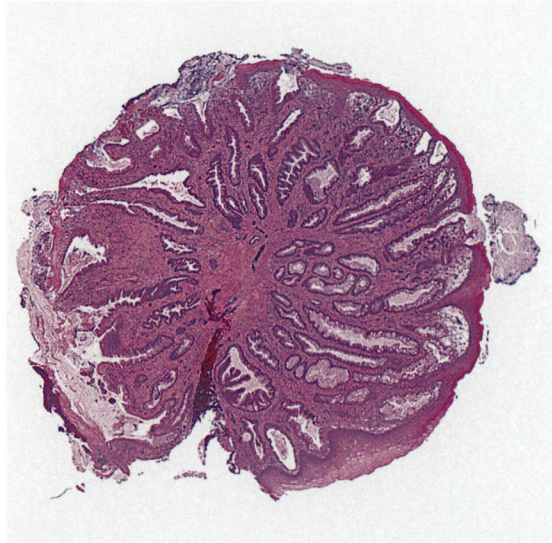

Figure 4-206: **Rectum. Inflammatory Cloacogenic Polyp.** Typical inflammatory cloacogenic polyp with glandular mucosa partially covered by squamous epithelium, partial erosion, mucofibrinous cap, epithelial hyperplasia, mucosal fibrosis, and hypertrophied mucosal muscle fibers.

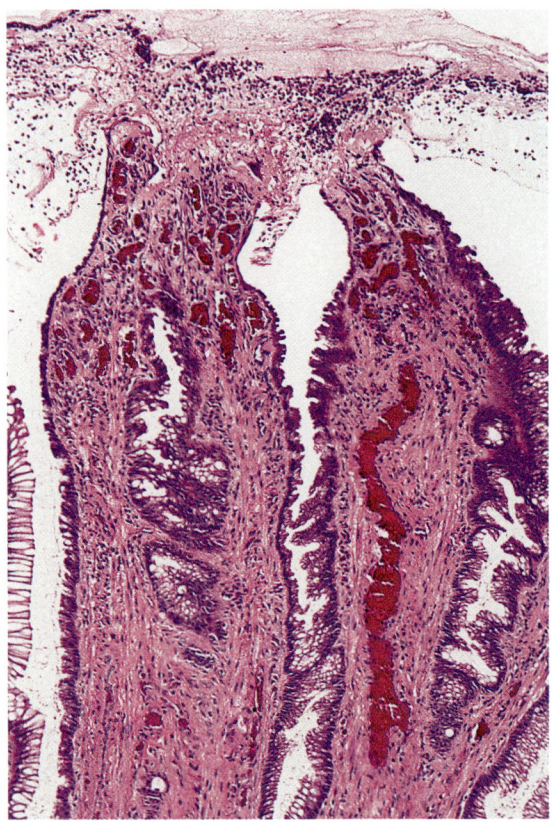

Figure 4-207: **Rectum. Inflammatory Cloacogenic Polyp.** Higher magnification illustrates erosion, mucofibrinous cap, hypertrophied mucosal muscle fibers, and glandular proliferation.

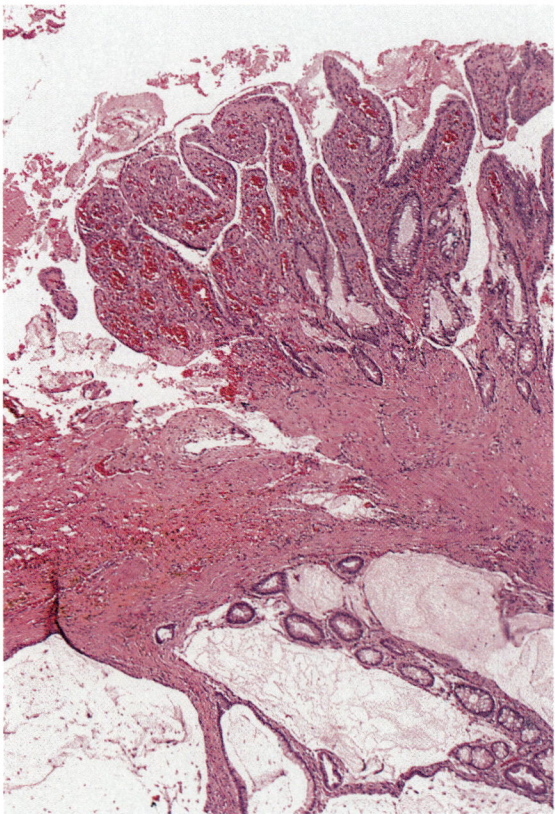

Figure 4-208: **Rectum. Rectal Prolapse, Colitis Cystica Profunda.** Chronic ulcer, hyperplastic fibrotic mucosa, displaced submucosal cystic colonic mucosa.

BARIUM GRANULOMA AND OLEOGRANULOMA

- Morphology .... In *barium granulomas*, the stroma is filled with histiocytes. The barium is fine, light gray, and somewhat birefringent under polarized light. Often there is a foreign body giant cell reaction. *Oleogranuloma,* or *paraffinoma,* is a reaction to oily substances introduced into the anal canal. The oil is removed by processing. Characteristically, there are clear spaces and a foreign body giant cell reaction.

- Endoscopic features .... Barium granuloma may appear as white plaques, nonspecific ulceration, and ulceration with induration suggestive of malignancy. In oleogranuloma, indurated, ulcerated masses are most commonly found in the anorectal area.

- Clinical features .... Rectal discomfort, hematochezia.

- Differential diagnosis...... Histologic: Pseudolipomatosis (insufflation artifact) can simulate oleogranuloma, but is largely confined to the lamina propria. Oleogranuloma usually affects submucosa as well. Pseudolipomatosis does not have a giant cell reaction.

  Endoscopic: Other inflammatory conditions and infiltrating malignancies.

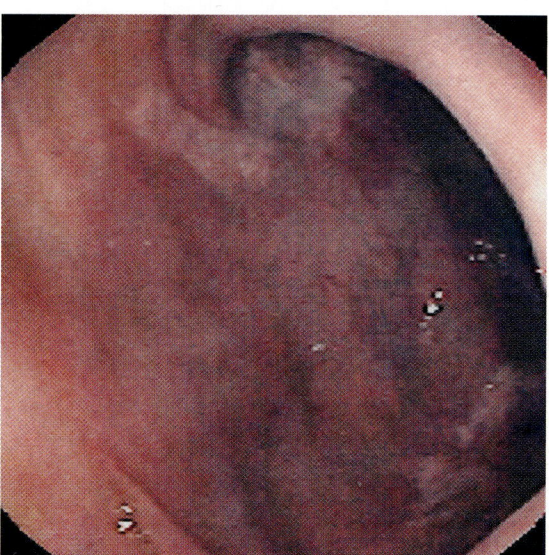

Figure 4-209: **Colon, Distal Transverse. Barium Granuloma.** At the upper and lower portions of the photo, there are irregular patches of white mucosa.

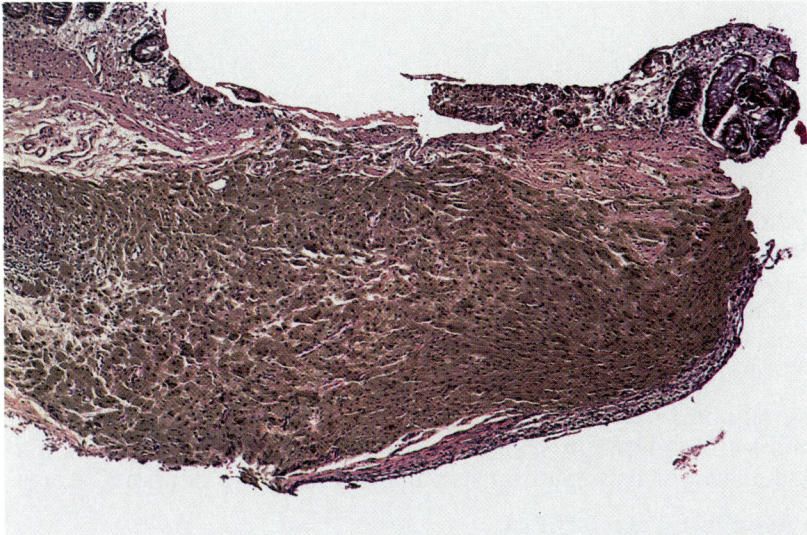

Figure 4-210: **Colon. Barium Granuloma.** Large submucosal collection of histiocytes containing refractile but poorly birefringent brown pigment.

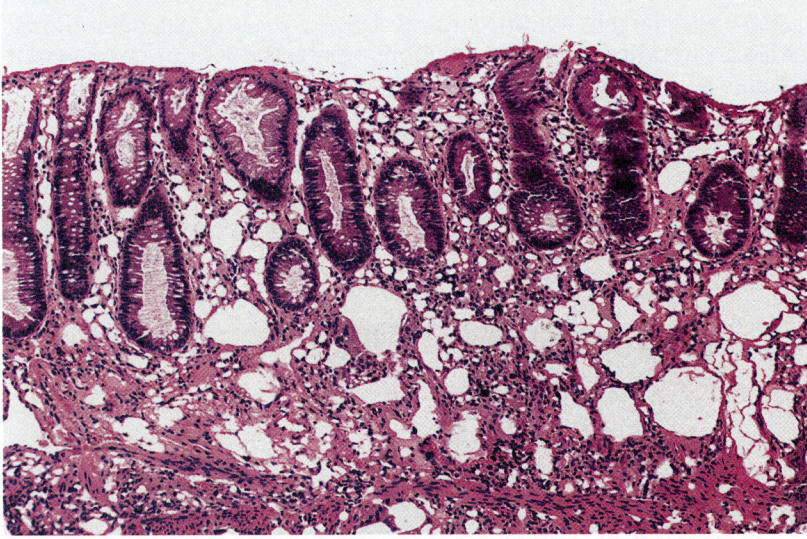

Figure 4-211: **Rectum. Oleogranuloma.** Irregular, clear, round spaces in the mucosa and submucosa.

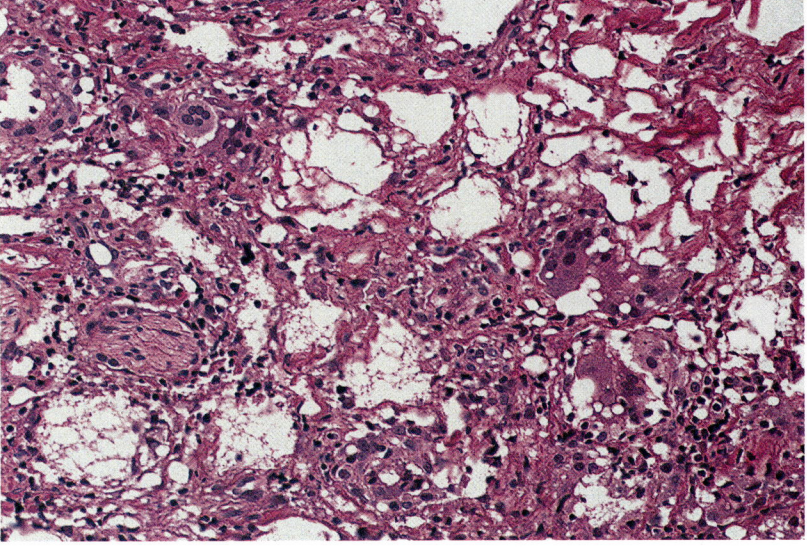

Figure 4-212: **Rectum. Oleogranuloma.** Irregular, clear spaces, multinucleated giant cell reaction, chronic inflammation, and fibrosis in submucosa.

HYPERTROPHIED ANAL PAPILLA/SKIN TAG

- Morphology .... Squamous mucosa with a fibrovascular core from the region of the anal papilla. Also termed *fibroepithelial polyp*.
- Endoscopic features .... Hypertrophied anal papillae are incidental findings. They are white-to-yellow polypoid lesions within the dentate line that vary in size from minute to 1 cm.
- Clinical features .... None.
- Differential diagnosis ...... Endoscopic: Hemorrhoids, cloacogenic polyp, inflammatory anal tags due to Crohn's disease.

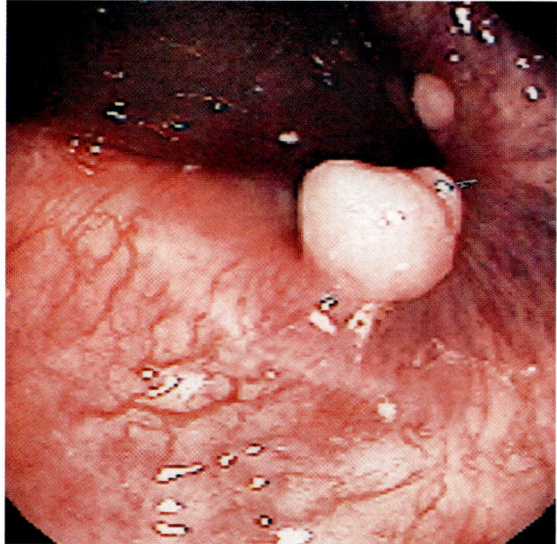

Figure 4-213: **Anal Canal. Hypertrophied Anal Papillae.** Retroflexed view within the rectum. Two whitish polyps are located at the dentate line.

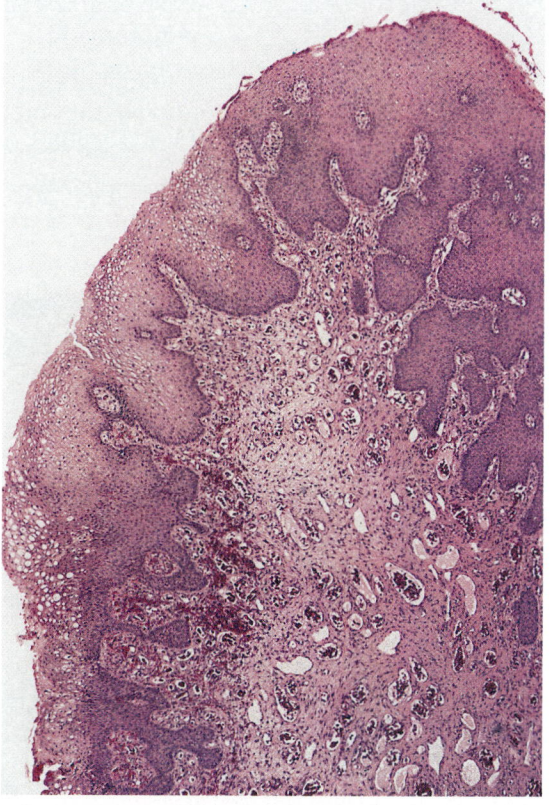

Figure 4-214: **Anal Canal. Hypertrophied Anal Papilla.** Polypoid, thickened squamous mucosa with fibrovascular stroma.

INFLAMMATORY POLYPS

- Morphology .... *Pseudopolyps* are residual islands of mucosa in areas of ulceration. *Inflammatory polyps* are focally expanded lesions due to mucosal inflammation, regeneration, and repair. *Postinflammatory polyps* are usually elongated, filiform, and branching, with a muscular core; the mucosa may be inflamed or normal. Single inflammatory or postinflammatory polyps result from isolated mucosal injury; numerous filiform postinflammatory polyps are often the result of a single severe mucosal injury. Multiple inflammatory polyps are usually the consequence of inflammatory bowel disease. In quiescent inflammatory bowel disease, the polyps often are more inflamed than the surrounding mucosa. Epithelial proliferation in the crypts may be intense.

- Endoscopic features .... Inflammatory polyps vary from isolated to innumerable crowded lesions that may branch and completely bridge the lumen. Coalescence, branching, and bridging are distinctive for inflammatory polyps. If sampled, they bleed more readily than other polyp types.

- Clinical features .... Active or quiescent inflammatory bowel disease. The polyps themselves are asymptomatic.

- Differential diagnosis ...... Histologic: Peutz-Jeghers polyp and juvenile polyp. Inflammatory polyps, although they may have a muscular core, lack the arborizing muscular strands of Peutz-Jeghers polyps.

    Endoscopic: Hyperplastic, hamartomatous, and neoplastic polyps.

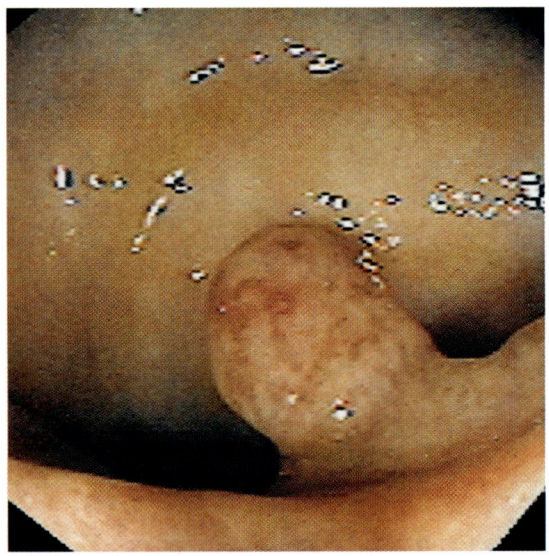

Figure 4-215: **Colon, Sigmoid. Inflammatory Polyp in Inflammatory Bowel Disease.** Discrete, small polyp on short, broad pedicle; surface features nonspecific.

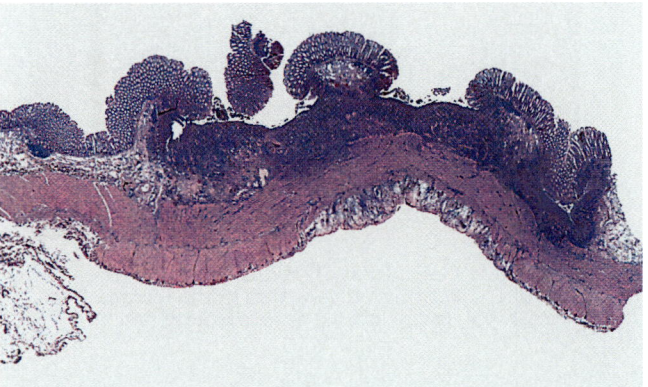

Figure 4-216: **Colon. Pseudopolyps in Ulcerative Colitis.** Ulcers interspersed with residual polypoid mucosa.

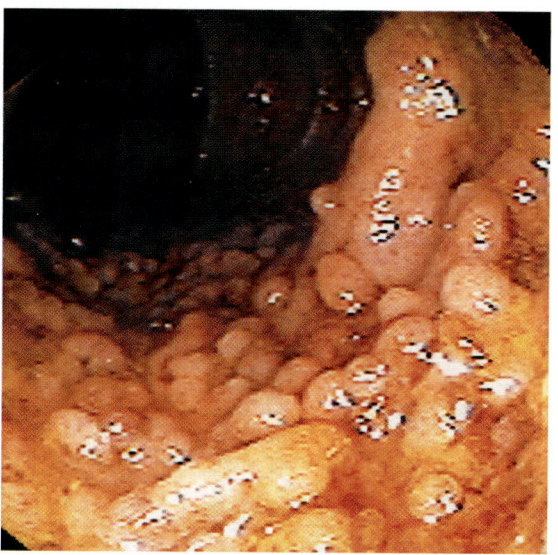

Figure 4-217: **Colon, Transverse. Inflammatory Polyps in Inflammatory Bowel Disease.** Multiple crowded, diminutive sessile polyps. There is also coalescence with formation of larger polyps.

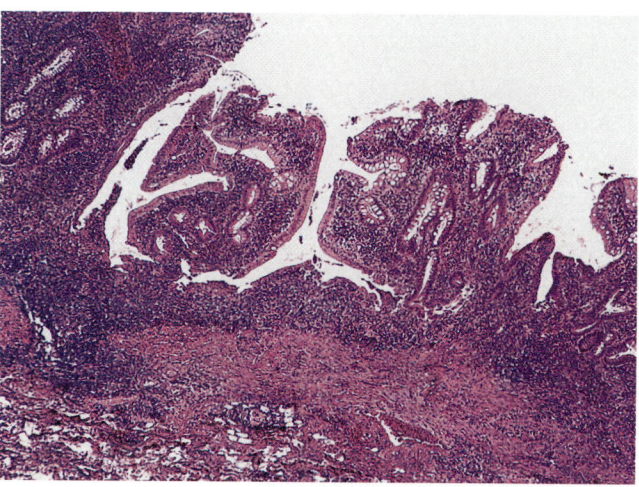

Figure 4-218: **Colon. Inflammatory Polyps in Ulcerative Colitis.** Chronic mucosal inflammation with architectural distortion and polyp formation.

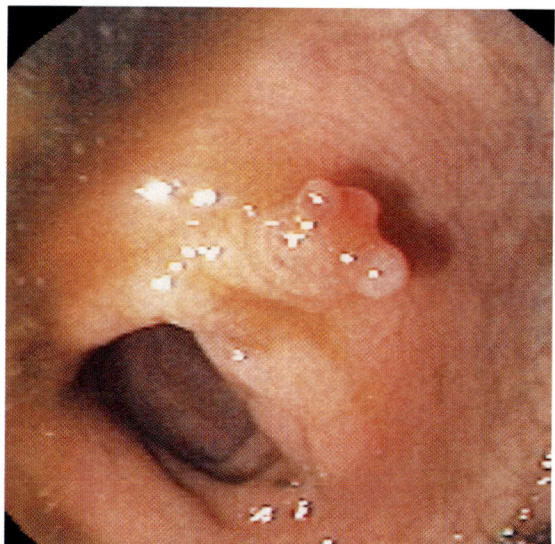

Figure 4-219: **Colon, Sigmoid. Inflammatory Polyp.** Isolated small polyp with distinctive branching.

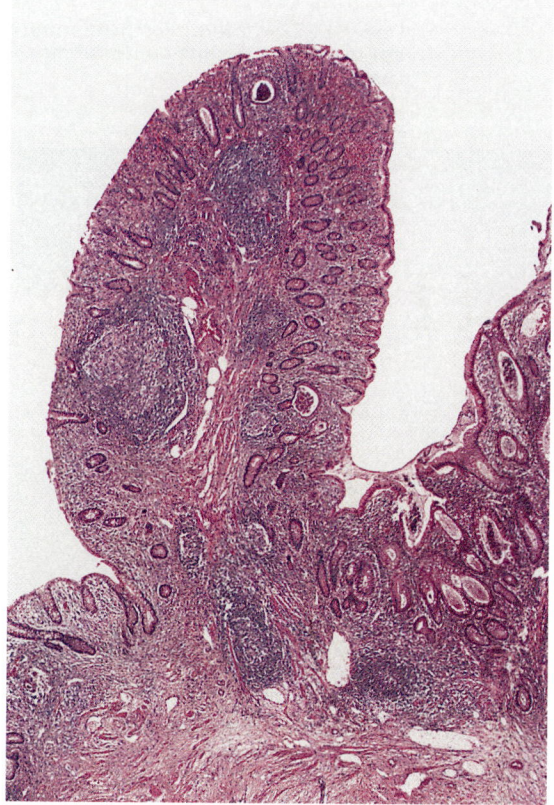

Figure 4-220: **Colon. Inflammatory Polyp in Inflammatory Bowel Disease.** Polyp with smooth muscle core in chronic active colitis. Crypt abscesses and lymphoid hyperplasia.

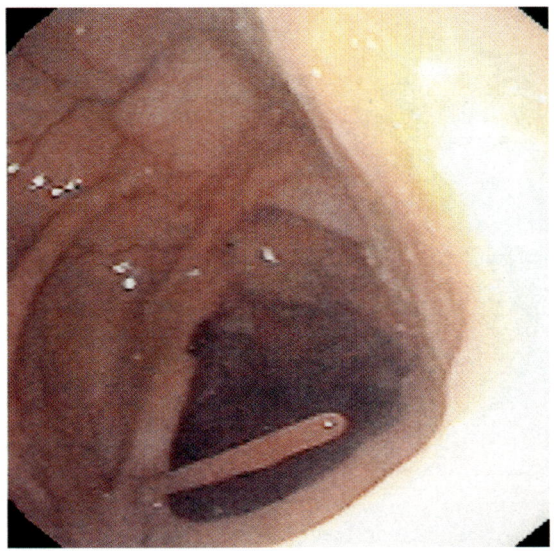

Figure 4-221: **Colon, Transverse. Postinflammatory Polyp in Quiescent Inflammatory Bowel Disease.** Long, thin polyp atypical for hyperplastic or adenomatous polyp and suspicious for inflammatory polyp.

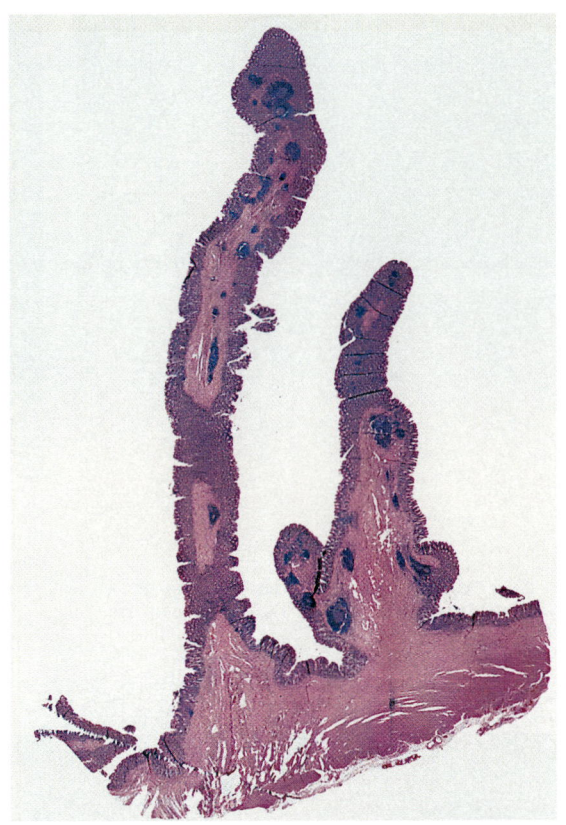

Figure 4-222: **Colon. Postinflammatory Polyps.** Filiform polyps with submucosal cores.

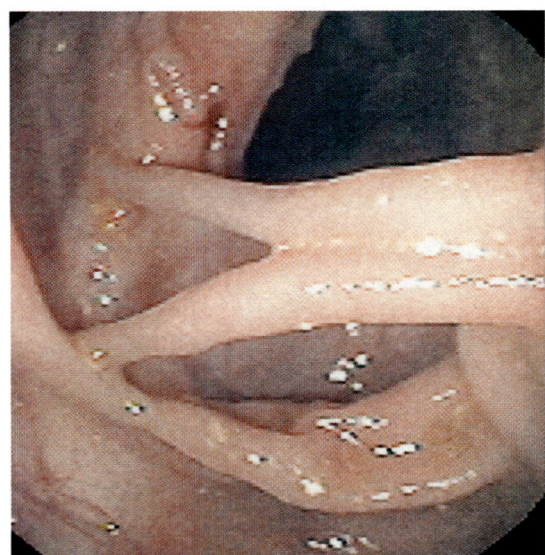

Figure 4-223: **Colon, Transverse. Postinflammatory Polyp in Quiescent Inflammatory Bowel Disease.** Long, Y-shaped inflammatory polyp bridging the bowel lumen.

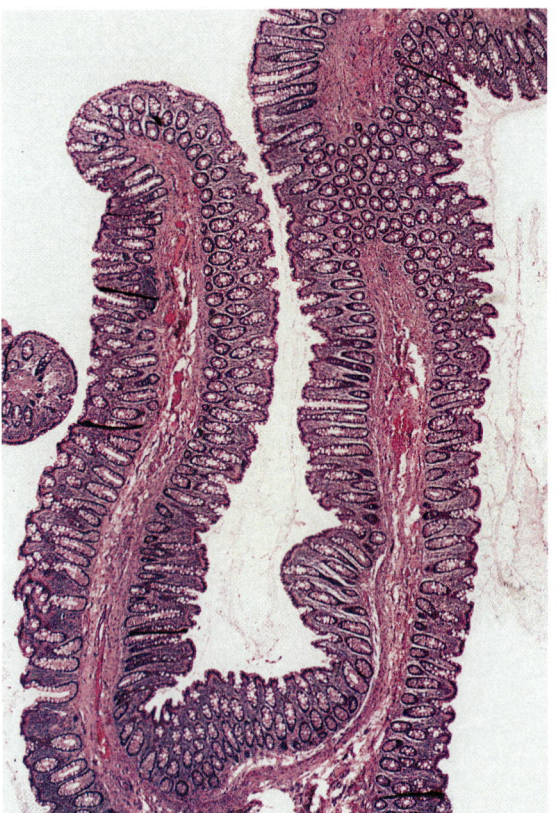

Figure 4-224: **Colon. Postinflammatory Polyps.** Branched filiform polyps with normal mucosa and submucosal core.

HYPERPLASTIC POLYP

- Morphology .... In hyperplastic polyps, the regenerative zone in the lower third of the crypts appears basophilic because of nuclear crowding and stratification. Maturation occurs towards the surface. This contrasts with adenomas, where dysplasia appears on the surface and then extends down the crypt. Failure of the surface epithelium to undergo apoptosis and desquamation at a normal rate produces a hyperplastic polyp. The epithelial cells pile on the surface along the length of the crypt, creating a serrated, longitudinal profile and star shape in cross sections. There are combined but discrete hyperplastic and adenomatous polyps, and serrated adenomas in which there is a subtle, intermingled combination of features of hyperplastic polyp and adenoma (see page 376). The latter, often mistaken for hyperplastic polyps, have the biological potential of adenomas.

- Endoscopic features .... Hyperplastic polyps are white or bland-appearing lesions, usually scattered through the rectum and sigmoid, that range in size from minute (1 or 2 mm) to large (up to 2 cm in diameter). High-resolution video endoscopy yields distinct surface features. The hyperplastic polyp has a pitted surface appearance representing an exaggeration of the pitted or honeycombed mucosal crypt pattern. When vital stains (e.g., methylene blue) or contrast stains (e.g., indigo carmine) are used, surface features are accentuated, as represented in figure 4-229.

- Clinical features .... None.

- Differential diagnosis ...... Histologic: Adenoma.

    Endoscopic: Adenoma, lymphoid nodule. The endoscopic differential diagnosis can be improved with high-resolution video endoscopy and surface staining.

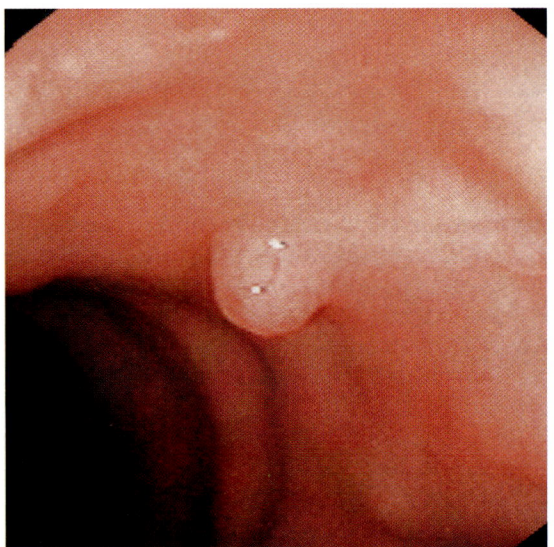

Figure 4-225: **Rectum. Hyperplastic Polyp.** Diminutive polyp with nonspecific features. It is not possible to distinguish a hyperplastic polyp from an adenoma.

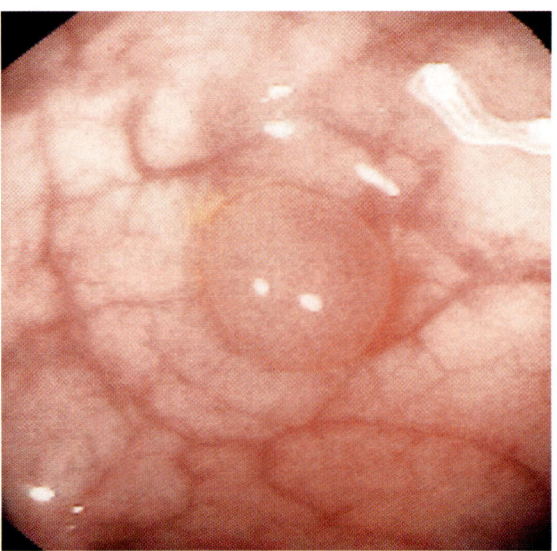

Figure 4-226: **Colon, Rectosigmoid. Hyperplastic Polyp.** Discrete, diminutive polyp without distinctive features.

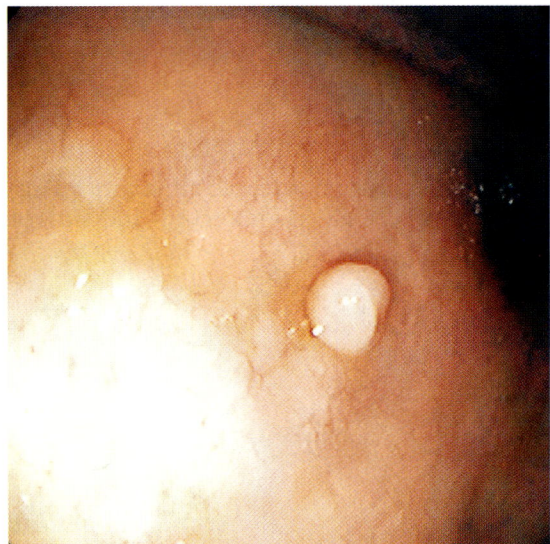

Figure 4-227: **Colon. Hyperplastic Polyp.** Diminutive polyp under normal endoscopic resolution. High-resolution video endoscopy along with mucosal contrast staining helps distinguish this from an adenoma (see Fig. 4-229).

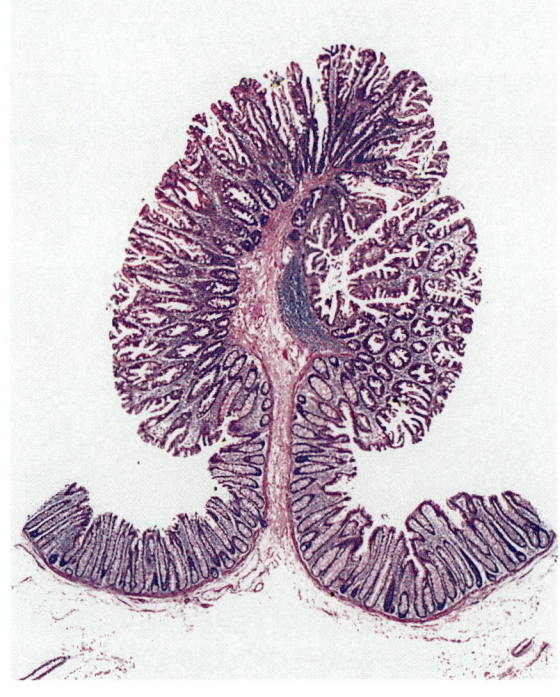

Figure 4-228: **Colon. Hyperplastic Polyp.** Crypts are elongated and superficially serrated.

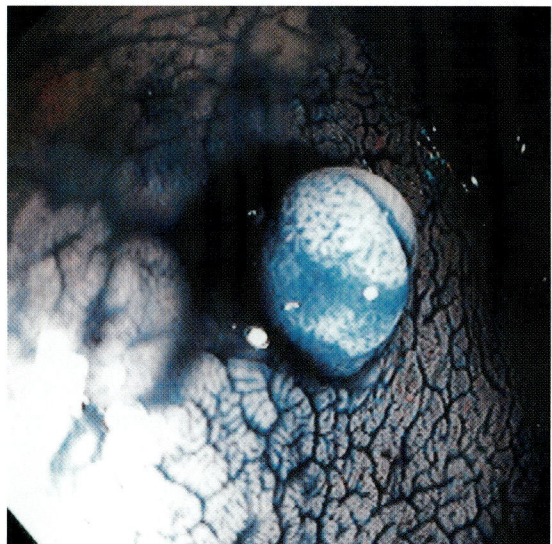

Fgure 4-229: **Colon. Hyperplastic Polyp.** Indigo carmine contrast staining viewed with a high-resolution instrument. Stained diminutive polyp has uniform pitted appearance. The pit pattern is similar to the pit pattern of the surrounding contrast-stained mucosal surface.

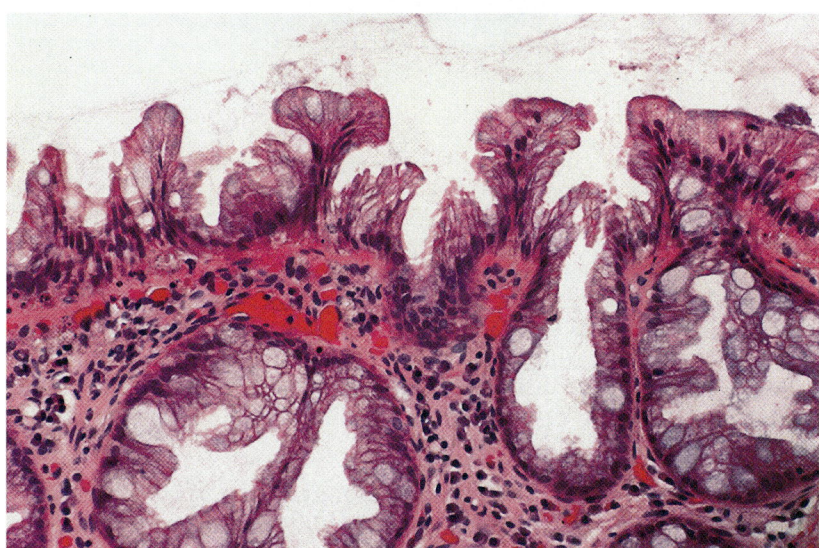

Figure 4-230: **Colon. Hyperplastic Polyp.** Surface epithelium is tufted and free of basophilia. Nuclei are small, regular, and evenly spaced.

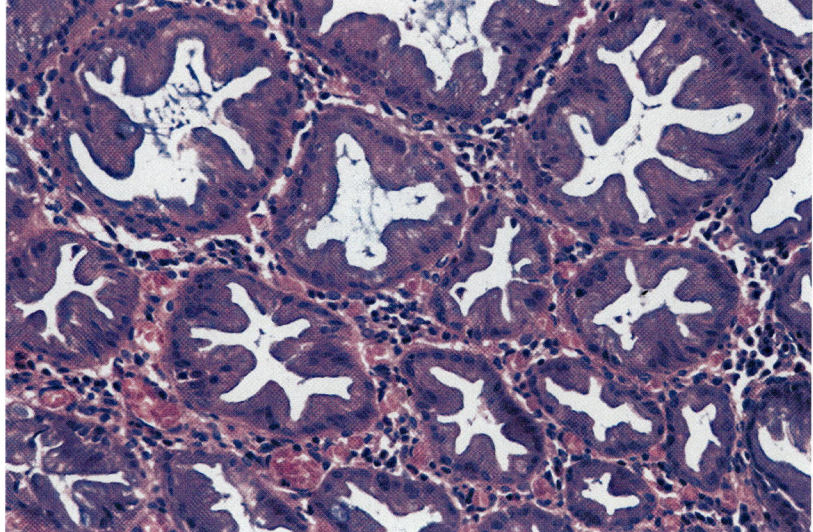

Figure 4-231: **Colon. Hyperplastic Polyp.** Star-shaped crypts on cross section due to piling-up of mature epithelium. No evidence of dysplasia.

COMBINED ADENOMA/HYPERPLASTIC POLYP

- Morphology .... Histologically, there are mingled but distinct areas of adenoma and hyperplastic polyp, often with an abrupt interface.

- Endoscopic features .... The combined adenoma/hyperplastic polyp is without distinctive endoscopic features, unless the surface is viewed with high-resolution chromoscopy. With contrast stains and high-resolution colonoscope (high-resolution chromoscopy), the hyperplastic portion has a characteristic pitted appearance and the adenomatous portion has deeper grooves or a sulciform pattern, as seen in figure 4-233.

- Clinical features .... Combined adenoma/hyperplastic polyps are relatively infrequent. They should be treated as adenomas.

- Differential diagnosis ...... Histologic and endoscopic: Hyperplastic polyp.

SERRATED ADENOMA

- Morphology .... Hyperplastic polyp architecture, but with dysplasia. Dysplasia may range from subtle to high-grade. A serrated adenoma has the biologic potential of an adenoma and should be distinguished from an innocuous hyperplastic polyp. Attention to nuclear detail, number, and location of mitotic figures is necessary for diagnosis.

- Endoscopic features .... Serrated adenoma has no special features. Surface erosion, as in any polyp of significant size ($\geq$ 2cm), should raise the possibility of severe dysplasia or carcinoma.

- Clinical features .... Serrated adenomas are relatively infrequent. They should be treated as adenomas.

- Differential diagnosis ...... Histologic and endoscopic: Hyperplastic polyp.

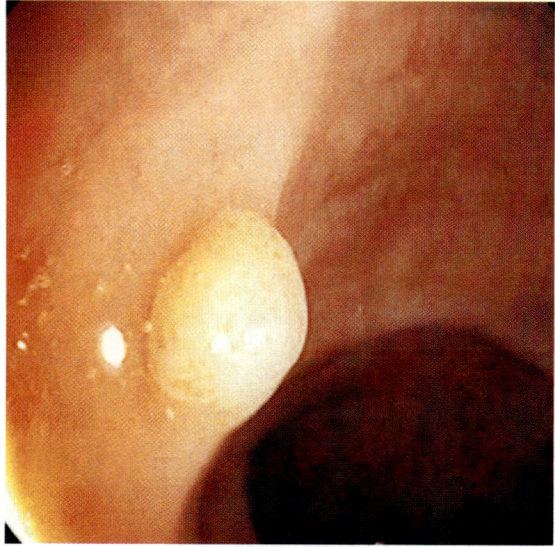

Figure 4-232: **Colon. Combined Adenoma/Hyperplastic Polyp.** A diminutive sessile polyp viewed with a high-resolution colonoscope. The surface pattern of the polyp can be seen, but is not distinctive in the absence of dye staining (chromoscopy).

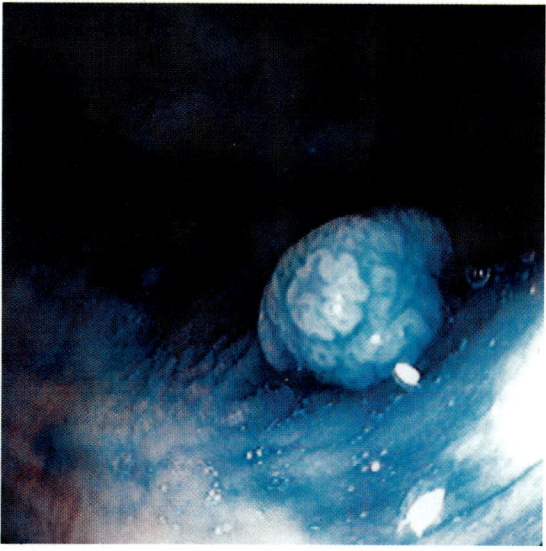

Figure 4-233: **Colon. Combined Adenoma/Hyperplastic Polyp.** The same polyp following contrast staining (indigo carmine) and viewed with a high-resolution colonoscope. The bulk of the polyp has the distinctive pitted appearance of a hyperplastic polyp, with the exception of the central portion, where the pattern is serrated or sulciform, distinctive for adenomatous tissue.

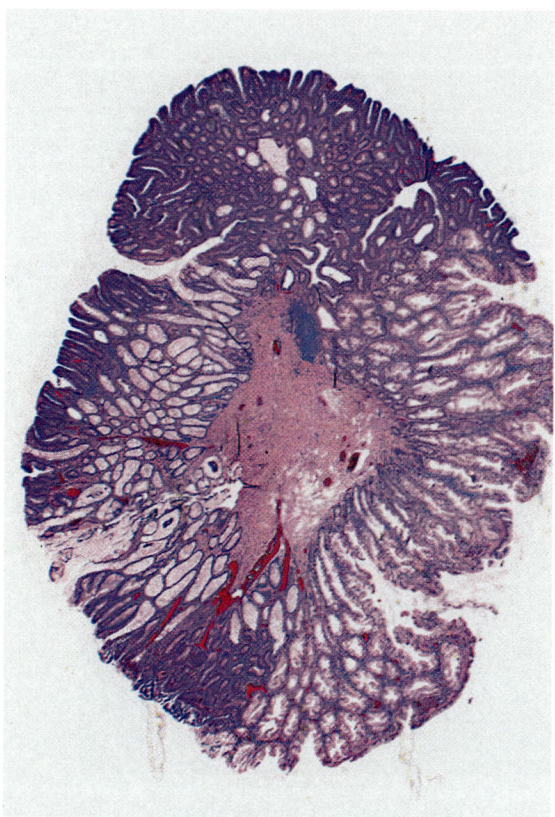

Figure 4-234: **Rectum. Combined Adenoma/Hyperplastic Polyp.** Basophilic adenomatous change contrasts with lighter hyperplastic areas.

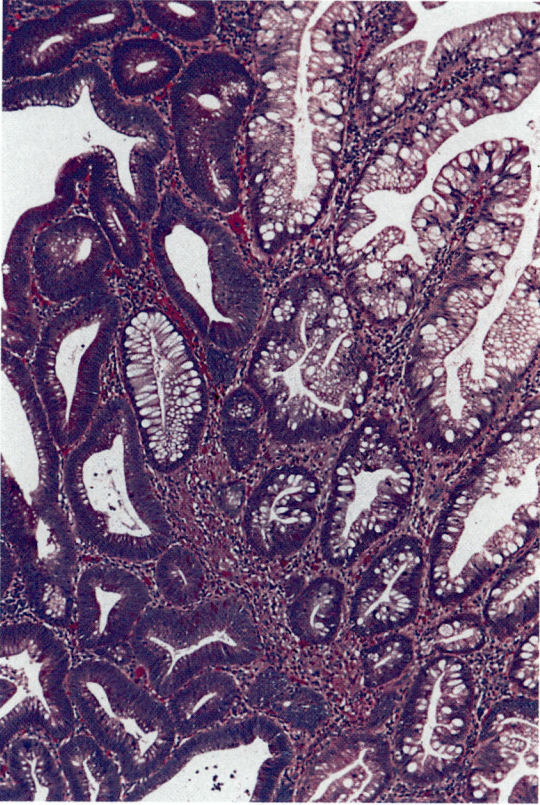

Figure 4-235: **Rectum. Combined Adenoma/Hyperplastic Polyp.** Border between adenomatous (blue) and hyperplastic (pale) components.

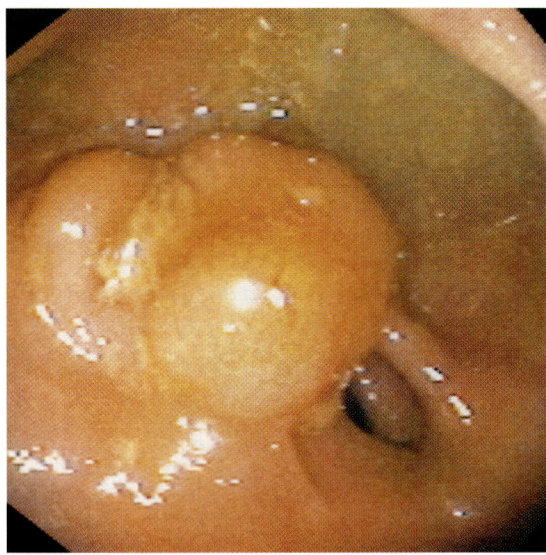

Figure 4-236: **Colon, Transverse. Serrated Adenoma.** Large sessile polyp with erosion.

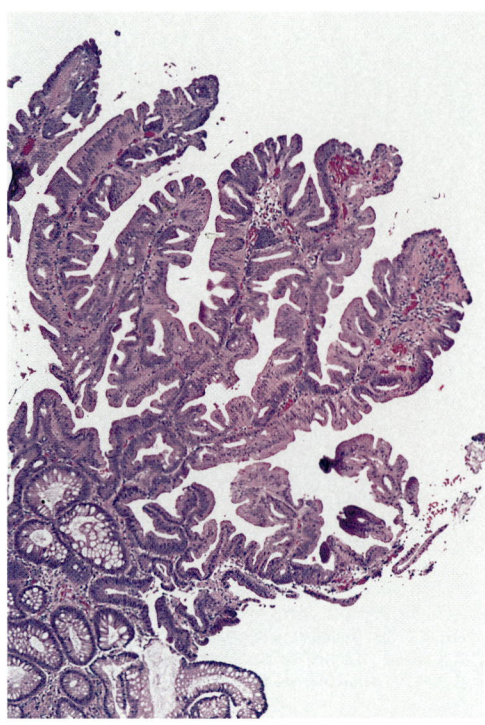

Figure 4-237: **Colon, Sigmoid. Serrated Adenoma.** Villous adenoma with serrated crypts.

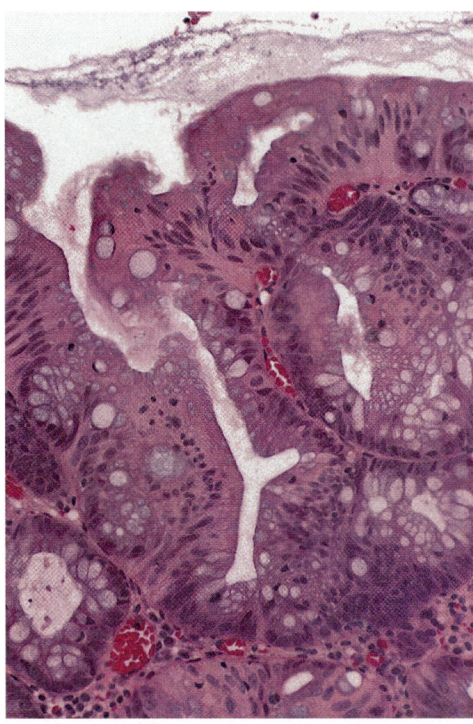

Figure 4-238: **Colon. Serrated Adenoma.** Mild dysplasia and superficial mitotic figures in serrated epithelium. Resembles hyperplastic polyp.

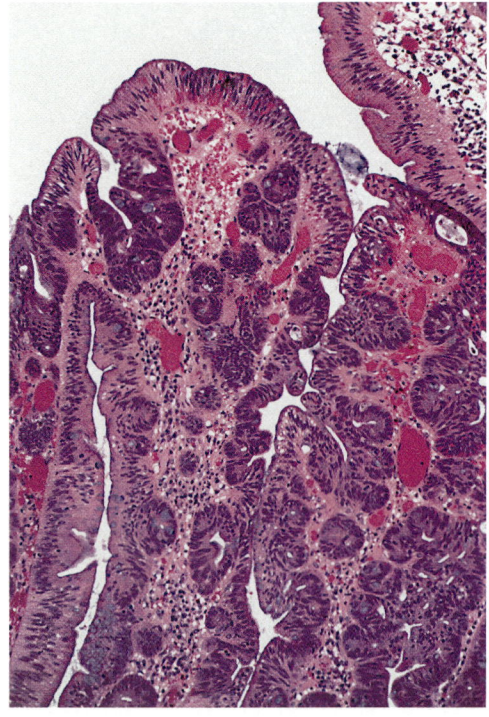

Figure 4-239: **Colon. Serrated Adenoma.** High-grade dysplasia in serrated epithelium.

JUVENILE POLYP

- Morphology .... These polyps may be single or multiple, inherited or sporadic. Single polyps are sporadic. Surface erosion leads to bleeding. Because of their lack of muscle, they can autoamputate when twisted. Dysplasia and carcinoma rarely occur in sporadic juvenile polyps, but are relatively common in juvenile polyposis.
- Endoscopic features .... The polyp is typically large, pedunculated, and friable.
- Clinical features .... These polyps are usually found in children and young adults. The polyps may give rise to GI blood loss in the form of periodic rectal outlet bleeding and, when they are multiple, iron deficiency anemia.
- Differential diagnosis ...... Histologic: Regenerative atypia may simulate dysplasia.

    Endoscopic: Inflammatory polyps, hyperplastic polyps, Peutz-Jeghers polyps, and adenomas.

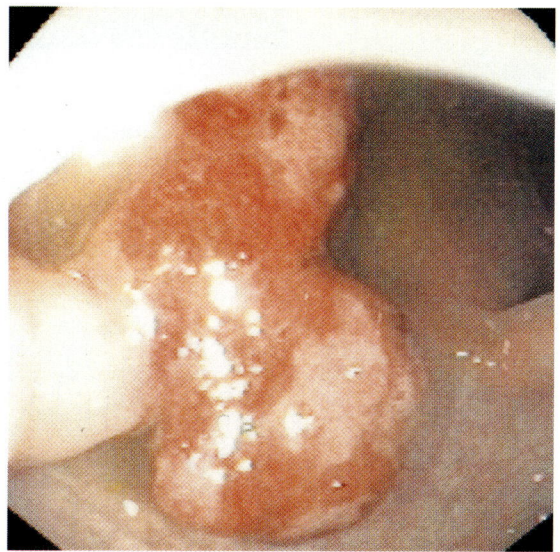

Figure 4-240: **Colon, Sigmoid. Juvenile Polyp.** Large, bilobed, pedunculated polyp with hemorrhagic surface.

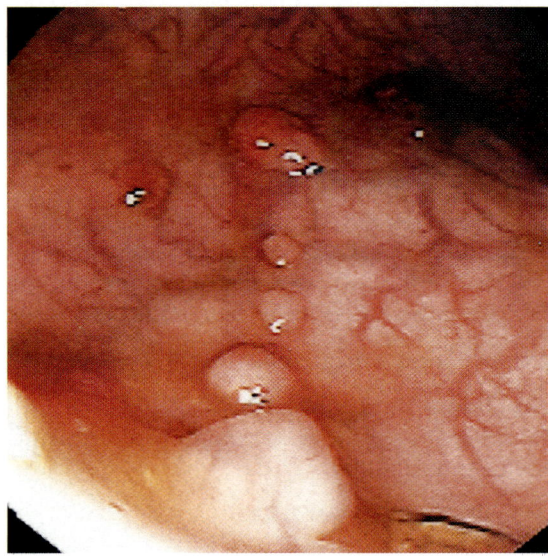

Figure 4-241: **Rectum. Juvenile Polyps.** Multiple sessile polyps of varying size, ranging from diminutive up to 1 cm. The largest polyp in the upper portion of the photograph has a hemorrhagic surface.

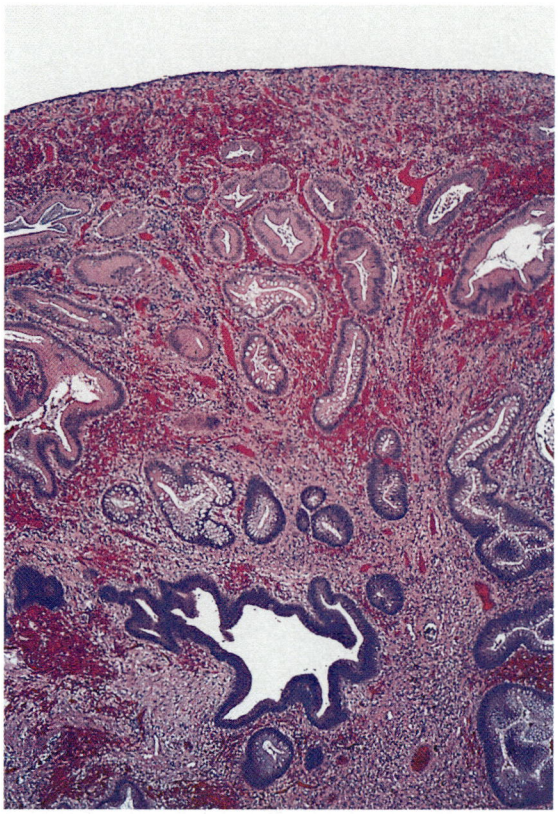

Figure 4-242: **Colon. Juvenile Polyp.** Expanded, inflamed lamina propria with cystic glandular dilatation, epithelial hyperplasia, regenerative epithelial atypia, surface erosion, and granulation tissue. The dilated basophilic gland is atypical, but its location in the basal proliferative zone and its association with an overlying erosion make regenerative atypia more likely than dysplasia.

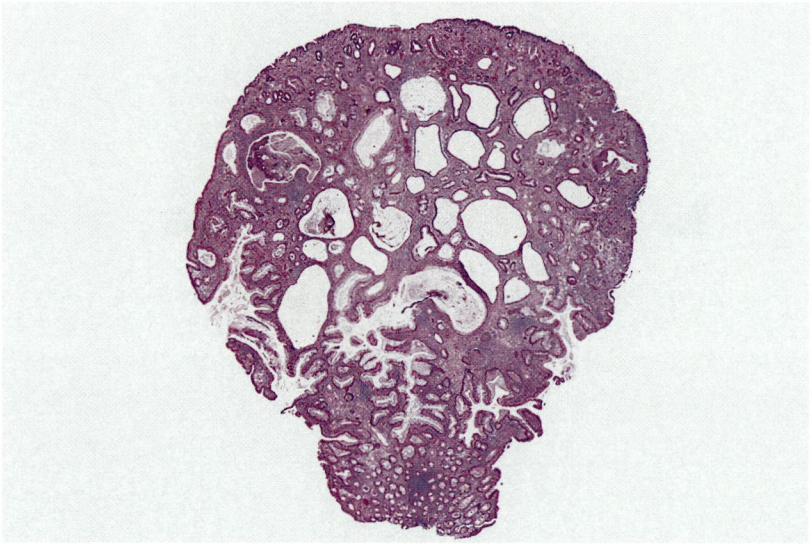

Figure 4-243: **Colon. Juvenile Polyp.** Round polyp with expanded lamina propria, cystic glandular dilatation, and erosion of the surface epithelium.

PEUTZ-JEGHERS POLYP

- **Morphology** — The polyps are usually lobulated with extensions of muscularis mucosae arborizing in the polyp head. Surface erosions may result when they are the lead point of an intussusception. Mucin pools in the submucosa are due to pseudoinvasive herniation.

- **Endoscopic features** — The Peutz-Jeghers polyp tends to be large and multilobulated, with hemorrhagic surface features. The polyps are typically on long stalks. When multiple, their stalks may be intertwined.

- **Clinical features** — About half are inherited and half occur sporadically. Syndromic Peutz-Jeghers polyps are generally discovered at an early age. Sporadic polyps occur at any age. Peutz-Jeghers polyps, when present in the colon, give rise to GI blood loss anemia. In the small intestine, in addition to chronic anemia, they may cause intermittent small bowel obstruction due to intussusception. Peutz-Jeghers syndrome is a precancerous condition, but the polyps are not a frequent site of cancer.

- **Differential diagnosis** — Endoscopic: Inflammatory polyps, juvenile polyps that have prolapsed.

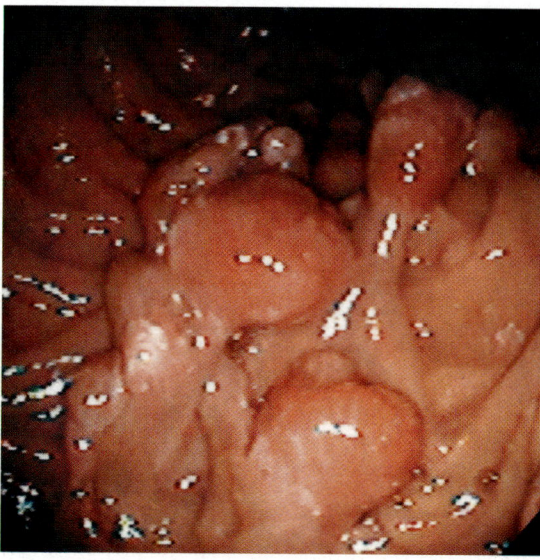

Figure 4-244: **Colon. Peutz-Jeghers Polyp.** A large cluster of multilobed, intertwined polyps.

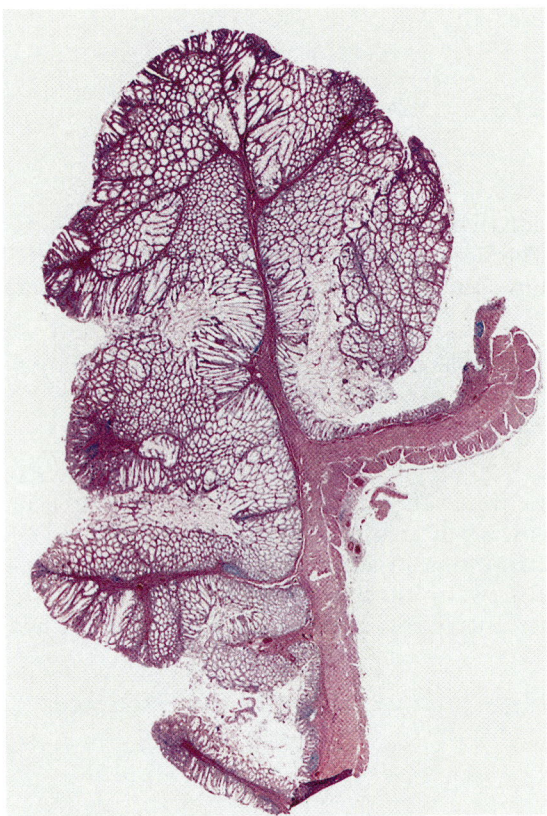

Figure 4-245: **Colon. Peutz-Jeghers Polyp.** Lobular polyp with arborizing muscularis mucosae.

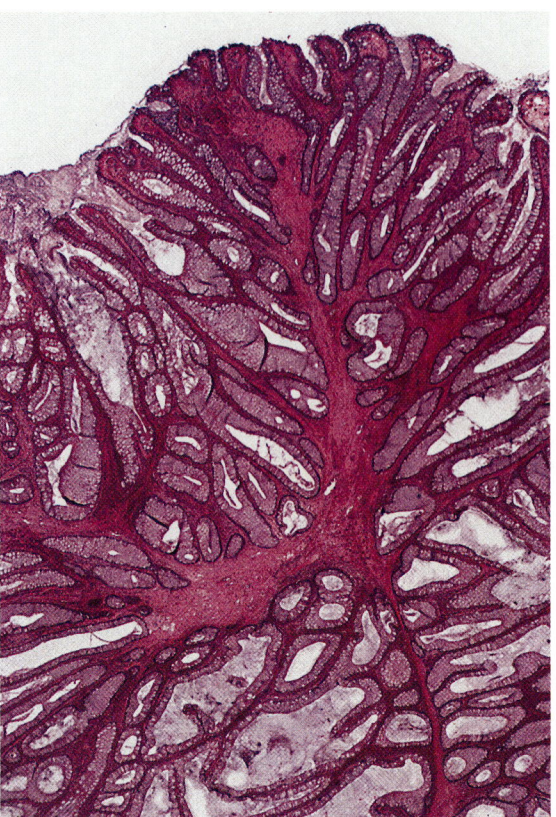

Figure 4-246: **Colon. Peutz-Jeghers Polyp.** Elongated but mature glands, without expansion of the lamina propria, overlie bands of muscularis mucosae.

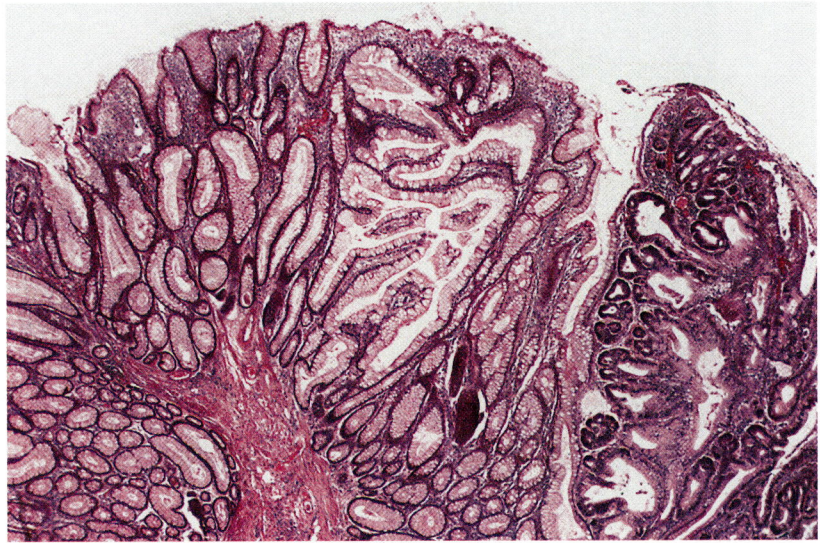

Figure 4-247: **Colon. Peutz-Jeghers Polyp with Dysplasia.** Dysplastic basophilic epithelium in one lobule.

COWDEN SYNDROME

- Morphology .... Polyps in Cowden syndrome are hamartomatous and heterogeneous. They may include fibrous and inflammatory tissue, can resemble juvenile polyps, and may have ganglioneuromatous components.
- Endoscopic features .... The colorectal polyps of Cowden syndrome are multiple and of varying size. They may be sessile or pedunculated with broad pedicles. The surface features can have a villiform pattern and a soft mucoid texture on probing and biopsy.
- Clinical features .... Cowden syndrome is an autosomal-dominant clinical syndrome in which there is a propensity for breast and thyroid cancer. The polyps do not become malignant.
- Differential diagnosis ...... Histologic: Inflammatory polyps, juvenile polyps, ganglioneuromas.

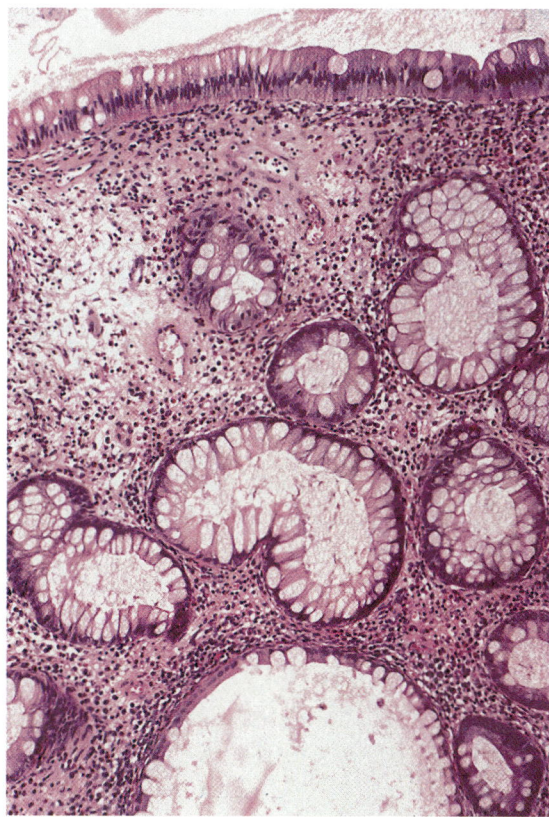

Figure 4-248: **Colon. Inflammatory-Type Polyp Associated with Cowden Syndrome.** Inflammatory cells expand lamina propria. Crypts dilated. Resembles inflammatory and juvenile polyps.

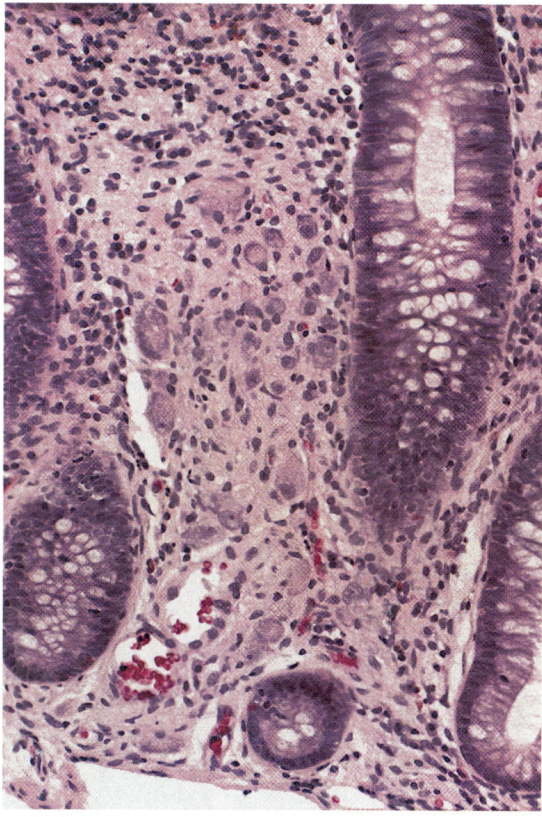

Figure 4-249: **Colon. Ganglioneuroma Associated with Cowden Syndrome.** Ganglion cells in expanded lamina propria.

GANGLIONEUROMA

- Morphology .... Ganglioneuromas consist of compact, interlacing bundles of Schwann and ganglion cells that infiltrate between crypts. Ganglion cells may be intermixed singly or in clusters. S-100 protein reacts strongly with the stroma.

- Endoscopic features .... These polyps, when solitary, are indistinguishable from adenomatous polyps. When multiple, they are diffusely distributed through the colon and vary in size, shape, and appearance.

- Clinical features .... Ganglioneuromas may be sporadic or syndromic. They occur more frequently in the large intestine than do neurofibromas and schwannomas. Solitary polypoid ganglioneuromas are not associated with a syndrome and occur at any age, but are most commonly found in patients less than 20 years old. Multiple ganglioneuromas and diffuse ganglioneuromatosis are associated with MEN 2b, tuberous sclerosis, Cowden syndrome, familial adenomatous polyposis, juvenile polyposis, and Hirschsprung and von Recklinghausen diseases.

- Differential diagnosis ...... Endoscopic: When isolated, adenomas; when multiple, tuberous sclerosis, Cowden syndrome, familial adenomatous polyposis, juvenile polyposis, and von Recklinghausen disease.

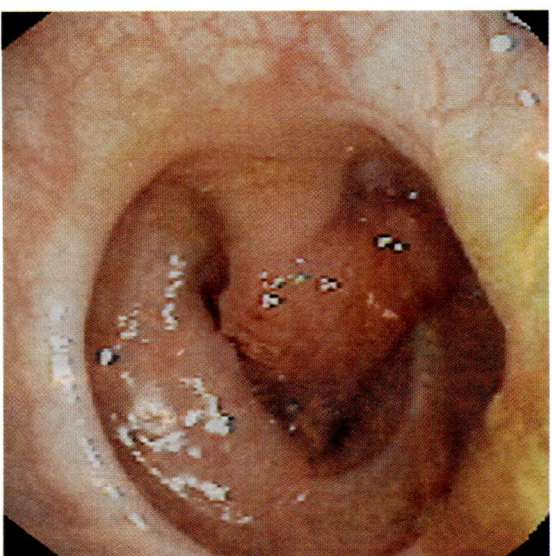

Figure 4-250: **Colon, Sigmoid. Ganglioneuroma.** Large, pedunculated polyp without distinctive features.

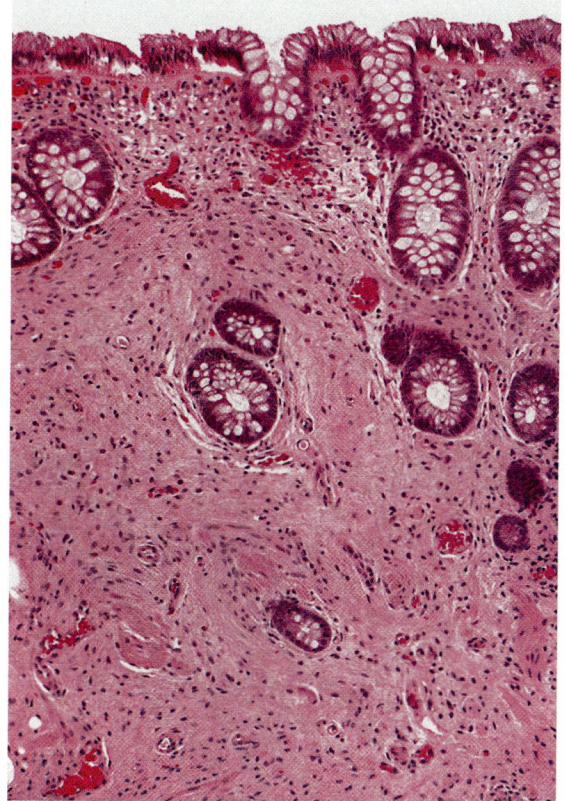

Figure 4-251: **Colon. Ganglioneuroma.** Lamina propria expanded by eosinophilic spindle cells and stroma that separate crypts.

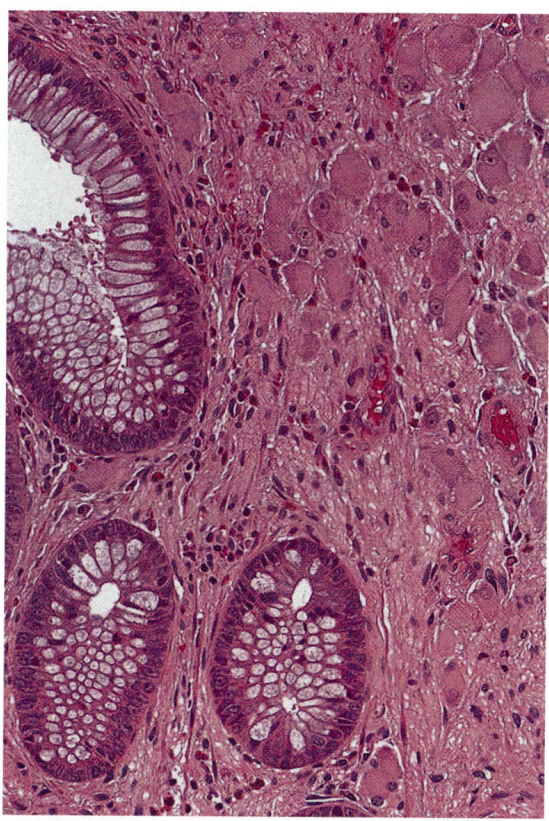

Figure 4-252: **Colon. Ganglioneuroma.** Cluster of ganglion cells and spindle cells in lamina propria.

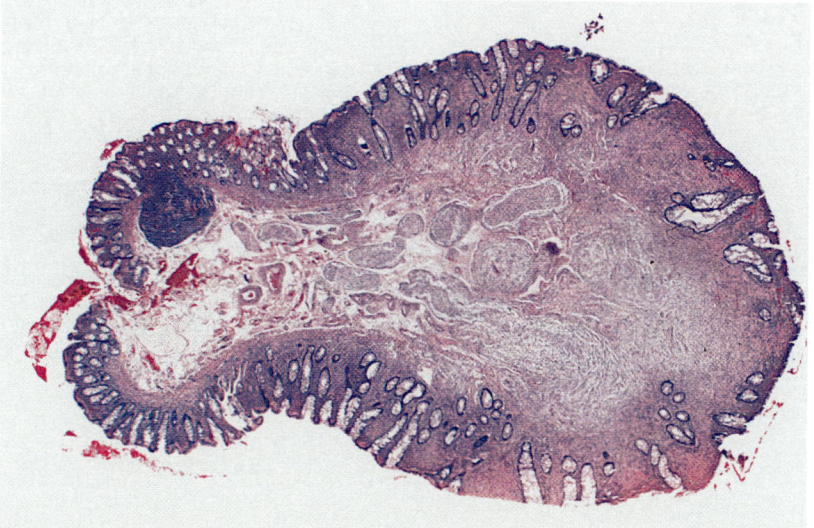

Figure 4-253: **Colon. Ganglioneuroma.** Pedunculated lesion with eosinophilic stroma in mucosa and submucosa, separating glands and replacing lamina propria.

CRONKHITE-CANADA POLYPS

- Morphology .... The entire gastrointestinal tract can be involved in Cronkhite-Canada syndrome. While biopsy samples of the colon can be indistinguishable from juvenile polyposis or inflammatory polyposis, the clinical features are very different.
- Endoscopic features .... Nodular mucosal appearance due to carpeting with innumerable diminutive polyps.
- Clinical features .... Severe protein-losing enteropathy with diarrhea, weight loss, alopecia, and nail changes. Gastrointestinal symptoms may precede dermatological lesions.
- Differential diagnosis ...... Histologic: Inflammatory polyps and juvenile polyposis. Similar changes are seen in some patients with systemic lupus erythematosus.

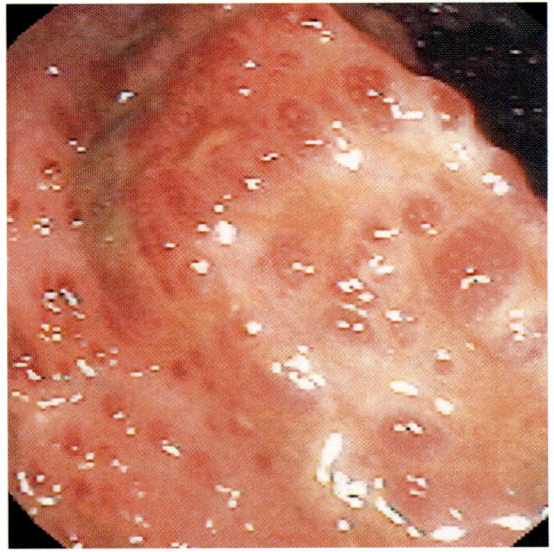

Figure 4-254: **Rectum. Cronkhite-Canada Polyps.** Innumerable atypical, sessile, intensely erythematous polyps.

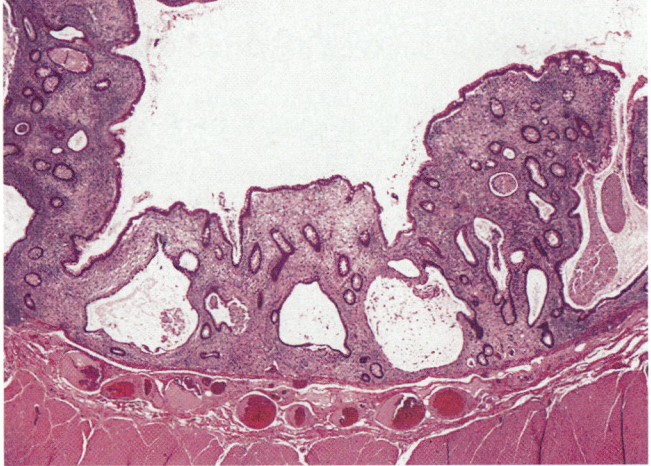

Figure 4-255: **Colon. Cronkhite-Canada Polyps.** Expanded edematous and chronically inflamed lamina propria forming poorly defined sessile nodules. Dilated crypts filled with mucin. Biopsies would resemble juvenile polyps.

GRANULAR CELL TUMOR

- Morphology .... Usually involves the submucosa and lamina propria. Composed of round and spindle cells with small central nuclei and abundant granular cytoplasm. May resemble signet-ring cell carcinoma because of the abundant eosinophilic cytoplasm. The nesting pattern can be mistaken for carcinoid tumor and, when spindled, schwannoma. Positive for S-100 protein on immunostaining.
- Endoscopic features .... Rarely encountered submucosal nodule of variable size, typically in the rectum.
- Clinical features .... No distinctive clinical presentation.
- Differential diagnosis ...... Histologic: Leiomyoma of the muscularis mucosae, signet-ring cell carcinoma, carcinoid tumor, schwannoma.

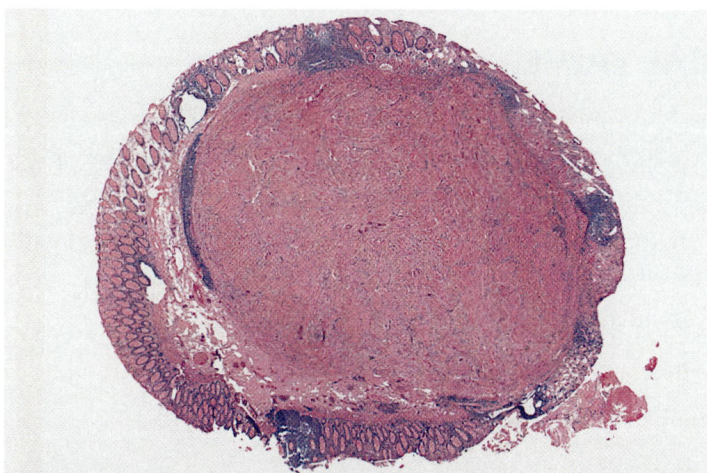

Figure 4-256: **Rectum. Granular Cell Tumor.** Round submucosal nodule composed of nests and fascicles of cells with abundant eosinophilic cytoplasm.

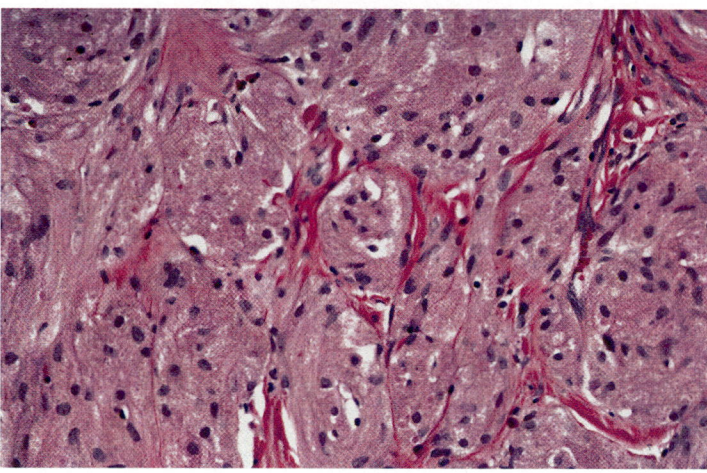

Figure 4-257: **Rectum. Granular Cell Tumor.** Nests of round and oblong cells with small nuclei and abundant granular eosinophilic cytoplasm.

LIPOMA

- Morphology .... Lipomas are easily overlooked on biopsy. Rarely, multiple or massive and associated with other lipomatous masses in the abdomen (lipomatous polyposis). On biopsy, an ulcerated lipoma may exhibit atypical cells and be mistaken for a smooth muscle/stromal neoplasm, metastatic malignancy, or vascular lesion (hemangioma, Kaposi sarcoma). Even when atypical, gastrointestinal lipomas have no malignant potential, in contrast to retroperitoneal lipomatous tumors.

- Endoscopic features .... Lipomas are more commonly encountered in the colon and rectum than in the stomach or esophagus. They are submucosal, vary in size from 1 to 3 cm, and usually have a characteristic yellow hue and exhibit the "pillow" sign when probed (Fig. 4-259).

- Clinical features .... None. Lesions are incidentally encountered.

- Differential diagnosis ...... Histologic: Lipohyperplasia of the ileocecal valve. When ulcerated, stromal/smooth muscle neoplasm, vascular tumors.

LIPOHYPERPLASIA OF ILEOCECAL VALVE

- Morphology .... Lipohyperplasia of the ileocecal valve is characterized by expansion of the submucosa that surrounds the valvular "spine" of the muscularis propria.

- Endoscopic features .... Prominent smooth, rounded enlargement of the ileocecal valve covered with intact, normal-appearing mucosa. "Pillow" sign present.

- Clinical features .... None. These are incidentally encountered.

- Differential diagnosis ...... Histologic: Lipoma.

    Endoscopic: Any submucosal neoplasm.

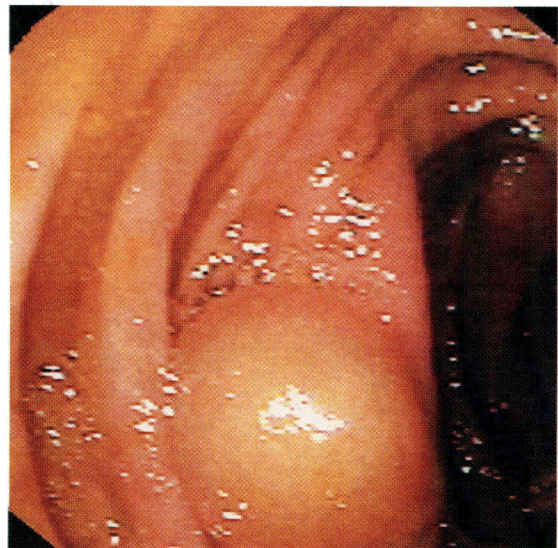

Figure 4-258: **Colon, Ascending. Lipoma.** A smooth, well-rounded submucosal nodule (see Fig. 4-259).

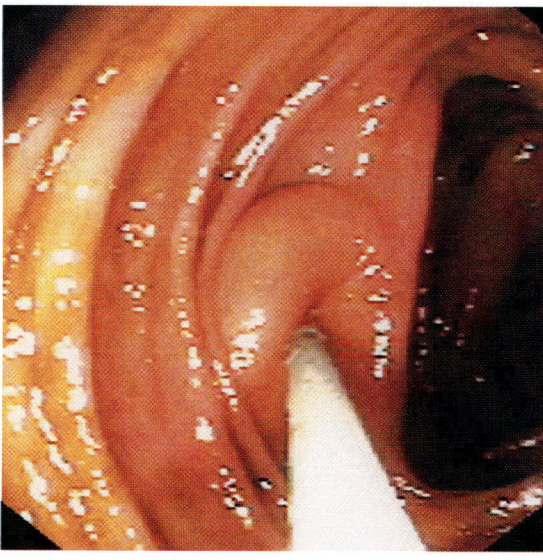

Figure 4-259: **Colon, Ascending. Lipoma.** "Pillow" sign. Probing of submucosal nodule results in collapse with indentation, characteristic of a lipoma.

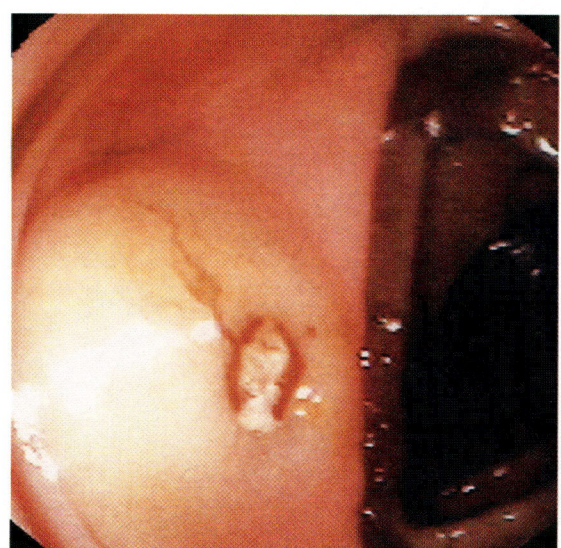

Figure 4-260: **Colon, Ascending. Lipoma.** The overlying mucosa of this submucosal nodule has been removed with standard pinch avulsion biopsy forceps, resulting in the diagnostic extrusion of fat.

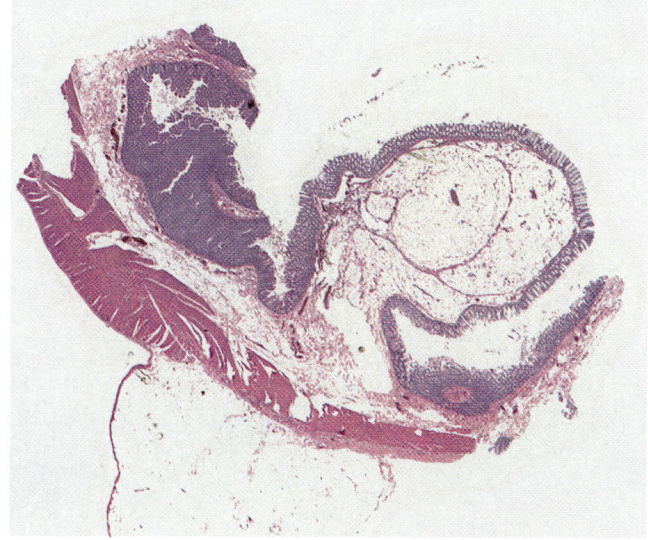

Figure 4-261: **Rectum. Lipoma.** Polypoid protrusion of mature submucosal fat.

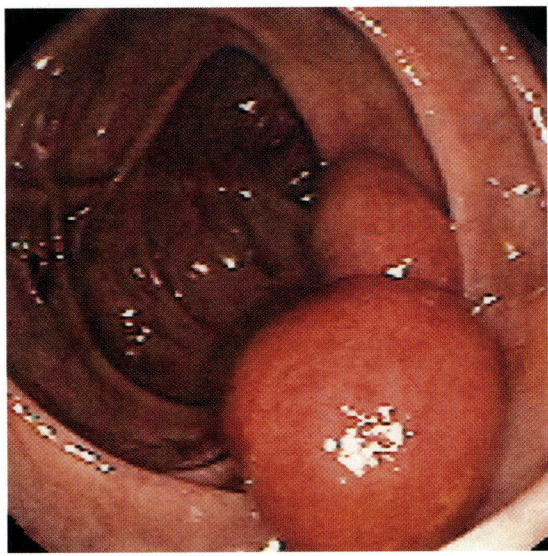

Figure 4-262: **Ileocecal Valve. Lipohyperplasia.** Focal nature resembles lipoma.

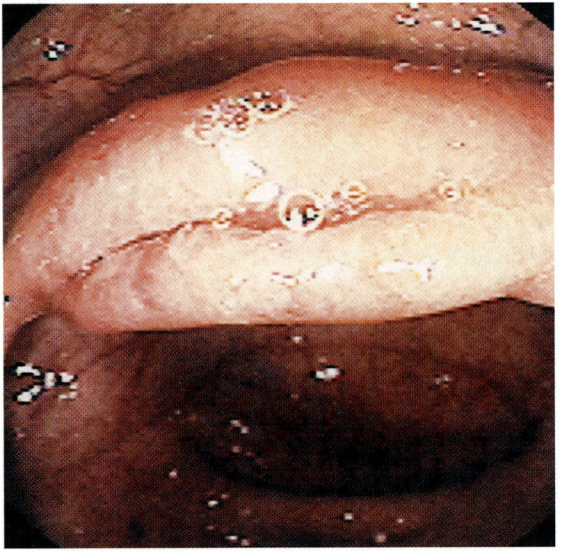

Figure 4-263: **Ileocecal Valve. Lipohyperplasia.** Irregular thickening at the ileocecal valve, typical of lipohyperplasia.

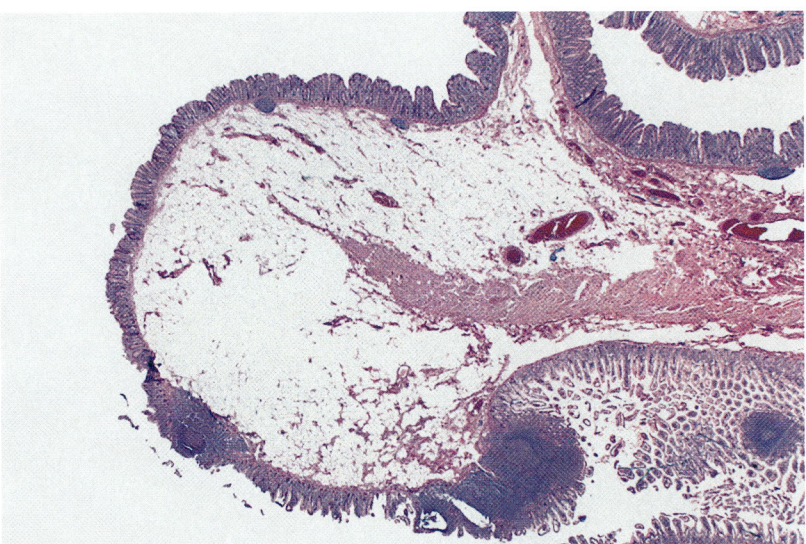

Figure 4-264: **Ileocecal Valve. Lipohyperplasia.** Submucosal fat surrounds the muscular "spine" at the ileocecal valve. Villous ileal mucosa on one side, colonic mucosa on the other.

ADENOMAS

- Morphology .... Dysplasia in an adenoma begins abruptly on or near the surface and grows along crypts toward the base. New crypts bud from the surface and become elongated and irregular, branched, or cystic. In *tubular adenomas*, dysplastic epithelium spreads downward and the surface remains relatively smooth. Lobulation reflects the underlying innominate groove architecture. *Villous adenomas* grow on delicate stromal fronds. *Tubulovillous adenomas* display combinations of these architectural patterns, with villous and tubular components accounting for more than 20% of the polyp. The greater the villous component, the greater the tendency for malignant change. The spectrum of dysplasia may be classified as low- or high-grade, based on nuclear cytologic changes and degree of nuclear stratification, which is limited to the lower half of the epithelium in low-grade dysplasia and reaches the glandular lumen in high-grade dysplasia. While grading adenomas is not universal, it does serve to standardize terminology and alert the clinician that in particular patients the process may be more aggressive, warranting closer observation. Adenomas show a localized inflammatory reaction in the lamina propria. For this reason, it is inappropriate to make a separate diagnosis of colitis based on inflammation in an adenoma.

- Endoscopic features .... Adenomas vary from minute, flat lesions to large sessile and pedunculated polyps. Larger lesions typically are friable. Minute and diminutive lesions can be more confidently identified with the use of chromoscopy. Villous and tubulovillous adenomas may be very large sessile polyps when discovered, and are commonly found in the cecum, proximal ascending colon, and rectum. They can exceed 5 cm in size and cover the entire rectum. The villous adenoma has a distinctive appearance when flat and sprawling. Unlike the more typical pedunculated tubular adenomas, which may be erythematous and friable, these polyps have a bland surface appearance.

- Clinical features .... Most adenomas are encountered incidentally during colorectal cancer surveillance, or during the evaluation of heme-positive stools.

- Differential diagnosis ...... Endoscopic: Hyperplastic, inflammatory, Peutz-Jeghers, and juvenile polyps. Carcinomatous degeneration is suspected when there is erosion or ulceration associated with large sessile polyps.

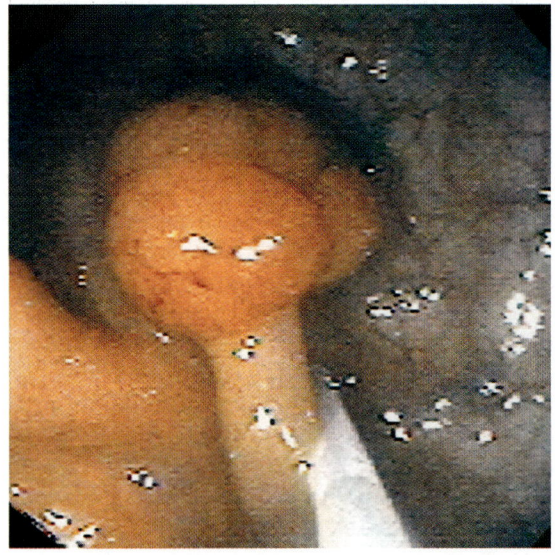

Figure 4-265: **Colon, Sigmoid. Tubular Adenoma.** Typical-appearing multilobed, pedunculated polyp with a long, well-defined stalk.

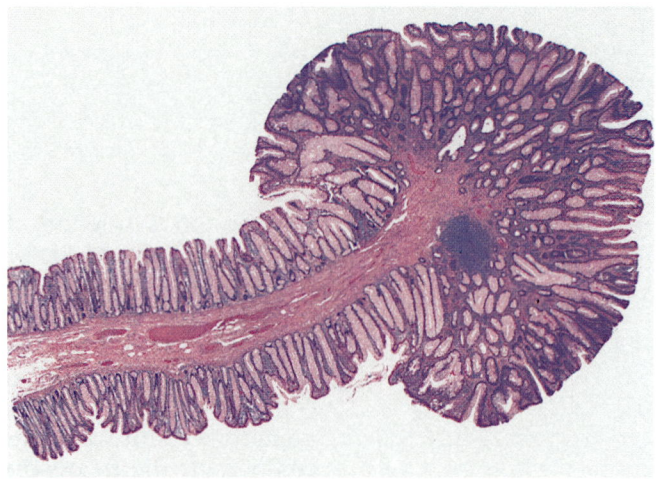

Figure 4-266: **Colon. Tubular Adenoma.** Hyperchromatic, basophilic dysplastic epithelium limited to polyp head. Abrupt transition to normal mucosa of stalk.

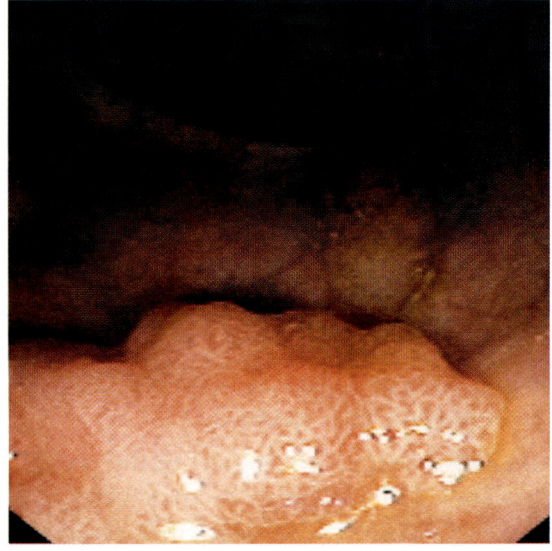

Figure 4-267: **Rectum. Villous Adenoma.** Flat, nodular, sessile polyp with distorted surface features.

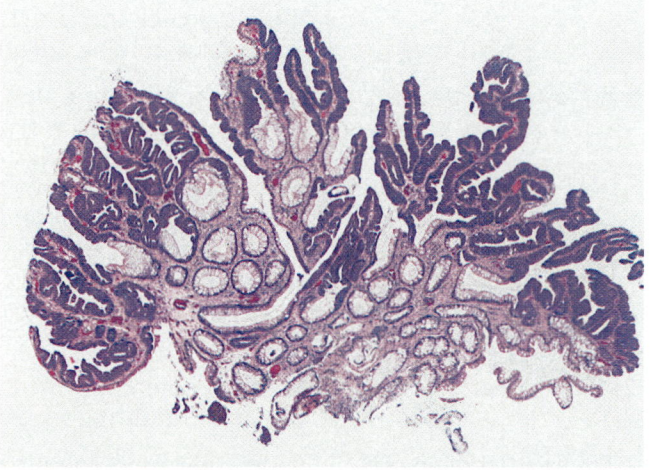

Figure 4-268: **Rectum. Villous Adenoma.** Sessile polyp with dysplasia confined to surface of delicate villous fronds.

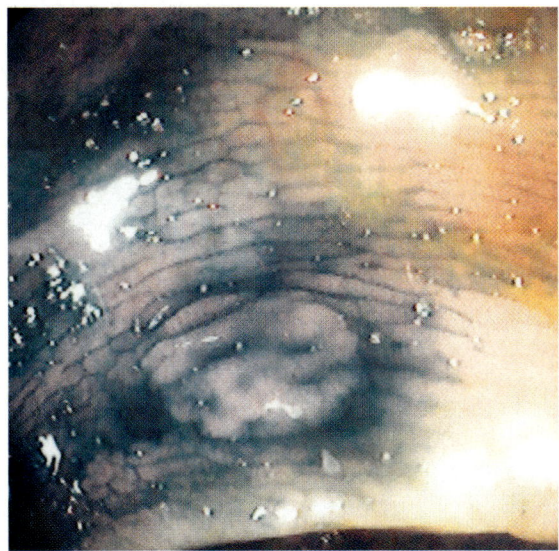

Figure 4-269: **Colon. Tubular Adenoma.** Diminutive sessile polyp, well-outlined by contrast staining (indigo carmine).

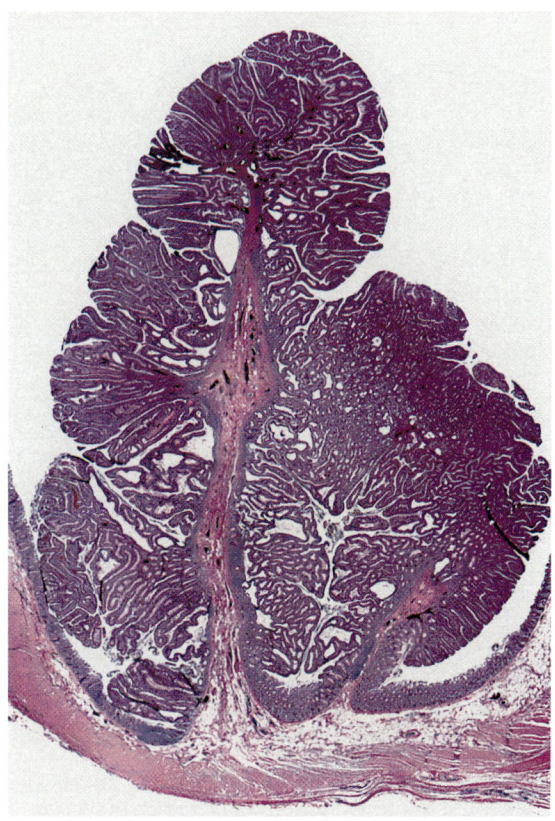

Figure 4-270: **Colon. Tubulovillous Adenoma.** Lobulated with multiple stalks. Combination of villous and tubular components.

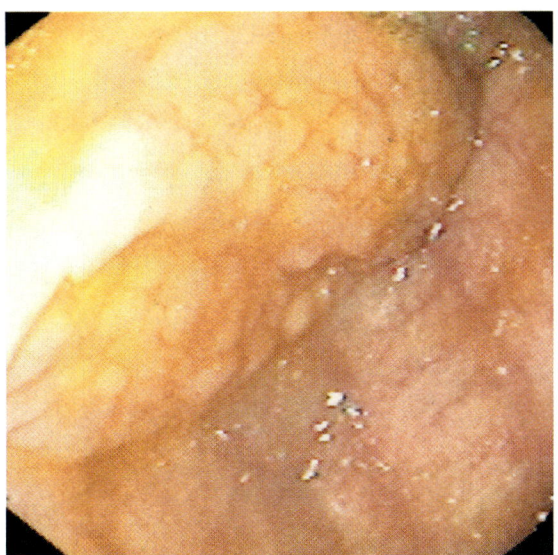

Figure 4-271: **Cecum. Villous Adenoma.** Large, flat, sprawling nodular polyp with bland surface appearance, characteristic of a villous adenoma.

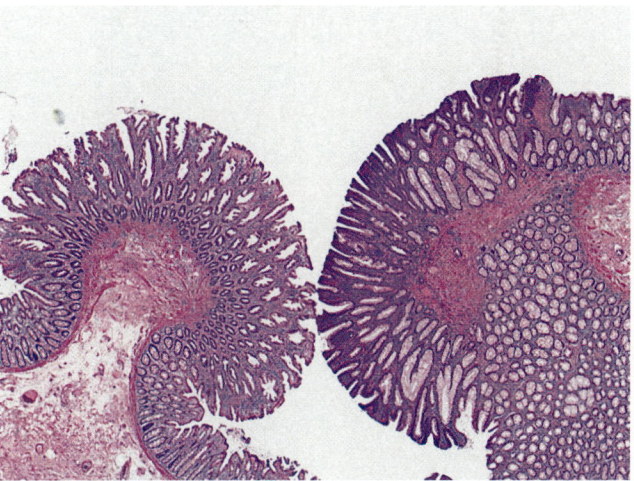

Figure 4-272: **Colon. Tubular Adenoma and Hyperplastic Polyp.** Small tubular adenoma (right) and hyperplastic polyp (left). No distinguishing macroscopic features. Crowded, hyperchromatic, basophilic surface epithelium and distorted, branched crypts of tubular adenoma contrast with tufted, serrated surface epithelium, basophilic crypt bases, and uniform, evenly spaced crypts of hyperplastic polyp.

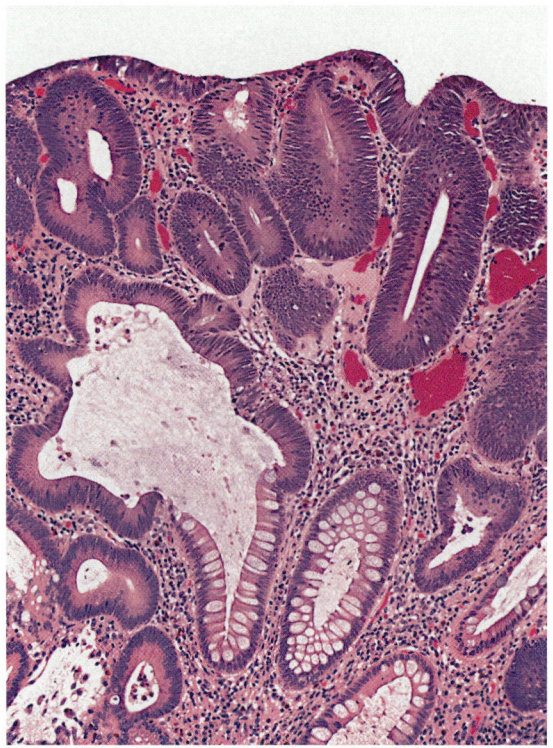

Figure 4-273: **Colon. Tubular Adenoma.** Dysplastic epithelium in upper portion of dilated crypt; abrupt change to normal epithelium in lower crypt. Active chronic inflammation in lamina propria.

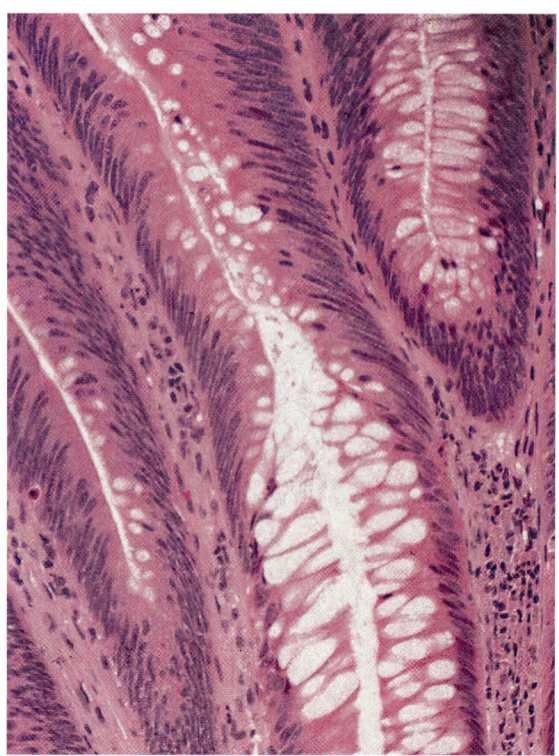

Figure 4-274: **Colon. Tubular Adenoma, Low-Grade Dysplasia.** Sharp interface between normal and dysplastic epithelium. Dysplastic nuclei stratified and polarized to lower half of the epithelial layer.

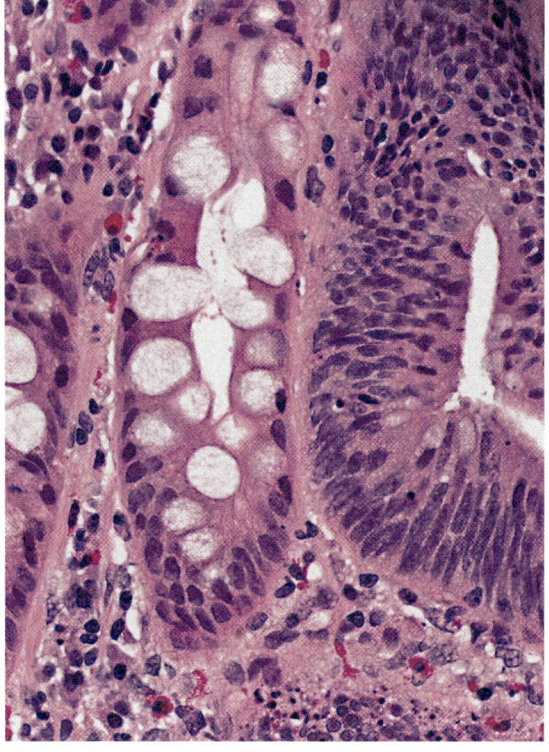

Figure 4-275: **Colon. Tubular Adenoma, High-Grade Dysplasia.** Dysplastic nuclei stratified throughout the epithelial layer to luminal surface contrast with nondysplastic crypt.

ADENOMA WITH PSEUDOINVASION

- Morphology .... Pseudoinvasive herniation most commonly occurs in pedunculated adenomas in the sigmoid. The appearance is a stalked polyp with a submucosal bolus of glands and lamina propria associated with pools of mucin, hemorrhage, and hemosiderin. It may be difficult to distinguish pseudoinvasion from true invasion. Features that favor pseudoinvasion include the presence of a bolus of glands with lamina propria, the absence of desmoplasia, and the presence of hemorrhage and hemosiderin. Points favoring a diagnosis of adenocarcinoma include extensive dysplastic glandular proliferation lining a mucin-filled cavity, the presence of dysplastic epithelium floating in mucin, desmoplasia, haphazardly scattered, isolated glands, and the absence of lamina propria around glands. Invasive adenocarcinoma may arise in an adenoma with pseudoinvasion.

- Endoscopic features .... There are no distinctive endoscopic features. The presence of ulceration should raise suspicion of carcinoma.

- Clinical features .... None is specific.

- Differential diagnosis ...... Histologic: Adenocarcinoma.

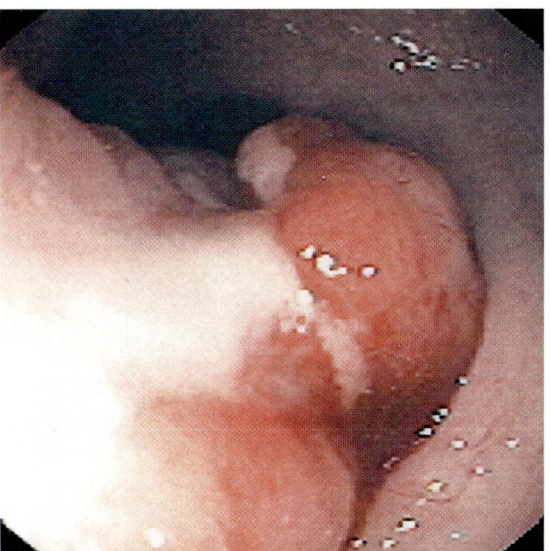

Figure 4-276: **Colon, Sigmoid. Tubular Adenoma with Pseudoinvasion.** Ulcerated polyp on a short, broad stalk. The mucosa at the base of the stalk appears edematous as well as erythematous. There is an area of mucosal hemorrhage contiguous to the small ulcer involving the polyp in the foreground.

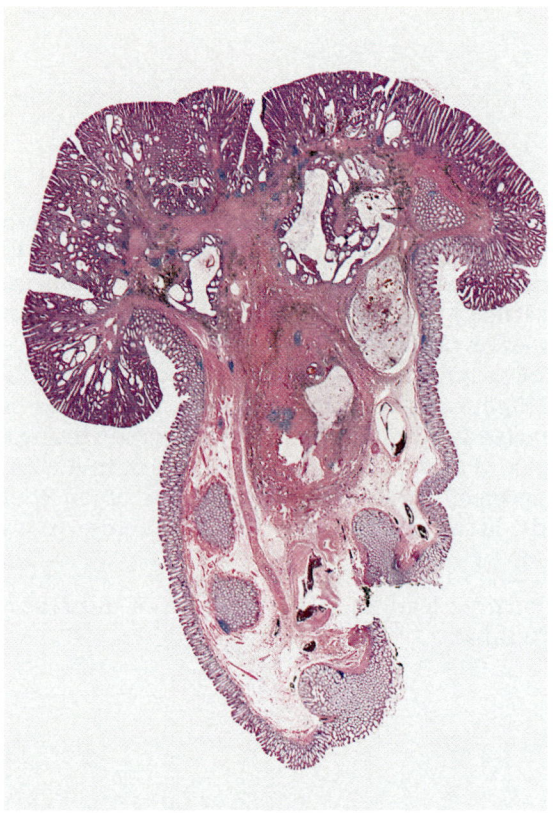

Figure 4-277: **Colon. Tubular Adenoma with Pseudoinvasion.** Several groups of cystic dysplastic glands in submucosa surrounded by hemorrhage and hemosiderin. Stalk is broad.

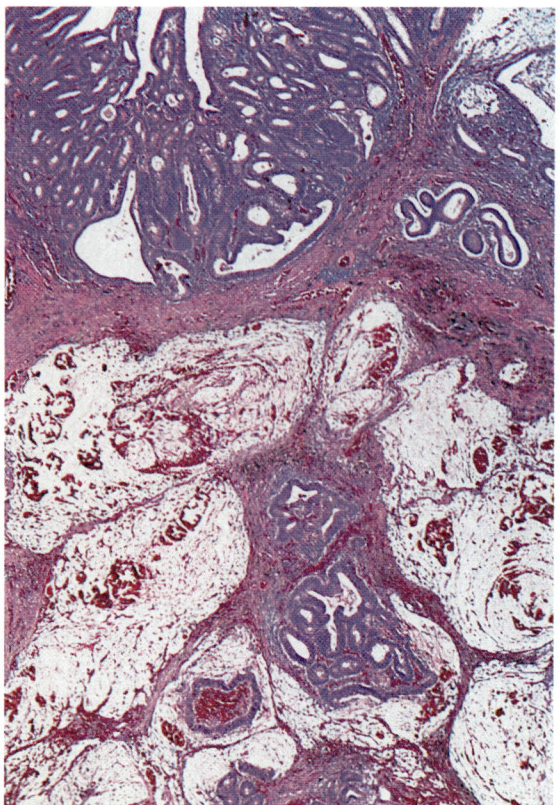

Figure 4-278: **Colon. Tubular Adenoma with Pseudoinvasion.** Submucosal focus of dysplastic glands with lamina propria, surrounded by mucin pools containing fresh hemorrhage.

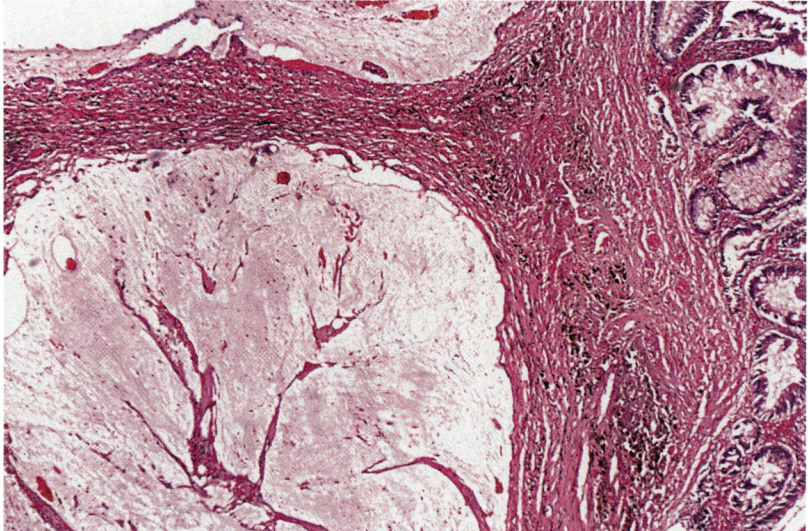

Figure 4-279: **Colon. Tubular Adenoma with Pseudoinvasion.** Acellular mucin pool in submucosa surrounded by fibrous tissue and hemosiderin.

FAMILIAL ADENOMATOUS POLYPOSIS

- Morphology .... These colorectal adenomas do not differ from those seen in nonpolyposis patients; most are tubular with low-grade dysplasia. Endoscopically normal mucosa commonly contains microscopic foci of dysplastic glands. The risk of adenocarcinoma is 100%, unless colectomy is performed. Polyposis with extraintestinal, mainly mesenchymal, manifestations define Gardner syndrome, which shares common chromosomal defects. Most important of these is mesenteric fibromatosis, which is often more infiltrative and aggressive than in nonpolyposis patients.

- Endoscopic features .... FAP syndrome presents with innumerable colorectal polyps. There are more than 100 and often around 1000 colonic adenomas. Usually the colon is carpeted with polyps ranging from millimeters to centimeters in size, typically dispersed throughout the entire colon and rectum. Attenuated forms may be associated with fewer polyps and a more proximal location. In some patients, the rectum can be involved with sheetlike adenomatous transformation. In these cases there is no true polypoid appearance, but rather a subtle change to the mucosa that can easily be missed in the presence of stool, fluid, and debris.

- Clinical features .... Colorectal polyps tend to develop at puberty, and by age 25, 80% of patients have polyps. Surveillance of the gastrointestinal tract for additional adenomas is necessary following colectomy as there may be adenomas in the small bowel, particularly in the duodenum near the ampulla and in the stomach. In the stomach, numerous fundic gland polyps occur. First-degree relatives should be screened endoscopically or with genetic testing.

- Differential diagnosis ...... Endoscopic: Sporadic adenomas and other polyposis syndromes.

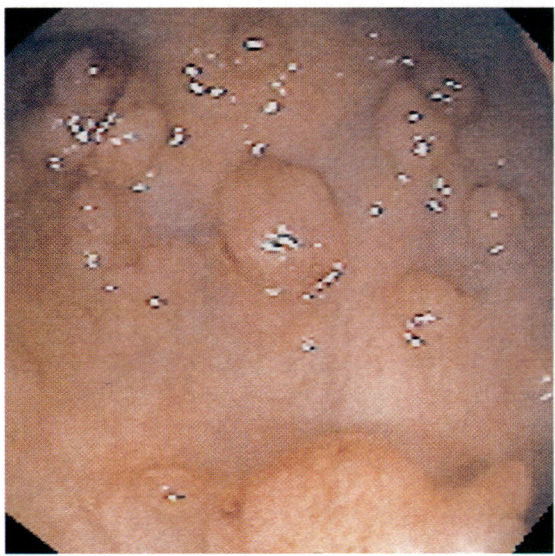

Figure 4-280: **Rectum. Familial Adenomatous Polyposis.** Multiple polyps varying in size, all of which are < 1 cm in diameter.

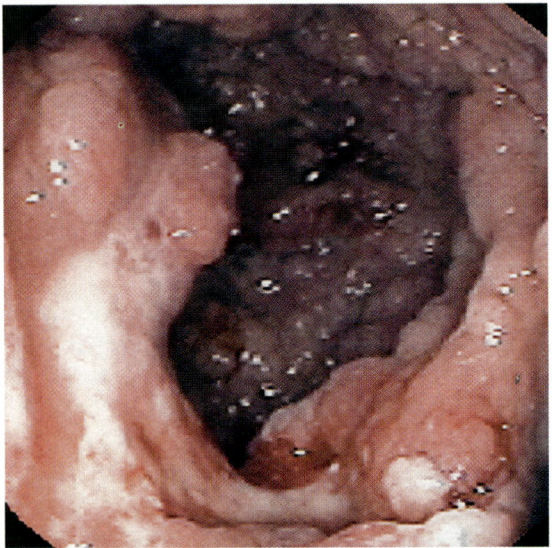

Figure 4-281: **Rectum. Familial Adenomatous Polyposis.** Multiple polyps of varying size and a large, irregularly shaped, ulcerated polyp in the foreground, suspicious for malignancy.

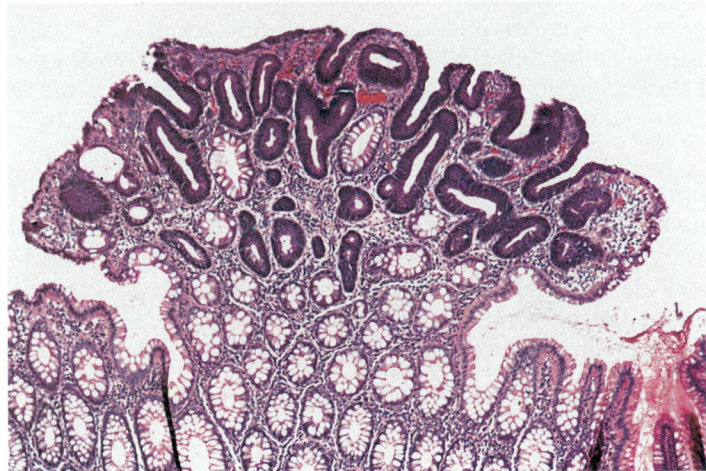

Figure 4-282: **Colon. Familial Adenomatous Polyposis.** Small tubular adenoma. Dysplasia in upper part of lesion.

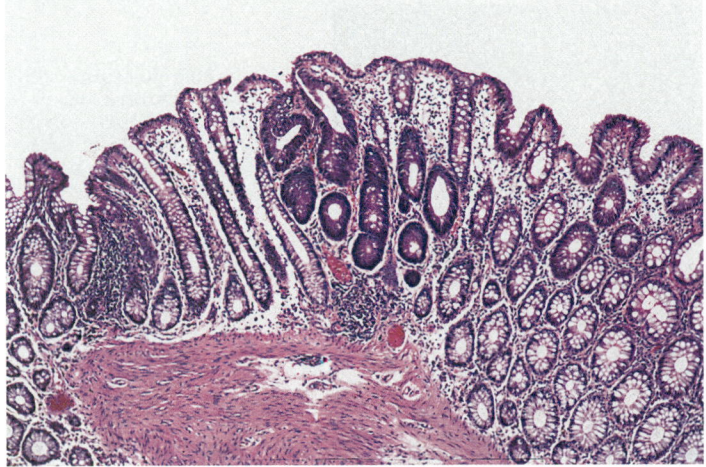

Figure 4-283: **Colon. Familial Adenomatous Polyposis.** Microscopic tubular adenoma (center), not likely to be visible on endoscopic examination. Several dysplastic crypts at right.

FLAT ADENOMA

- Morphology .... Flat adenomas (no more than 50% thicker than the surrounding mucosa) are difficult to detect endoscopically and may be misinterpreted as lymphoid aggregates or hyperplastic polyps. They tend to have higher grades of dysplasia than usual adenomas and may contain invasive carcinoma, despite their small size. On biopsy, their deep margin must be demonstrated to avoid missing an invasive component.

- Endoscopic features .... The classic flat adenoma is diminutive and easily overlooked. The lesion may be slightly raised or depressed relative to the mucosa and erythematous or bland in appearance. Their identification is enhanced by the use of chromoscopy (e.g. contrast staining with indigo carmine). These polyps are ideally removed using mucosectomy techniques, allowing the lesion to be isolated by creating a submucosal saline cushion via direct injection (Fig. 4-286), and then snare excision (Fig. 4-287).

- Clinical features .... Prevalent in the Japanese population and in patients with HNPCC syndrome.

- Differential diagnosis ...... Endoscopic: Hyperplastic polyp, lymphoid aggregate.

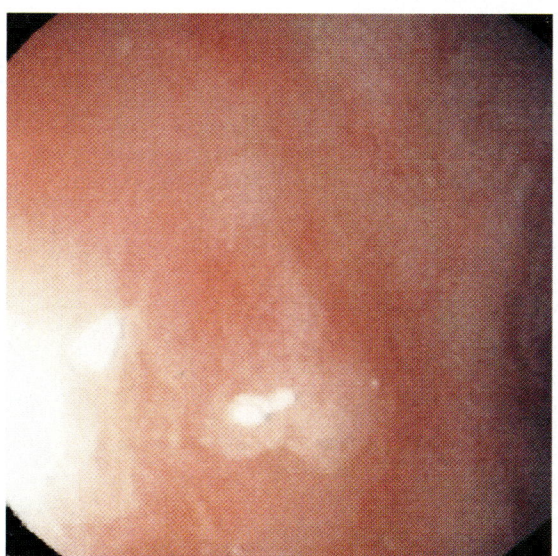

Figure 4-284: **Colon, Transverse. Flat Adenoma.** Diminutive, flat nodular change to the mucosa.

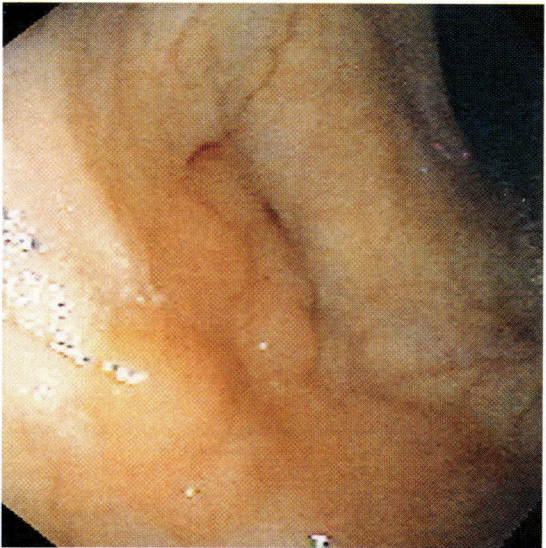

Figure 4-285: **Colon, Sigmoid. Flat Adenoma.** Small sessile, slightly nodular polyp.

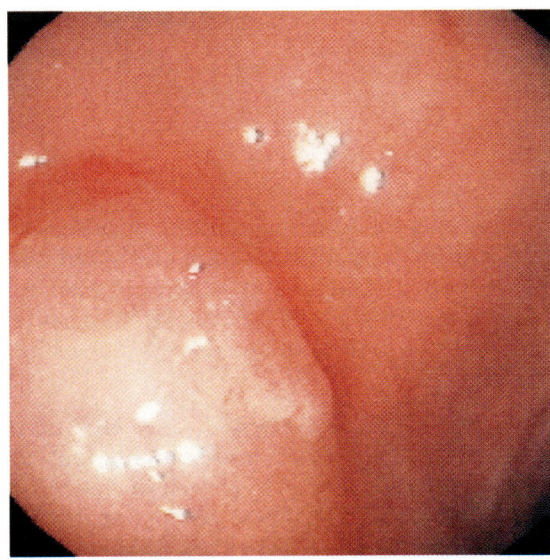

Figure 4-286: **Colon, Transverse. Flat Adenoma.** Flat adenoma sitting atop discrete submucosal saline fluid cushion.

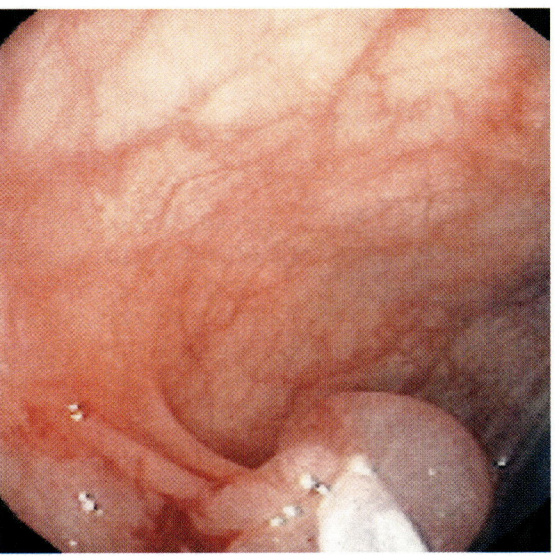

Figure 4-287: **Colon, Transverse. Flat Adenoma.** The isolated adenoma is easily snared because of the fluid cushion.

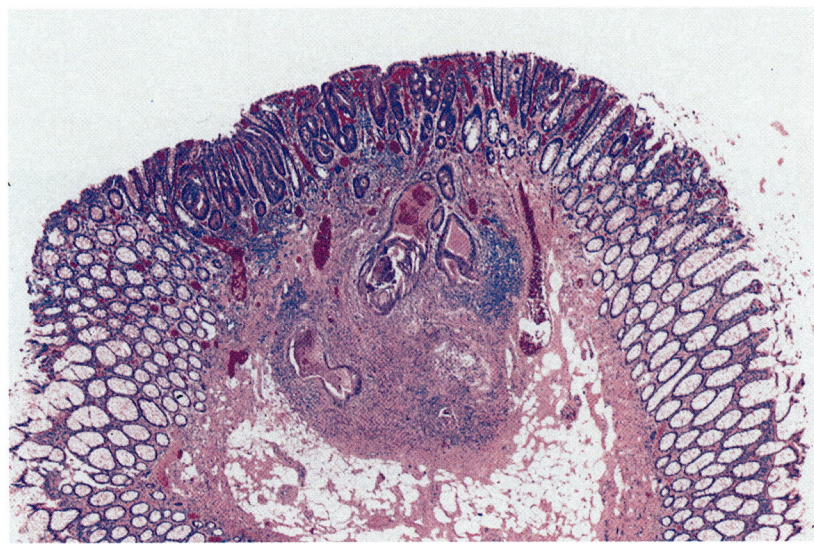

Figure 4-288: **Colon, Sigmoid. Adenocarcinoma Arising in Flat Adenoma.** Small, thin focus of dysplasia in flat mucosa overlying invasive adenocarcinoma.

ADENOCARCINOMA ARISING IN AN ADENOMA

- Morphology .... Adenocarcinoma usually develops in the center of the head of an adenoma. It is often pale, granular, and hard in comparison to the surrounding adenoma. Adenocarcinoma is usually associated with high-grade dysplasia. Although small, irregular nests or individual epithelial cells indicate invasion, a desmoplastic stromal reaction, if present, is an important indication of submucosal invasion. Adenocarcinomas confined to the mucosa of the head of the polyp (intramucosal adenocarcinoma) have no metastatic potential. Adenocarcinomas invasive into the submucosa of the core of the polyp have metastatic potential. The chance that an adenocarcinoma arising in the head of a pedunculated polyp has already metastasized to regional lymph nodes depends on tumor grade, the presence or absence of obvious vascular invasion, and the depth of invasion. If the advancing edge of a pedunculated tumor is more than 2 mm from the line of resection, is well-or moderately differentiated with no vascular invasion, polypectomy should be sufficient treatment. Submucosal invasion in a sessile polyp usually requires segmental resection.

- Endoscopic features .... Endoscopically evident lobules on the polyp surface disappear as the carcinoma grows. Malignant polyps are more commonly large (> 2 cm), firm, and ulcerated. A large sessile polyp with a discoid or saddle-shaped appearance suggests malignancy. The inability to raise a large sessile polyp above the surrounding mucosa with submucosal saline injection (nonlift sign) suggests invasive malignancy.

- Clinical features .... Occult blood-positive stools, iron deficiency anemia, family history for colorectal neoplasia.

- Differential diagnosis ...... Histologic: Pseudoinvasion.

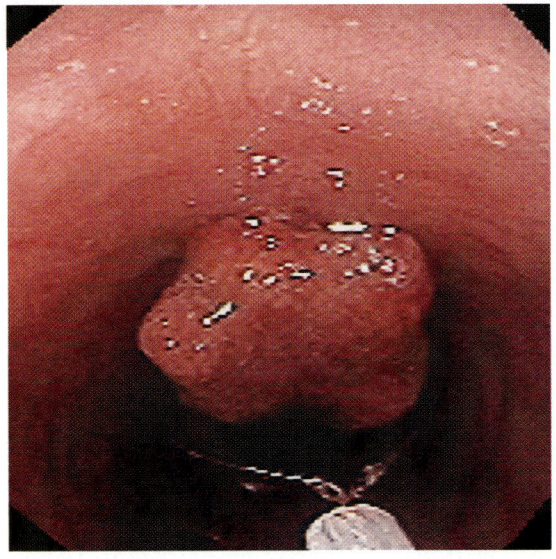

Figure 4-289: **Colon, Sigmoid. Adenocarcinoma Arising in an Adenoma.** Large, firm polyp (2 cm) with short base of attachment.

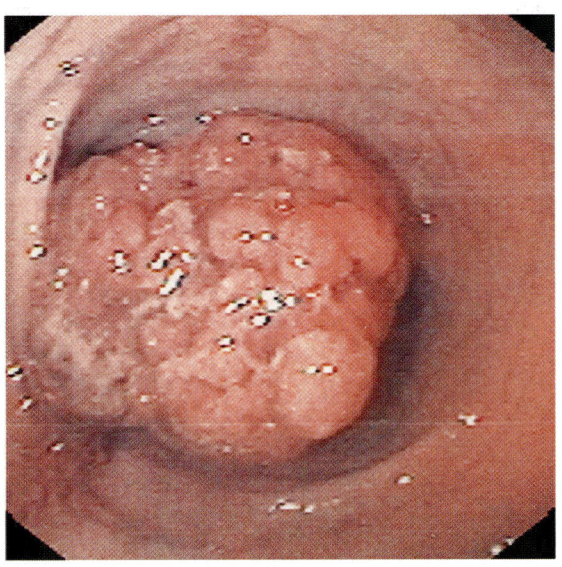

Figure 4-290: **Colon, Splenic Flexure. Adenocarcinoma Arising in an Adenoma.** Large polypoid mass spanning 2 haustral folds, with an area of necrosis at the lower left portion of the polyp.

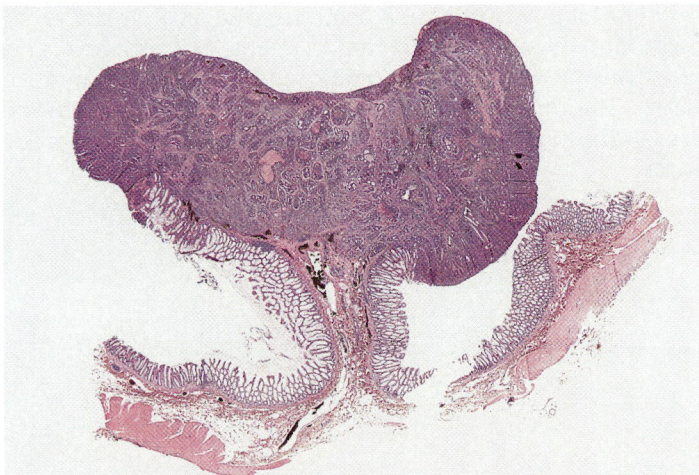

Figure 4-291: **Rectum. Adenocarcinoma Arising in an Adenoma.** Adenocarcinoma fills the polyp. Upper portion of stalk is invaded. Residual adenoma at the periphery.

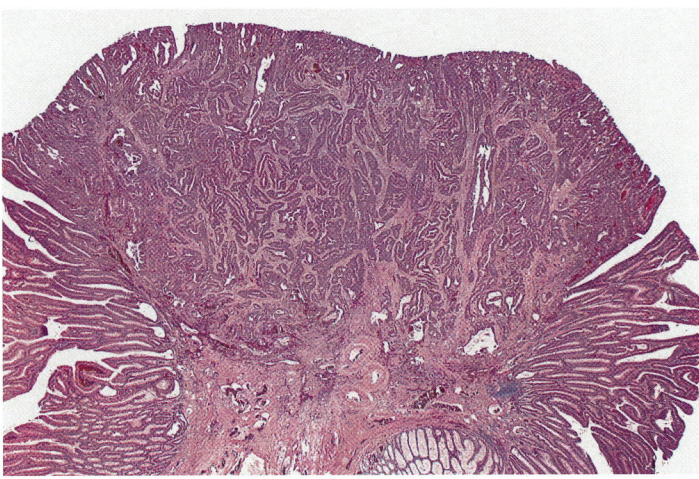

Figure 4-292: **Colon. Adenocarcinoma Arising in an Adenoma.** Desmoplastic stroma surrounds infiltrating glands. Residual adenoma on each side.

ADENOCARCINOMA

- Morphology .... Adenocarcinomas of the large intestine usually arise in adenomas. Submucosal invasion may elicit a desmoplastic response that can extend toward the mucosa and replace the lamina propria. Anatomic extent (stage) is the most important prognostic factor. Biopsy samples from adenocarcinomas with villous features may be too superficial to be diagnostic. It may be necessary to biopsy both the edge and ulcerated areas of adenocarcinomas for a definitive diagnosis of invasion. Most large bowel carcinomas are well- or moderately differentiated and form glandular structures.

- Endoscopic features .... Adenocarcinoma may present as an ulcerated sessile polyp, often saddle-shaped. When removal is attempted, particularly when saline is injected into the submucosa prior to snare resection, they do not lift up, a feature that suggests invasive malignancy. Advanced adenocarcinoma is usually a circumferential or partially circumferential mass that is firm, ulcerated, and friable, and often partially obstructing. Blood, fresh or altered, is commonly present, reflecting the tendency to bleed spontaneously.

- Clinical features .... Overt or occult bleeding, change in bowel habits or caliber of stool. Adenocarcinoma arising in a patient of less than 40 years should raise the suspicion of a hereditary cancer syndrome such as hereditary nonpolyposis colon cancer (HNPCC) and familial adenomatous polyposis (FAP).

- Differential diagnosis ...... Endoscopic: Diverticulitis of the cecum or ascending colon. Ulcerated nodular amyloidosis, lymphoma, and metastatic carcinoma.

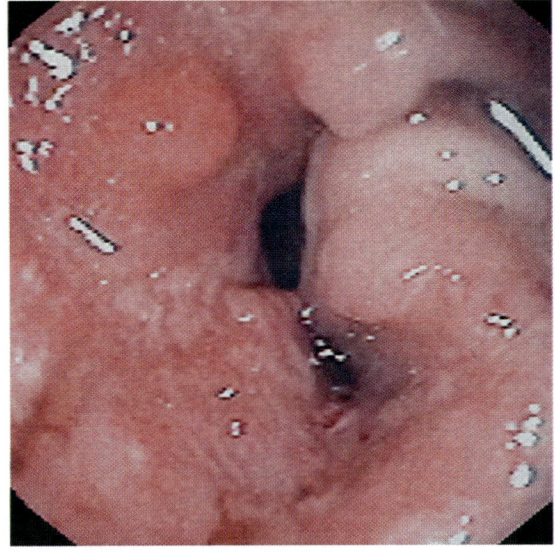

Figure 4-293: **Cecum. Adenocarcinoma.** Circumferential obstructing "napkin ring"-type neoplasm with some spontaneous bleeding and a suggestion of ulceration within the obscured lumen.

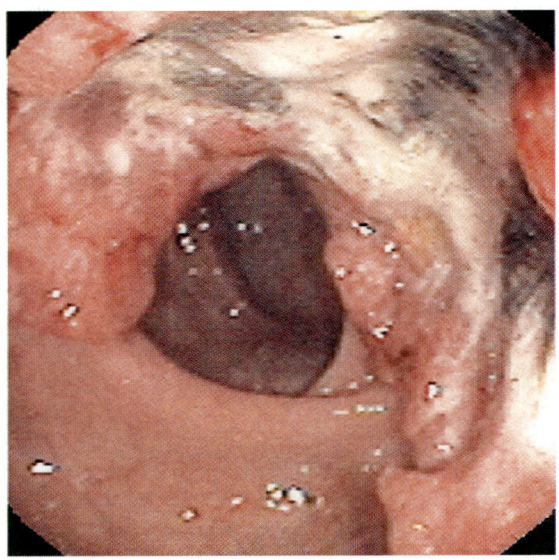

Figure 4-294: **Rectum. Adenocarcinoma.** Near circumferential, obstructing, ulcerated neoplasm with exophytic friable margins.

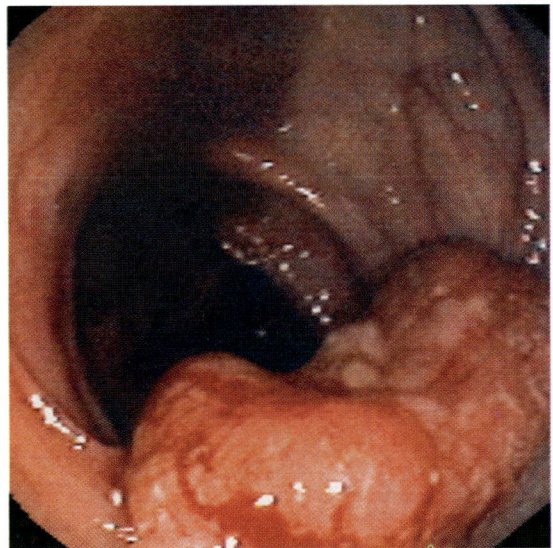

Figure 4-295: **Colon, Ascending. Adenocarcinoma.** Large sessile, partially circumferential polypoid mass with central necrotic and ulcerated area, friability, and spontaneous bleeding. Saddle shape is suggestive of malignancy.

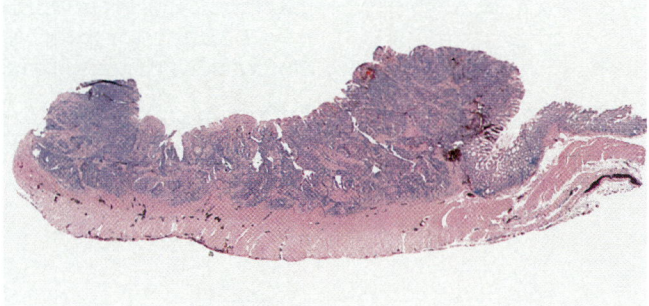

Figure 4-296: **Colon. Adenocarcinoma.** Saucer-shaped adenocarcinoma with raised edges extends into submucosa, T1.

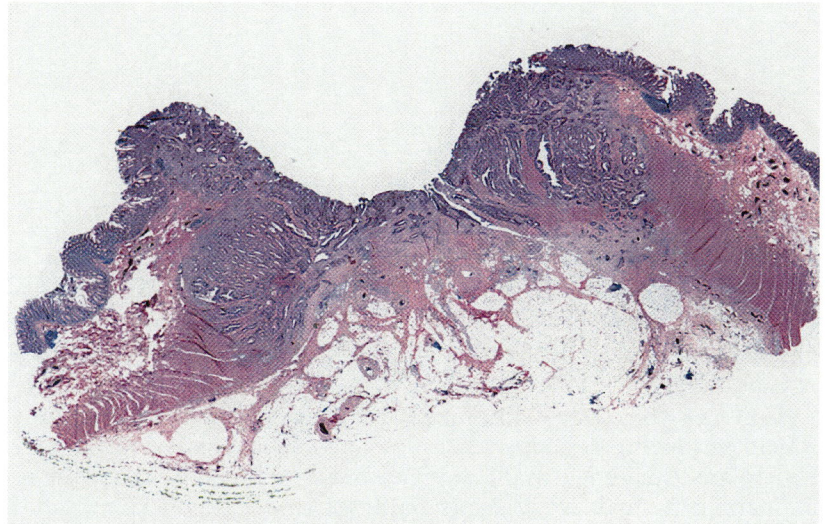

Figure 4-297: **Colon. Adenocarcinoma.** Centrally ulcerated tumor with heaped-up margins has invaded through muscularis propria into desmoplastic pericolic stroma, T3.

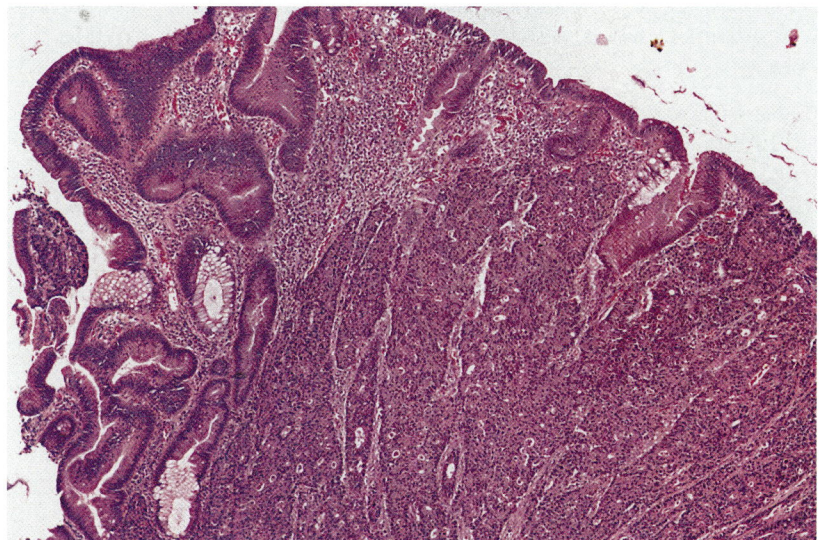

Figure 4-298: **Colon. Adenocarcinoma.** Sheets of moderately differentiated adenocarcinoma and remnants of an adenoma at the uneroded edge of a tumor. No desmoplasia in this field.

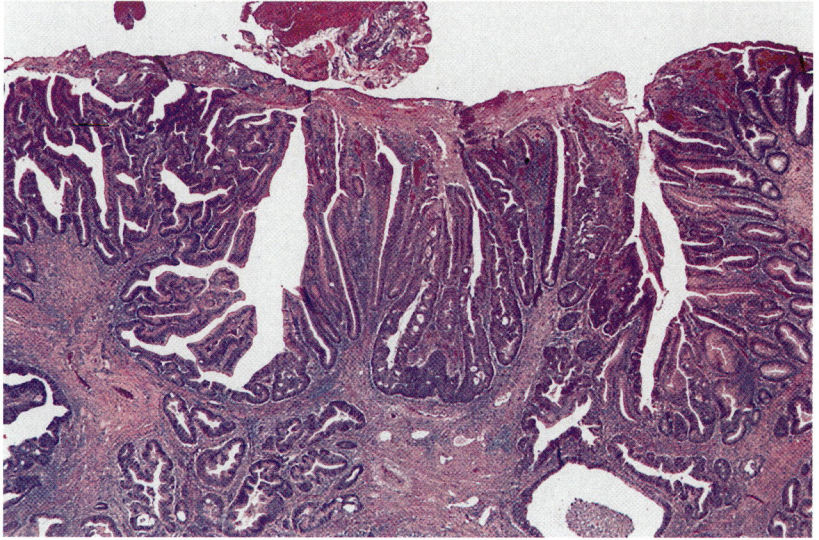

Figure 4-299: **Colon. Adenocarcinoma.** Well-differentiated adenocarcinoma with well-formed glands and an eroded surface.

CARCINOMA VARIANTS

MUCINOUS ADENOCARCINOMA

- Morphology .... The term *mucinous* is used to describe an adenocarcinoma that contains a substantial amount (over 50%) of mucin within the tumor mass. It corresponds to tumors with grossly visible mucin. ("Mucinous" is not synonymous with "mucin-producing.") Biopsy samples may be difficult to interpret because there are usually few malignant cells scattered in abundant mucin. The malignant cells may be well-differentiated and cytologically bland, making it difficult to distinguish mucinous adenocarcinoma from displaced colonic epithelium, e.g., pseudoinvasion and colitis cystica profunda—benign conditions in which mucin may also be abundant and located in the submucosa.

- Endoscopic features .... There are no distinctive endoscopic features that would predict a mucinous adenocarcinoma. These lesions may present as typical malignancies—exophytic, obstructing, friable, and ulcerated. They may also appear as atypical obstructing polypoid lesions with exudative ulceration as opposed to cavitating ulceration.

- Clinical features .... Anemia, hematochezia, diarrhea.

- Differential diagnosis...... Histologic: Pseudoinvasive adenoma, colitis cystica profunda.

  Endoscopic: When ulcerated, lymphoma, metastatic disease.

SIGNET-RING CELL AND SMALL CELL CARCINOMAS

- Morphology .... *Signet-ring cell carcinomas* occur as both primary or metastatic tumors. They may be associated with abundant extracellular mucin. Metastases most commonly are from the stomach and less frequently from the breast (signet-ring cell variant of lobular carcinoma). Immunostaining for cytokeratin 7 and 20 and BRST 2 may be useful in determining primary site.

  Small cell carcinomas are rare and also can be primary or metastatic. Primary colorectal small cell carcinomas frequently arise in association with an overlying adenoma or adenocarcinoma. They have morphologic and immunohistochemical features similar to those found in the lung.

- Differential diagnosis...... Histologic: Metastatic carcinoma.

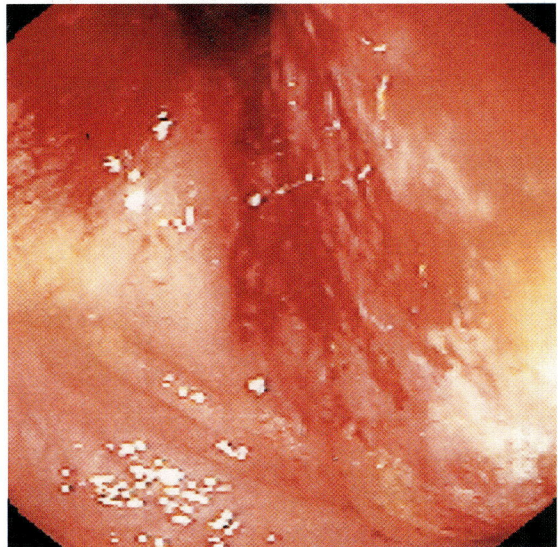

Figure 4-300: **Rectum. Mucinous Adenocarcinoma.** Flat, stenosing rectal mass with atypical pattern of ulceration.

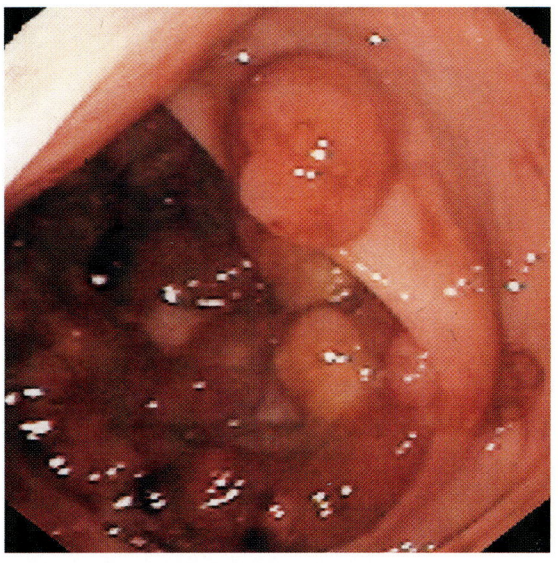

Figure 4-301: **Cecum. Mucinous Adenocarcinoma.** Cecal mass with nodular appearance and central ulceration.

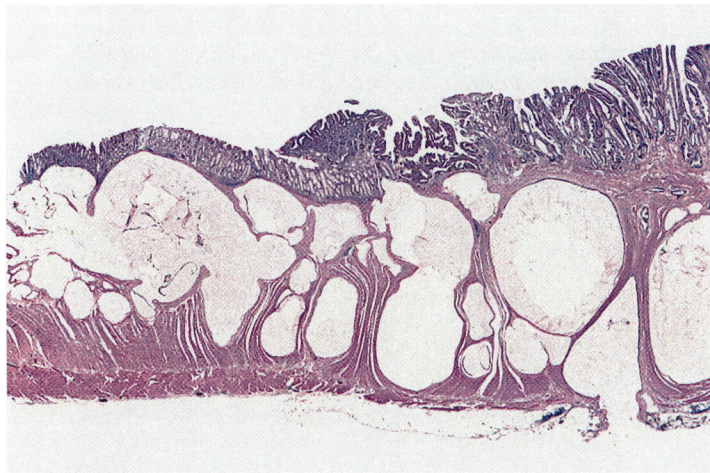

Figure 4-302: **Colon. Mucinous Adenocarcinoma.** Villous adenoma overlies pools of mucin with small clusters of malignant cells.

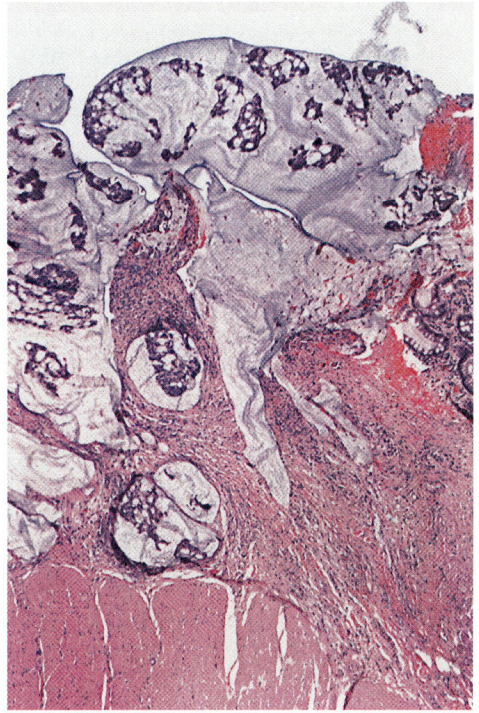

Figure 4-303: **Colon. Mucinous Adenocarcinoma.** Clusters of malignant epithelial cells float in mucin pools that infiltrate into deep submucosa up to the muscularis propria.

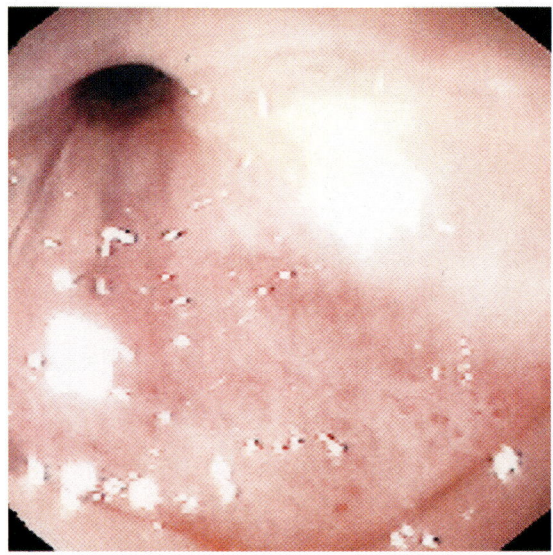

Figure 4-304: **Colon. Sigmoid. Signet-Ring Cell Carcinoma.** Narrow, constricted lumen with congested, dusky mucosa and focal superficial erosions. Suspicious for malignancy.

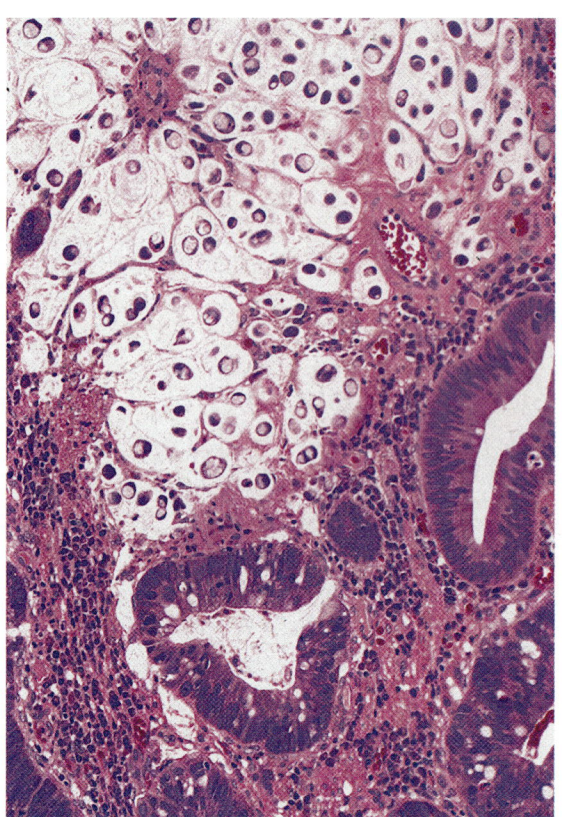

Figure 4-305: **Colon. Signet-Ring Cell Carcinoma.** Signet-ring cells float in mucin amongst remnants of an adenoma.

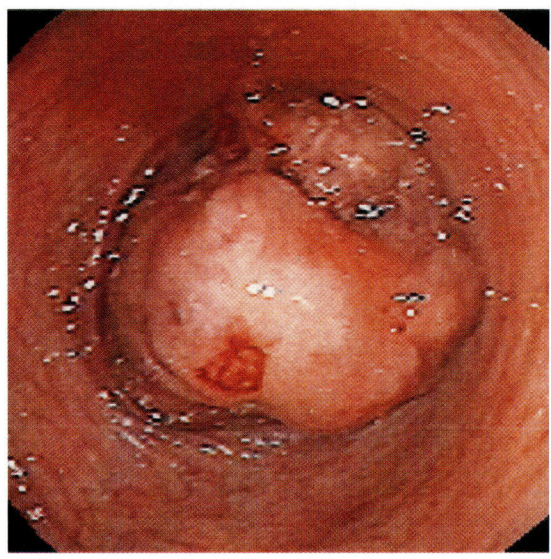

Figure 4-306: **Colon, Transverse. Small Cell Carcinoma.** The lumen is completely filled with a hemorrhagic, ulcerated neoplasm. Biopsy showed fragments of adenoma; resection revealed underlying small cell carcinoma.

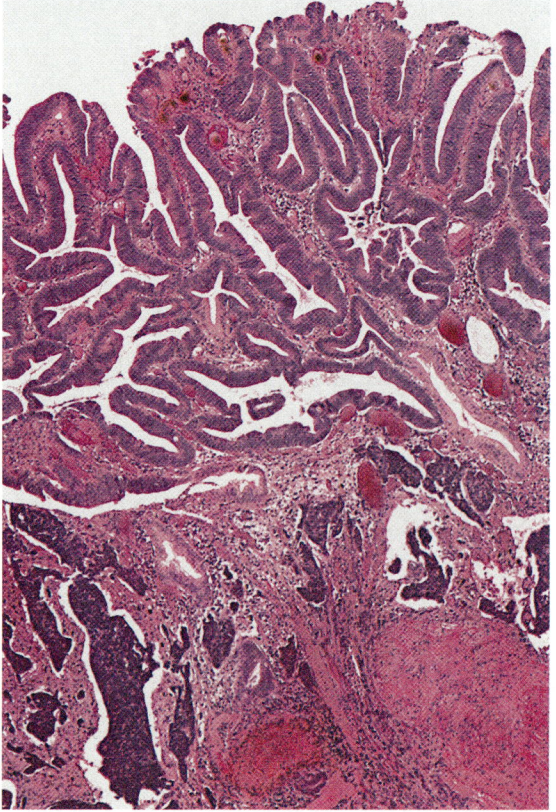

Figure 4-307: **Colon. Small Cell Carcinoma.** Small cell carcinoma invades the wall beneath a tubulovillous adenoma.

RECURRENT ADENOCARCINOMA

- **Endoscopic features** .... Recurrent malignancy is typically located at or near an anastomosis. The presentation may be an obvious ulcerated neoplasm that compromises the lumen, infiltrates the submucosa, and causes nodularity at, or proximal or distal to, the anastomosis, and extrinsic compression.
- **Clinical features** .... Low-lying recurrences may cause perineal pain. With mucosal involvement, obstruction and/or bleeding may be the first sign.
- **Differential diagnosis** ...... Endoscopic: Nonspecific postoperative anastomotic nodularity and ulceration. Benign ulcers are more common with ileocolonic than with colocolonic anastomoses.

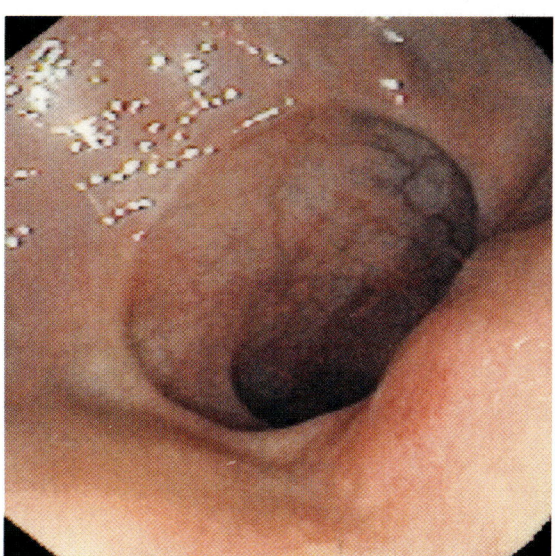

Figure 4-308: **Colon. Recurrent Adenocarcinoma.** A ringlike anastomosis is in the central background portion of the photograph. In the foreground on the right, the mucosa is elevated and thickened. There is focal erythema.

METASTATIC TUMORS

- Morphology .... Distinguishing a metastasis from a primary in a biopsy sample may be difficult. Features that support a metastasis include the lack of surface epithelial dysplasia and the presence of the bulk of the tumor in the submucosa, with only focal mucosal involvement. Immunohistochemical studies, particularly cytokeratins 7 and 20 and S-100 and HMB-45 (for melanoma), may be helpful in suggesting a primary site. Metastatic lesions are often multiple. Carcinomas that commonly metastasize to the GI tract include lung, stomach, breast, and ovary, and melanoma.

- Endoscopic features .... Although metastatic carcinoma can resemble a primary colorectal carcinoma endoscopically, the mucosa may lack the irregular nodularity, ulceration, and granular appearance common to primary carcinomas.

- Clinical features .... Hematochezia and obstruction.

- Differential diagnosis ...... Histologic and endoscopic: Primary colorectal carcinoma, carcinoid tumor, lymphoma, sarcoma, and melanoma.

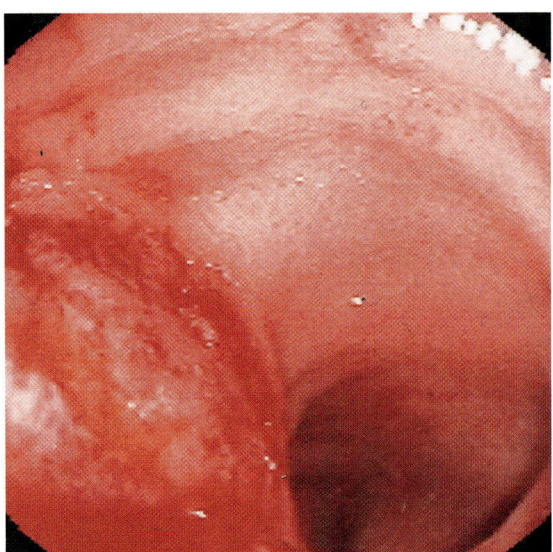

Figure 4-309: **Colon, Sigmoid. Metastatic Squamous Cell Carcinoma.** A soft, sessile, polypoid, ulcerated, and friable mass with spontaneous bleeding. Surface features are atypical for an adenoma or carcinoma arising in the colon.

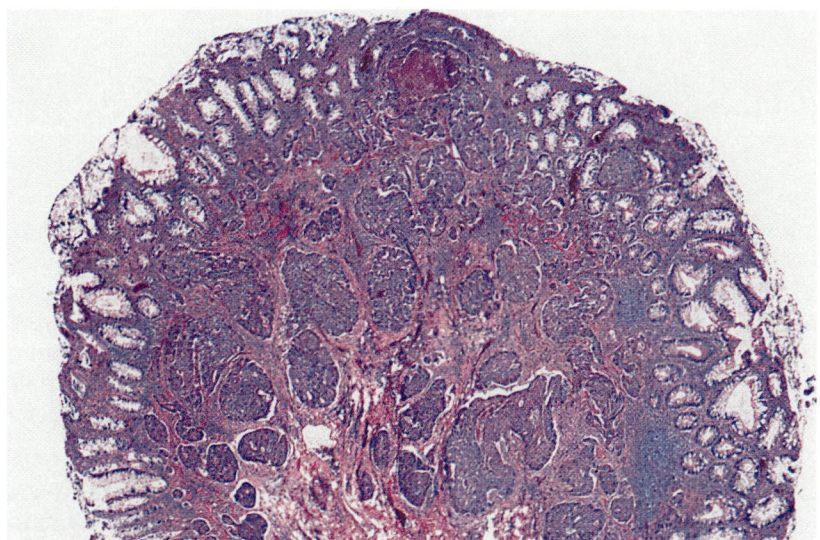

Figure 4-310: **Colon. Metastatic Adenocarcinoma.** Polypoid lesion with metastatic adenocarcinoma in submucosa and mucosa, particularly in lymphatics.

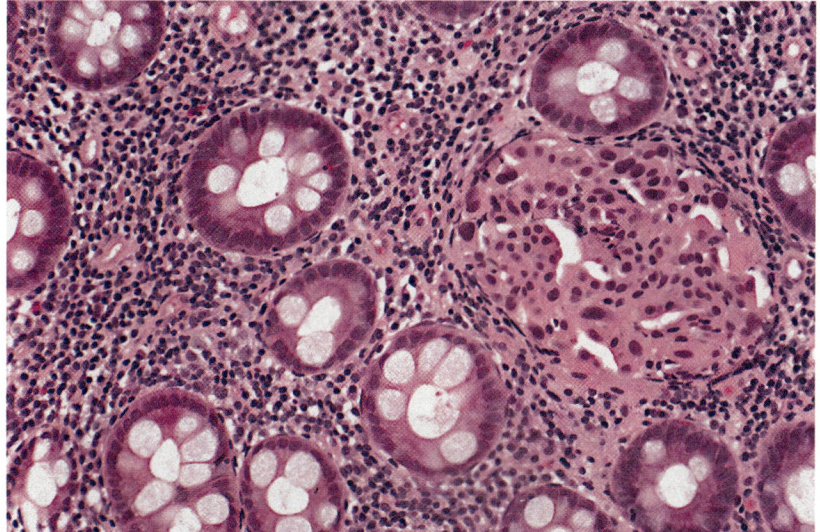

Figure 4-311: **Colon. Metastatic Carcinoma.** Carcinoma compatible with transitional cell carcinoma in a mucosal vessel.

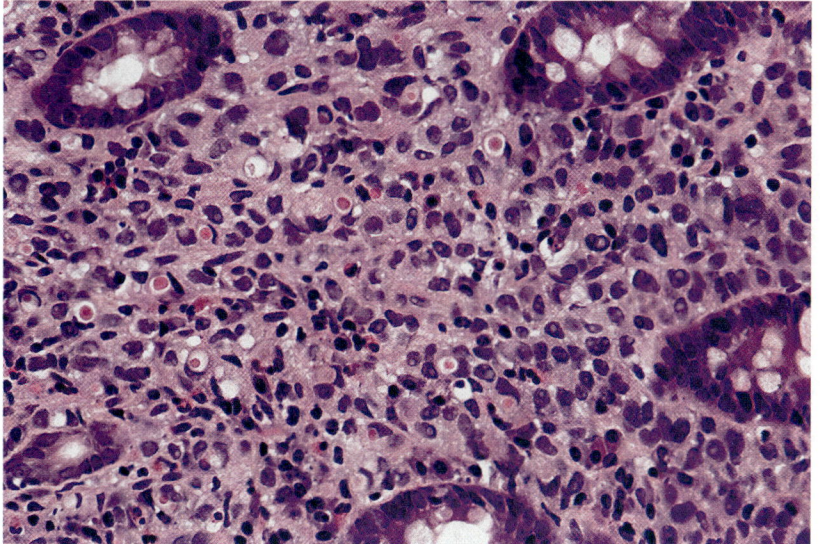

Figure 4-312: **Colon. Metastatic Breast Carcinoma.** Compact small cells with scant cytoplasm and eccentric nuclei fill lamina propria, separating glands. Occasional signet-ring cells with opaque eosinophilic cytoplasmic mucin surrounded by a clear space (so-called bull's-eye).

CARCINOID TUMOR

- Morphology .... Carcinoids are uncommon in the colon, but relatively frequent in the rectum. Tumors are usually small, and only a few cells may be present in shallow mucosal biopsy specimens. The small sample size and variety of histologic patterns can lead to difficulty in distinguishing carcinoids from adenocarcinoma. Carcinoids in the rectum are sometimes negative for chromogranin, but more frequently positive for prostatic acid phosphatase (PAP). In a male patient, it is important to perform an immunostain for PSA on a rectal carcinoid. PSA should be negative in all GI carcinoids.

- Endoscopic features .... Carcinoids are usually nonspecific small polyps that on close inspection are submucosal and sometimes have a distinctive yellow hue. They are encountered in the ileum, often during an evaluation for unexplained bleeding and symptoms of obstruction. Carcinoids of the appendix usually involve the tip and are not diagnosed endoscopically, unless they project into the cecum.

- Clinical features .... Rectal carcinoids are generally incidental findings. In the terminal ileum, these lesions may be associated with unexplained bleeding and, less often, obstruction. Large lesions (> 2 cm) are likely to be associated with metastasis and, when the liver is involved, may produce the carcinoid syndrome.

- Differential diagnosis ...... Endoscopic: In the rectum, adenoma and leiomyoma; in the terminal ileum, leiomyoma, lymphoma, adenocarcinoma, and metastatic tumors.

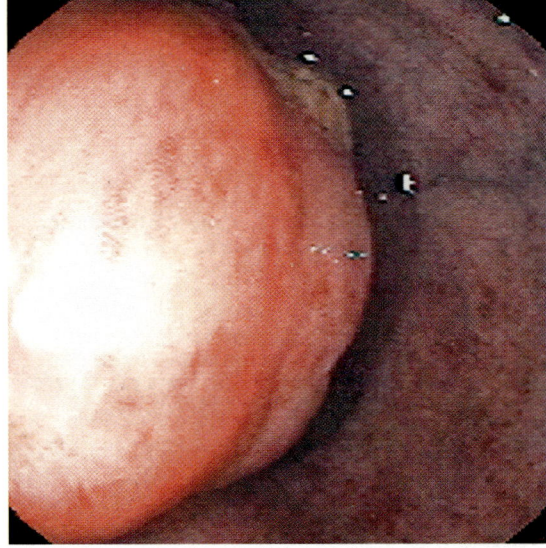

Figure 4-313: **Ileocecal Valve. Carcinoid.** Large, smooth, polypoid neoplasm obscures ileocecal valve. May have arisen in ileum and prolapsed into colon.

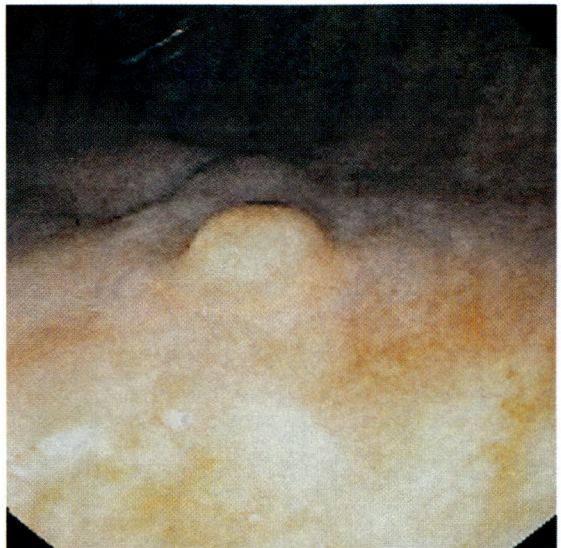

Figure 4-314: **Rectum. Carcinoid.** Small rectal carcinoid appearing as a distinctive yellow submucosal nodule.

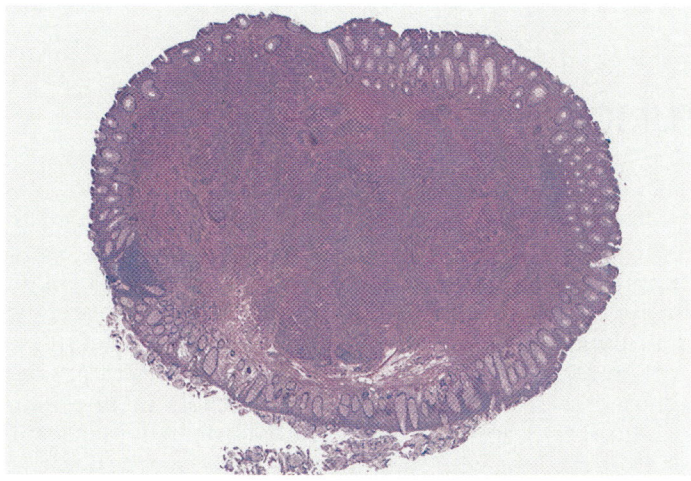

Figure 4-315: **Rectum. Carcinoid.** Bulk of tumor in submucosa with only focal mucosal infiltration. Normal colonic mucosa.

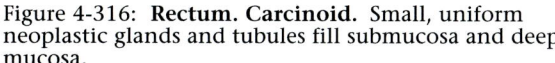

Figure 4-316: **Rectum. Carcinoid.** Small, uniform neoplastic glands and tubules fill submucosa and deep mucosa.

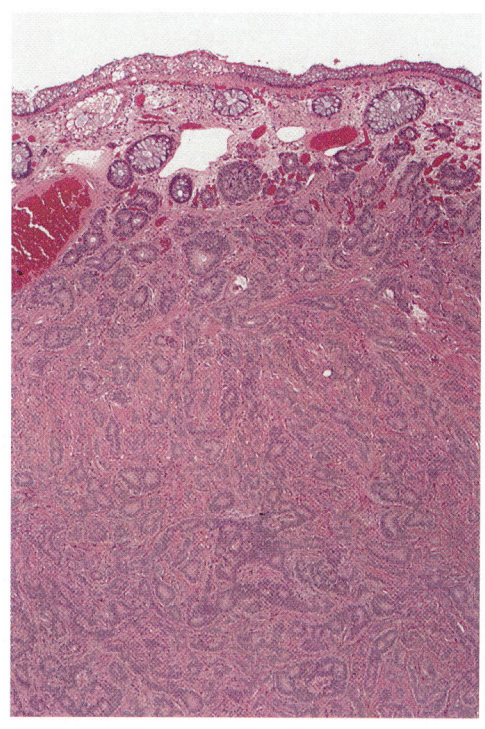

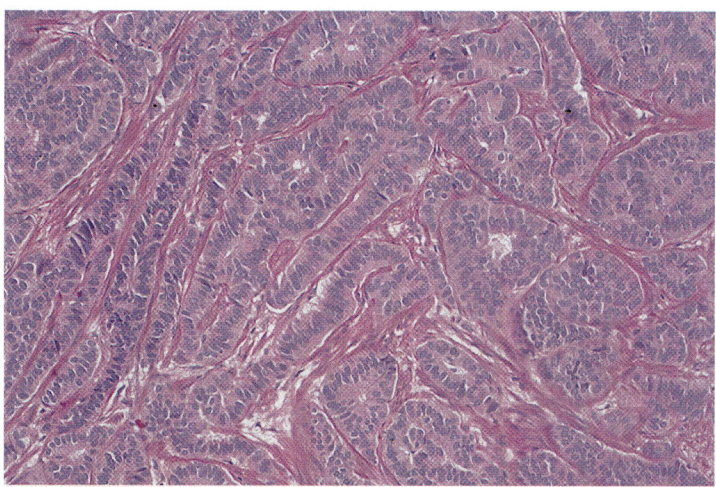

Figure 4-317: **Rectum. Carcinoid.** Tumor cells with pale chromatin and inconspicuous nucleoli, mainly arranged in a trabecular pattern, often a feature of rectal carcinoids.

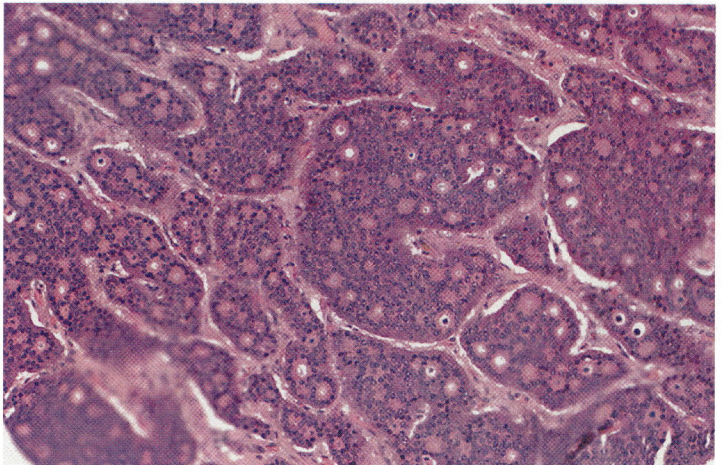

Figure 4-318: **Rectum. Carcinoid.** Insular growth pattern with gland or rosettelike structures typical of midgut carcinoids.

SMOOTH MUSCLE/STROMAL TUMORS

- Morphology .... Smooth muscle/stromal tumors of the colon are rare. They are difficult to diagnose on mucosal biopsy because of their submucosal location. Small smooth muscle tumors arising from the muscularis mucosae are benign. Predicting the behavior of larger neoplasms is difficult; mitotic index is the best indicator. Small biopsy sample size generally precludes a definitive diagnosis, unless the mitotic rate is high. Tumors removed at biopsy are probably best diagnosed as smooth muscle/stromal tumors of uncertain malignant potential, until they are resected and fully evaluated. Metastatic large cell carcinoma from the lung with spindle cell features may be negative for cytokeratin, express only vimentin, and simulate a leiomyosarcoma.

- Endoscopic features .... Leiomyoma presents as a submucosal nodule or mass. The main differential for this lesion is a lipoma; the latter typically has a yellow hue (see page 389). Leiomyomas may be indistinguishable from leiomyosarcomas which are larger (>2 cm) and often have irregular ulcers, in contrast to the smooth contour and small central ulceration more typical of leiomyomas.

- Clinical features .... Leiomyomas are incidental, or may be discovered because of acute and chronic bleeding as the lesion becomes ulcerated and erodes a significant-sized vessel. Leiomyosarcomas in an advanced stage may present with bowel obstruction, blood loss, or locally metastatic disease.

- Differential diagnosis ...... Histologic: Bizarre reactive stromal cells in an ulcer, spindle cell squamous carcinoma, and spindled renal cell carcinoma.

    Endoscopic: Submucosal neoplasms such as lipoma, carcinoid, and metastases. When mucosa is involved, adenocarcinoma.

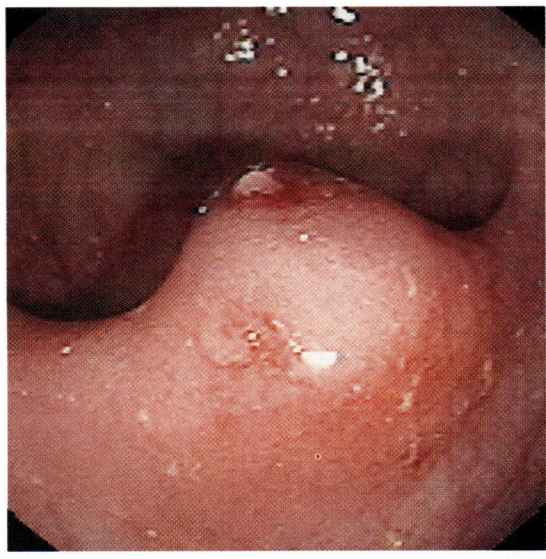

Figure 4-319: **Rectum. Leiomyoma.** Small submucosal nodule with central umbilicated ulceration containing exudate and blood. The centrally located ulcer is characteristic for an intramural neoplasm such as a leiomyoma.

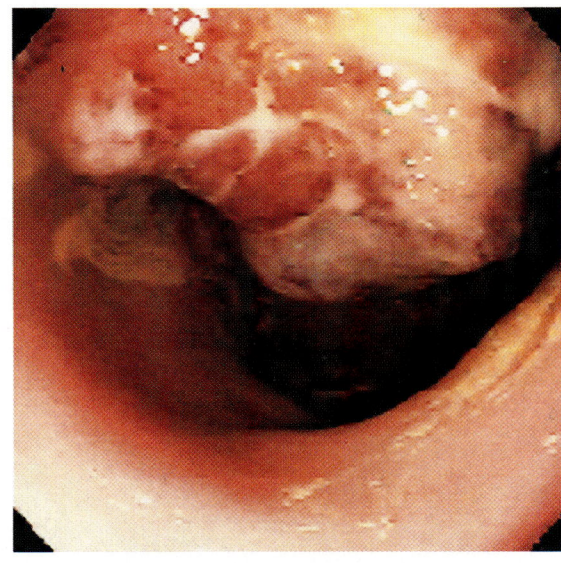

Figure 4-320: **Rectum. Leiomyosarcoma/Stromal Tumor.** Large, exophytic sessile neoplasm with ulceration, exudate, and spontaneous bleeding. The lesion, although focal, compromises the lumen.

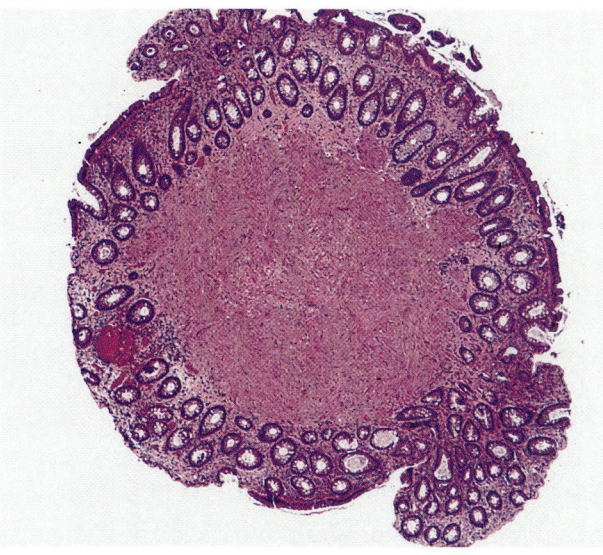

Figure 4-321: **Rectum. Leiomyoma.** Whorling, interlacing fascicles of smooth muscle arise from muscularis mucosae and form a nodule, creating a small polyp.

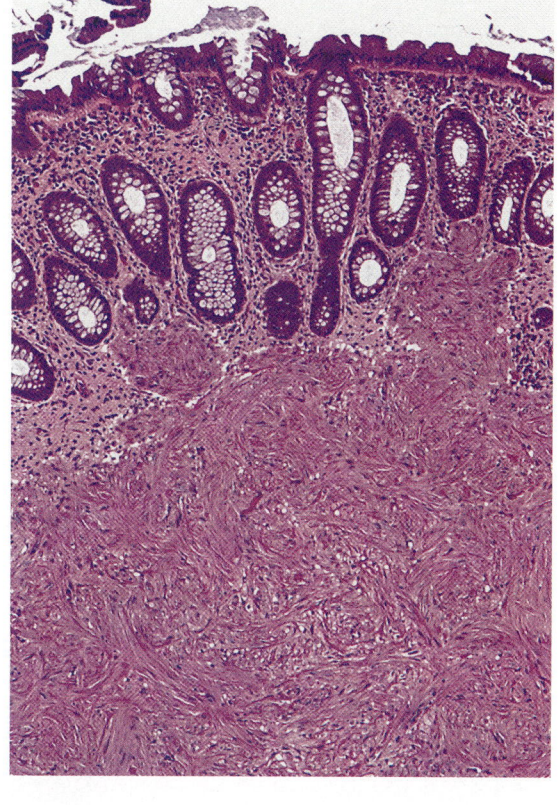

Figure 4-322: **Rectum. Leiomyoma.** Higher magnification of Fig. 4-321. The tumor extends focally into the lamina propria, displacing but not destroying glands.

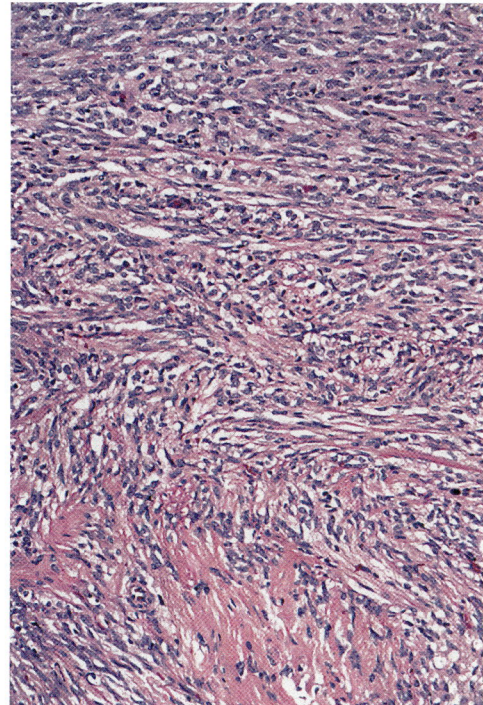

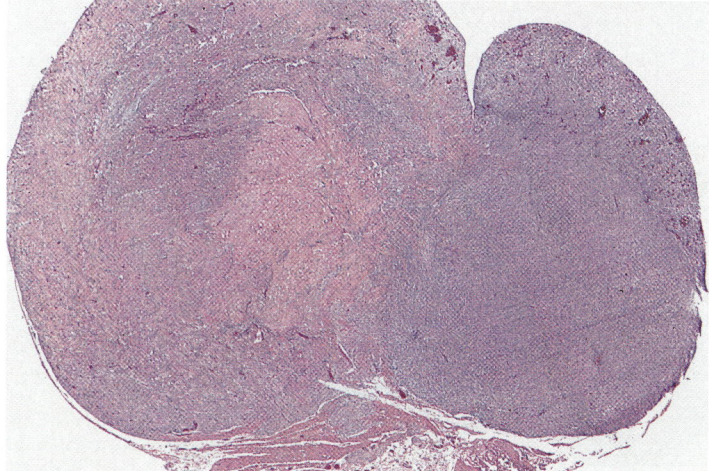

Figure 4-324: **Colon. Leiomyosarcoma/Stromal Tumor.** A large, multinodular stromal tumor replaces the muscularis propria and forms a polypoid mass.

Figure 4-323: **Colon. Leiomyosarcoma/Stromal Tumor.** Interlacing fascicles of spindle cells with blunt-ended nuclei, eosinophilic cytoplasm, and mitotic activity.

KAPOSI SARCOMA

- Morphology .... Because Kaposi sarcoma is usually located in the submucosa, biopsies of endoscopically obvious lesions, if too superficial, can fail to show the lesion. Biopsy samples may be misinterpreted as granulation tissue of an ulcer, smooth muscle tumor, or hemangioma. Spindle cells can be confused with reactive fibrosis, other stromal neoplasms, or even crush artifact. A vascular lesion from a patient with AIDS should be considered Kaposi sarcoma until proven otherwise. CD31 is positive in cases of Kaposi sarcoma.

- Endoscopic features .... On endoscopic examination, early lesions resemble hemorrhages. Larger lesions appear as dome-shaped erythematous masses or nodules.

- Clinical features .... Kaposi sarcoma involving the colon is usually asymptomatic. Kaposi sarcoma involves the small bowel more frequently than the colon, where it may cause abdominal pain, intussusception, and bleeding.

- Differential diagnosis ...... Histologic: Benign and malignant vascular or stromal neoplasms and granulation tissue.

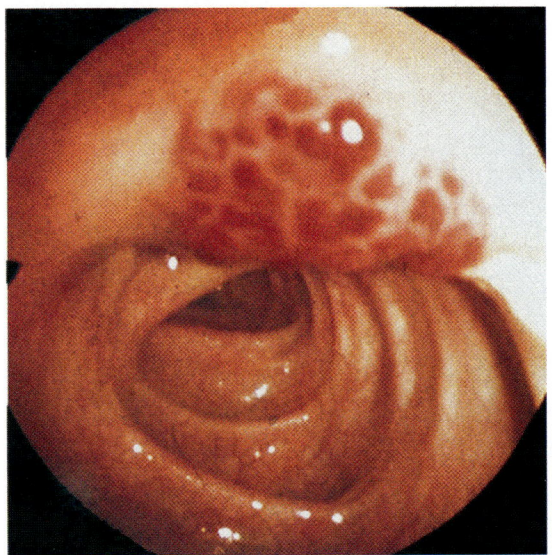

Figure 4-325: **Colon. Kaposi Sarcoma.** Discrete, slightly irregular deep red nodule typical of Kaposi sarcoma.

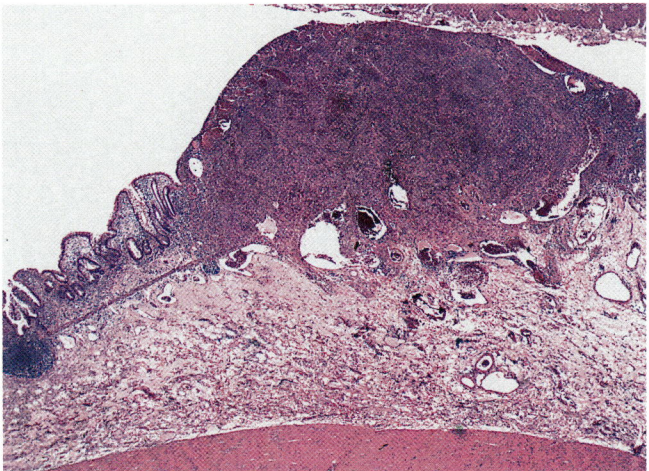

Figure 4-326: **Colon. Kaposi Sarcoma.** Spindle cell neoplasm forming a dome-shaped nodule in submucosa and mucosa. See Fig. 3-221 for histologic appearance at higher magnification.

MALIGNANT LYMPHOMA

- Morphology .... Distinguishing lymphoma from reactive lymphoid hyperplasia on mucosal biopsy can be difficult. A diffuse, atypical lymphoid infiltrate and crypt destruction are features that raise suspicion of lymphoma. Identification of germinal centers, tingible body macrophages, mixed inflammation, and a mixture of B and T cells (by immunohistochemistry) favor a reactive process. Lymphomas of the colon and rectum are rare. A lymphoid mass in the rectal area of a young patient is usually lymphoid hyperplasia (rectal tonsil). A large cell lymphoma may be confused with undifferentiated carcinoma or melanoma. While most diagnoses can be made on formalin-fixed tissue, frozen tissue for immunostains, flow cytometry, and gene rearrangement may be necessary for precise classification. When the biopsy shows lymphoma or lymphoid infiltrates suspicious for lymphoma, a hematopathologist may be helpful regarding current classification and terminology, need for additional studies, requirements for staging, and therapeutic options.

- Endoscopic features .... Lymphoma may present as a discrete polypoid mass, a broader ulcerating and obstructing neoplasm, a subtle mucosal thickening, nodularity, or irregular, shallow ulceration.

- Clinical features .... Obstruction and bleeding.

- Differential diagnosis ...... Histologic: Reactive lymphoid hyperplasia, undifferentiated carcinoma, melanoma, cecal diverticulitis, and tuberculosis.

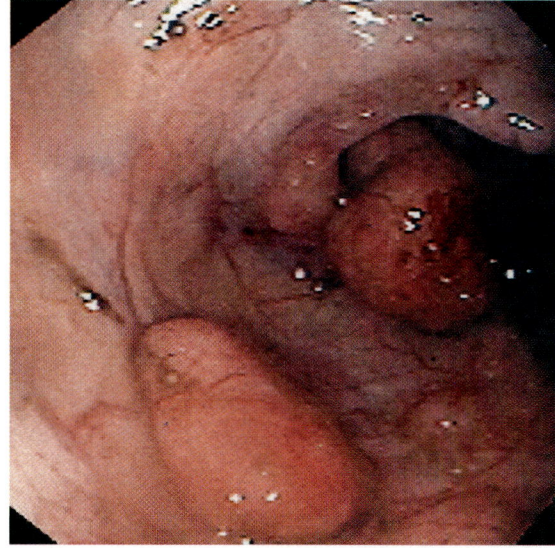

Figure 4-327: **Colon. Malignant Lymphoma.** Smooth, sessile polypoid nodules with surface hemorrhage. Intact mucosa and mucosal vessels favor a submucosal lesion. Friability suggests malignancy.

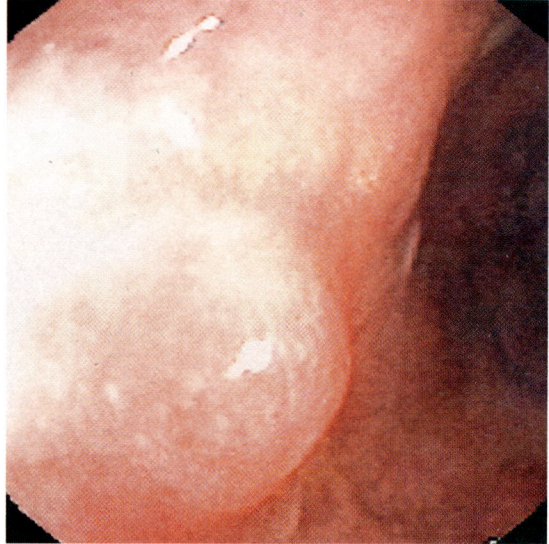

Figure 4-328: **Rectum. Malignant Lymphoma.** Thickened nodular mucosa with subtle, shallow, irregular ulceration.

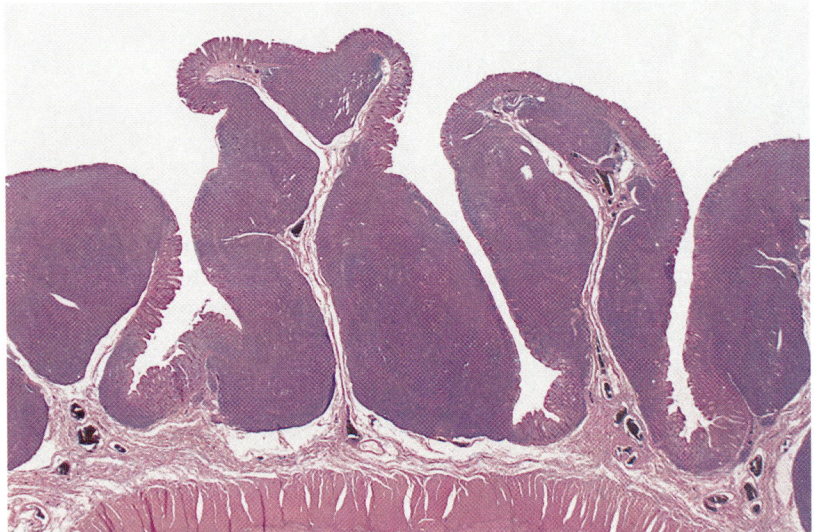

Figure 4-329: **Colon. Malignant Lymphoma (Malignant Lymphomatous Polyposis).** Multinodular lymphoid mucosal and submucosal infiltrates form polyps.

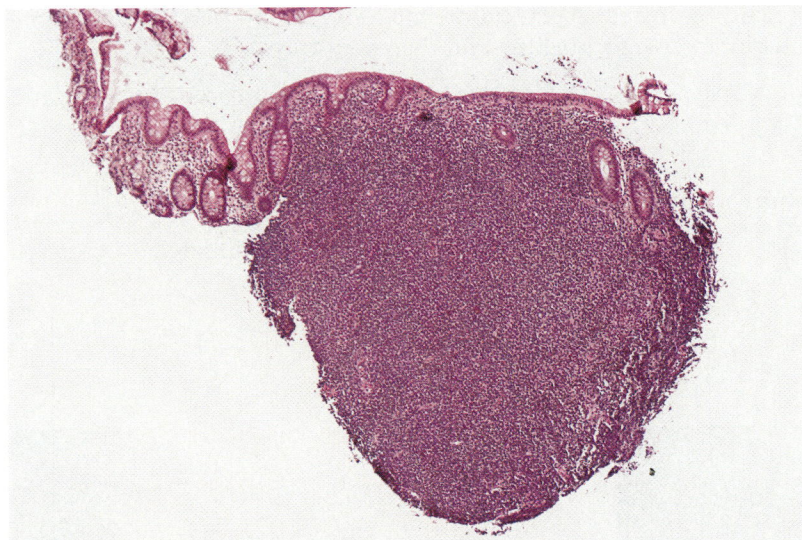

Figure 4-330: **Colon. Malignant Lymphoma.** Mucosal biopsy specimen with dense lymphoid nodule, no germinal center, and loss of crypts.

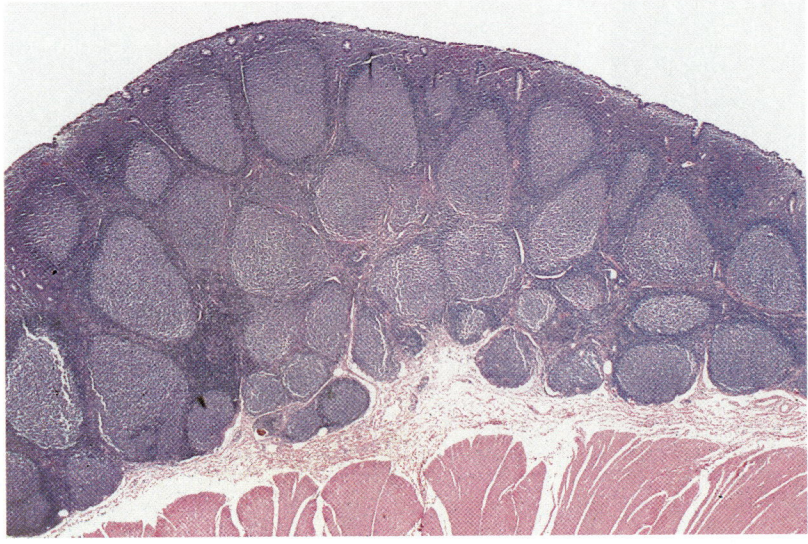

Figure 4-331: **Colon, Sigmoid. Malignant Lymphoma, Follicle Center Cell Type.** Numerous monotonous giant follicles without reactive features replace mucosa and partially fill submucosa.

MALIGNANT MELANOMA

- **Morphology** .... Melanoma may be primary in the anorectal area or metastatic anywhere in the colon. Biopsies demonstrate a large cell infiltrate, which on routine histology cannot be distinguished from large cell lymphoma or undifferentiated carcinoma, unless melanin is obvious. A diagnosis of primary melanoma is clear-cut if melanoma cells are arising from the squamous surface epithelium. Metastatic melanoma may not be suspected clinically when diagnosed on mucosal biopsy. The histologic appearance varies; the cells may be epithelioid, spindled, and plasmacytoid. While melanin pigment is frequently present, immunohistochemical studies for HMB-45 and S-100 protein are often required for diagnosis. Iron pigment can resemble melanin.

- **Endoscopic features** .... Malignant melanoma in the colon and rectum may present as a nonspecific ulcerating neoplasm or a distinctive pigmented mass. Anorectal melanomas often resemble thrombosed internal hemorrhoids.

- **Clinical features** .... GI blood loss and obstruction.

- **Differential diagnosis** ...... Histologic: Undifferentiated carcinoma, lymphoma, sarcoma.

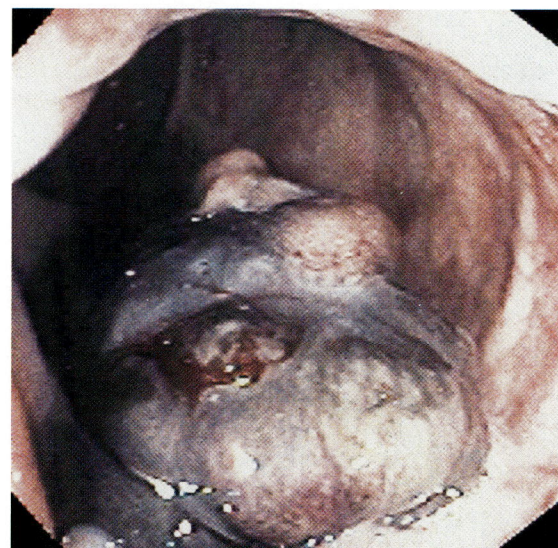

Figure 4-332: **Rectum. Primary Melanoma.** A discrete polypoid and heavily pigmented neoplasm occupies the rectum.

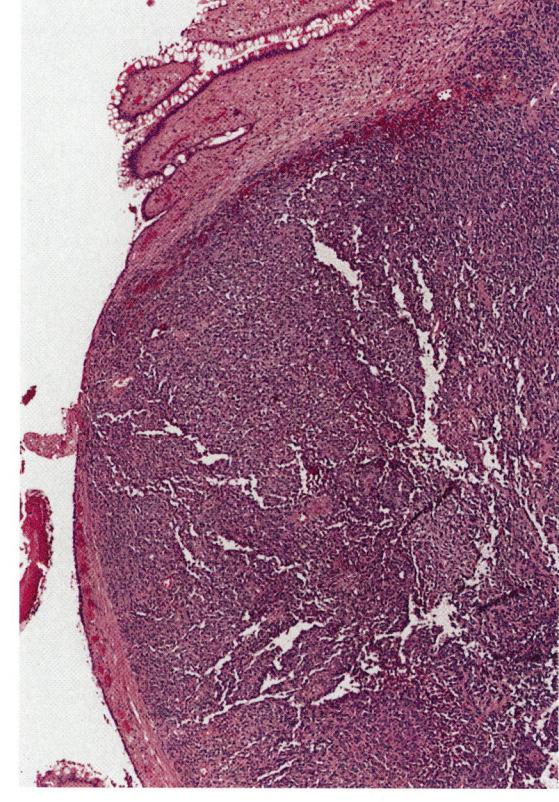

Figure 4-333: **Anorectal Junction. Primary Melanoma.** Large mass erodes anal mucosa and extends into rectum.

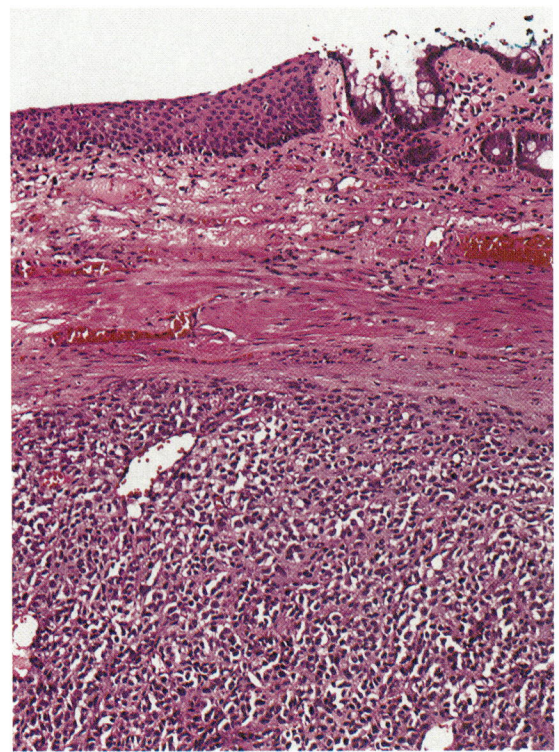

Figure 4-334: **Anorectal Junction. Primary Melanoma.** Nodule of large polygonal cells.

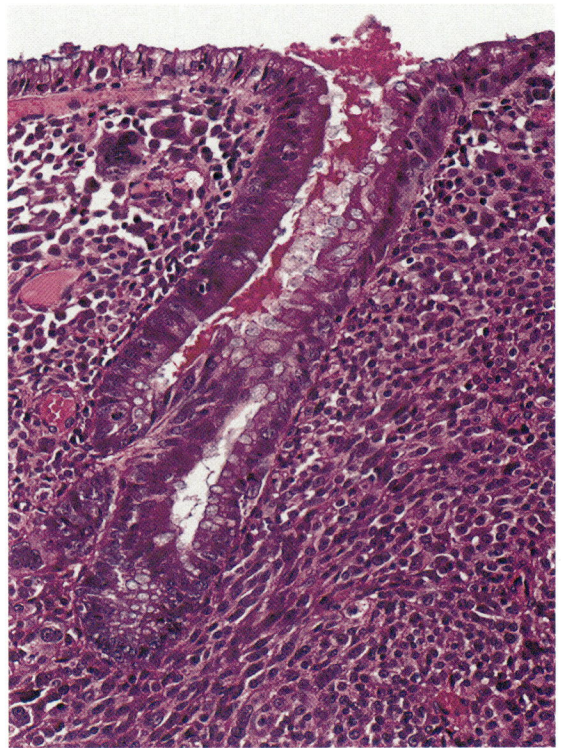

Figure 4-335: **Colon. Metastatic Melanoma.** Spindle and epithelioid cells infiltrate lamina propria.

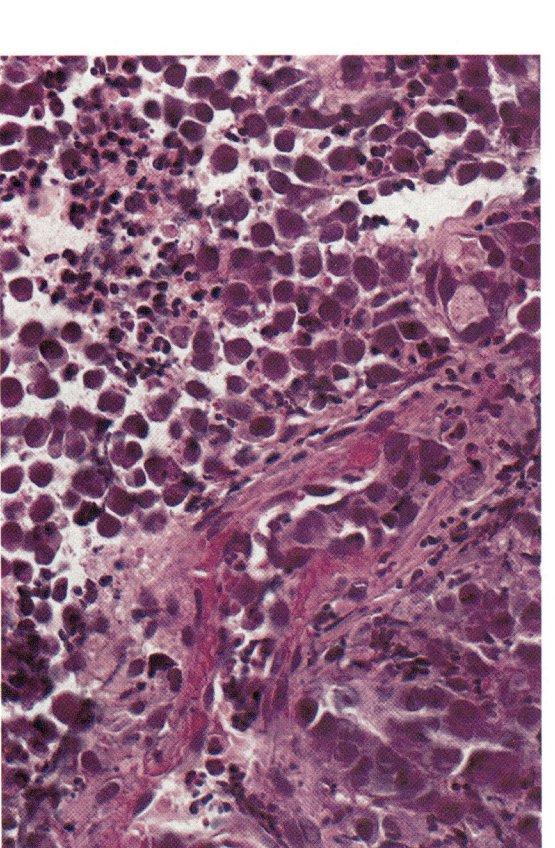

Figure 4-336: **Colon. Metastatic Melanoma.** Tumor cells with a plasmacytoid appearance.

SQUAMOUS LESIONS

- Morphology .... The most common squamous lesion in the anal canal is condyloma acuminatum. Squamous cell dysplasia and carcinoma and basal cell carcinoma occur much less frequently. The anorectal transition zone appears less mature than other areas of the anal canal; this can simulate dysplasia.

    Squamous cell (cloacogenic) carcinomas arise from transitional epithelium of the anal canal, often appear largely undifferentiated, and grow in sheets and nests. The mitotic rate is brisk. The cells usually are small and basaloid, but squamous, transitional, and glandular differentiation occur. When undifferentiated small basaloid cells predominate, these tumors may resemble lymphomas or melanomas. Immunostains are useful for diagnosis. When differentiated elements predominate, cloacogenic carcinoma may be confused with basal or squamous cell carcinoma of anal skin (anal margin) and metastatic adenocarcinomas from contiguous or distant organs. Clinicopathologic correlation is necessary.

- Endoscopic features .... Condylomas are distinctive, small, squamous polyps in the perianal area that may become confluent. The diagnosis is made prior to entry into the anal canal. Squamous cell carcinoma is usually a nodule or an irregular ulcerated mass in the anal canal.

- Clinical features .... Perianal irritation, mucoid discharge, rectal outlet bleeding.

- Differential diagnosis ...... Histologic: Condyloma acuminatum versus squamous cell dysplasia and verrucous carcinoma. Basaloid squamous cell (cloacogenic) carcinoma versus basal cell carcinoma.

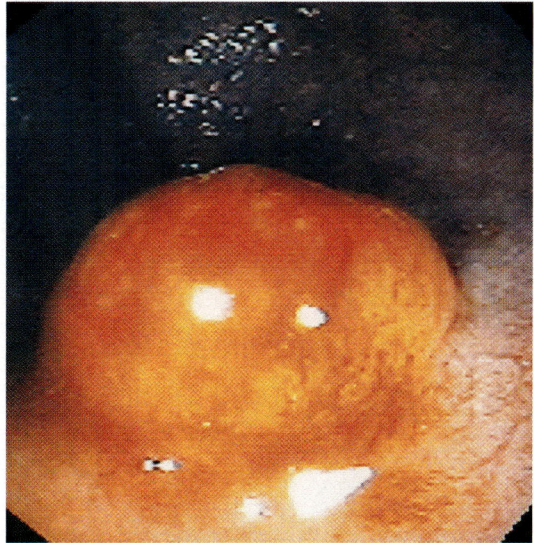

Figure 4-337: **Anorectal Area. Squamous Cell Carcinoma.** Sessile, friable, anorectal polyp, located just at the dentate line, seen on retroflexion.

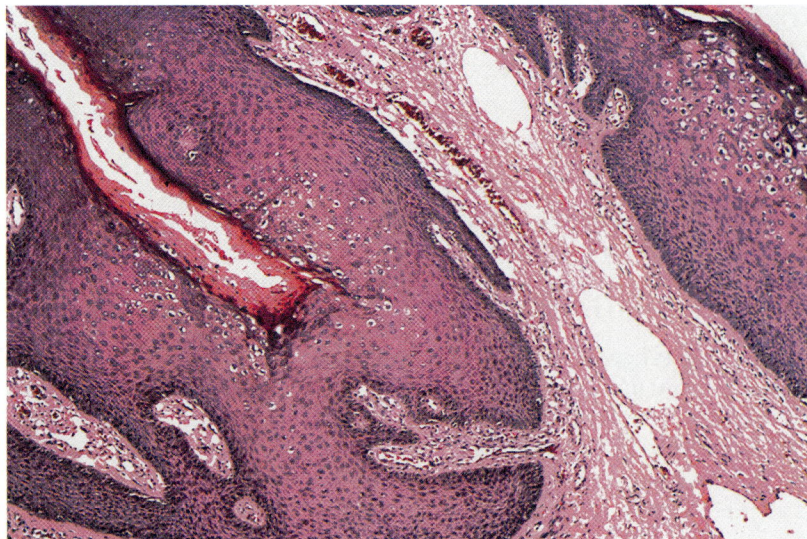

Figure 4-338: **Anal Margin. Condyloma Acuminatum.** Squamous mucosa with hyperkeratosis, and groups of vacuolated koilocytes typical of condyloma acuminatum.

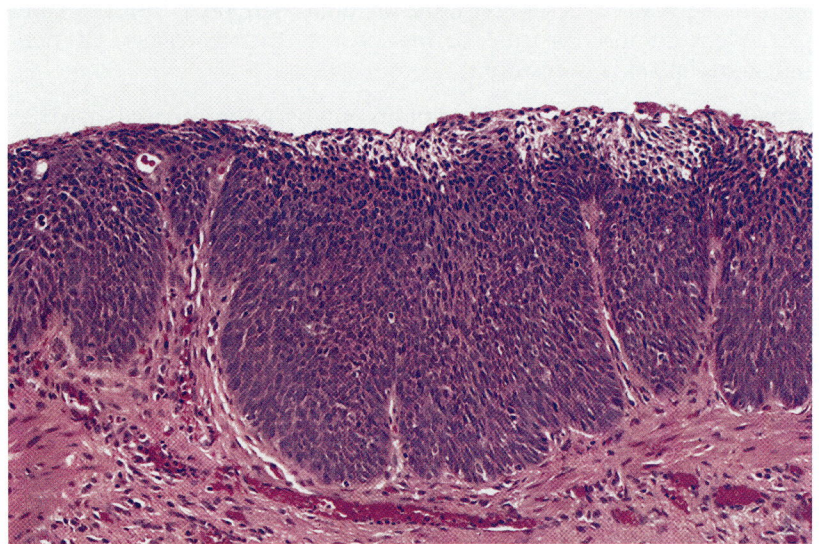

Figure 4-339: **Anal Canal. Squamous Cell Dysplasia, High-Grade.** Full-thickness squamous dysplasia.

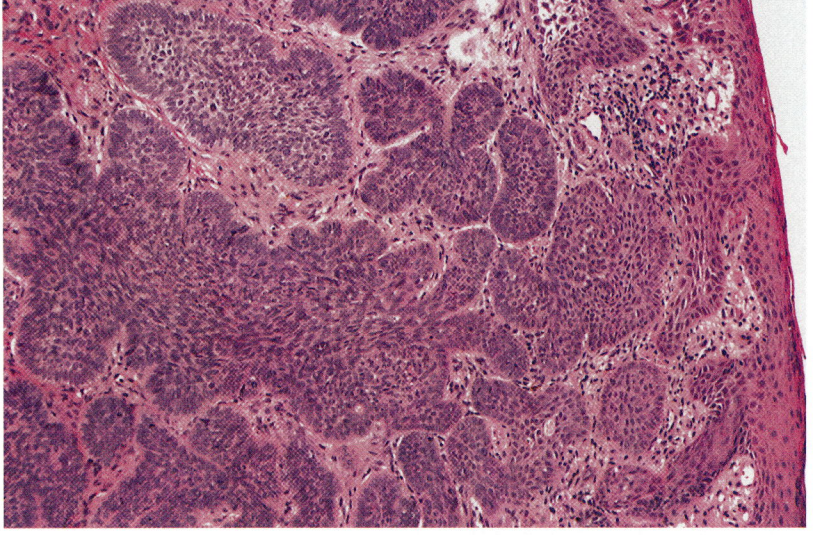

Figure 4-340: **Anal Margin. Basal Cell Carcinoma.** Islands of basaloid cells bud from overlying squamous epithelium.

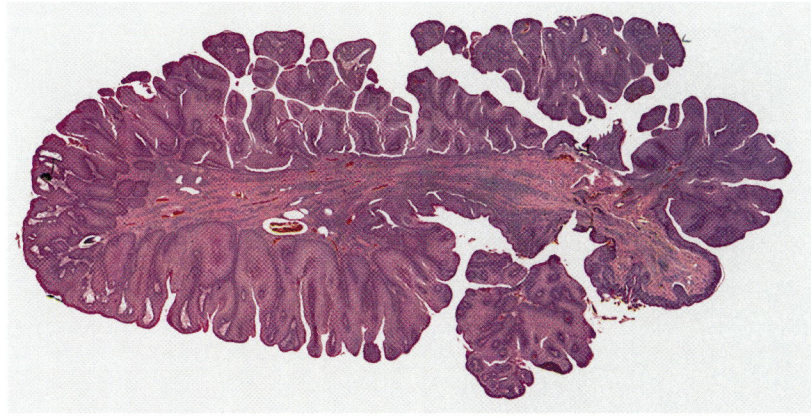

Figure 4-341: **Anal Canal. Condyloma Acuminatum.** Papillary proliferation of hyperplastic squamous epithelium.

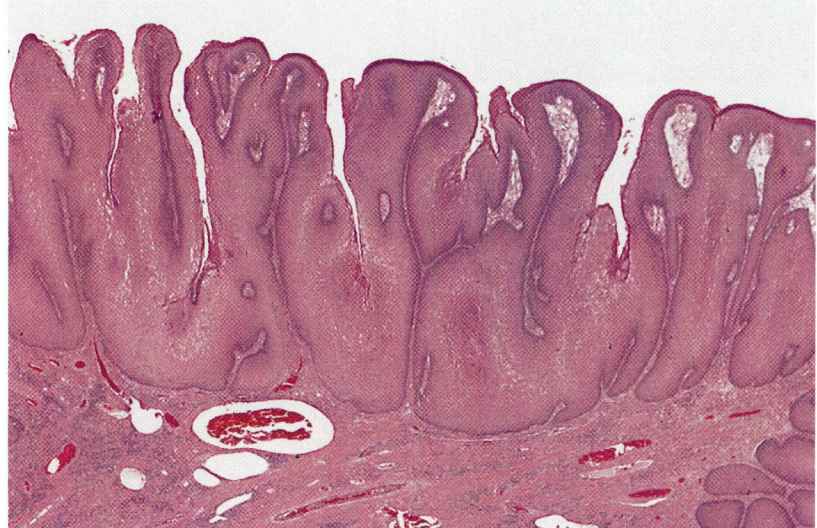

Figure 4-342: **Anal Canal. Condyloma Acuminatum.** Higher magnification of Fig. 4-341. Sharp uniform demarcation between condylomatous epithelium and stroma.

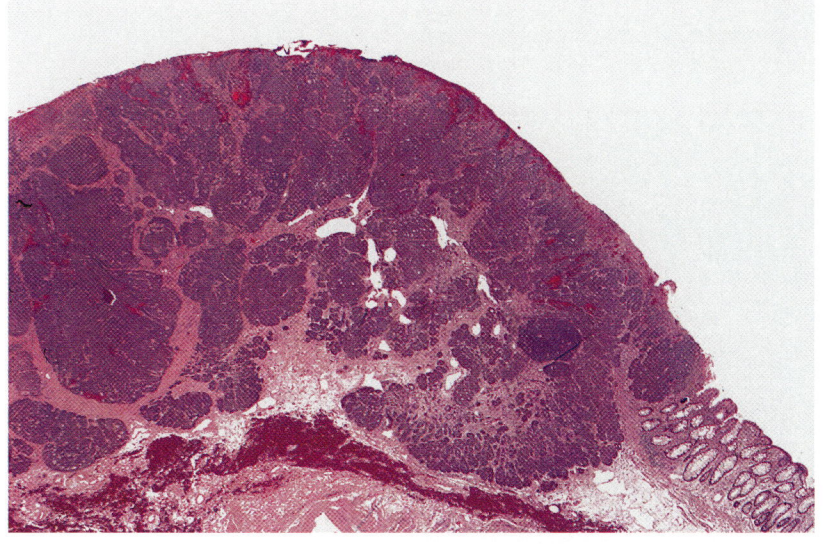

Figure 4-343: **Anal Canal. Squamous Cell (Cloacogenic) Carcinoma.** Undifferentiated basaloid cells replace surface epithelium and invade the stroma adjacent to rectal mucosa.

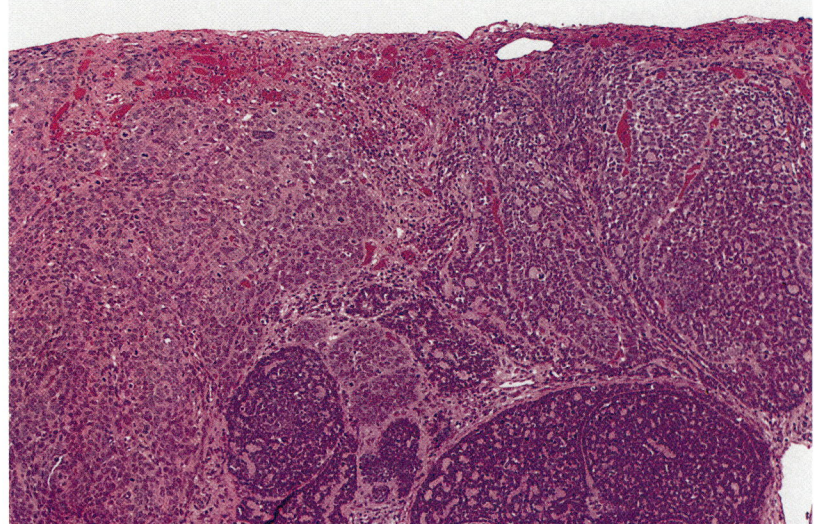

Figure 4-344: **Anal Canal. Squamous Cell (Cloacogenic) Carcinoma.** Basaloid cells with a brisk mitotic rate form nests and trabecular structures.

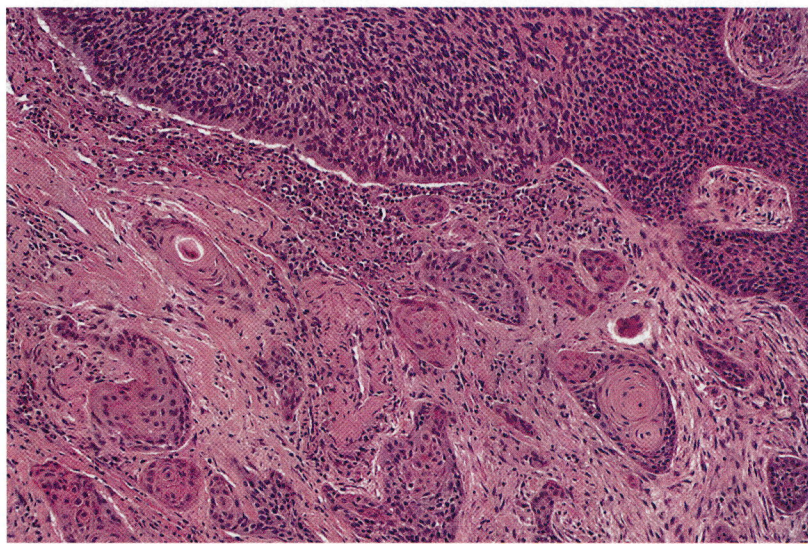

Figure 4-345: **Anal Canal. Squamous Cell (Cloacogenic) Carcinoma.** Undifferentiated and basaloid surface tumor. Invasive nests with obvious squamous differentiation.

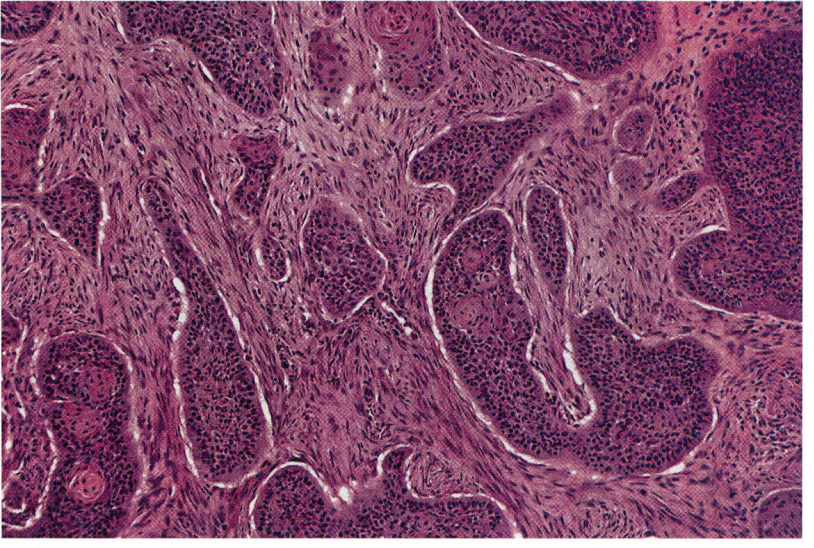

Figure 4-346: **Anal Canal. Squamous Cell (Cloacogenic) Carcinoma.** Islands of invasive, malignant squamous cells resemble squamous carcinoma of anal skin. Peripheral palisading suggests cloacogenic carcinoma.

Appendix 1

Selected Reference Texts

Gastroenterology:

Brandt LJ, Daum F, eds. *Clinical Practice of Gastroenterology*. Edinburgh, Scotland: Churchill Livingstone; 1998.

Sivak MV, Schleutermann DS. *Gastroenterologic Endoscopy*. Philadelphia, Pa: WB Saunders Co; 1999.

Sleisenger MH, Fordtran JS, Scharschmidt BF, Feldman M, eds. *Gastrointestinal Disease: Pathophysiology/ Diagnosis/Management*. 5th ed. Philadelphia, Pa: WB Saunders Co; 1993.

Wilcox CM. *Atlas of Clinical Gastrointestinal Endoscopy Companion to Sleisenger and Fordtrans's Gastrointestinal Disease*. Philadelphia, Pa.: WB Saunders Co; 1995.

Yamada T, Alpers DH, Owyang C, Powell DW, Silverstein FE, eds. *Textbook of Gastroenterology*. Philadelphia, Pa: JB Lippincott Co; 1991.

Pathology:

Blaser MJ, Smith PD, Ravdin JI, Greenberg HB, Guerrant RL, eds. *Infections of the Gastrointestinal Tract*. New York, NY: Raven Press; 1995.

Fenoglio-Preiser CM, Noffsinger AE, Stemmermann GN, Lantz PE, Linstrom MB, Rilke FO. *Gastrointestinal Pathology: An Atlas and Text*. 2nd ed. Philadelphia, Pa: Lippincott-Raven; 1999.

Lewin KJ, Riddell RH, Weinstein WM. *Gastrointestinal Pathology and Its Clinical Implications*. New York, NY: IGAKU-SHOIN Medical Publishers, Inc; 1992.

Ming S-C, Goldman H, eds. *Pathology of the Gastrointestinal Tract*. 2nd ed. Philadelphia, Pa: Lippincott-Williams & Wilkins Publishers; 1998.

Morson BC, Dawson IMP, Day DW, Jass JR, Price AB, Williams GT. *Morson & Dawson's Gastrointestinal Pathology*. 3rd ed. Oxford, England: Blackwell Scientific Publications; 1990.

Sternberg SS, ed. *Histology for Pathologists*. New York, NY: Raven Press; 1992.

Whitehead R, ed. *Gastrointestinal and Oesophageal Pathology*. 2nd ed. Edinburgh, Scotland: Churchill Livingstone; 1994.

Appendix 2

Mayo Clinic GI Working Group Abbreviations

Esophagus

Tissue sites/normal

SEM/NSEM	Squamous esophageal mucosa/Normal SEM
GEJM	Gastroesophageal junction-type mucosa
GCM	Gastric cardia-type mucosa
GFM	Gastric fundus-type mucosa

Pathology

AE	Active esophagitis
CUE	Chronic ulcerative esophagitis
HSEM	Hyperplastic squamous esophageal mucosa
SPEC	Specialized Barrett's mucosa
CWR	Consistent with reflux
CWR-G	Consistent with reflux if gastritis is excluded

Stomach

Tissue sites/normal

GCM/NGCM	Gastric cardia-type mucosa/Normal GCM
FM/NFM	Fundic-type mucosa/Normal FM
AFTZ/NAFTZ	Antral-fundic transition zone mucosa/Normal AFTZ
AM/NAM	Antral mucosa/Normal AM
AFM/NAFM	Antral and fundic mucosa/ Normal AFM
PCM/NPCM	Pyloric channel mucosa/Normal PCM

Pathology

Gastritis, Common Pattern

Acute Gastritis

ASG	Acute suppurative gastritis

Active Chronic, Chronic, and Atrophic Gastritis, Common Pattern.

Construct a standard diagnostic phrase in order listed (AM w ACG2, IM1, GA1, HP2)

1. Location – **GCM, FM, AFTZ, AFM, AM**
2. Inflammation-
   ACG1 (ACG2, ACG3)   Mild (moderate, severe) active chronic gastritis
   CG1 (CG2, CG3)   Mild (moderate, severe) chronic gastritis
3. Intestinal metaplasia-
   IM0 (IM1, IM2, IM3)   No (focal, moderate, extensive) intestinal metaplasia
4. Glandular atrophy-
   GA0 (GA1, GA2, GA3)   No (mild, moderate, severe) glandular atrophy
5. *H. pylori*-
   HP0, HP1, HP2, HP3   No (occasional, moderate, numerous) *Helicobacter pylori*

ATG   Chronic atrophic gastritis characterized by ___ (Construct a standard diagnostic phrase as above and add additional features such as metaplasia.)

Gastritis with Distinctive Features

LG   Lymphocytic gastritis characterized by active chronic inflammation in the lamina propria and a striking increase in intraepithelial lymphocytes in the foveolar and surface epithelium. Lymphocytic gastritis may be a hypersensitivity reaction to *H. pylori*. It is sometimes associated with celiac sprue or sprue-like changes. The hypertrophic form may present clinically as Menetrier's syndrome.

GG   Granulomatous gastritis. Findings are consistent with Crohn's disease, isolated granulomatous gastritis, infections, sarcoid, drug reactions, and foreign body reactions.

EG   Eosinophilic gastritis. Differential diagnosis includes a reaction to foods, drugs, or parasites, hypereosinophilic syndromes, and idiopathic eosinophilic gastritis.

HLG   Hypertrophic lymphocytic gastritis. One histologic pattern which may be seen in patients who present clinically as Menetrier's syndrome.

Reactive Gastropathy, Common Pattern, Acute and Chronic

AEG   Acute erosive gastropathy. Erosions are present but there is no significant inflammation or reactive foveolar hyperplasia. These lesions may reflect stress, shock, alcohol, drugs, or other nonspecific etiologies.

RG-FM (or –AFM -AFTZ, *AFM*-AM)
     Consistent with reactive gastropathy. Fundic (or antral and fundic, antral-fundic transition zone, antral) mucosa shows reactive foveolar hyperplasia, negligible inflammation, and no *Helicobacter pylori*. These changes suggest chemical-type injury such as can be seen with nonsteroidal anti-inflammatory drugs, alcohol, and bile reflux (in the setting of gastroenteric anastomosis).

RGE-FM (or -AFM, -AFTZ, *AFM*-AM)
Consistent with reactive gastropathy with erosion. Fundic (or antral and fundic, antral-fundic transition zone, antral) mucosa shows reactive foveolar hyperplasia, negligible inflammation, erosion, and no Helicobacter pylori. These changes suggest chemical type injury such as can be seen with nonsteroidal anti-inflammatory drugs, alcohol, and occasionally bile reflux.

RGU-FM (or -AFM, -AFTZ, *AFM* -AM)
Consistent with reactive gastropathy with ulcer. Fundic (or antral and fundic, antral-fundic transition zone, antral) mucosa shows ulceration in a background of reactive foveolar hyperplasia, relatively little inflammation, and no Helicobacter. These changes suggest "chemical" type injury such as can be seen with non-steroidal anti-inflammatory drugs, alcohol, and occasionally bile reflux.

Reactive Gastropathy, Distinctive Patterns

RG-BR-AM (or –AFM, -AFTZ, -AFM, FM)
Reactive gastropathy with features suggestive of bile reflux. In addition to the common features of reactive gastropathy (reactive foveolar hyperplasia, little inflammtion and no *Helicobacter pylori*), there are epithelial subnuclear vacuoles.

RG-RC-AM (or –AFM, -AFTZ ,-AFM, FM)
Reactive gastropathy with features suggestive of radiation or chemotherapy effect. In addition to the common features of reactive gastropathy (reactive foveolar hyperplasia, little inflammtion and no *Helicobacter pylori*), there is cellular atypia (nuclear enlargement, vacuolization, macronucleoli).

RG-CONG-AM (or –AFM, -AFTZ, -AFM, FM)
Reactive gastropathy with superficial vascular ectasia. This finding occurs in congestive gastropathy due to portal hypertension, watermelon stomach, and scleroderma.

HRG
Hypertrophic gastropathy. A histologic pattern that may be seen in patients with Menetrier's syndrome. There is massive foveolar hyperplasia, glandular atrophy, edema, but little inflammation.

Miscellaneous descriptors

CONG	Congestive gastropathy
WS	Watermelon stomach
SVE	Superficial vascular ectasia
SVEetc.	Superficial vascular ectasia. This finding occurs in congestive gastropathy, watermelon stomach, and in scleroderma.
OMFT	Organizing microvascular fibrin thrombus
RFH	Reactive foveolar hyperplasia
GX	Gastric xanthelasma
PYLM	Pyloric (antral) metaplasia
PANM	Pancreatic metaplasia
ECH	Endocrine cell hyperplasia

Small Bowel

Tissue sites/normal

DM/NDM　　Duodenal mucosa/Normal duodenal mucosa
SBM　　　 Small bowel mucosa
IM/NIM　　Ileal mucosa/Normal ileal mucosa
JM/NJM　　 Jejunal mucosa/Normal jejunal mucosa

Pathology

Malabsorption

NSBM
　　Small bowel mucosa without diagnostic abnormality. Villi and plasma cells are present. No evidence of Whipple's (PAS), celiac sprue, or *Giardia*.

MPCS
　　Malabsorption pattern with total villous atrophy, consistent with celiac sprue. There is surface epithelial degeneration with increased intraepithelial lymphocytes, total villous atrophy, crypt hyperplasia, and chronic inflammation. These changes are compatible with celiac sprue; however, other conditions such as hypersensitivity reactions to other proteins (soy, milk), severe bacterial overgrowth, chronic malnutrition, etc. can show similar changes.

MPBO
　　Malabsorption pattern with partial villous atrophy. There is partial villous atrophy, crypt hyperplasia, and chronic inflammation. These changes are nonspecific, but may reflect conditions such as early or partially treated celiac sprue, bacterial overgrowth, hypersensitivity reaction to nongluten proteins, tropical sprue, or protein calorie malnutrition.

Nonspecific Inflammation

Duodenum

AD1 (AD2, AD3)
　　Mild (moderate, severe) acute duodenitis
ACD1 (ACD2, ACD3)
　　Mild (moderate, severe) active chronic duodenitis
ACDW1 (ACDW2, ACDW3)
　　Mild (moderate, severe) active chronic duodenitis without granulomas or specific features

Small Bowel, NOS

ASB1 (ASB2, ASB3)
　　Mild (moderate, severe) acute enteritis
ACSB1 (ACSB2, ACSB3)
　　Mild (moderate, severe) active chronic enteritis
ACSBW1, ACSBW2, ACSBW3
　　Mild (moderate, severe) active chronic enteritis without granulomas or specific features

Terminal ileum

FAI
    Focal acute ileitis consistent with aphthous lesion
AI1 (AI2, AI3)
    Mild (moderate, severe) acute ileitis
ACI1 (ACI2, ACI3)
    Mild (moderate, severe) active chronic ileitis
ACI1 etc. (ACI2 etc., ACI3 etc.)
    Mild (moderate, severe) active ileitis of uncertain duration. Histologic features are nonspecific. Consider Crohn's disease, infections, and NSAIDs.
ACIW1 (ACIW2, ACIW3)
    Mild (moderate, severe) active chronic ileitis without granulomas or specific features.
ACIW1 etc. (ACIW2etc., ACIW3etc.)
    Mild (moderate, severe) active chronic ileitis without granulomas or specific features. Consider Crohn's disease, infections, and NSAIDs.

Pouch
ACPW1, ACPW2, ACPW3
    Mild (moderate, severe) active chronic pouchitis without granulomas or specific features

Inflammation with Particular Features

EEC-SB   Eosinophilic enteritis. Differential diagnosis includes a reaction to food, drugs, or parasites, hypereosinophilic syndromes, and idiopathic eosinophilic enterocolitis.

GE   Granulomatous enteritis. Consider Crohn's disease, infection, and sarcoidosis.

Colon

Tissue Sites/normal

CM/NCM   Colonic mucosa/Normal colonic mucosa
SM/NSM   Squamous mucosa/Normal squamous mucosa
ATZ/NATZ   Anal transition zone/Normal anal transition zone.

Anatomic Sites

ASC   Ascending colon
HF   Hepatic flexure
PTV   Proximal transverse
DTV   Distal transverse
SF   Splenic flexure
PD   Proximal descending
DD   Distal descending

SIG   Sigmoid
REC   Rectum

Pathology

Acute Colitis

AC   Acute colitis consistent with acute self-limited colitis or infectious origin (including *C. difficile*). Also consider drugs.

PSC   Acute colitis with pseudomembranes. These changes may be due to *C. difficile*, other toxin-producing bacteria, or acute ischemia.

AISC   Consistent with acute ischemic colitis. There is edema and hemorrhage in the lamina propria and superficial epithelial necrosis. These changes may be due to vascular disease, low perfusion states, verotoxin-producing *E. coli* 0157:H7, other toxin-producing bacteria, or rarely drugs.

FAC   Focal acute colitis.

FACCD   Focal acute colitis consistent with aphthous ulcer. Aphthous ulcers may be seen in infectious colitis (especially *Yersinia*) or in Crohn's disease. Also consider drug reaction.

Active Chronic/Chronic Crypt Destructive Colitis (Add diagnosis or Differential Diagnosis as appropriate.)

Desciptive Diagnosis

ACC1 (ACC2, ACC3)   Mild (moderate, severe) active chronic crypt destructive colitis

ACCW1 (ACCW2, ACCW3)
    Mild (moderate, severe) active chronic crypt destructive colitis without granulomas or specific features

ICC   Inactive chronic crypt destructive colitis

CC   Inactive chronic crypt destructive colitis without granulomas or specific features.

CAC   Minimal crypt architectural changes only. Consistent with inactive chronic colitis or other quiescent crypt destructive process.

Clinicopathologic Diagnosis

CWIBD   Consistent with chronic idiopathic inflammatory bowel disease of undetermined subtype

CWIBD/CUC	Consistent with chronic idiopathic inflammatory bowel disease. There are no features inconsistent with chronic ulcerative colitis
CWCD	Consistent with Crohn's disease.
CWCDI	Consistent with Crohn's disease or granulomatous infection (mycobacteria, fungus, *Yersinia*).
CWCUC	Consistent with chronic ulcerative colitis
CWCUCI	The changes are consistent with chronic ulcerative colitis. Prolonged bacterial or other infections can produce similar histologic changes.

Chronic Destructive Colitis without Crypt Destruction

ACC-NC	Active chronic colitis without evidence of crypt destruction and lacking features of lymphocytic or collagenous colitis. Consistent with chronic colitis of undetermined type, including very mild chronic idiopathic inflammatory bowel disease.
COCO	Collagenous colitis. Mild chronic active colitis without crypt architectural distortion. Collagen is deposited around the absorptive capillary complex beneath the surface epithelium.
LC	Suggestive of lymphocytic colitis. Mild chronic active colitis without crypt architectural distortion or collagen deposition. Intraepithelial lymphocytes are increased. These changes are consistent with lymphocytic colitis; however, the diagnosis requires clinicopathologic correlation. Some patients with lymphocytic colitis may go on to develop collagenous colitis. Some have celiac sprue or sprue-like small bowel changes. Also consider drug reaction.
NOCC	No evidence of collagenous or lymphocytic colitis
EEC-C	Eosinophilic colitis. The differential diagnosis includes a reaction to food, drugs, or parasites, hypereosinophilic syndromes, and idiopathic eosinophilic enterocolitis.
GC	Granulomatous colitis. Consider Crohn's disease, infections (fungal, AFB, *Yersinia, Salmonella*), sarcoidosis, and drug reactions.

Colopathy

CONC
    Congestive colopathy. The capillaries and venules in the lamina propria are prominent, ectatic, and have thickened sclerotic walls. These features are seen in portal hypertension, portal venous outflow obstruction, and rarely in patients with scleroderma in the absence of portal hypertension.

common pattern 84
H pylori, H heilmanii 84
loss of acid secretion, B12 92
metaplasia 92
pernicious anemia 92
visible submucosal vascular network 92
watermelon stomach 92, 117
Chronic ileitis 179
Chronic ischemia 363
Chronic nondestructive colitis 290
   autoimmune process 329
   celiac sprue 329
   collagenous colitis 329
   drug reaction 329
   ischemia 329
   lymphocytic colitis 329
Chronic venous hypertension 281
Churg-Strauss 95
Cirrhosis 115
   portal hypertensive colopathy 344
Clostridium 292
Cloxacillin 35
Cobblestoning, Crohn's 190
Cocaine 292
   ischemia 227
Coccidioides 292
Colitis
   active chronic destructive 312, 316
   acute 289, 290, 292
   amebic 292, 298, 300
   chronic nondestructive 290, 329
   Crohn's 305, 312
   collagenous 290, 329, 330
   granulomatous 325
   indeterminate 290
   lymphocytic 212, 267, 290, 329, 330
   ulcerative 280, 290, 312, 316, 319
Colitis cystica profunda 366
Collagen vascular disease 230
Collagenous colitis 290, 329, 330
Collagenous sprue 227
   vs ischemia 227
Combined adenoma/hyperplastic polyp 376
Common variable immunodeficiency
   Giardia 208
   IgA immunodeficiency 208
Condyloma acuminatum 421
Congestive colopathy. 348
Congestive erythema 78
Congestive gastropathy
   portal hypertension 85
   scleroderma 85
   watermelon stomach 85
Connective tissue diseases 224
Corticosteroids 35
Cowden syndrome 383, 384
Crohn's disease 88, 98, 181, 186, 190, 210, 227, 266, 280, 286, 312, 325, 335, 338, 342, 351

adenocarcinoma 321
aphthous ulcer 322, 323
cobblestone pattern 323
colitis 18, 38, 84, 265, 290
granuloma 190, 324
ileal ulcers/erosions 186
ischemia 227
lymphoid hyperplasia 210
rake ulcers 322, 323
Cronkhite-Canada polyp 143, 145
   inflammatory polyps 386
   juvenile polyposis 386
Cronkhite-Canada syndrome 216
Crow's feet 284, 362
Crypt distortion 317
Crypt epithelial apoptosis 332
Crypt hyperplasia 181
Cryptococcus 292
Cryptosporidia 122, 176, 193, 196, 292, 296
Cystic fibrosis 353
Cytomegalovirus 18, 33, 181, 184, 186, 199, 227, 292, 298, 299, 310
   esophagitis 31, 32
   ischemia 122, 227
   ulceration 122, 335

D

DALM 287, 318, 319
Deferoxamine 292
Dermatomyositis 40, 230
Diaphragms
   NSAIDs 186, 335
   tuberculosis 186
Dicloxacillin 35
Dieulafoy lesion 131
Digitalis 292
Diversion colitis 290, 334
Diverticula 11, 12, 174, 234, 338, 339
   Crohn's disease 338
   Zenker diverticulum 11
Diverticular disease-associated colitis 290
Drug reaction 224, 290, 306, 325, 329
Drugs 84, 85, 95, 101, 103
Duodenitis
   neutrophils 182
Dye staining 46, 58, 399
   indigo carmine 373, 375
   Lugol's iodine 2, 48, 49, 50
   methylene blue 2, 46, 58, 373
   toluidine blue 2
Dysmotility disorders 40, 356
   achalasia 40
   dermatomyositis 40
   scleroderma 40
Dysphagia 36, 53
Dysplasia 46, 143, 149, 310
   atypia indefinite for 51, 52
   Barrett's esophagus 46

chromoscopy 46, 149
grading 49
reactive atypia 46, 149
regenerative atypia 149
squamous 46, 58
stomach 149
ulcerative colitis 318
variations 48
vital dye staining 46, 149
Dysplasia-associated lesion/mass (DALM) 287, 318, 319

E

E coli 0157:H7 292
E vermicularis (pinworm) 302
Ectopic gastric mucosa 13, 42, 58, 61
Endocrine cell hyperplasia
 chromogranin 136
 micronests 135
Endometriosis 361, 362
Endoscopic examination 18
 brush cytology 2
 chromoscopy 2
 dye staining 2
 esophagus 2
 hiatal hernia 78
 jumbo biopsy forceps 2
 large intestine 280
 mucosectomy 2
 pinch avulsion biopsy forceps 2
 small intestine 174
 stomach 78
Endoscopic ultrasound 78
Enlarged rugal folds
 H pylori 119
 infiltrating carcinomas 119
 metastatic carcinoma 119
 Zollinger-Ellison (ZE) syndrome 119
Enteroadherent *E coli* 297
Enterochromaffinlike cell (ECL cell)
 hyperplasia 135
Enterococcus 181
Enterocytozoon bieneusi 197
Enteropathy-associated T-cell
 lymphoma 269
Eosinophilic colitis 292, 331
 drug allergy 291
 food allergy 291
 idiopathic eosinophilic enteritis 291
 parasitic infestation 291
 vasculitis 291
Eosinophilic enteritis 181
 edema 188
 inflammatory fibroid polyp 188
 ulceration/erosions 188
Eosinophilic esophagitis 18, 26, 27
 hypersensitivity 26
 idiopathic 26

parasites 26
pill-induced 26
reflux 26
Eosinophilic gastritis 84
 allergic reactions 95
 Churg-Strauss 95
 drugs 95
 parasites 95
Eosinophils
 inflammatory fibroid polyp 147, 248
 amphetamines 292
Ergotamines
 ischemia 227
Erosion 90, 103, 104, 107, 181, 182, 184, 305
Erythema 78, 303
 angiodysplasia 78
 congestive erythema 78
 hemorrhagic erythema 78
 portal hypertensive gastropathy 78
 radiation angiectasias 78
 reactive gastropathy 106
 watermelon stomach 78
Esophageal gland duct 44
Esophageal varices 16
Esophagitis 18, 26
 Candida 18
 Crohn's 18
 cytomegalovirus 18, 32
 endoscopic examination 18
 eosinophilic 18, 26, 27
 grading 19
 granulomatous esophagitis 18
 herpesvirus 18
 histologic findings 18
 pill esophagitis 18
 reflux 18, 19
 squamous cell 18
 squamous cell carcinoma 18
Esophagus
 amyloid 41
 bizarre stromal cells 33
 Candida 14
 capillary hemangioma 69
 chemical injury 34
 diverticula 11, 12
 dysmotility disorders 40
 fibrovascular polyp 70
 glycogenic acanthosis 14, 15
 granular cell tumor 72
 hiatal hernia 8, 10
 high-grade dysplasia 47
 histology 3
 inflammatory polyps 23, 24
 inlet patch 13
 Kaposi sarcoma 69
 leiomyoma 75
 lipoma 75
 low-grade dysplasia 47

melanoma 65
metastatic breast carcinoma 67
metastatic small cell carcinoma 67
pancreatic metaplasia 3
pill esophagitis 35
radiation injury 37
reflux 8
ring 10
rings, webs, hernias 8
Schatzki ring 8
scleroderma 41
signet-ring cell carcinoma 56
squamous cell carcinoma 62
squamous dysplasia 60
squamous papilloma 23, 25
stromal tumors 74
ulceration 11
varices 16
vascular lesions 68
webs 10
Z line 2, 3
Estrogen 292
  ischemia 227

F

Familial adenomatous polyposis 260, 263, 265, 384
  adenocarcinoma 397
  colectomy 397
  Gardner syndrome 397
  mesenteric fibromatosis 397
  fundic gland polyp 141
Fibrosing colopathy 353
  chronic colitis 353
  cystic fibrosis 353
  ischemic colitis 353
Fibrovascular polyp 70, 71
Filiform polyps 372
Fistula 38
Flat adenoma 399
Folate deficiency 310
Forceps
  jumbo biopsy 2
  pinch avulsion biopsy 2, 280
Foreign body, esophagus 84
Foreign material, esophagus 38
Foveolar hyperplasia 103, 105, 119
Foveolar metaplasia 242
Friability 312
Fundic gland polyp 141

G

Gangliocytic paraganglioma 254
Ganglioneuroma 384
  Cowden syndrome 384
  familial adenomatous polyposis 384
  Hirschsprung disease 384
  juvenile polyposis 384

MEN 2b 384
  tuberous sclerosis 384
  von Recklinghausen disease 384
Ganglionic blocking agents 292
Gastric heterotopia 13
  Barrett's esophagus 13
  inlet patch 13
  hyperplastic polyp 247
Gastric hyperplastic polyp 247
  juvenile polyp 145
Gastritis
  active chronic 84, 88, 92
  acute 84, 87
  Crohn's 88
  H pylori 84, 87, 88
  atrophic 117
  chronic 84, 92
  lymphocytic 84, 212
  granulomatous 84
  varioliform 88, 89
Gastropathy 84, 113, 165
  dysplasia 113
GERD 11
Giardia lamblia 176, 193, 194, 208,
GIST 165, 271, 388, 414
Glomus tumor 165, 169
Glutaraldehyde 292
Glycogenic acanthosis 14, 15
  Candida 14
Goatee 263, 264
Goblet cell metaplasia 42, 47, 118
Gold 292
Graft-versus-host reaction 291
  crypt epithelial apoptosis 332
  graft-versus-host pattern 291
  immunosuppression 291
  viral infections 291
Granular cell tumor 73, 387
  squamous cell carcinoma 72
  squamous hyperplasia 72
Granuloma 181
  histoplasmosis 190
  yersiniosis 190
  sarcoid 190
  tuberculosis 190
Granulomatous colitis 325
  Crohn's disease 325
  drug reactions 325
  histoplasmosis 325
  schistosome 325
  tuberculosis 325
  Yersina granulomas 325
Granulomatous esophagitis 18, 38, 39
  Crohn's 38
  foreign material 38
  fungal infection 38
  sarcoid 38
  tuberculous 38

Granulomatous gastritis 84
    collagen vascular disorder 98
    Crohn's 98
    drug reaction 98
    fungal 98
    parasitic 98
    sarcoid 98
    spirochetal 98
    tuberculosis 98
    vasculitis 98
    Crohn's, sarcoid, idiopathic, fungi, mycobacteria, 84

H

H heilmanii 84, 88, 91
H pylori 84, 87, 88, 91, 95, 122, 161, 184
    mosaic pattern 161
Hamartomatous polyps 145, 363
    juvenile 145
    Peutz-Jeghers 145
    Cowden 383
Haustral folds 282
Helminths 292
Hemangiomas 68, 221, 272, 344, 388
Hemocystic spot 16, 17
Hemorrhagic enteropathy 226
    ischemia, mechanical obstruction 226
    mesenteric venous thrombosis 226
    overanticoagulation 226
    small vessel vasculitis 226
    superior mesenteric artery 226
Hemorrhagic erythema 78
Hemorrhoids/varices 349
Henoch-Schoenlein vasculitis
    Campylobacter jejuni 224
    E coli 224
    IgA deposition 224
    streptococcus 224
Herpes esophagitis 30
Herpesvirus 18, 299
Heterotopic gastric mucosa
    duodenum 242
Hiatal hernia 8, 10, 78
High-resolution video endoscopy 373, 377
Hirschsprung disease 356, 384
Histiocyte infiltrates 294
Histology
    esophagus 3
    large intestine 281
    small intestine 175
    stomach 79
Histoplasma capsulatum 204, 292, 298, 326, 327
HNPCC syndrome 399
Hollow visceral myopathy 230, 356
Hypergastrinemia 135
Hyperosmolar solutions 292
Hyperplastic foveolae 168

Hyperplastic polyp 117, 141, 393
    Cronkhite-Canada polyp 143
    dysplasia 143
    watermelon stomach 143
    gastric heterotopia 247
    large intestine 373
    stomach 143
    with adenoma 376
Hypertonic enemas 292
Hypertrophic gastropathy and gastritis
    foveolar hyperplasia 119
    lymphocytic gastritis 119
    Zollinger-Ellison (ZE) syndrome 119
    Menetrier disease 85
Hypertrophic lymphocytic gastritis 84
    Menetrier disease 84
Hypertrophied anal papilla 369
Hypogammaglobulinemia
    lymphoid hyperplasia 208
Hypovolemia/low-flow states 290

I

IgA deposition 224
IgA immunodeficiency 208
Ileal ulcers and lesions
    carcinoids 186
    Crohn's disease 186
    leiomyomas 186
    lymphoma 186
    NSAIDs 186
Immunosuppressed patients 197, 198, 204, 272
    cryptosporidia 196
    giardiasis 194
Indeterminate colitis 290
Indigo carmine 373, 375
Inflammatory cloacogenic polyp 366
    adenocarcinoma 363
    chronic ischemia 363
    hamartomatous polyps 363
    mucinous adenocarcinoma 363
    quiescent ulcerative colitis 363
Inflammatory fibroid polyp 147, 188, 248
Inflammatory polyps 23, 24, 386
Inflammatory polyps, esophagus
    adenocarcinomas of the cardia 23
    gastric hyperplastic polyps 23
    hyperplastic polyp 23
    squamous papillomas 23
Inlet patch 13
    gastric heterotopia 13
Innominate grooves 281
Insufflation artifact 293, 367
    lipoma 293
    xanthelasma 293
Intestinal metaplasia 92, 93, 94, 111, 149
    xanthelasma 111
Intraepithelial lymphocytosis 181
Intussusception 232

adenomas 232
carcinomas 232
inflammatory fibroid polyps 232
lipomas 232
Meckel diverticula 232
Peutz-Jeghers polyp 232
stromal tumors 232
Peutz-Jeghers polyp 145
Inverted appendix 362
cecal adenoma 362
endometriosis 362
Iodine 58
Iron 239
Iron sulfate 35
Ischemia
large intestine 281, 290, 292, 306, 329, 335, 342, 353
C difficile 307
chronic crypt destructive colitis 307
drug reactions 307
E coli 0157:H7 307
early 290
emboli 307
hypovolemic/low-flow states 307
mesenteric artery occlusion 307
mild 306
rectal prolapse 307
Shigella verotoxin 307
thrombotic states 307
thumbprinting 307
vasculitis/vasculopathy 307
verotoxin-producing *E coli* infection 307
small intestine
collagenous sprue 227
Crohn's disease 227
hypotension 227
mechanical obstruction 226
peripheral vascular disease 227
cytomegalovirus gastropathy 122
ergotamine 227
estrogen 227
NSAIDs 227
viruses 227
stomach 103, 122
Isospora belli 193, 176, 198

J

Jumbo biopsy forceps 2
Juvenile polyp 379
gastic hyperplastic polyp 145
Cronkite-Canada polyp 145
Juvenile polyposis 216, 379, 384, 386

K

Kaposi sarcoma 68, 69, 221, 272, 274, 416, 388
Kayexalate 292
Koch pouch 237

L

L-tryptophan 292
Leiomyosarcoma/stromal sarcoma 74, 165, 168
Leiomyoma 74, 75, 414
Leishmania 204, 298
"Leopard- skin" pattern 337
Leukemia 115, 161
mosaic pattern 161
Linear erosions 186
Linitis plastica 160, 161
mosaic pattern 161
signet-ring cell carcinoma 159
Lipid-filled histiocytes 294
Lipofuscin 337
Lipohyperplasia of the ileocecal valve 388
Lipoma
esophagus 75, 170
large intestine
vs hemangioma 388
vs insufflation artifact 293
vs smooth muscle/stromal neoplasm 388
vs metastatic malignancy 388
stomach 165
Lugol's iodine 2, 58, 59, 60
Lupus erythematosus 386
Lymphangiectasia 176, 218,
punctate, white spots 219
Lymphangioma 275
Lymphatics, dilated 174
Lymphocytic colitis 212, 267, 290, 330, 329
Lymphocytic gastritis 84, 212
autoimmune 84
celiac sprue 95
gliaden hypersensitivity 84
H pylori 95
Menetrier 95
T-lymphocytes 95
hypertrophic gastropathy 119
Lymphoid hyperplasia 90, 208, 267
Crohn's disease 210
rectal tonsil 357
terminal ileum 357
Lymphoid nodules 174, 175, 280, 286
Lymphoma
enteropathy-associated T-cell lymphomas 184, 267
extranodal marginal zone (MALT) 161, 267, 270
follicle center cell 267, 270
large cell 267, 276, 419
carcinoma 161
large intestine 357, 417
mucosal mosaic pattern 161
small intestine 267
celiac sprue 267
large cell 267
stomach 88, 115, 153, 161, 179
T-cell 267

Lysosomal debris 337

M

Malabsorption 212
    autoimmune disorders 212
    celiac sprue 212
    lymphocytic colitis 212
    lymphocytic gastritis 212
    peptic duodenitis 212
    protein calorie malnutrition 212
    tropical sprue 212
    bacterial overgrowth 212
Malabsorption pattern 181
Mallory-Weiss tear 11
MALT lymphoma 161, 267
Meckel diverticulum 232
    pancreatic heterotopia 252
Melanoma, malignant 64, 277, 239
    anal 349
Melanosis coli 337
Melanosis duodeni 239
Menetrier disease 84, 85, 95, 119, 143, 161
    mosaic pattern 161
Mesenteric artery occlusion 307
    ischemia, large intestine 307
Mesenteric venous thrombosis 226
Metastatic tumors
    esophagus 66
    large intestine 410
    small intestine 276
    stomach 171
Methotrexate 292
Methyldopa 292
Methylene blue 2, 46, 58, 373
Methysergide 292
Micronests, endocrine 135
Microsporidia 176, 193, 197, 298, 300
Mosaic pattern 115, 159, 160
    H pylori 115
    H pylori infection 161
    leukemia 115, 161
    linitis plastica 161
    lymphoma 115, 161
    Menetrier disease 161
    portal hypertensive gastropathy 115, 161
    signet-ring cell carcinoma 159, 160
Mucinous adenocarcinoma 250, 363, 406
Muciphage 153
Mucosa-associated lymphoid tissue (MALT)
    lymphoma 161, 267
Mucosal atrophy 227
Mucosal magnification 180
Mucosectomy 2, 78, 280, 399
Mucous neck cells 82
Multiple endocrine neoplasia (MEN)
    syndromes 135, 384
Muscular dystrophy syndromes 356
Mycobacteria 84

Mycobacterium avium-intracellulare 201, 294
Myeloma 354
Myoepithelial hamartoma 139
    pancreatic heterotopia 139

N

Narcotics 292
Neurofibroma 257
Neurogenic tumors, stomach 165
Nonsteroidal anti-inflammatory drugs 35
Normal esophagus
    squamocolumnar junction 5
Normal ileum mucosal pattern 193, 292
    Cryptosporidium 193
    Giardia lamblia 193
    Isospora 193
    Isospora belli 193
    Microsporidia 193
Normal small intestine 176
    Peyer patches 179
Normal stomach 82
    chief cells 82
    eosinophils 82
    lymphocytes 82
    mucous neck cells 82
    plasma cells 82
NSAIDs 35, 85, 101, 103, 182, 184, 292, 303
    CMV ulcers 335
    Crohn's disease 335
    diaphragm strictures 335
    ileal ulcers/erosions 186
    ileocolitis/ulcers 335
    ischemia 227, 335
    ischemic ulcers 335
    ulcers of T-cell lymphoma 335
    ulcers and erosions, small intestine 186
Nutcracker esophagus 40

O

Odynophagia 31, 35, 36, 38
Oleogranuloma 367
Oral contraceptives 35, 292
Osler-Weber-Rendu (hereditary hemorrhagic
    telangiectasia 132, 221, 344
Oxyntic glands 80

P

Pancreatic enzymes 35
Pancreatic heterotopia
    adenomyoma 139
    central umbilication 139
    Meckel diverticulum 252
    myoepithelial hamartoma 139
Pancreatic metaplasia 3, 7, 139
Paneth cells 94, 175, 281, 288
Papilla of Vater 176, 178
Paraffinoma 367

Parasites   26, 84, 95, 207
   seeds   301
   starch grains   301
Patterns of injury
   large intestine   289
   small intestine
      inflammation   181
         intraepithelial lymphocytosis   181
         malabsorption syndrome   181
         NSAID injury   181
         peptic disease   181
   stomach   84
Peptic disease   181, 182
Peptic duodenitis   212
   malabsorption   212
Peptic ulcer   127, 154
Peripheral vascular disease
   ischemia   227
Peutz-Jeghers polyp   145
   intussusception   232
   mucinous adenocarcinoma   250
   pseudoinvasive herniation   250, 381
Peyer patches   179, 180, 204, 210
Phenothiazines   292
Phlebectasias   174, 344
Pigments   239
Pill esophagitis   35
   cloxacillin   35
   corticosteroids   35
   dicloxacillin   35
   iron sulfate   35
   location   35
   nonsteroidal anti-inflammatory drugs   35
   oral contraceptives   35
   pancreatic enzymes   35
   potassium chloride   35
   quinidine   35
   tetracycline   35
Pinch avulsion-type biopsy forceps   2, 280
Plaques, esophagus
   Candida   14
   glycogenic acanthosis   14
   topical anesthetic   14, 28
Pneumatosis coli   359, 360
Polyarteritis nodosa   224
Polyposis
   familial adenomatous   260, 263
   juvenile   216, 379, 384, 386
Portal hypertension   85, 103
Portal hypertensive colopathy   344, 346
   hepatic arteriovenus fistula   291
   portal hypertension due to cirrhosis   291
   portal vein or tributary obstruction   291
Portal hypertensive enteropathy   221
Portal hypertensive gastropathy   78, 85, 103, 161, 115
   cirrhosis   115
   ectasia   115
   obstruction   115
   portal vein thrombosis   115
   prolapse   115
   sclerosis   115
   mosaic pattern   161
Postinflammatory polyps   312, 370
Potassium chloride   35, 292
Pouchitis   237
Presbyesophagus   40
Prostatic adenocarcinoma   172
Protein calorie malnutrition   181
   malabsorption   212
Protein-losing enteropathy   216
Pseudoepitheliomatous hyperplasia   61
   esophagus   61
   granular cell tumor   72
   squamous cell carcinoma   61
Pseudo-obstruction   230
Pseudoinvasive herniation   250, 381, 395
Pseudolipomatosis   367, 293
Pseudomembranous colitis   290, 292
   antibiotics   306
   bacterial toxins   306
   C difficile   306
   drug reaction   306
   mild ischemia   306
Pseudopolyps   370
Push enteroscopy   174
Pyloric metaplasia   93, 186, 242

Q

Quiescent ulcerative colitis   363
Quinidine   35

R

Radiation effect   114
Radiation enteritis   227
Radiation injury   36, 113, 114
   angiectasias   78
   bizarre stromal cells   36
   chemotherapy effect   310
   cytomegalovirus   310
   dysphagia   36
   dysplasia   310
   folate deficiency   310
   hematemesis   36
   ischemia   36
   malignancy   310
   malignant cells   36
   melena   36
   proctopathy   344
   stricture   36
   ulcers   36
Rake-type ulcer   190
Raynaud phenomenon   117
Reactive atypia
   dysplasia   51, 149
Reactive gastropathy

alcohol 103
antrum 103
bile reflux 85, 103, 108
chemotherapy 85, 103
dysplasia 106
erosions 103, 104, 107
erythema 106
foveolar hyperplasia 103
inflammation 103
ischemia 103
NSAID 85, 103
portal hypertension 103
radiation 85, 103
repair 103
stomal polypoid hyperplasia 103
underlying mass 103
uremia 85, 103
versus gastritis 103
Reactive lymphoid hyperplasia 417
Reactive proliferation 46
Rectal prolapse 307, 364
occult 291
polyp 365
syndrome 363
ulcer 365
Rectal tonsil 357
Red ring sign 280, 286
Red wale marking 16
Reflux esophagitis 8, 18, 26, 42
basal cell hyperplasia 21
esophagitis 18, 19, 20, 22, 53
re-epithelialization 21
stricture 22
Regenerative atypia 52, 46
dysplasia 149
Ring 10
Schatzki A ring 8
Schatzki B ring 8

S

Salicylates 292
Salmonella 181, 204, 305
Sarcoid 38, 84, 98, 327
granulomas 190, 325
Schatzki ring 8, 9
Schistosomiasis 325, 328
Schwannoma 74, 165, 169, 387
lymphoid follicles 256
Scleroderma 40, 41, 85, 117, 230, 356
Seed 302
Serrated adenoma 376, 378
Shigella 292
verotoxin 290
Short-chain fatty acids 334
Short-segment Barrett's esophagus 42
Signet-ring cell carcinoma
esophagus 55, 56
large intestine 387, 406
mosaic pattern 159
small intestine 276, 294
stomach 111, 112, 155
linitis plastica 159
xanthelasma 111, 159
Skin tag 369
Small cell carcinoma 61, 63, 406
Smooth muscle/stromal tumors (GISTs) 165, 271, 388, 414
Solitary or multiple idiopathic ulcer 292
Solitary rectal ulcer 364
Sonde enteroscopy 174
Spirochetes 84
Spirochetosis 292, 297
Sprue, see Celiac sprue
Squamocolumnar junction 5
Squamous cell carcinoma 18, 44, 61, 62, 63, 72, 410
basaloid variant 63
granular cell tumor 72
small cell carcinoma variant 61, 63
ulcer, esophagus 61
Squamous dysplasia 58, 59, 60
ectopic gastric mucosa 58
Lugol's iodine 58, 59, 60
Squamous island 45
Squamous lesions, large intestine 421
Squamous papilloma 23, 25
verrucous carcinoma 23
Steroids 292
Stomal polypoid hyperplasia 108, 143
Streptococcus 84, 87
Stricture 22, 36, 53
Barrett's esophagus 53
radiation injury 36
reflux 22
Stricture/anastomosis, large intestine
Crohn's disease 342
ischemic colitis 342
Stromal tumors 74, 165, 168, 232
glomus tumor 165
leiomyoma 74, 165
leiomyosarcoma 74, 165
lipoma 74, 165
schwannoma 74, 165
Strongyloides 122, 207
Submucosal vascular pattern 94, 280, 285
Subnuclear vacuoles 108, 109
Sulfasalazine 292
Sulfur 239
Superior mesenteric artery occlusion 226
Surgical enteroscopy 174
Syphilis 292
Systemic bacterial infections 292
Systemic fungal infections 181, 186
Systemic lupus erythematosus 386

T

T-cell lymphoma 267
Telangiectasia 344
Terminal ileitis 181
Tetracycline 35
Thumbprinting 307
    ischemia, large intestine 307
Toluidine blue 2
Topical anesthetic 28
Transitional cell carcinoma 411
Transverse colon
    triangular haustral configuration 283
Tricyclic antidepressants 292
Tropheryma whippelii
    Whipple disease 201
Tropical sprue
    malabsorption 212
Tuberculosis 38, 122, 181, 186, 190, 292, 325, 327
Tuberous sclerosis 384
Tubular adenoma 391, 393
Tubulovillous adenoma 391
Typhoid 204

U

Ulcer 31, 38, 61, 104, 122, 181, 184, 280, 312
    esophagus
        Barrett's esophagus 53
        chemical injury 34
        Crohn's 38
        cytomegalovirus esophagitis 31, 122
        Herpes 30, 31
        muciphages 153
        pill 31
        radiation injury 36
        reflux 31
    colon 291
        cytomegalovirus 291
        drug reaction 291
        NSAIDs 291
        stercoral 291
        vasculitis 291
    small intestine 206
        T-cell lymphoma 335
    stomach, benign
        bizarre stromal cells 125
        peptic ulcer 78, 127, 153
    stomach, malignant 153
        adenocarcinoma 153
        benign peptic ulcers 153
        lymphoma 153
        muciphages 153
        xanthelasma 153
Ulcerative colitis 280, 290, 312, 316, 319
Ultrasound, gastric 78
Uremia 85, 101, 103

V

Vaccinia 227
Varicella 200
Varices
    esophagus 16
        grading 16
        hemocystic spots 16, 17
        red wale 16
    large intestine 350
    stomach 132
Varioliform gastritis 88, 89
Vascular ectasia 221
    angiodysplasia 221
    arteriovenous malformations 221
    chronic venous hypertension 221
    inflammatory masses 221
    neoplastic masses 221
    portal hypertension 221
    telangiectasia 221
    vascular tumors 221
Vascular lesions 68
    angiosarcoma 272, 274
    arteriovenous malformations 344
    hemangioma 68, 272, 344, 388
    hemorrhagic 344
    Kaposi sarcoma 68, 221
    Osler-Weber-Rendu syndrome (hereditary phlebectasias 344
    radiation proctopathy 344
Vascular malformation 221, 346, 347
    stomach 132
Vasculitis 84, 224, 226
    Behcet syndrome 351
    ischemia 351
Vasculopathy 290
Venereal agents 292
Venous hypertension 281
Verotoxin-producing *E coli* infections 290, 307
Villous adenoma 286, 391
Villous flattening (atrophy) 181, 208
Vincristine 292
Vinyl chloride 272
Viral gastroenteritis 267
Viral infections
    adenovirus 199
    cytomegalovirus 31, 32, 184, 186, 199, 227, 335
    herpesvirus 18, 30, 298, 299
    vaccinia 227
    varicella 200
Visible vessel 78, 128, 131, 184
Vital dye stain 2, 46, 58, 373
von Recklinghausen disease 384

W

Watermelon stomach 78, 85, 92, 117, 143
    angiectasias 117
    fibrin microthrombi 117
    hyperplastic polyps 117
    intestinal (goblet cell) epithelium 118
    Raynaud phenomenon 117
    scleroerma 117
Webs 8, 10
Wenger-Angritt stain 91
Whipple Disease 201, 294
Worms 207

X

Xanthelasma 112, 153, 159, 174, 293, 294
    bile reflux 111
    insufflation artifact 293
    intestinal metaplasia 111
    signet-ring cell carcinoma 111

Y

Yersinia 181, 186, 292, 328

Z

Z line 2, 5, 6, 7, 42
    Barrett's esophagus 42
Zenker diverticulum 11
Zollinger-Ellison (ZE) syndrome 119, 135
    hypertrophic gastropathy 119